Obesity

Related Titles

The Liver: Oxidative Stress and Dietary Antioxidants
(ISBN: 9780128039519)

HIV/AIDS: Oxidative Stress and Dietary Antioxidants
(ISBN: 9780128098530)

Gastrointestinal Tissue: Oxidative Stress and Dietary Antioxidants
(ISBN: 9780128053775)

Aging: Oxidative Stress and Dietary Antioxidants
(ISBN: 9780124059337)

Diabetes: Oxidative Stress and Dietary Antioxidants
(ISBN: 9780124058859)

Obesity
Oxidative Stress and Dietary Antioxidants

Edited by

Amelia Marti del Moral
Department of Nutrition, Food Sciences and Physiology
School of Pharmacy and Nutrition, University of Navarra
IdiSNA, Navarra Institute for Health Research
Pamplona, Spain

Center of Biomedical Research in Physiopathology of Obesity and
Nutrition (CIBEROBN) Institute of Health Carlos III
Madrid, Spain

Concepción María Aguilera García
Department of Biochemistry and Molecular Biology
Institute of Nutrition and Food Technology
Center of Biomedical Research, University of Granada
Granada, Spain

Center of Biomedical Research in Physiopathology of Obesity and
Nutrition (CIBEROBN) Institute of Health Carlos III
Madrid, Spain

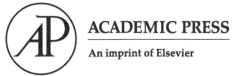

ACADEMIC PRESS

An imprint of Elsevier

Academic Press is an imprint of Elsevier
125 London Wall, London EC2Y 5AS, United Kingdom
525 B Street, Suite 1650, San Diego, CA 92101, United States
50 Hampshire Street, 5th Floor, Cambridge, MA 02139, United States
The Boulevard, Langford Lane, Kidlington, Oxford OX5 1GB, United Kingdom

Library of Congress Cataloging-in-Publication Data
A catalog record for this book is available from the Library of Congress

British Library Cataloguing-in-Publication Data
A catalogue record for this book is available from the British Library

ISBN: 978-0-12-812504-5

For information on all Academic Press publications visit our website at
https://www.elsevier.com/books-and-journals

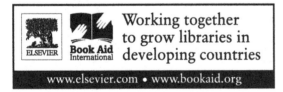

Working together
to grow libraries in
developing countries

www.elsevier.com • www.bookaid.org

Publisher: Mica H. Haley
Acquisition Editor: Tari K. Broderick
Editorial Project Manager: Ana Claudia A. Garcia
Production Project Manager: Mohanapriyan Rajendran
Cover Designer: Matthew Limbert

Typeset by TNQ Technologies

Contents

8. Inflammatory and Oxidative Stress Markers in Skeletal Muscle of Obese Subjects

Victoria Catalán, Gema Frühbeck and Javier Gómez-Ambrosi

9. Evaluation of Oxidative Stress in Humans: A Critical Point of View

Josep A. Tur, Antoni Sureda and Antoni Pons

List of Contributors

Itziar Abete, Department of Nutrition, Food Science and Physiology, Faculty of Pharmacy and Nutrition, University of Navarra, Pamplona, Spain; Biomedical Research Centre Network in Physiopathology of Obesity and Nutrition (CIBERobn), ISCIII, Madrid, Spain

Concepción M. Aguilera, University of Granada, Granada, Spain; IBS (Instituto de Investigación Biosanitaria de Granada), Granada, Spain; CIBERobn (Centro de Investigación Biomédica en Red, Fisiopatología de la obesidad y nutrición), Carlos III Health Institute, Madrid, Spain

J. Alfredo Martínez, Department of Nutrition, Food Science and Physiology, Faculty of Pharmacy and Nutrition, University of Navarra, Pamplona, Spain; Biomedical Research Centre Network in Physiopathology of Obesity and Nutrition (CIBERobn), ISCIII, Madrid, Spain; Navarra Institute for Health Research (IdiSNA), Pamplona, Spain

Lucia Alonso-Pedrero, University of Navarra, Pamplona, Spain; IdiSNA (Instituto de Investigación Sanitaria de Navarra), Pamplona, Spain

M. Angeles Zulet, Department of Nutrition, Food Science and Physiology, Faculty of Pharmacy and Nutrition, University of Navarra, Pamplona, Spain; Biomedical Research Centre Network in Physiopathology of Obesity and Nutrition (CIBERobn), ISCIII, Madrid, Spain; Navarra Institute for Health Research (IdiSNA), Pamplona, Spain

Augusto Anguita-Ruiz, University of Granada, Granada, Spain

Miguel Arredondo-Olguín, Universidad de Chile, Santiago, Chile

M. Vanessa Bullón-Vela, Department of Nutrition, Food Science and Physiology, Faculty of Pharmacy and Nutrition, University of Navarra, Pamplona, Spain

Rafael A. Casuso, University of Granada, Granada, Spain

Victoria Catalán, Clínica Universidad de Navarra, Pamplona, Spain; Centro de Investigación Biomédica en Red-Fisiopatología de la Obesidad y Nutrición (CIBEROBN), Instituto de Salud Carlos III, Pamplona, Spain; Instituto de Investigación Sanitaria de Navarra (IdiSNA), Pamplona, Spain

Elia Escasany, Universidad Rey Juan Carlos, Madrid, Spain

Xavier Escoté, Centre for Nutrition Research, University of Navarra, Pamplona, Spain

Elisa Felix-Soriano, Centre for Nutrition Research, University of Navarra, Pamplona, Spain

Marta Fernández-Galilea, Centre for Nutrition Research, University of Navarra, Pamplona, Spain; Center for Applied Medical Research, University of Navarra, Pamplona, Spain

Gema Frühbeck, Clínica Universidad de Navarra, Pamplona, Spain; Centro de Investigación Biomédica en Red-Fisiopatología de la Obesidad y Nutrición (CIBEROBN), Instituto de Salud Carlos III, Pamplona, Spain; Instituto de Investigación Sanitaria de Navarra (IdiSNA), Pamplona, Spain

Ángel Gil, University of Granada, Granada, Spain; IBS (Instituto de Investigación Biosanitaria de Granada), Granada, Spain; CIBERobn (Centro de Investigación Biomédica en Red, Fisiopatología de la obesidad y nutrición), Carlos III Health Institute, Madrid, Spain

Javier Gómez-Ambrosi, Clínica Universidad de Navarra, Pamplona, Spain; Centro de Investigación Biomédica en Red-Fisiopatología de la Obesidad y Nutrición (CIBEROBN), Instituto de Salud Carlos III, Pamplona, Spain; Instituto de Investigación Sanitaria de Navarra (IdiSNA), Pamplona, Spain

Carolina Gomez-Llorente, University of Granada, Granada, Spain

Pedro González-Muniesa, Centre for Nutrition Research, University of Navarra, Pamplona, Spain; CIBERobn, Institute of Health Carlos III, Madrid, Spain; IdiSNA, Navarra Institute for Health Research, Pamplona, Spain

Jesús R. Huertas, University of Granada, Granada, Spain

Adriana Izquierdo-Lahuerta, Universidad Rey Juan Carlos, Madrid, Spain

Paulina López-López, Universidad de Chile, Santiago, Chile

Amelia Marti del Moral, University of Navarra, Pamplona, Spain; IdiSNA (Instituto de Investigación Sanitaria de Navarra), Pamplona, Spain; CIBERobn (Centro de Investigación Biomédica en Red, Fisiopatología de la obesidad y nutrición), Carlos III Health Institute, Madrid, Spain

Leyre Martínez-Fernández, Centre for Nutrition Research, University of Navarra, Pamplona, Spain

Gema Medina-Gómez, Universidad Rey Juan Carlos, Madrid, Spain

Maria D. Mesa-Garcia, University of Granada, Granada, Spain

Lydia Morell-Azanza, University of Navarra, Pamplona, Spain; IdiSNA (Instituto de Investigación Sanitaria de Navarra), Pamplona, Spain

María J. Moreno-Aliaga, Centre for Nutrition Research, University of Navarra, Pamplona, Spain; CIBERobn, Institute of Health Carlos III, Madrid, Spain; IdiSNA, Navarra Institute for Health Research, Pamplona, Spain

Ana Ojeda-Rodriguez, University of Navarra, Pamplona, Spain; IdiSNA (Instituto de Investigación Sanitaria de Navarra), Pamplona, Spain

Josune Olza, University of Granada, Granada, Spain; IBS (Instituto de Investigación Biosanitaria de Granada), Granada, Spain; CIBERobn (Centro de Investigación Biomédica en Red, Fisiopatología de la obesidad y nutrición), Carlos III Health Institute, Madrid, Spain

Belén Pastor-Villaescusa, University of Granada, Granada, Spain

Álvaro Pejenaute, University of Navarra, Pamplona, Spain

Julio Plaza-Diaz, University of Granada, Granada, Spain

Antoni Pons, University of the Balearic Islands & CIBEROBN, Palma de Mallorca, Spain

Oscar D. Rangel-Huerta, University of Oslo, Oslo, Norway

Loreto Rojas-Sobarzo, Pontificia Universidad Católica de Chile, Santiago, Chile

Francisco J. Ruiz-Ojeda, University of Granada, Granada, Spain

Azahara I. Rupérez, University of Zaragoza, Zaragoza, Spain

Estefania Sanchez Rodriguez, University of Granada, Granada, Spain

Antoni Sureda, University of the Balearic Islands & CIBEROBN, Palma de Mallorca, Spain

Josep A. Tur, University of the Balearic Islands & CIBEROBN, Palma de Mallorca, Spain

Guillermo Zalba Goñi, University of Navarra, Pamplona, Spain; IdiSNA, Navarra Institute for Health Research, Pamplona, Spain

About the Editors

Amelia Marti del Moral is Professor of Physiology at the Department of Food Science and Physiology of the University of Navarra. She is the director of the Navarra Study Group for Childhood Obesity (GENOI) and the Children Obesity Group of the Spanish Society of Obesity. She has published more than 250 scientific articles with a factor H of 42. She has supervised 15 doctoral theses which have received both national (Royal Academy of Doctors) and international (Ibero-American Academy of Pharmacy, Best Thesis Award of the European Society of Obesity) prizes. Her research has been honored with the Silver Medal of the British Nutrition Society, the Merck & Daphne Award, and the Be Alsajara Award for Excellence, among other awards. In 2017 she edited *Telomeres, Diet and Human Disease: Advances and Therapeutic Opportunities*, published by CRC Press.

Concepción M. Aguilera is a Professor in the Department of Biochemistry and Molecular Biology at the University of Granada in Spain. She leads the research on childhood obesity as a member of the Research Excellence Group BIONIT. Currently she is leading various projects in genetics, particularly on the evaluation of genetic and epigenetic markers and their association with obesity and prepubertal metabolic changes related to early onset of metabolic syndrome. Professor Aguilera has published more than 75 scientific articles and supervised ten PhD theses. Currently she is secretary of the Institute of Nutrition and Food Technology at the University of Granada and the Iberomerican Nutrition Foundation, an institution supported by the International Union of Nutritional Sciences, and secretary of the Spanish Society of Nutrition.

Preface

This volume contains 13 contributions from a panel of experts, ranging from basic science to relevant clinical work concerning the role of oxidative stress and antioxidants in obesity.

Oxidative stress is a feature of obesity or weight-related metabolic syndrome which centers on or around molecular and cellular processes. Although a dysfunction in energy balance is the central feature of these conditions, oxidative stress can also arise from nutritional imbalance over a spectrum of time frames before the onset of obesity or weight-related metabolic syndrome. The major aim of the present book is to provide an in-depth review of our current knowledge on oxidative stress and human obesity, and examine the role of antioxidants in obesity and associated comorbidities. It also points to future directions in research on oxidative stress damage, telomere length as a marker of oxidative stress, and/or antioxidant supplementation.

The first part of the volume (Chapters 1—8) focuses on the effect of inflammation and oxidative stress on the human body, specifically covering damage to adipose tissue, vascular endothelia, liver, kidney, and skeletal muscle of obese subjects. In Chapters 1 and 2 a general overview of the relationship between obesity and oxidative stress and the evidence on the genetic basis of these conditions are presented.

A review of the evidence on the potentially therapeutic usage of natural antioxidants for obesity-related disease is presented in the second part of this volume (Chapters 9—13), ranging from vitamin C and selenium to polyphenols and antioxidant food. The last chapter offers a critical view on antioxidant supplements as angels or demons.

There is a fundamental need to understand the processes inherent in the oxidative stress in subjects who are obese.

The text is intended to furnish the reader with a general view of the state of the art in this novel area of research. We will be satisfied if the multidisciplinary nature of these proceedings informs and stimulates readers. It is our hope that the volume will encourage further research and understanding of all aspects of this intriguing and complex field of "obesity, oxidative stress, and antioxidants."

The editors express their gratitude to the authors of the chapters, and to Elsevier for having made possible the publication of this volume.

Chapter 1

Oxidative Stress and Inflammation in Obesity and Metabolic Syndrome

Francisco J. Ruiz-Ojeda[1], Josune Olza[1,2,3], Ángel Gil[1,2,3] and Concepción M. Aguilera[1,2,3]

[1]University of Granada, Granada, Spain; [2]IBS (Instituto de Investigación Biosanitaria de Granada), Granada, Spain; [3]CIBERobn (Centro de Investigación Biomédica en Red, Fisiopatología de la obesidad y nutrición), Carlos III Health Institute, Madrid, Spain

1. INTRODUCTION

Obesity is a worldwide public health problem that has been increasing in the last decades. According to the World Health Organization, obesity and overweight are defined as "abnormal or excessive fat accumulation that may impair health." Increased consumption of highly caloric foods, without an equal increase in energy expenditure, mainly by physical activity, leads to an unhealthy increase in weight; decreased levels of physical activity will result in an energy imbalance and will lead to weight gain. Worldwide obesity has more than doubled since 1980. In 2014, more than 1.9 billion adults 18 years and older were overweight, and of these over 600 million were obese. Thus 30% of adults aged 18 years and over were overweight in 2014 and 13% were obese. In addition, 41 million children under the age of five were overweight or obese in 2014. Thus the problem is twice as important than in the 1980s, and about 13% of the population is estimated to be obese [1].

Obesity is a well-known risk factor for insulin resistance (IR) and the development of type 2 diabetes (T2D). Diabetes is associated with complications such as cardiovascular diseases (CVDs), nonalcoholic fatty liver disease (NAFLD), retinopathy, angiopathy, and nephropathy, which consequently lead to higher mortality risks. Obesity-associated diabetes is hence a major public health problem, and paucity of available medication against IR requires the validation of new therapeutic targets [2]. Deaths from CVD and diabetes accounted for approximately 65% of all deaths, and general adiposity and mainly abdominal adiposity are associated with increased risk of death for all these disorders. Adiposity is also associated with a state of low-grade chronic inflammation, with increased tumor necrosis factor (TNF)-α and interleukin (IL)-6 releases, which interfere with adipose cell differentiation and the action pattern of adiponectin and leptin until the adipose tissue (AT) begins to be dysfunctional. Accordingly, the subjects present IR and hyperinsulinemia, probably the first step of a dysfunctional metabolic system. Subsequent to central obesity, IR, hyperglycemia, hypertriglyceridemia, hypoalphalipoproteinemia, hypertension, and fatty liver are grouped in the so-called metabolic syndrome (MetS) [3]. With regard to MetS, overnutrition leads to Kuppfer cell activation, chronic inflammation, hepatic steatosis, and eventual steatohepatitis and cirrhosis. Similarly, in the vascular intima, overnutrition-induced hyperlipidemia leads to oxidized low-density lipoprotein (LDL) formation and uptake in macrophages leading to foam cell formation and vascular inflammation. The cross-talk between metabolism and inflammation is also demonstrated by immunomodulatory corticosteroids that also have strong effects on host protein and carbohydrate metabolism [4].

In subjects with MetS an energy balance is critical to maintain a healthy body weight, mainly limiting high energy density foods. The first factor to be avoided in the prevention of MetS is obesity; the percentage of fat in the diet has traditionally been associated with the development of obesity. However, it is well established that the type of fat consumed could be more decisive than the total amount of fat consumed when we only look at changes in body composition and distribution of AT. Additionally, IR is a feature of MetS and is associated with other components of the syndrome. The beneficial impact of fat quality on insulin sensitivity (IS) was not seen in individuals with a high fat intake (>37% of energy). Other dietary factors that can influence various components of MetS, like postprandial glycemic and insulin

Obesity. https://doi.org/10.1016/B978-0-12-812504-5.00001-5

levels, triacylglycerols (TAGs) and high-density lipoprotein (HDL) cholesterol levels, weight regulation and body composition, as well as fatty liver, are the glycemic load and the excess of fructose, and amount of dietary fiber content of food eaten. The increased levels of TAG associated with hypoalphalipoproteinemia are a feature of IR and MetS, and increase cardiovascular risk regardless of LDL cholesterol levels [3,4].

AT is the main organ for energy storage, but also AT itself can be seen as an endocrine organ that plays a critical role in immune homeostasis. In healthy people, AT represents about 20% of the body mass in men and about 30% in women. In obesity, it expands tremendously and may constitute more than 50% of the body mass in morbidly obese individuals. AT produces and releases a variety of adipokines and cytokines, including leptin, adiponectin, resistin, and visfatin, as well as TNF-α and IL-6, among others [5]. Proinflammatory molecules produced by AT have been implicated as active participants in the development of metabolic disease. Furthermore, AT macrophages (ATMs) are prominent sources of proinflammatory cytokines, which can block insulin action in AT, skeletal muscle, and liver autocrine/paracrine signaling and cause systemic IR via endocrine signaling, providing a potential link between inflammation and IR [6].

2. OXIDATIVE STRESS, OBESITY, AND METABOLIC SYNDROME

Another critical factor that is involved in the pathogenesis of metabolic diseases is oxidative stress. Oxidative stress is a state of imbalance between the oxidative and antioxidative systems of cells and tissues, resulting in the production of excessive oxidative free radicals and reactive oxygen species (ROS) [7] caused either by exposure to damaging agents, or limited capabilities of endogenous antioxidant systems [8]. The components of the MetS as well as their comorbidities lead to the progression of prooxidative status contributing to the damage of biomolecules that are highly reactive and can stimulate cell and tissue dysfunctions, leading to the development of metabolic diseases [7]. High levels of circulating glucose and lipids can result in excessive energy substrates for metabolic pathways in adipose and nonadipose cells, increasing the production of ROS; if ROS are not well controlled, they can damage proteins, lipids, sugars, and DNA [8,9].

It is well known that mitochondria are the most critical sites for ROS production, because an excess supply of electrons to the electron transport chain can produce very high levels of ROS [10]. In addition to the range of pathologies that it can cause, this increase in ROS production can also damage the mitochondria, affecting the cellular redox signaling, indicating that this organelle can be an important target in the treatment of those pathologies [11].

A large quantity of epidemiological as well as in vivo and in vitro studies have suggested that obesity and redox alteration are interconnected through mutual mechanisms. It is hypothesized that oxidative stress is one of the links between fat accumulation-derived alterations and the appearance of a cluster of health problems including adipokine secretion alteration, inflammation, and IR (Fig. 1.1).

ROS have been involved in the adipogenesis (proliferation and differentiation) process, indicating its participation in the development of metabolic diseases through various mechanisms including chronic adipocyte inflammation, fatty acid oxidation, overconsumption of oxygen and accumulation of cellular damage, diet, and mitochondrial activity. Obesity can cause oxidative stress through the activation of intracellular pathways such as nicotinamide adenine dinucleotide phosphate (NADPH) oxidase (NOX), oxidative phosphorylation in mitochondria, glycoxidation, protein kinase C, and polyol [12]; it can also deregulate the synthesis of adipokines such as adiponectin, visfatin, resistin, leptin, plasminogen activator inhibitor-1 (PAI-1), and TNF-α and IL-6. Both TNF-α and IL-6 increase the activity of NOX and the production of superoxide anions [13]. Indeed it seems that obesity is the connection between oxidative stress and inflammation although it is not easy to confirm which one antecedes the other. It has also been observed that oxidative stress controls food intake and body weight by upholding some effects on hypothalamic neurons with impact on satiety and hunger [14].

Different studies in obese subjects have reported low levels of antioxidant molecules, oxidized-LDL (ox-LDL) and thiobarbituric acid reactive substances (TBARSs) as well as increased activities of antioxidant enzymes [13]. Additionally, high levels of protein oxidation have been correlated with the presence of AT, IR, and inflammation [15].

2.1 Biomarkers of Oxidative Stress

The direct quantification of ROS is a valuable biomarker that can reflect the disease process [8]; however, their measurement in biological systems has been complex given their short half-life and instability, which makes it a significant challenge to perform an accurate assessment of these species [16]. For this reason, different methods have been developed for measuring stable markers that reflect a systemic or tissue-specific oxidative stress [17].

Lipids, proteins, and DNA are the most common molecules that are modified when ROS levels increase in the organism. These modifications can have a direct effect on the function of target molecules or can just reflect a local degree of

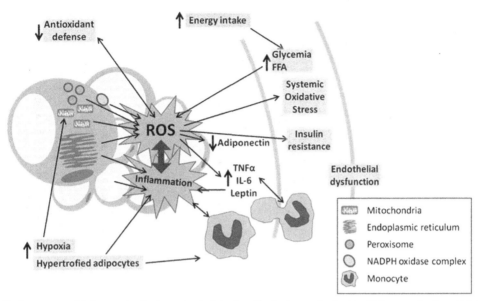

FIGURE 1.1   Oxidative stress and inflammation in the context of obesity. Obesity is associated with a high energy intake, which increases glycemia and circulating FFA. These increase ROS in the cells due to the overactivation of mitochondrial electron transport chain and the endoplasmic reticulum. The obesity associated fat accumulation leads to inflammation, hypertrophied adipocytes, and hypoxia. Moreover, oxidative stress worsens inflammation and alters adipokine secretion. Many of these phenomens activate the monocyte infiltration in adipose tissue that worsens the inflammatory processes. Hypoxia also increases glucose uptake and thus mitochondrial function, further contributing to ROS production. Through these mechanisms, ROS contribute to the development of insulin resistance, systemic oxidative stress, and endothelial damage. *FFA*, free fatty-acids; *IL-6*, interleukin 6; *NADPH*, nicotinamide adenine dinucleotide phosphate; *ROS*, reactive oxygen species; *TNFα*, tumor necrosis factor alpha.

oxidative stress; these modifications influence the clinical applicability of markers because the functional significance or the causal role of oxidative modifications on biological functions is essential for the validity of a biomarker. Thus it is important to take this into account when choosing a valid biomarker, the type of sample, and the characteristics of the individual under investigation. Table 1.1 summarizes the main biomarkers of oxidative stress studied in human obesity and MetS.

2.1.1 Lipid Oxidation Products

Lipid oxidation end product determination is an extensively used marker of oxidative stress. Cell membranes are susceptible to lipid peroxidation due to the presence of polyunsaturated fatty acids (PUFAs) that make them highly susceptible to oxidative damage in the presence of ROS or free radicals [18]. Enzymatic reactions, which oxidize arachidonic acid (AA) into prostaglandins, prostacyclin, thromboxane, and leukotrienes, can also produce lipids peroxidation through the activity of lipooxygenase and cyclooxygenase (COX) [8]. Primary products of lipid peroxidation are unstable hydroperoxides that decompose to various secondary products, among which are stable aldehydes, malondialdehyde (MDA), and 4-hydroxynonenal (HNE) [19]. These last compounds represent the most investigated end products of lipid oxidation [20] together with F2-isoprostane 15(S)-8-iso-prostaglandin F2a (15(S)-8-iso-PGF2a) [21].

2.1.1.1 Malondialdehyde, Alkenals, and Alkadienes Enclose Thiobarbituric Acid Reactive Substances

Although TBARS is the oldest methodology to determine these products, it is still widely used. This methodology has been criticized for its low sensitivity and selectivity since several MDA-unrelated species from biological samples can react with TBA, and some artifactual generation of MDA during the assay has been raised [22]. In the last few years, several innovations have been introduced to improve the specificity of the test and to reduce known bias. The combination of spectrophotometric and fluorometric technologies with high-performance liquid chromatography (HPLC) has increased the sensitivity of the test, and more recently gas chromatography coupled with mass spectroscopy (GC−MS)-based methods have been developed [17]. These methods have been demonstrated to be specific and more sensitive than the batch TBARS assays. Much evidence has been published in patients with metabolic diseases where plasma MDA and TBARS have been positively correlated with obesity in clinical studies [23]. It has also been shown that plasma glucose and insulin levels are positively associated with MDA levels in patients with T2D and IR compared with healthy volunteers [21]. Likewise,

TABLE 1.1 Main Biomarkers of Oxidative Stress in Obesity and Metabolic Syndrome Studies

Oxidative Stress Biomarkers	Analysis Methodology/Sample	Alteration
Lipid Oxidation Products		
Malondialdehyde, alkenals, and alkadienes (TBARS)	Spectrophotometry, GC–MS, HPLC/plasma	↑ Obesity, T2D, IR, and dislipidemia
4-hydroxynonenal	GC–MS, HPLC, immunoassay/plasma	↑ Obesity
F2-isoprostanes	GC–MS, HPLC, immunoassay/orine/blood	↑ Obesity and visceral fat
Protein Oxidation		
Protein carbonyls	HPLC, immunoassay/plasma	↑ Obesity, T2D, IR, and adiposity
Advanced oxidation protein products	Spectrophotometry	↑ Obesity, T2D, IR, and hypertrigliceridemia
Advanced lipoxigenation and glycation end products	Immunoassay, spectrofluorimetric, MS	↑ Obesity, T2D, and IR
Nitrotyrosine (3-NO-Tyr)	ELISA, HPLC, GC–MS/MS, LC–MS/MS/blood	↑ Obesity and MetS
Oxidized low-density lipoproteins	Immunoassay	↑ Waist circumference and MetS
DNA Oxidation		
7,8-dihydroxy-8-oxo-2′-deoxyguanosine	Immunoassay, HPLC, HPLC-ECD GC–MS/orine	
Antioxidant Defense System		
Glutathione peroxidases	Activity by spectrophotometry/adipose tissue	↑ Obesity and IR
Catalases	Activity by spectrophotometry/erythrocyte	↓ Obesity and IR
Paraoxonases	Activity by spectrophotometry/serum	↓ Obesity, NAFLD, and IR because of lower HDLc
Peroxiredoxins	Activity by spectrophotometry/adipose tissue	↓ Obesity
Superoxide dismutases	Activity by spectrophotometry/adipose tissue and plasma	↑ ↓ Obesity and IR

GC/MS, gas chromatography coupled with mass spectroscopy; *HPLC*, high-performance liquid chromatography; *IR*, insulin resistance; *LC/MS*, liquid chromatography coupled with mass spectroscopy; *MetS*, metabolic syndrome; *MS*, metabolic syndrome; *NAFLD*, nonalcoholic fatty liver disease; *T2D*, type 2 diabetes; *TBARS*, thiobarbituric acid reactive substance.

different studies in humans and animals have demonstrated that a dyslipidemic state is associated with higher levels of plasma MDA, and reduction of these plasmatic lipid levels is associated with the reduction of MDA.

2.1.1.2 4-Hydroxynonenal

4-HNE is mainly formed by n-6 fatty acid oxidation, and high concentrations of this compound have been shown to trigger well-known pathways such as induction of caspases and release of cytochrome c from mitochondria. The most frequently used methods to determine 4-HNE are GC−MS, HPLC, and by immunological techniques using polyclonal or monoclonal antibodies against 4-HNE-protein conjugates [8,20]. 4-HNE is derived from fatty acids such as linoleic and AAs. The content of these fatty acids in the body depends on the composition of the diet. In obesity higher levels of 4-HNE have been reported [24]. A recent study in obese subjects observed higher concentrations of 4-HNE per unit of intramuscular triglycerides [13].

2.1.1.3 F2-Isoprostanes

Isoprostanes (IsoPs) are prostaglandin-like molecules produced in vivo from AA by a free radical catalyzed mechanism and do not need COXs for their synthesis. They are stable products released into circulation before the hydrolyzed form is excreted in urine. Many end products are generated, but the main focus has been aimed at F2-IsoPs. F2-IsoPs are unaffected by lipid content in the diet, and thus their measurement in biological fluids (mainly urine) as well as exhaled breath condensate can provide an estimation of total body production. Different methodologies have been used for its analysis such as GC−MS, HPLC/GC−MS, GC-tandem, and more recently some immunoassay techniques have been developed and the results have shown that urine samples correlate well with MS techniques while plasma samples show some discrepancies [17].

IsoPs have advantages over other oxidative stress markers. These molecules are chemically stable, they are unaffected by lipid content in the diet, they are specific products of peroxidation, they are formed in vivo, and they are detectable in tissues and biological fluids [25]. Several studies have demonstrated that subjects with obesity and/or diabetes have elevated levels of IsoP in blood as well as in urine. Results from the Framingham study have demonstrated the correlation between body mass index (BMI) and urinary levels of IsoP. Another study observed that subjects with android obesity had higher IsoP than subjects with gynoid obesity [25], indicating that individuals with central adiposity have higher oxidative stress.

2.1.2 Protein Oxidation

Proteins represent broad targets for radicals and oxidants in biological systems. These compounds damage side-chain and backbone sites. The modifications that occur result in increased side-chain hydrophilicity, side-chain and backbone fragmentation, aggregation via covalent cross-linking or hydrophobic interactions, protein unfolding and altered conformation, altered interactions with biological partners, and modified turnover [26]. Some of these actions are reversible, such as oxidation, while others such as carbonylation, nitrosylation, breaking of the histidine and tryptophan rings, and hydrolysis of the peptide bond in the presence of proline are irreversible [8].

Although their formation has been associated with several diseases, markers of protein oxidation are not as extensively used as lipid oxidation parameters and are usually determined in combination with them [17]. Protein oxidation markers can be determined in blood or urine, but also in tissues or cells for more accurate information. Different techniques have been used for their determination, but more methodologies are needed to identify and quantify specific protein oxidative modifications.

2.1.2.1 Protein Carbonyls

Carbonylation is an irreversible protein modification induced by ROS. It can be produced by oxidative cleavage of the backbone of the protein or by the attack of ROS radicals to some specific amino acids in the side chains such as lysine, arginine, proline, or threonine [15]. Protein carbonyls are the most widely used markers to measure oxidative protein damage, generally by colorimetric or ELISA methods. However, HPLC is also used for its determination. Protein carbonyl levels increase with age and are elevated in several pathologic conditions including obesity and diabetes. Different studies have demonstrated a positive correlation between protein carbonyls and BMI in obese subjects as well as in subjects with MetS. In a recent study, higher concentrations of protein carbonyl were observed in the subcutaneous AT of obese subjects, which was associated with the degree of adiposity and plasma free fatty acids. Other studies have demonstrated a positive correlation between protein carbonyl and homeostatic model assessment (HOMA) index. High levels of protein carbonyl in patients with T2D and even higher levels in those with cardiovascular complications have also been reported. Likewise, patients with hyperlipidemia have reported higher levels of protein carbonyl [15]. It has been observed that reduction of body weight by surgery, caloric restriction, physical activity, or pharmacologic treatments provoke a reduction in protein carbonyls.

2.1.2.2 Advanced Oxidation Protein Products

Hypochlorous acid oxidized proteins, especially albumin, produce advanced oxidation protein products (AOPPs) including protein aggregates by disulphide bridges and/or tyrosine cross-linking. AOPPs are novel protein biomarkers of oxidative damage and a novel class of inflammatory mediators. These products can promote oxidative stress and inflammation and thus participate in many pathophysiological disease processes including those present in obesity and diabetes [27]. AOPPs can be detected through spectrophotometric techniques. It has been observed that in obese subjects central obesity, high levels of triglycerides, and altered glucose metabolism are correlated with elevated levels of plasma AOPP. Likewise, higher AOPP levels have been associated with resistin, TNF-α, and IL-6 in obese subjects with T2D. Moreover, higher levels of AOPP have been observed in obese adolescents compared with their lean counterparts [15].

2.1.2.3 Advanced Lipoxigenation and Glycation End Products

Functional groups of proteins can react with several products resulting from the ROS-induced oxidation of PUFAs and carbohydrate, generating advanced peroxidation end products (advanced lipoxigenation end products [ALEs]) and advanced glycation end products (AGEs), respectively [28]. These products increase with aging. When there is an overproduction of ROS induced by hyperglycemia the AGE pathway is activated [29]. AGEs can induce a signal transduction cascade leading to an inflammatory response [30].

The determination of these products is mainly through specific antibodies, immunoassays, or spectrofluorimetric methods. Additionally, MS techniques have been used with excellent results. Some studies have demonstrated that AGE accumulation in AT is associated with IR in obesity. It has also been proposed that AGEs can precede the onset of T2D and their accumulation in these patients can result from different biochemical reactions in different signaling pathways [31].

2.1.2.4 Nitrotyrosine

3-nitrotyrosine (3-NO-Tyr) is the main product of tyrosine oxidation. It is formed after the substitution of a hydrogen by a nitro group in the phenolic ring of the tyrosine residues. The determination of 3-NO-Tyr can be performed by ELISA, chromatography methods, and HPLC; however, the most reliable analytical approach in terms of sensitivity and accuracy is currently stable-isotope dilution tandem mass spectrometry coupled with gas chromatography (GC−MS/MS) or liquid chromatography (LC−MS/MS) [21]. An association between increased circulating levels of 3-NO-Tyr and cellular oxidative stress markers has been observed in patients with MetS [14].

2.1.2.5 Oxidized Low-Density Lipoproteins

Oxidation of LDLs is increased in atherosclerosis. These molecules are an easy target for denaturalization by a variety of oxidative processes, which result in functional and structural modification of these molecules [27]. Ox-LDLs are deposited on the vessel walls and lead to the formation of foam cells, promoting an oxidative environment that induces the infiltration of mononuclear cells into the vascular wall and contributing to the pathogenesis of vascular dysfunction observed in the first stages of atherosclerosis. It is usually measured by immunoassay; however, this has been criticized because of the heterogeneity of oxidation products, the low specificity of the antibodies, and the low concordance among assays [8]. The modification of LDL into ox-LDL is mainly due to the oxidative condition that is present during metabolic disorders. Different studies have demonstrated increased levels of ox-LDL in patients with MetS, which is associated with higher risk of CVDs such as atherosclerosis and myocardial infarction. The increasing oxidation of LDL in plasma has been associated with the early onset of atherosclerosis and it can progress to the development of atherosclerotic lesions. It has also been reported that in patients with MetS that high ox-LDLs are associated with low concentration of HDL-c and higher oxidative stress [7]. Several studies have reported that LDL oxidation heightened with an increasing waist circumference, higher C reactive protein (CRP) concentrations, and the quantity of LDL molecules [14].

2.1.3 DNA Oxidation

The induction of DNA oxidation by ROS leads to several DNA modifications such as nucleotide oxidation, strand breakage, loss of bases, and adduct formation. Either the nucleotides or the sugars can react with the oxidants and generate different products, with 7,8-dihydroxy-8-oxo-2′-deoxyguanosine the most common (8oxodG) [8]. The DNA damage can also be produced indirectly by the oxidation of other molecules. The best techniques to measure 8oxodG are HPLC with electrochemical detection (HPLC-ECD) and HPLC/GC−MS; however, some immunoassays with specific antibodies have shown to be suitable methods to measure 8oxodG in urine.

2.2 Antioxidant Defense System

Antioxidants can be divided into enzymatic antioxidants and nonenzymatic antioxidants. The enzymatic antioxidants are either primary or secondary enzymes. The primary enzymes are glutathione peroxidase (GPX), catalase (CAT), and superoxide dismutase (SOD), which prevent the formation or neutralize free radicals. Likewise, peroxiredoxins (PRDXs) neutralize small amounts of peroxides; these enzymes use their interior active site cysteine residues to reduce target molecules. The secondary enzymes such as glutathione reductase, which reduces oxidized glutathione; and glucose 6-phosphate dehydrogenase, which regenerates NADPH, play an indirect role, supporting other endogenous antioxidants [32].

Antioxidants can capture free radicals that are generated either by cellular metabolism or exogenous sources through the donation of hydrogen atoms of these molecules, breaking the chain reaction, which prevents attack on lipids, amino acids, and DNA, avoiding damage and loss of cell integrity [16]. The determination of these enzymes is widely used in clinical studies to evaluate the antioxidant defense system, and the methodologies used are mainly enzyme activity, protein content, or gene expression; however, the way the samples are collected and preserved is critical.

2.2.1 Glutathione Peroxidases

The GPX family is composed of at least six isoenzymes and constitutes one of the main antioxidant defense systems, using glutathione to degrade hydrogen peroxide [33]. GPX1 is the most abundant isoenzyme, ubiquitous in the intracellular fraction and formed by four 22-kDa subunits, each carrying one selenocysteine. Cellular and extracellular GPX activity was shown to be lower in the AT of obese rats [34].

2.2.2 Catalase

CAT is one of the most important antioxidant enzymes in the cell, located in the peroxisomes. It degrades any hydrogen peroxide that exceeds the physiological levels. CAT expression was increased after caloric restriction in obese mice [35], and its erythrocyte activity was lower in children with IR and obesity [36,37].

2.2.3 Paraoxonases

The paraoxonase (PON) family consists of three antioxidant isoenzymes. PON1 and PON3 are expressed mainly in the liver and kidneys and are found bound to HDLs in the circulation. They inhibit the lipid peroxidation of the LDL and HDL particles in plasma. PON2 is a more ubiquitous membrane-bound form that is found in a variety of tissues. Regarding alterations in PON expression in obesity, only one study has been conducted, in pigs, where PON3 mRNA expression in fat tissue was positively correlated with subcutaneous, visceral, and total body fat weight, indicating a role for PON3 in obesity [38].

2.2.4 Peroxiredoxins

PRDXs are a family of six thioredoxin-dependent peroxidases that degrade H_2O_2 in the cell. Recent studies have clearly shown that PRDXs contribute to ROS signaling, regulating cell proliferation, differentiation, and apoptosis. PRDX3 is located exclusively in the mitochondria, where it scavenges up to 90% of the H_2O_2 produced in this organelle, followed by scavenging by GPX1 and GPX4 [39]. Taking into account that mitochondrial respiration is the principal ROS producer, PRDX3 is considered highly important in terms of antioxidant defense and redox status regulation. PRDX3 levels have been observed to be decreased in the AT of obese mice and humans [40].

2.2.5 Superoxide Dismutases

The three members of the SOD family are the first line of defense against ROS, eliminating the strong superoxide radical and producing H_2O_2 that can then be degraded by CAT, GPX, and PRDX. CuZn-SOD (SOD1) is a homodimer localized in the cytosol, manganese-dependent superoxide dismutase (Mn-SOD) (SOD2) is a tetramer localized in the mitochondria, and the extracellular tetramer CuZn-SOD (SOD3 or extracellular (EC)-SOD) is localized exclusively in extracellular spaces. Mn-SOD is one of the most important antioxidant enzymes because most superoxide is produced in the mitochondria [41].

EC-SOD levels have been observed to increase in the white and brown AT and in the plasma of obese mice. In the same study, TNFα and IL-1β levels were also observed to be higher in white AT, which could be interpreted as an adaptation by the AT to the enhanced oxidative stress associated with obesity [42]. However, in a study of T2D patients, EC-SOD levels were shown to be reduced and inversely related to BMI and HOMA-IR [43].

3. INFLAMMATION, OBESITY, AND METABOLIC SYNDROME

The MetS and T2D are metabolically associated and there is a strong relationship between abdominal obesity and T2D. The pathophysiology of MetS is complex where the IS reduction is implicated in the development of T2D. Cellular and humoral inflammation is located not only in AT, more particularly in visceral adipose tissue (VAT), but also in skeletal muscle, liver, and pancreatic islets, which may explain both IR and β-cell progressive failure [44]. The complex cross-talk between adipocytes and macrophages is demonstrated by the ability of preadipocytes to differentiate into macrophages and possibly also macrophages to differentiate into preadipocytes [4].

Abdominal obesity corresponds to a subclinical inflammatory condition that promotes the production of proinflammatory factors involved in the pathogenesis of IR. Inflammatory cytokines, including TNF-α, have been shown to promote IR, and altered expression of adipokines in obese AT is thought to be an important link between obesity and IR. Moreover, the metabolically unhealthy obese phenotype seems to be associated with an increased activation of the nucleotide-binding oligomerization domain, leucine-rich repeat and pyrin domain containing 3 (NLRP3) inflammasome in macrophages infiltrating VAT, and a less promising inflammatory profile compared with the metabolically healthy obese phenotype. Indeed, an increased secretion of IL-1β, increased expression of IL-1β and NLRP3, increased number of ATMs, and decreased number of regulatory T has been found in the VAT of metabolically unhealthy obese patients compared with metabolically obese patients and lean subjects. In macrophages derived from VAT, both caspase-1 activity and IL-1β levels are higher in metabolically unhealthy obese patients than metabolically healthy patients [45]. Fig. 1.2 summarizes the main cytokines and adipokines secreted by AT, specifically the alterations regarding inflammation in the subjects with obesity and MetS.

Macrophages are mononuclear phagocytes and key to the innate immune response to pathogens. Macrophages maintain tissue homeostasis and function by scavenging debris, pathogens, and apoptotic or necrotic cells. Circulating monocytes differentiate into diverse resident macrophages found in almost all tissues including ATM. Each macrophage phenotype has a specialized function and maintains the local tissue microenvironment and inflammatory tone. Upon activation, macrophages release cytokines and chemokines that initiate an inflammatory response. The suppressor of cytokine signaling (SOCS) family regulates this response via feedback inhibition targeting the Janus kinase (JAK) pathway, a signaling cascade that transduces signals from cytokines and regulates cell proliferation and IS. Toll-like receptors (TLRs) are evolutionarily conserved pathogen-associated molecular pattern receptors that recognize potential pathogens and mount an immune response. The SOCS family regulates this response via feedback inhibition targeting the JAK pathway, a signaling cascade that transduces signals from cytokines and regulates cell proliferation and IS [4,44,45].

MicroRNA (miRNA) is small noncoding RNA molecules that regulate gene expression by binding to messenger RNA. Some miRNA such as miRNA-155 is released by inflammatory macrophages in response to danger signals such as TLR ligands and lipopolysaccharide (LPS). miRNA-155 represses SOCS leading to JAK signaling and increased inflammation. Proinflammatory miRNA from inflammatory macrophages such as this are balanced by antiinflammatory cytokines such as protection, which is involved with the resolution of inflammation and tissue healing [4].

Metaflammation is the process whereby excess nutrients promote chronic low-grade inflammation. Unlike the acute, intense, and rapidly resolving inflammation in response to infection and injury, low-grade chronic tissue stress is associated with a physiologic adaptive immune response called para-inflammation. This para-inflammation upsets recruitment of monocytes and tissue macrophages, which are the center of the interaction between metabolism and inflammation. Additionally, the regulation of chronic para-inflammation may contribute to disease progression. Consequently, the MetS appears due to chronic low-grade inflammation that causes IR in metabolically healthy obesity, and MetS is a metabolic disorder, but also a chronic systemic syndrome is characterized by elevated TNF-α and macrophage infiltration into AT [4]. Therefore, macrophages are central to immunometabolism, obesity associated tissue remodeling, and the development of adiposity-based chronic disease comorbidities including chronic systemic inflammation, MetS, obesity-related IR, NAFLD, and T2D [46].

Macrophages regulate adipogenesis and angiogenesis in response to environmental, nutritional, and physical stimuli through interactions with preadipocytes. Macrophages secrete platelet-derived growth factor, which promotes preadipocyte

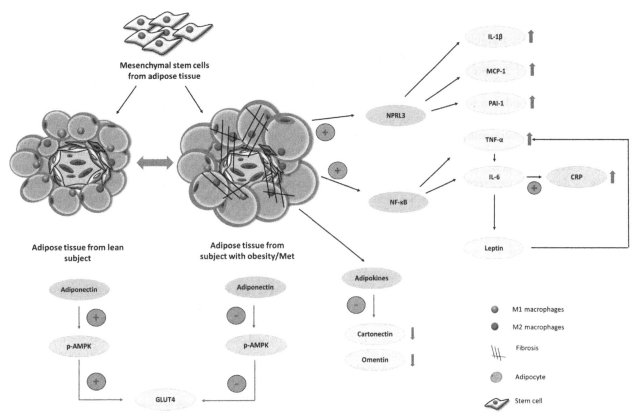

FIGURE 1.2 Inflammation biomarkers linking to obesity and metabolic diseases. *AMPK*, adenosine monophosphate kinase; *CRP*, C-reactive protein; *GLUT4*, glucose transporter 4; *IL1β*, interleukin 1-beta; *IL6*, interleukin 6; *MCP1*, monocyte chemotactic protein-1; *NF-κB*, nuclear factor kappa-light-chain-enhancer of activated B cells; *NPRL3*, nitrogen permease regulator-like 3; *PAI-1*, plasminogen activator inhibitor 1; *TNFα*, tumor necrosis factor alpha.

survival leading to AT hyperplasia and maintenance of IS. Conversely, M1 macrophages induce IR, which is reviewed later. In lean tissue, M2 macrophages interact with preadipocytes by releasing factors that promote survival and maintain adequate angiogenesis. Peroxisome proliferator activator receptor (PPAR)-γ, which is a family of nuclear proteins that regulate adipocyte gene expression and function, promotes primary human monocytes to differentiate into an M2 phenotype. M2 macrophages maintain IS by secreting the antiinflammatory cytokine IL-10. Macrophage-specific deletion of the PPAR-γ receptor impairs M2 macrophage activation and decreases expression of genes involved in oxidative phosphorylation in liver and muscle tissue, which is associated with decreased IS in these tissues [4].

It has also been well established that inflammation is essential for repair, remodeling, and even renewal of tissues, including those with critical metabolic function. These responses also need to be temporally and spatially regulated to maintain homeostasis, including metabolic homeostasis, otherwise they will be uniformly damaging when sustained. These considerations aside, the immunological aspect of metabolic regulation in a multicellular organism could be framed in its most fundamental form by examining a highly conserved relationship between a potent and pleiotropic immune mediator TNF, a pathogen sensing system (TLRs), and a powerful metabolic hormone (insulin) [47].

3.1 Biomarkers of Inflammation

Various biomarkers of inflammation have been shown to be associated with a higher risk to develop T2D mellitus and CVD. Among those markers, CRP, especially high-sensitive CRP, has been the most extensively studied [44]. Furthermore, soluble adhesion molecules such as eselectin, vascular cell adhesion molecule-1 (VCAM-1), and intercellular adhesion molecule-1 (ICAM-1) are molecular markers for endothelial dysfunction, an early marker of atherosclerosis. And, the cytokines released by AT such as TNF-α, IL1β, IL6, adipsin, C3, and acylation stimulating protein (ASP), leptin, adiponectin, p-selectin, monocyte chemoattractant protein-1 (MCP1), resistin, C1qTNF-related proteins (CTRPs), visfatin, omentin, and PAI-1, which are described in detail.

3.1.1 Tumor Necrosis Factor-α

TNF-α is a key cytokine that intervenes in acute and chronic phase inflammation inducing inflammation, apoptosis, tumor necrosis, and cachexia. TNF-α is mainly produced by M1-macrophages, but also by many other immune cells as well adipocytes, which also express TNF-α receptors. Besides its role in inflammation, TNF-α has now been implicated in energy homeostasis and the development of obesity-induced MetS and T2D mellitus. TNF-α increases secretion in AT of proinflammatory molecules such as IL-6, MCP-1, leptin, and PAI-1, thus contributing to inflammatory conditions linked to obesity. In obese individuals, an increase in the production of TNF-α by adipocytes was observed, which positively correlates with IR and T2D mellitus. In AT and liver, TNF-α suppresses the expression of genes involved in the storage of free fatty acids and increases expression of genes involved in the de novo synthesis of cholesterol and fatty acids. The increase of serum fatty acids has been shown to induce IR in multiple tissues. Furthermore, TNF-α also impairs insulin signaling by decreasing the expression of the insulin-sensitive glucose transporter 4 and insulin receptor substrate-1 (IRS-1), suppresses tyrosine phosphorylation of IRS-1, and enhances serine phosphorylation of IRS-1 (increasing degradation of insulin receptors) [47,48].

3.1.2 Interleukin-1β

IL-1β is a major proinflammatory cytokine produced by macrophages. In AT, macrophages produced IL-1β via activated NLRP3 inflammasome. IL-1β is also released by nonfat cells from AT, and this secretion is enhanced in obesity. This cytokine is a promoter of AT inflammation in obesity. IL-1β induces hypertrophic adipocyte cell death that launches the inflammatory cascade, leukocyte and macrophage recruitment, and macrophage lipid accumulation. Scientific evidence suggests that IL-1β is key linking obesity-associated inflammation to IR and pathogenesis of T2D. Recently the implication of IL-1β in pancreatic beta-cell demise that precedes diabetes development was demonstrated in rodent models. Also, various works showed the role of IL-1β in the macrophage-adipocyte cross-talk, which blocks insulin action in human AT (inhibition of insulin signaling and glucose metabolism in human adipocytes). Furthermore, studies have demonstrated that IL-1β also limit hyperplastic (AT) expansion, promoting ectopic fat accumulation (and decreasing subcutaneous fat storage), thus favoring liver steatosis and obesity-associated morbidity [49].

3.1.3 Interleukin-6

IL-6 is a cytokine involved in regulation of the hematopoiesis, immune response, and acute and chronic phase inflammation. This cytokine secreted by T cells, macrophages, adipocytes, and AT matrix together with TNF-α plays a key role in the development of IR and atherosclerosis, pathologies related to obesity and MetS. Up to 35% of circulating IL-6 is produced by AT and increased with the expansion of AT, particularly visceral AT. IL-6 promotes the production by macrophages and T cells of proinflammatory CRP, associated with increased risk of diabetes, hypertension, and CVD [48].

3.1.4 Adipsin, C3, and Acylation Stimulating Protein

Adipsin (complement factor D) is a serine protease synthesized by adipocytes. This enzyme activates the alternative pathway of the complement, triggering the natural defense against infections. It is implicated in the enzymatic production of C3adesArg or ASP, a complement protein that intervenes in systemic energy balance regulation (lipid and glucose metabolism). Studies in humans show that adipsin is associated with IR, dyslipidemia, MetS, and CVD. Adipsin concentrations are elevated in obese individuals, abdominal obesity, and MetS. Complement component 3 (C3) is an immune protein produced mainly by the liver, but also by AT. This protein plays a main role in the activation of both classical and alternative complement pathways. C3 is cleaved by spontaneous hydrolysis or by C3 convertase enzyme complex in catalytic C3b and smaller anaphylatoxin fragment C3a. C3b forms a complex with factor B (also produced by AT), which is cleaved by adipsin generating noncatalytic Ba fragment and C3bBb complex, which is the alternative pathway C3 convertase that acts enzymatically on additional molecules of C3, amplifying the complement cascade. C3a is a potent chemoattractant and plays a large role in the immune response. C3a induces the production of proinflammatory IL-6 and TNF-α, leading to attract and activate T cells, mast cell degranulation, and macrophage activation, amplifying obesity-induced inflammation. C3a is cleaved to remove its carboxy-terminal arginine to generate C3adesArg (or ASP), a molecule with lowered inflammatory function but, as already mentioned, a metabolic effector. High circulating C3 levels have been positively associated with pathological states, such as MetS and its phenotypes (abdominal obesity, hyperglycemia, IR, dyslipidemia), T2D mellitus, CVD, and hypertension. In fact, numerous investigations reported up to a threefold increased risk of MetS and its associated metabolic perturbations in subjects with high C3 levels.

Some authors showed that C3 concentrations in the top 50th percentile may increase the risk of metabolic perturbations. Also, an increase in C3 concentrations was found after fasting or fat uptake. Postprandial phase, insulin, and chylomicrons are among the most potent stimulators of AT production of C3 and subsequent activation of the alternate complement pathway, leading to the formation of C3a and ASP (C3adesArg). Since MetS is characterized by fasting and postprandial hypertriglyceridemia and hyperinsulinemia, this may explain the abnormal increments in C3 concentrations in MetS. This, in turn, aggravates the metabolic disorders of this syndrome. C3/ASP system has been recognized as a regulator of AT fatty acid metabolism. C3/ASP is a stimulator of fatty acid trapping and triglyceride synthesis in human adipocytes. Also, it diminishes lipolysis and release of free fatty acids from adipocytes. C3/ASP also promotes glucose transport in adipocytes and insulin secretion from pancreatic β-cells. Increased C3/ASP levels in the MetS counteract the insulin-resistant states, acting as a backup system for postprandial free fatty acids uptake [50,51].

3.1.5 Leptin

Leptin is a polypeptide secreted by adipose cells, and is a mediator of long-term regulation of energy balance through the central nervous system (CNS) [21]. Leptin suppresses food intake by inhibiting orexigenic neuropeptides and stimulating anorexigenic ones, and increases energy expenditure. This peptide has structural homology to helical cytokines, such as IL-2. Its receptors, found both in cells of the CNS and in the periphery, belong to the cytokine receptor class I superfamily, such as the IL-6 receptor. As already mentioned, leptin secretion increases with the expansion of AT, particularly visceral AT, and was found to be high in MetS and obesity. Leptin correlates with many parameters of MetS including waist circumference, glucose level, insulin level, IR, and triglyceride level. This peptide promotes proliferation of proinflammatory cells and cytokines, as well as endothelial cell growth and angiogenesis. In monocytes, leptin promotes the production of proinflammatory TNF-α and IL-6. In macrophages, leptin stimulates the production of chemoattractant molecules MIP-1α (macrophage inflammatory protein), MIP-1β, and regulated on activation normal T cell expressed and secreted (RANTES), which promotes the recruitment and activation of multiple immune cells [52,53].

3.1.6 P-Selectin

P-selectin is a protein produced by activated platelets and endothelial cells that functions as a cell adhesion molecule. P-selectin plays an essential role in the initial recruitment of leukocytes and in the recruitment and aggregation of platelets to the site of injury during inflammation. Increased levels of this protein have been associated with MetS. Indeed, P-selectin expression and secretion have also been associated with increased visceral AT, low HDL cholesterol, high oxidized LDL, and elevated fasting glucose. An increased of P-selectin is known to be involved in the attachment of circulating leukocytes to the vascular endothelium, contributing to the early development of atherosclerotic lesions [54].

3.1.7 Monocyte Chemotactic Protein-1

MCP-1 is a cytokine produced in AT that recruits monocytes, macrophages, T cells, and dendritic cells to the sites of inflammation. During obesity development higher levels of MCP-1 promote accumulation of monocytes in arteries and macrophage infiltration of AT, which triggers production of proinflammatory mediators including MCP-1. Increments in MCP-1 level were associated with visceral obesity-related complications such as IR and neointimal formation with the development of atherosclerosis [48].

3.1.8 Plasminogen Activator Inhibitor-1

PAI-1 is a serine protease inhibitor that arrests fibrinolysis via inhibition of the tissue-type plasminogen activator. PAI-1 is secreted by several tissues, including adipocytes and other cells of AT. Serum levels of PAI-1 are increased in MetS (obesity, visceral adiposity, and IR) and in response to TNF-α. Scientific evidence suggested that high levels of PAI-1 are necessary to the development of obesity and its comorbidities. This protein is implicated in angiogenesis and atherogenesis and therefore in the development of CVD related to obesity [48].

3.1.9 Resistin

Resistin is a cysteine-rich peptide secreted by adipocytes, immune cells, and epithelial cells. High levels of resistin were found in MetS. This proinflammatory cytokine causes the resistance of peripheral tissues to insulin and is considered by many researchers as a possible link between obesity and T2D mellitus. Resistin promotes the secretion of TNF-α and IL-6 by mononuclear cells. Furthermore, resistin counteracts the effects of antiinflammatory adiponectin on vascular endothelial cells by enhancing leukocyte adhesion to this endothelium. This peptide increases the expression of the VCAM-1 and MCP-1, the key processes in early atherosclerotic lesion formation [55].

3.1.10 Visfatin

Visfatin is an adipokine mainly produced by visceral fat. This protein is a proinflammatory mediator, recognized as a pre-B-cell enhancing factor, which also interferes with insulin-receptor signaling. Some studies have shown higher plasma visfatin levels associated with MetS. Information suggests that this cytokine is related to IR and chronic inflammatory reaction that contributes to the development of MetS. However, these findings regarding implications of visfatin in metabolic disorders associated with MetS and obesity are still inconclusive [56].

3.2 Adipose Tissue and Antiinflammatory Proteins

3.2.1 Adiponectin

Adiponectin is an antiinflammatory adipokine exclusively produced in differentiated adipocytes of white AT and secreted at high levels into the circulating bloodstream. This protein shares strong homology in its primary sequence with complement factor C1q. Adiponectin expression is higher in subcutaneous than in visceral fat. Its multiple metabolic functions include decrease of intracellular triglyceride content in liver and skeletal muscle (through the increase in fatty acid oxidation), decrease of gluconeogenesis in liver, increase of glucose uptake in skeletal muscle, increment in IS, antiinflammatory effects, and antiatherogenic effects. Antiatherogenic properties of adiponectin are due to the inhibition of endothelial expression of adhesion molecules (VCAM-1 and ICAM-1), the attenuation of smooth muscle cell proliferation, suppression of the transformation of macrophages into foam cells, vasodilatation via increase of nitric oxide production in endothelial cells, and stimulation of angiogenesis. Adiponectin also diminishes the infiltration of CD4$^+$ T cells into atherosclerotic lesions via the suppression of chemoattractants in macrophages [26]. Antiinflammatory effects of adiponectin are also modulated via switch of macrophages from the proinflammatory M1-like phenotype that secretes proinflammatory cytokines (TNF-α, IL-1β, IL-6, and MCP-1) to antiinflammatory M2-like phenotype that produce antiinflammatory IL-10, further inhibition of TLR-mediated nuclear factor kappa-light-chain-enhancer of activated B cell (NF-κB) activation in macrophages. Several clinical studies have demonstrated a close association between low plasma adiponectin concentration with obesity, T2D mellitus, CVD, and MetS and its related disorders (low HDL cholesterol and high triglyceride levels). Indeed, some authors consider this multifunctional protein as a key molecule in the pathogenesis of MetS. Adiponectin expression is higher by the functional adipocytes of subcutaneous fat of lean organisms. However, its expression is downregulated in the dysfunctional adipocytes of subjects with obesity. Studies in rodents and humans showed that circulating adiponectin decreased in obesity (negative correlation with the accumulation of body fat, particularly visceral fat) and inflammatory states (TNF-α, IL-1β, and interferon gamma (IFN-γ)), and is positively correlated with IS. Consistent with these findings, an increase in adiponectin level was observed associated with IS improvement and reduction in inflammatory markers, such as CRP and IL-6, after weight loss in overweight individuals. Furthermore, the absence of adiponectin in adiponectin-deficient mice was associated with vascular alterations and abnormal metabolic profiles, independently of diet or body weight [53,57].

3.2.2 C1qTNF-Related Proteins

CTRPs are adiponectin produced mainly by adipocytes that share structural similarities with C1q complement factor. CTRPs are also multifunctional proteins involved in metabolism, cell differentiation and apoptosis, and innate immunity. Similar to adiponectin, several CTRPs have hypoglycemic effects and antiinflammatory functions. CTRP-3 or cartonectin is an antiinflammatory protein produced by mature adipocytes that modulates the immune system by suppressing the NF-κB signaling pathway. Cartonectin suppresses TLR stimulation in macrophages and adipocytes. Also, it inhibits monocyte-derived macrophage recruitment via macrophage migration inhibitory factor, MCP-1, or C−C motif chemokine ligand-4. Cartonectin promotes the secretion of adiponectin in adipocytes. Deficiencies of cartonectin were related to increments in the expression of proinflammatory adipokines and reduction in adiponectin expression in preadipocytes. CTRP-12 or adipolin is an adipokine also produced by adipocytes. Adipolin is the CTRP protein that shows lesser sequence identity to adiponectin. This adipokine diminishes inflammatory responses in fat tissues and promotes IS through activation of insulin signaling in the liver and AT, where it suppresses gluconeogenesis and enhances glucose uptake [58]. Adipolin attenuates macrophage infiltration and reduces the expression of proinflammatory cytokines (TNFα, IL-1β, and MCP-1) in response to stimulation with LPS or TNF-α. Adipolin expression in white fat tissue and serum adipolin levels are decreased in obesity, with the increment in waist circumference and in hyperglycemia. Clinical trials confirmed a negative correlation between adipolin levels and obesity and T2D. Recent studies indicate that adipolin expression during obese conditions is suppressed via upregulation of KLF3 and downregulation of KLF15. KLF3 and KLF15 are Krüppel-like factor proteins that bind DNA repressing (KLF3) or activating (KLF15) transcription of adipolin. Furthermore, a study in rodents showed that obese states enhance the cleavage of full adipolin through induction of furin endopeptidase in AT, increasing levels in the bloodstream of the lesser active cleaved adipolin. CTRP9 is also abundantly expressed in AT. CTRP9 can form heterotrimers with adiponectin and share adiponectin receptors. Recent studies indicated that circulating CTRP9 levels decrease in obesity. Research also showed that CTRP9 protein promotes glucose uptake induced by insulin and fat oxidation in skeletal muscle. Like adiponectin, CTRP9 exerts antiatherogenic properties via inhibition of vascular smooth muscle cell proliferation, and nitric oxide–mediated vasodilatation. Several reports indicate that CTRP9 can protect against the development of obesity-linked metabolic dysfunction and CVD. Other CTRPs with metabolic and antiinflammatory functions, such as CTRP6 and CTRP1, are profusely produced by adipocytes; however, no decreases in its concentrations associated with BMI was observed. CTRP6 can induce the expression of antiinflammatory cytokine IL-10 in human monocyte-derived macrophages. It also increases fatty acid oxidation in skeletal muscle cells. CTRP1, secreted by AT in response to infections and cytokines, has many metabolic adiponectin-like functions [58].

3.2.3 Omentin

Omentin (or intelectin-1) is an adipocytokine that is highly expressed in visceral fat tissue and in omentum (visceral peritoneum). Reduced levels of this antiinflammatory protein are associated with obesity-related metabolic dysfunction. Circulating omentin levels are indeed significantly reduced in obese individuals or individuals with increased waist circumstance and in obesity-linked metabolic disorders such as IR, glucose intolerance, dyslipidemia, elevated blood pressure, and T2D mellitus. In vitro studies carried out in human adipocytes revealed that omentin improves insulin-stimulated glucose transport. Furthermore, recent research showed the close relationship between serum omentin levels and cardiovascular health. This adipokine exerts a protective effect in the vasculature. Omentin attenuates vascular inflammation and atherogenesis at the level of endothelial cells and smooth muscle cells. Omentin diminishes monocyte adhesion to endothelial and smooth muscle cells and promotes vasodilation and endothelial cell differentiation and survival [54].

4. CONCLUSIONS AND FUTURE PERSPECTIVES

In conclusion, imbalance of oxidative stress and inflammatory components contributes to the development of obesity and MetS-linked pathologies such as IR, T2D, or CVD. Although initially all these inflammatory processes and metabolic disturbances start within the AT, they can finally derive in a chronic systemic inflammation, affecting the physiology and metabolism of different tissues such as skeletal muscle, liver, and brain, among others. Thereby, the control of inflammation and oxidative stress in MetS, as well as obesity, may be an outcome in the control of many of the pathologies related to these. In this regard, further knowledge concerning the immune function of AT may contribute to finding better alternatives for treatment or prevention of MetS-related disorders.

REFERENCES

[1] World Health Organization (WHO). Obesity and overweight. 2016. http://www.who.int/mediacentre/factsheets/fs311/en/.

[2] Morigny P, Houssier M, Mouisel E, Langin D. Adipocyte lipolysis and insulin resistance. Biochimie 2016;125:259−66.

[3] Paniagua JA. Nutrition, insulin resistance and dysfunctional adipose tissue determine the different components of metabolic syndrome. World J Diabetes 2016;7(19):483−514.

[4] Thomas D, Apovian C. Macrophage functions in lean and obese adipose tissue. Metabolism 2017;120:143.

[5] Trayhurn P, Wood IS. Adipokines: inflammation and the pleiotropic role of white adipose tissue. Br J Nutr 2007;92:347.

[6] Steckhan N, Hohmann CD, Kessler C, Dobos G, Michalsen A, Cramer H. Effects of different dietary approaches on inflammatory markers in patients with metabolic syndrome: a systematic review and meta-analysis. Nutrition 2016;32(3):338−48.

[7] Rani V, Deep G, Singh RK, Palle K, Yadav UC. Oxidative stress and metabolic disorders: pathogenesis and therapeutic strategies. Life Sci 2016;148:183−93.

[8] Marrocco I, Altieri F, Peluso I. Measurement and clinical significance of biomarkers of oxidative stress in humans. Oxid Med Cell Longev 2017;2017:6501046.

[9] McMurray F, Patten DA, Harper ME. Reactive oxygen species and oxidative stress in obesity-recent findings and empirical approaches. Obesity (Silver Spring) 2016;24(11):2301−10.

[10] Matsuzawa-Nagata N, Takamura T, Ando H, Nakamura S, Kurita S, Misu H, et al. Increased oxidative stress precedes the onset of high-fat diet-induced insulin resistance and obesity. Metabolism 2008;57:1071−7.

[11] Balaban RS, Nemoto S, Finkel T. Mitochondria, oxidants, and aging. Cell 2005;120:483−95.

[12] Savini I, Catani MV, Evangelista D, Gasperi V, Avigliano L. Obesity-associated oxidative stress: strategies finalized to improve redox state. Int J Mol Sci 2013;14:10497−538.

[13] Manna P, Jain SK. Obesity, oxidative stress, adipose tissue dysfunction, and the associated health risks: causes and therapeutic strategies. Metab Syndr Relat Disord 2015;13(10):423−44.

[14] Spahis S, Delvin E, Borys JM, Levy E. Oxidative stress as a critical factor in nonalcoholic fatty liver disease pathogenesis. Antioxid Redox Signal 2017;26(10):519−41.

[15] Hopps E, Caimi G. Protein oxidation in metabolic syndrome. Clin Invest Med 2013;36(1):E1−8.

[16] Francisqueti FV, Chiaverini LC, Santos KC, Minatel IO, Ronchi CB, et al. The role of oxidative stress on the pathophysiology of metabolic syndrome. Rev Assoc Med Bras (1992) 2017;63(1):85−91.

[17] Knasmüller S, Nersesyan A, Misík M, Gerner C, Mikulits W, Ehrlich V, Hoelzl C, Szakmary A, Wagner KH. Use of conventional and -omics based methods for health claims of dietary antioxidants: a critical overview. Br J Nutr 2008;99(E Suppl. 1):ES3−52.

[18] Negre-Salvayre A, Auge N, Ayala V, Basaga H, Boada J, Brenke R. Pathological aspects of lipid peroxidation. Free Radic Res 2010;44(10):1125−71.

[19] Nair U, Bartsch H, Nair J. Lipid peroxidation-induced DNA damage in cancer-prone inflammatory diseases: a review of published adducts types and levels in humans. Free Radic Biol Med 2007;43:1109−20.

[20] Sousa BC, Pitt AR, Spickett CM. Chemistry and analysis of HNE and other prominent carbonyl-containing lipid oxidation compounds. Free Radic Biol Med 2017;111:294−308.

[21] Tsikas D. What we-authors, reviewers and editors of scientific work-can learn from the analytical history of biological 3-nitrotyrosine. J Chromatogr B Analyt Technol Biomed Life Sci 2017;1058:68−72.

[22] Domijan AM, Ralić J, Radić Brkanac S, Rumora L, Žanić-Grubišić T. Quantification of malondialdehyde by HPLC-FL − application to various biological samples. Biomed Chromatogr 2015;29(1):41−6.

[23] Srikanthan K, Shapiro JI, Sodhi K. The role of Na/K-ATPase signaling in oxidative stress related to obesity and cardiovascular disease. Molecules 2016;21(9):E1172.

[24] Picklo MJ, Long EK, Vomhof-DeKrey EE. Glutathionyl systems and metabolic dysfunction in obesity. Nutr Rev 2015;73(12):858−68.

[25] Czerska M, Zieliński M, Gromadzińska J. Isoprostanes - a novel major group of oxidative stress markers. Int J Occup Med Environ Health 2016;29(2):179−90.

[26] Davis M. Protein oxidation and peroxidation. Biochem J 2016;473(Pt 7):805−25.

[27] Ou H, Huang Z, Mo Z, Xiao J. The characteristics and roles of advanced oxidation protein products in atherosclerosis. Cardiovasc Toxicol 2017;17(1):1−12.

[28] Delgado-Andrade C. Carboxymethyl-lysine: thirty years of investigation in the field of AGE formation. Food Funct 2016;7(1):46−57.

[29] Niemann B, Rohrbach S, Miller MR, Newby DE, Fuster V, Kovacic JC. Oxidative stress and cardiovascular risk: obesity, diabetes, smoking, and pollution: part 3 of a 3-part series. J Am Coll Cardiol 2017;70(2):230−51.

[30] Song F, Schmidt AM. Glycation and insulin resistance: novel mechanisms and unique targets? Arterioscler Thromb Vasc Biol 2012;32:1760−5.

[31] Boyer F, Vidot JB, Dubourg AG, Rondeau P, Essop MF, Bourdon E. Oxidative stress and adipocyte biology: focus on the role of AGEs. Oxid Med Cell Longev 2015;2015:534873.

[32] Amir Aslani B, Ghobadi S. Studies on oxidants and antioxidants with a brief glance at their relevance to the immune system. Life Sci 2016;146:163−73.

[33] Margis R, Dunand C, Teixeira FK, Margis-Pinheiro M. Glutathione peroxidase family − an evolutionary overview. FEBS J 2008;275(15):3959−70.

[34] Asayama K, Nakane T, Dobashi K, Kodera K, Hayashibe H, Uchida N, Nakazawa S. Effect of obesity and troglitazone on expression of two glutathione peroxidases: cellular and extracellular types in serum, kidney and adipose tissue. Free Radic Res 2001;34:337−47.

[35] Lijnen HR, Scroyen I. Effect of vascular endothelial growth factor receptor 2 antagonism on adiposity in obese mice. J Mol Endocrinol 2013;50(3):319−24.

[36] Shin MJ, Park E. Contribution of insulin resistance to reduced antioxidant enzymes and vitamins in nonobese Korean children. Clin Chim Acta 2006;365(1−2):200−5.

[37] Rupérez AI, Olza J, Gil-Campos M, Leis R, Mesa MD, Tojo R, Cañete R, Gil A, Aguilera CM. Are catalase -844A/G polymorphism and activity associated with childhood obesity? Antioxid Redox Signal 2013;19(16):1970−5.

[38] Labrecque B, Beaudry D, Mayhue M, Hallé C, Bordignon V, Murphy BD, Palin MF. Molecular characterization and expression analysis of the porcine paraoxonase 3 (PON3) gene. Gene 2009;443(1−2):110−20.

[39] Chung KH, Lee DH, Kim Y, Kim TH, Huh JH, Chung SG, Lee S, Lee C, Ko JJ, An HJ. Proteomic identification of overexpressed PRDX 1 and its clinical implications in ovarian carcinoma. J Proteome Res 2010;9(1):451−7.

[40] Huh JY, Kim Y, Jeong J, Park J, Kim I, Huh KH, Kim YS, Woo HA, Rhee SG, Lee KJ, Ha H. Peroxiredoxin 3 is a key molecule regulating adipocyte oxidative stress, mitochondrial biogenesis, and adipokine expression. Antioxid Redox Signal 2012;16(3):229−43.

[41] Zelko IN, Mariani TJ, Folz RJ. Superoxide dismutase multigene family: a comparison of the CuZn-SOD (SOD1), Mn-SOD (SOD2), and EC-SOD (SOD3) gene structures, evolution, and expression. Free Radic Biol Med 2002;33(3):337−49.

[42] Nakao C, Ookawara T, Sato Y, Kizaki T, Imazeki N, Matsubara O, Haga S, Suzuki K, Taniguchi N, Ohno H. Extracellular superoxide dismutase in tissues from obese (ob/ob) mice. Free Radic Res 2000;33:229−41.

[43] Adachi T, Inoue M, Hara H, Suzuki S. Effects of PPARgamma ligands and C/EBPbeta enhancer on expression of extracellular-superoxide dismutase. Redox Rep 2004;9(4):207−12.

[44] Esser N, Paquot N, Scheen AJ. Inflammatory markers and cardiometabolic diseases. Acta Clin Belg 2015;70(3):193−9.

[45] Esser N, L'Homme L, De Roover A, Kohnen L, Scheen AJ, Moutschen M, et al. Obesity phenotype is related to NLRP3 inflammasome activity and immunological profile of visceral adipose tissue. Diabetologia 2013;56(11):2487−97.

[46] Nikolajczyk BS, Jagannathan-Bogdan M, Denis GV. The outliers become a stampede as immunometabolism reaches a tipping point. Immunol Rev 2012;249(1):253−75.

[47] Hotamisligil GS. Inflammation, metaflammation and immunometabolic disorders. Nature 2017;542(7640):177−85.

[48] Kershaw E, Flier J. Adipose tissue as an endocrine organ. J Clin Endocrinol Metab 2004;89:2548−56.

[49] Bing C. Is interleukin-1β a culprit in macrophage-adipocyte crosstalk in obesity? Adipocyte 2015;4:149−52.

[50] Chedraui P, Pérez-López F, Escobar G, et al. Circulating leptin, resistin, adiponectin, visfatin, adipsin and ghrelinlevels and insulin resistance in postmenopausal women with and without the metabolic syndrome. Maturitas 2014;79:86−90.

[51] Al Haj Ahmad RM, Al-Domi HA. Complement 3 serum levels as a pro-inflammatory biomarker for insulin resistance in obesity. Diabetes Metab Syndr 2016. https://doi.org/10.1016/j.dsx.2016.12.036.

[52] Fabersani E, Torres S, Valdez C. Fermented milks from small ruminant: effect on metabolism and immune status of mice fed mild caloric restricted diet. J Immunol Res 2014;(Suppl. 2):1−10.

[53] Scarpinelli E, Tjack J. Obesity and metabolic syndrome: an inflammatory condition. Dig Dis 2012;30:148−53.

[54] Dallmeier D, Larson M. Vasan metabolic syndrome and inflammatory biomarkers: a community-based cross-sectional study at the Framingham Heart Study. Diabetol Metab Syndr 2012;4(Suppl. 28):1−7.

[55] Singh V, Arora S, Goswami B. Metabolic syndrome: a review of emerging markers and management. Diabetes Metab Syndr Clin Res Rev 2009;3:240−54.

[56] Kim J, Kim SH, Im JA, Lee DC. The relationship between visfatin and metabolic syndrome in postmenopausal women. Maturitas 2010;67:67−71.

[57] Ohashi K, Shibata R, Murohara T. Role of anti-inflammatory adipokines in obesity-related diseases. Trends Endocrinol Metabol 2014;25:348−55.

[58] Enomoto T, Shibata R, Ohashi K. Regulation of adipolin/CTRP12 cleavage by obesity. Biochem Biophys Res Commun 2012;428:155−9.

Chapter 2

Genetics of Oxidative Stress and Obesity-Related Diseases

Azahara I. Rupérez[1] and Augusto Anguita-Ruiz[2]

[1]*University of Zaragoza, Zaragoza, Spain;* [2]*University of Granada, Granada, Spain*

1. INTRODUCTION

Obesity is one of the major preventable health conditions worldwide and it is well known that the presence of obesity increases the risk of cardiometabolic complications, insulin resistance, and ultimately, cardiovascular death risk. Thus the detailed characterization of the individual contributors to the progression and severity of these complications is essential for the establishment of efficient diagnostic and prevention strategies.

In the context of obesity, oxidative stress is involved in many of the physiopathological alterations that occur in obese adipose tissue. The main feature of obesity is fat accumulation, which can be derived from an excessive caloric supply and insufficient physical activity. Subsequent to the deposition of excessive energy storage, adipose tissue suffers from a variety of situations that start a vicious cycle of cellular and metabolic complications. First, the excessive nutrient supply and metabolic changes lead to adipocyte hypertrophy. Second, the accelerated mitochondrial activity generates an excess of reactive oxygen species (ROS). Third, adipocyte hypertrophy worsens and leads to hypoxia of the tissue, which further complicates the situation. And fourth, all of these processes favor that adipocytes and other cells from adipose tissue, including macrophages, enter a situation of low-grade inflammation, characterized by the secretion of cytokines and proinflammatory molecules, which further contribute to oxidative stress.

However, in addition to mechanical and physiopathological alterations that take place in complicated obesity, there are many regulatory points at the cellular level that are triggered in response to the disturbed metabolism. In this aspect, the broad and usually diffuse concept of oxidative stress plays a more important role than may be expected, as it will be evidenced in the present chapter. Besides the oxidation of many structural and regulatory macromolecules, ROS have greater consequences through their action on signaling pathways, which ultimately affect gene expression of many proteins. Many of the proteins and enzymes whose expression is affected belong to the cell's antioxidant defense system, whereas other are involved in the generation of oxidative stress, or in the regulation of the cellular redox homeostasis.

As a survival mechanism, cells have a complicated regulatory machinery that responds to oxidative stress in order to protect themselves against oxidative damage. Many of the responding mechanisms are ultimately based in the activation of transcription factors that act on gene expression of the effector target genes, either increasing or decreasing it. Due to this fact, understanding the action of the main transcription factors involved in redox homeostasis is essential to obtain a global vision of the consequences of a prolonged oxidative stress exposure situation.

Given the importance of specific proteins and enzymes in the maintenance of appropriate ROS levels, the effect of genetic variants on their function shall also be acknowledged and revised. Indeed, genetic variations such as single mutations and copy number variants (CNVs) may have a great impact on the gene product function and/or expression level. Specifically, variations affecting genes related with antioxidant defense, oxidative stress production, and redox regulation will be reviewed, as these enzymes have a crucial role in the response against increased ROS levels.

In addition to changes in the genome sequence, epigenetic mechanisms can also alter the function and levels of candidate gene transcripts and protein products. As the main epigenetic processes, posttranscription and postreplication regulatory points including microRNAs (miRs), DNA methylation, and histone acetylation, have been the most commonly

Obesity. https://doi.org/10.1016/B978-0-12-812504-5.00002-7

studied to date. The impact of epigenetic changes on oxidative stress—related genes in relation to obesity and its comorbidities is of great interest, since these processes have been proven to be modifiable by environmental and behavioral factors such as diet and exercise.

Interestingly, miRs have been shown to be involved in redox balance in the context of obesity. These molecules are also related to gene expression, but in a different regulatory level, since they act on mRNAs affecting their stability in different ways. Due to their importance and novelty in this field as potential candidates for diagnosis and evaluation of disease progression, their role on obesity complications such as oxidative damage in adipose tissue, the atherosclerotic vessel wall, or the liver will be carefully explained.

DNA methylation, usually referred to as epigenetic changes, has also been observed to play a role on redox regulation through its association with different components of the metabolic syndrome, frequently present in individuals with obesity. Similarly, histone acetylation has been observed to be another regulatory mechanism through which oxidative stress exerts its action in the context of obesity-derived metabolic abnormalities.

Finally, given the relationship between obesity and cancer, the potential mechanisms through which obesity-derived oxidative stress may contribute to increased tumor development are discussed.

2. GENE EXPRESSION OF ANTIOXIDANT ENZYMES

Many studies have been conducted to investigate the changes in gene expression of enzymes of the antioxidant defense system in the context of obesity and related diseases (Table 2.1). In general, it is expected that oxidative stress increases due to the inflammatory status and metabolic derangement, which then would lead to a higher expression of antioxidant enzymes that could tackle the problem. However, there are some exceptions to this sensible idea that complicate the mechanisms by which oxidative stress and its regulators act in the organism.

As a first example, the expression of **glutathione peroxidase (GPX)** 3 has been found to be decreased in adipose tissue and plasma of obese mice, which could be mediated by adipose tissue inflammation and hypoxia. In fact, treatment with antioxidants and rosiglitazone was able to restore *GPX3* expression improving the insulin resistance phenotype and attenuating the inflammatory gene expression pattern [1]. In a similar way, caloric restriction in obese mice also increased the mRNA expression of *GPX1* [2], although in this case *GPX1* knockout mice are surprisingly protected against high-fat diet (HFD)-induced insulin resistance and atherosclerosis [3]. In the case of GPX7, another study showed that its loss enhances oxidative stress [4] and adipocyte hypertrophy, and increases white adipose tissue mass by stimulating

TABLE 2.1 Changes in Expression of Antioxidant Enzymes in the Context of Obesity and Related Diseases

Gene	Disease Model	Observed Change
GPX1	Caloric restriction in mice	Increased expression [2]
	Knockout mice	Protection against HFD induced IR [3]
GPX3	Obesity in mice	Decreased expression (restored with antioxidants/rosiglitazone) [1]
GPX7	Knockout mice	OS and adipocyte hypertrophy [4,5]
CAT	Children with IR and obesity	Lower erythrocyte activity [6,7]
	Obesity in mice	Increased after caloric restriction [2]
	Mice	Increased after HFD [8]
PRDX3	Obesity in mice and humans	Decreased expression [9]
EC-SOD	Obesity in animal models	Increased expression [10]
	T2D in humans	Decreased expression [11]
	Induction in obesity in mice	Decreases OS and restores glucose tolerance [12]
MSRA	Rats	Decreased expression in VAT [15]
	Knockout HFD mice	IR [14]

CAT, catalase; *EC-SOD*, extracellular superoxide dismutase; *GPX*, glutathione peroxidase; *HFD*, high-fat diet; *IR*, insulin resistance; *MSRA*, methionine sulphoxide reductase A; *OS*, oxidative stress; *PRDX*, peroxiredoxin; *VAT*, visceral adipose tissue.

adipogenesis [5] in mice. Finally, human studies have shown lower erythrocyte GPX activity in young adults and pubertal children with obesity [6]. All these studies highlight the complexity of antioxidant enzyme's function and regulation.

In the case of **catalase** (CAT), it is a peroxisomal enzyme involved in clearance of excessive H_2O_2 levels, whose erythrocyte activity was found to be lower in children with insulin resistance and obesity [6,7]. In animal models its expression was increased after both caloric restriction in adipose tissue of obese mice [2] and high-fat feeding in mice hearts, although in this case CAT activity was decreased and thus, the change in expression could be a compensatory mechanism [8]. In any case, the available literature is not clear enough to understand CAT changes in expression and activity in the presence of obesity or its related situations.

Another antioxidant enzyme family is **peroxiredoxins** (PRDX). In obesity, PRDX3 has been observed to be decreased in adipose tissue of mice and humans with obesity, and its loss is associated with increased fat mass, insulin resistance, adipogenic and lipogenic gene expression, and oxidative stress in mitochondria [9].

Concerning the **superoxide dismutase** (SOD) family of antioxidant enzymes, the expression of extracellular SOD has been observed to be increased in animal models of obesity [10], but decreased and inversely associated with body mass index (BMI) and homeostasis model assessment of insulin resistance (HOMA-IR) in humans with type 2 diabetes (T2D) [11]. The induced overexpression of SOD1 or SOD2 in mice is only able to reduce oxidative stress and restore glucose tolerance without changing BMI [12].

In addition to enzymes that remove free radicals and oxidants, there are protein-repairing enzymes that participate in the regulation of protein-based signaling regulation. Indeed, protein oxidation is a reversible process through which oxidative stress acts, leading to insulin resistance or other metabolic alterations [13]. In this aspect, the disruption of **methionine sulphoxide reductase** A (MsrA) has an impact on protein signaling, since it provokes insulin resistance in HFD-fed $MSRA^{-/-}$ mice [14], and its activity is lower in visceral adipose tissue [15] (Table 2.1).

3. REACTIVE OXYGEN SPECIES RESPONSE MECHANISMS

Among the many agents involved in the regulation of oxidative balance, transcription factors are essential for an adequate cellular homeostasis. Transcription factors are needed for the induction of gene expression of ROS detoxifying and ROS responding enzymes involved in the cellular responses against oxidative stress (Fig. 2.1).

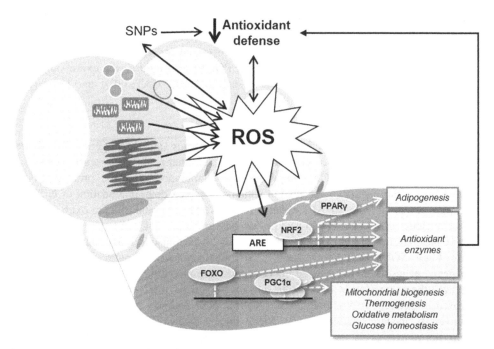

FIGURE 2.1   **Cellular response mechanisms against oxidative stress.** Schematic diagram of the cellular response against reactive oxygen species and oxidative stress in terms of gene expression regulated by transcription factors. *ARE*, antioxidant response element; *FOXO*, forkhead box O; *NRF2*, nuclear factor (erythroid-derived 2)-like 2; *PGC1α*, PPARγ coactivator 1 alpha; *PPARγ*, peroxisome proliferator-activated receptor gamma; *ROS*, reactive oxygen species; *SNPs*, single nucleotide polymorphisms.

3.1 Peroxisome Proliferator-Activated Receptor Gamma

The **peroxisome proliferator-activated receptor gamma** (PPARγ) is a master regulator of adipogenic differentiation and cell metabolism. It functions by binding to lipophilic ligands, such as polyunsaturated fatty acids, prostaglandin derivatives, and oxidized fatty acids, and creating a heterodimer with the retinod X receptor [16], which binds to the promoter of target genes with peroxisome proliferator response elements (PPREs). Its expression is increased in the adipose tissue of obese individuals [17]. PPARγ has been shown to have a role as a regulator of the antioxidant response to ROS, either by its own action or through activation of other transcription factors such as the nuclear factor (erythroid-derived 2)-like 2 (Nrf2), forkhead box O (FoxO) or the nuclear factor kappa-light-chain-enhancer of activated B cells. In fact, mice with lower PPARγ levels showed decreased *NRF2* expression, which indicates that this gene, tightly involved in redox homeostasis, is under transcriptional control of PPARγ. Moreover, both PPARγ and Nrf2 act synergistically on the expression of other target genes that share PPREs and antioxidant response element (ARE) sequences in their promoters, such as glutathione S-transferase (*GSTA2*), CAT, **heme oxygenase-1** (HO-1), and SOD2. In addition, PPARγ is involved either directly or indirectly in the expression of other antioxidant enzymes, since, For instance, adipose tissue-specific loss of an allele of *PPARγ*, with the subsequent loss of activity, was associated with a higher resistance to oxidative stress, which seemed to be partially mediated through the upregulation of ROS scavenging genes, including *GPX1*, glutathione reductase, *PRDX3*, *SOD2*, and *CAT*, together with the upregulation of the ROS responding transcription factor *FOXO3A* in adipose tissue [18]. Other enzymes whose expression is regulated by PPARγ are GPX3, uncoupling protein (UCP) 2, and endothelial nitric oxide (NO) synthase (eNOS), which is essential for endothelial vascular homeostasis.

However, the beneficial effects of reduced PPARγ activity are not clear, since another study showed that PPARγ activation decreased tumor necrosis factor alpha (TNF-α) or glucocorticoid-induced ROS production in human adipocytes [19]. Thus, although PPARγ has a role in ROS clearance, its paradoxical function warrants further investigation in order to clarify whether PPARγ activation decreases ROS production or increases ROS scavenging, especially in the context of disease. In general, it is mostly clear that balanced PPARγ activity is necessary for adequate cardiovascular and metabolic health.

3.2 PPARγ Coactivator 1 Alpha

The transcriptional coactivator **PPARγ coactivator 1 alpha** (PGC1α) acts on nuclear receptors such as PPARα and γ or FoxO1, together with other proteins and factors upon the sensing of increased oxidative stress derived from an enhanced oxidative metabolism, among other mechanisms [20]. It is involved in mitochondrial biogenesis, adaptive thermogenesis, oxidative metabolism, and glucose homeostasis. Of special interest is its role in the regulation of oxygen consumption and oxidative phosphorylation in the mitochondria. Indeed, it is essential for adipocyte browning and thermogenesis in brown adipose tissue. In parallel to these metabolic processes, PGC1α also induces the expression of ROS detoxifying enzymes in order to control the augmented ROS production, such as SOD2, CAT, GPX, and HO-1 [20,21].

3.3 Nuclear Factor (Erythroid-Derived 2)-Like 2

The **Nrf2** is a leucine zipper factor that controls the expression of numerous antioxidant genes through the ARE sequence located in their promoters. In addition, it is involved in the regulation of other responses against external stresses. The Nrf2 is itself mainly regulated by the Kelch-like ECH (Golgi apparatus membrane protein-like protein ECHIDNA)-associated protein 1 (KEAP1), whose binding facilitates the ubiquitination and proteasomal degradation of Nrf2, with a very rapid turnover [22]. When ROS levels increase, KEAP1 cysteine residues 151, 273, and 288 are oxidized and Nrf2 is released and translocated to the nucleus where it binds to a Maf protein and to the promoter of target genes. However, other redox independent regulatory mechanisms also exist. Some of the genes under transcriptional control of Nrf2 include GSTA2, glutathione reductase, CAT, SOD, or HO-1. Moreover, Nrf2 also regulates adipogenesis by the modulation of the expression of adipogenic genes such as reduced nicotinamide adenine dinucleotide phosphate (NADPH) quinone oxidoreductase, and even the expression of PPARγ. In relation to obesity, it has been observed that *NRF2* and *KEAP1* expression are increased in differentiated adipocytes and that the Nrf2 pathway is enriched in individuals with high fat percentages [23]. Conversely, the targeted disruption of *NRF2* protects against HFD-induced obesity and insulin resistance in mice [24] and impairs adipogenesis through the inhibition of CCAAT/enhancer-binding protein beta expression. However, the role of Nrf2 in adipogenic differentiation is not simple, since other authors have observed lower Nrf2 levels in the nuclei of differentiating adipocytes in vitro, which could otherwise lead to the appropriate ROS levels needed for the process.

Finally, another aspect that further complicates the role of Nrf2 is the tissue where it exerts its regulatory functions. The mentioned studies have not yet clarified this issue, and thus tissue-specific knockout models are needed for the adequate description of Nrf2 function in obesity.

3.4 Forkhead Box O

The **FoxO** transcription factor family includes the ubiquitous forms FoxO1a, FoxO3a, FoxO4, and FoxO6 in humans. FoxO proteins transduce the inhibitory signal of insulin or insulin-like growth factor 1 (IGF1) and are involved in the regulation of cell metabolism and cell death and proliferation, as well as in the activation of gene expression of many antioxidant enzymes [25]. For this reason, their alteration is related to cancer and short lifespan. The action of FoxO factors is exerted through the insulin responsive element present in the promoter of target genes. Upon presence of insulin or IGF1 signaling, the FoxO factors are phosphorylated. At this stage, some FoxO factors are translocated to the cytoplasm, which leads to their inactivation and lower gene expression of their target genes, whereas others (FoxO1 and FoxO6) suffer a conformational change and/or bind to the protein 14-3-3, which impairs the binding of FoxO to the DNA. In addition, FoxO proteins are also sensitive to other regulatory mechanisms such as acetylation. In diabetes, it has been observed that FoxO is permanently present in the nucleus where it constantly activates its target genes, resulting in an abnormal insulin signaling. It is worth highlighting the action of these transcription factors on the protection against ROS damage. FoxO3a, for example, regulates the expression of human manganese-dependent superoxide dismutase (MnSOD) (SOD2) and CAT. In the same way, FoxO4 is involved in the expression of SOD2, FoxO1a in that of SOD1, and both activate the expression of CAT and GPX. Similarly, PRDX3 and PRDX5 are also regulated by FoxOs, together with thioredoxin (Trx2) and thioredoxin reductase, which are needed to regenerate active PRDX. In addition, FoxOs also regulate the expression of metal ion chelators, as metallothioneins, ceruloplasmin, and selenoprotein, which prevent the formation of aggressive ROS derivatives such as the hydroxyl radical. In diabetic subjects, FoxO6 levels and activity are increased in the liver as a result of a maintained insulin stimulation, which leads to a perturbed very low-density lipoprotein and triglyceride (TG) production that contributes to hypertriglyceridemia [26].

4. GENETIC VARIANTS

Genetic variants are changes or differences in the DNA sequence between individuals or populations. These can be single nucleotide variations in a single position, also named single nucleotide polymorphisms (SNPs), or structural variants, which include CNVs, deletions or insertions (indels), block substitutions, or inversions (Fig. 2.2). SNPs are the most

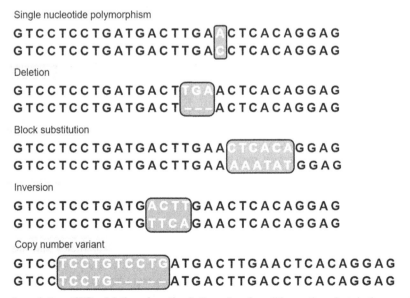

FIGURE 2.2 Types of genetic variations (SNPs, deletions, insertions). Examples of possible genetic variants in the genomic sequence. Changes are shown in terms of comparison of a standard unaltered sequence (above) with a modified or mutated sequence (below). *SNPs*, single nucleotide polymorphisms.

common type of genetic variants, since the human genome contains at least 11 million of these polymorphisms. Depending on the frequency of the minor allele of an SNP in a population, this can be a common variant ($\geq 1\%$) or a rare variant ($<1\%$) (Fig. 2.2).

In the context of oxidative stress–related diseases, SNPs can affect the function of certain antioxidant enzymes, subsequently increasing the risk of a number of diseases such as cancer. In the same way, SNPs in the genes coding these enzymes and other factors implicated in ROS regulation have also been associated with obesity and its related diseases [27].

One possible explanation for this relationship could be the presence of SNPs, which affect expression and activity of antioxidant enzymes and can contribute to cellular oxidative stress and cell dysfunction by altering signaling cascades or damaging macromolecules by oxidation.

4.1 Antioxidant Defense System Genes

4.1.1 Glutathione Peroxidases

GPXs comprise a total of eight genes and isoenzymes in humans. Most degrade H_2O_2 using glutathione as a cofactor, whereas GPX7 acts as an oxidative stress sensor/transducer in the regulation of ROS accumulation.

SNPs associated with obesity and insulin resistance have been described for *GPX1* and *GPX7* genes (Table 2.2). In the case of *GPX1*, this gene harbors a missense SNP at nucleotide 594 that results in the substitution of proline for leucine at codon 198 of the protein (Pro198Leu; rs1050450). Many studies have shown the Leu allele to be associated with oxidative stress, central obesity, and insulin resistance. Indeed, male Leu allele (T) carriers have higher metabolic syndrome prevalence, seen as higher waist–hip ratios, TG and insulin circulating concentrations, HOMA of β-cell function, and systolic and diastolic blood pressures [28]. In women, the T allele has also been associated with higher body fat mass and higher insulin circulating concentrations and greater values of HOMA-IR [29]. Regarding T2D, the Leu allele has been associated with cardiovascular disease [30] and Leu carriers also present worse outcomes in DNA damage and higher levels of lipoperoxides and malondialdehyde (MDA) in low-density lipoproteins (LDLs) [31]. Moreover, the combination of this SNP with the CNV Ala5/Ala6 at codon 7-11 decreases the activity of the enzyme by 40% in vitro [30]. The authors of this study concluded that the Leu allele is associated with lower GPX activity, and this could be the reason why Leu carriers display worse outcomes in obesity phenotypes.

In *GPX7*, the A allele of SNP rs835337 (G/A) has been associated with lower BMI, higher GPX7 expression in abdominal adipose tissue, and lower serum MDA concentrations in adults. The hypothesized mechanism of the conferred protection against obesity is an impaired adipogenesis by the lower ROS levels present in A allele carriers [32].

4.1.2 Catalase

This peroxisomal enzyme, previously described in terms of its gene expression, harbors a number of variants in its promoter that have shown significant associations with obesity. The three SNPs rs769214 (-844A/G), rs7943316 (-89T/A), and rs1049982 (-20C/T) located in the *CAT* regulatory region have been individually associated with a higher risk of childhood obesity in Spanish children [6]. Moreover, these polymorphisms were also associated with higher weight, BMI Z-Score, and circulating levels of adipocyte fatty acid-binding protein. However, the SNPs were not associated with CAT activity, although the **haplotype** formed by the three variants had been associated with lower CAT expression in human cells exposed to oxidative stress in another study [33]. In addition, another variant, rs1001179, has revealed conflicting results regarding its association with lower CAT activity, which some have observed but others have not. Altogether, findings indicate that CAT activity and expression may be affected by genetic variants, which could contribute to oxidative stress in the cell and subsequently, obesity-derived metabolic complications.

4.1.3 Paraoxonases

Paraoxonases (PON) in humans comprise a family of three antioxidant enzymes with different functions. PON1 and PON3 circulate in the blood stream bound to high-density lipoprotein (HDL) particles and are expressed in liver and kidneys. They are involved in the protection of plasma LDL and HDL particles against oxidation. In contrast, PON2 is bound to the cellular membrane and is present in a more ubiquitous manner. Although their activity is influenced by a wide variety of factors, including obesity itself in addition to diet, age, sex, and drugs, the greater cause of variation is the presence of genetic variants in their protein coding sequence. In this sense, the *PON1* gene harbors the missense SNPs Q192R (rs662) and L55M (rs854560), which have been deeply studied. In particular, the 192RR genotype is associated

TABLE 2.2 Genetic Variants of Oxidative Stress Related Genes Associated With Obesity and Its Related Diseases

Gene	Variant	Population	Association
GPX1	rs1010450 (Pro198Leu)	Male adults	Metabolic syndrome and IR [28]
		Female adults	Fat mass, IR [29]
		Adults—T2D	CVD [30]
		Adults	Lipoperoxides and MDA [31]
	rs1010450 + CNV Ala5/Ala6	Adults—T2D	40% lower GPX activity in vitro [30]
GPX7	rs835337	Adults	Lower BMI, higher GPX7 expression [32]
CAT	rs769214	Children	Obesity [6]
	rs7943316	Children	Obesity [6]
	rs1049982	Children	Obesity [6]
	rs769214/rs7943316/rs1049982	Human cell model	Lower CAT expression [33]
PON1	rs662	Adults	Higher PON activity [34]
	rs854560	Adults	Higher PON levels [35]
	rs854566	Children	Lower obesity risk and higher PON lactonase activity [36]
PRDX3	rs3740562/rs2271362/rs7768/rs3377	Adults—HFD	Higher BMI [37]
SOD2	rs4880	Elderly	Obesity risk [39]
		Children	NAFLD (ns) [42]
		Healthy adults	Inflammation [43]
		Young healthy adults	Lower DNA damage [44]
MSRA	rs7826222	Adults	Obesity [45]
		Male adults	T2D [46]
	rs473034	Children	Obesity [48]
	rs516175	Asian adults	BMI Z-Score [49]
UCP2	rs659366	Adults	Obesity and T2D [52]
	rs660339	Adults	Obesity and T2D [52]

Continued

TABLE 2.2 Genetic Variants of Oxidative Stress Related Genes Associated With Obesity and Its Related Diseases—cont'd

Gene	Variant	Population	Association
UCP3	rs3781907	Adults	Obesity and T2D [52] [53]
P22phox	rs9932581	Phagocytes – hypertensive adults	Higher p22phox expression and NADPH oxidase activity
		Adults	IR [54] [55]
	rs4673	Adults—T2D	Lower IMT and 8-OHdG [41]
		Adults	Lower IR [56]
		Adults—hypertension	Higher IR and WC [57]
	rs7195830	Female adults	Obesity [58]
	rs12709102	Female adults	Obesity [58]
	rs1049255	Adults—T2D	CVD [41]
MPO	rs2333227	Adults	T2D [60]
PPARG	rs1801282	Adults	Obesity [61]
		Adults—IR	T2D [62]
		Adults - Obesity	T2D [63]
		Adults—T2D	Lower BP and MI [64]
		Adults – Chinese	NAFLD [65]
	rs72551362	Adults	IR, DM, hypertension [68]
PGC1A	rs8192678	Adults—obesity	IR [69]
		Female adults	Lower BMI and VAT [70]
		Adults—Chinese	Higher HOMA-IR, insulin [71]
		Adults—obesity	IR [72]
		Male adults—T2D	Lower adiponectin concentrations [73]
NRF2	rs6721961	Male adults	Lower T2D risk [75]
FOXO3A	−343−1582C/T	Korean adults	Higher BMI [76]

BMI, body mass index; CAT, catalase; CNV, copy number variant; CVD, cardiovascular disease; FOXO3A, forkhead box O 3 A; GPX, glutathione peroxidase; HFD, high-fat diet; HOMA-IR, homeostasis model assessment of insulin resistance; IMT, intima media thickness; IR, insulin resistance; MDA, malondialdehyde; MPO, myeloperoxidase; MSRA, methionine sulphoxide reductase A; NADPH, nicotin- amide adenine dinucleotide phosphate; NAFLD, nonalcoholic fatty liver disease; NRF2, nuclear factor (erythroid-derived 2)-like 2; ns, nonsignificant; P22phox, human neutrophil cytochrome b light chain; PGC1A, PPARγ coactivator 1 alpha; PON, paraoxonase; PPARG, peroxisome proliferator-activated receptor gamma; PRDX, peroxiredoxin; SOD, superoxide dismutase; T2D, type 2 diabetes; UCP, uncoupling protein; VAT, visceral adipose tissue.

with a higher PON-paraoxonase activity, and 55LL carriers display increased serum PON1 concentrations [34,35]. However, the association between these alleles and obesity has yielded mostly negative results, except for one study that found an association between the 192R allele and obesity in Portuguese women. In contrast, a novel intronic SNP, rs854566, was found to be associated with higher PON-lactonase activity and lower obesity risk in prepubertal Spanish children [36].

4.1.4 Peroxiredoxins

PRDXs degrade H_2O_2 in different cell compartments, as mentioned earlier. Until now, only one study has investigated the association between PRDX3 genetic variants and obesity in the context of an HFD used with the aim of generating high ROS production. In that study rs3740562 (A/G), rs2271362 (C/T), rs7768 (G/C), and rs3377 (A/C) were significantly associated with BMI only in the group of HFD, and rs1553850 (A/T) was not. The haplotype formed by the five variants T-G-C-C-C was also associated with an increased BMI [37]. These findings indicate a role for PRDX3 genetic variations and an interaction between these SNPs and dietary fat intake in association with BMI and obesity risk.

Since PRDX3 is located in the mitochondria, a key organelle tightly involved in the metabolic disruption triggered by the excessive nutrient supply present in obesity, its role in the association between oxidative stress and obesity complications is of special interest. Certainly, future studies will be valuable for the elucidation of the underlying mechanisms.

4.1.5 Superoxide Dismutases

The SOD family degrades the superoxide radical $O_2^{\cdot-}$ and is the first line of defense against ROS. The variant rs4880 (C/T) in MnSOD, which generates a change from alanine to valine in the 16th aminoacidic position, has been widely studied. The Val allele has been associated with lower MnSOD activity through its arrest in the inner mitochondrial membrane, which results in an increased susceptibility to oxidative stress and mitochondrial dysfunction due to excessive ROS levels [38]. Although both homozygous genotypes, AlaAla and ValVal, have been associated with a variety of diseases, probably due to an imbalance in oxidative stress either by excess or defect in ROS levels, the Val allele has been linked to a higher obesity risk in the elderly [39] and to a higher diabetes and cardiovascular disease risk in several studies [40,41]. Similarly, the ValVal genotype was more frequent among obese children with nonalcoholic steatohepatitis than in those without the disease, although the difference was not significant [42]. This allele has also been related to inflammation, seen as higher concentrations of interleukin (IL)-1, IL-6, TNF-α, and interferon gamma, and lower levels of IL-10 [43]. However, opposite results have also been observed, since Val allele carriers of a healthy cohort displayed lower DNA damage levels [44]. It has been suggested that this discrepancy may be due to the interaction between the SNP and the disease with environmental factors such as diet and plasma antioxidant capacity. Further studies are required to clarify the nature of these associations, although it is clear that MnSOD is an essential enzyme in the regulation of ROS, so that metabolic complications are avoided.

4.1.6 Methionine Sulphoxide Reductase A

MsrA is a 26 kDa protein localized in the cytosol and mitochondria involved in the repair of oxidized proteins by reducing the methionine-S-sulphoxide epimers back to methionine, using Trx2 as a cofactor. Several loci in the *MSRA* gene have been associated with visceral obesity, such as rs7826222 (also named rs545854), that has been found to be positively associated with obesity in Hispanic and Caucasian populations [45] and T2D risk in men [46], despite having given negative results in other studies conducted in Asian populations [47]. Other *MSRA* SNPs are rs473034 and rs516175, which have been associated with extreme childhood obesity [48] and BMI Z-score in Singaporeans [49], respectively.

4.1.7 Uncoupling Proteins

UCPs are a family of anion carrier membrane proteins found in mitochondria. While UCP1 is found only in brown fat mitochondria, and UCP3 is mostly present in skeletal muscle and heart, UCP2 is the most ubiquitous form, found in a wide variety of tissues [50]. Regarding the functions of these proteins, UCP1 has a thermogenic action in brown adipose tissue, where it leaks protons through the inner mitochondrial membrane, uncoupling adenosine triphosphate synthesis, resulting in rapid oxygen and energy consumption and heat production. However, UCP2 and UCP3 are expressed in a much lesser content and display other actions such as protection against ROS, export of fatty acids, and regulation of insulin secretion [51]. Concerning their ROS protection role in mitochondria, both UCP2 and UCP3 act by decreasing the membrane potential, which ameliorates the generation of superoxide and other ROS derivatives. The association between these proteins and obesity and metabolic syndrome has been observed through different genetic association studies. In UCP2, different genetic variations have been associated with obesity and related diseases. An indel has been found to be associated with BMI in four studies conducted in different ethnic groups and SNPs -866G/A (rs659366) and Ala55Val (rs660339) have been associated with obesity and T2D risk in different populations [52]. As for UCP3, different SNPs including rs3781907 have been associated with BMI, body composition measures, and T2D in other studies [53]. Regarding the regulatory function of UCP2 on insulin secretion, the association between the variant -866G/A and T2D has also been described. Interestingly, this SNP increases UCP2 transcription and is associated with an impaired insulin sensitivity and β-cell function and earlier and severe diabetes.

4.2 Prooxidant Enzyme Genes

4.2.1 Nicotinamide Adenine Dinucleotide Phosphate Complex

The NADPH oxidase complex generates $O_2^{\cdot-}$ and, subsequently, other ROS such as H_2O_2 in the cell. This function is not limited to the phagocyte respiratory burst, but is also involved in the regulation of signaling mechanisms. Hormones such as insulin, as well as cytokines, act on NADPH oxidase stimulating ROS production as signal transducers. Interestingly, the SNP -930A/G (rs9932581) in the promoter of the human neutrophil cytochrome b light chain (*p22phox*) gene, a subunit of NADPH oxidase, was found to be associated with higher *p22phox* expression and NADPH oxidase activity in phagocytic cells from hypertensive patients carrying the GG genotype [54]. This variation resulted in an increased the risk of insulin resistance seen as higher HOMA-IR and insulin, but not with obesity, in a cohort of Spanish GG carriers [55]. Another SNP in the *p22phox* subunit, 242C/T (rs4673), has been associated with lower intima media thickness and 8-hydroxy-2′-deoxyguanosine (8-OHdG) values, as well as higher cardiovascular disease risk in T2D patients carrying the T allele [41]. Conversely, nondiabetic T allele carriers are protected against insulin resistance and exhibit lower HOMA-IR and fasting plasma insulin values [56]. The CC genotype confers protection against diabetes mellitus and obesity through an association with lower fasting plasma glucose levels and waist circumference in hypertensive patients [57]. Finally, SNPs rs7195830 (C allele), rs12709102 (T allele), and 640A/G (rs1049255) have also been associated with a higher risk of obesity in women [58] and cardiovascular disease in T2D patients [41], respectively.

4.2.2 Myeloperoxidase

Myeloperoxidase (MPO) is a heme-peroxidase involved in pathogen destruction being produced by neutrophils and monocytes. It generates ROS contributing to the degradation of microorganisms and to cellular homeostasis [59]. This enzyme is thought to be implicated in the beginning and progression of cardiovascular disease, and it is indeed found to be at higher circulating levels in obese adults and children. Regarding its genetic variations, rs2333227 (G/A) has been associated with higher MPO activity and higher risk for T2D [60].

4.3 Genetic Variants in Transcription Factors

Although the presented transcription factors are per se regulators of gene expression of antioxidant enzymes, their activity and expression is also affected by single mutations and other genetic variations in or near their sequence in the genome.

4.3.1 Peroxisome Proliferator-Activated Receptor Gamma

The genetic variants of PPARγ have been extensively studied due to the importance of this TF in the regulation of adipogenesis and metabolism in adipose tissue. The most known polymorphism in *PPARG* is the missense variant Pro12Ala (rs1801282), whose Ala allele has been associated with obesity in a metaanalysis including nearly 50,000 subjects [61]. However, the same allele has also been observed to be linked to lower T2D risk, higher insulin sensitivity, and lower BMI, as well as higher weight loss through exercise-based interventions [62,63]. Moreover, the Ala allele of this SNP has also been associated with lower risk of myocardial infarction and lower blood pressure [64]. In contrast, the Pro allele has been associated with a higher risk of nonalcoholic fatty liver disease (NAFLD) in Chinese, showing a positive significant interaction with smoking [65]. The reason for these protective actions of the Ala allele has been hypothesized to rely on a higher resistance of Ala carriers against oxidative stress, observed through higher antioxidant gene expression and adipose tissue FoxO3a levels [66]. However, Pro individuals have also been observed to display higher PPARγ expression in adipose tissue [67]. As for other variants, rs72551362 (Val290Met) and rs72551363 (Phe388Leu) are examples of loss-of-function SNPs, which have been associated with different conditions such as lipodystrophy, insulin resistance, and hypertension, since they generate an inactive form of the transcription factor [68].

4.3.2 PPARγ Coactivator 1 Alpha

Given the relevance of this molecule in the regulation of oxidative balance, many studies have investigated the potential association between its genetic variants and metabolic diseases. For example, SNP rs8192678 located in the *PGC1α* gene results in an amino acid substitution of glycine to serine at position 482 (Gly482Ser) and has been associated with higher HOMA-IR in obese nondiabetic subjects [69] and with lower BMI, waist and hip circumference, and total body fat, but only in women [70]. However, this SNP has not been found to be associated with obesity or T2D in overweight nondiabetic Chinese individuals, although it was associated with high insulin, HOMA-IR, and thiobarbituric acid reactive substances in hyperglycemia [71], although a low calorie diet was able to decrease the observed insulin resistance in Ser allele carriers according to another study [72]. Since adiponectin is under the transcriptional control of PPARγ, which is a target of PGC1α, the effects of the Gly482Ser variant on adiponectin plasma levels were also investigated to find that in T2D men, but not women, carriers of this SNP have lower adiponectin concentrations [73]. In this study, authors suggested that the causative SNP could be in linkage disequilibrium with the common Gly482Ser variant, which agrees with another study that determined that neither the Gly482Ser nor Trp612Met variants of PGC1α affected the functionality of the protein regarding its coactivator activity on PPARγ2 [74]. Thus, results indicate that the true functional variant in PGC1α has yet to be described.

4.3.3 Nuclear Factor (Erythroid-Derived 2)-Like 2

The NRF2 transcription factor regulates cellular responses in response to oxidative stress and other endogenous and exogenous stresses. And it is also involved in the regulation of gene expression during adipocyte differentiation. Its role in obesity and related diseases has been also studied, with knockout models shown to be protected against obesity and its comorbidities [24]. As for genetic variants in this gene, the rs6721961 (C/A) has been negatively associated with diabetes in men, with AA carriers showing lower glucose concentrations [75].

4.3.4 Forkhead Box O

Although most research regarding this transcription factor family is related with longevity, there has been at least one study that has shown a relationship between the FoxO3a SNP -343−1582C/T and BMI in Korean adults [76].

5. MICRORNAS

MiRs are highly conserved small noncoding RNAs ranging from 18 to 24 ribonucleotides in length that act as key posttranscriptional regulators of gene expression. By inducing mRNA degradation or blocking translation, miRs are involved in important cell processes such as cell growth, cell differentiation, and apoptosis, and their dysregulation has been proposed as one of the main triggers of carcinogenesis. Many other complex diseases aside from cancer have also been linked to alterations in miRs such as obesity, metabolic syndrome, and specifically, one of their joint features, oxidative stress.

Because the redox state in adipose tissue is a potentially useful therapeutic target for obesity, in this section, recent insights regarding the role of miRs as regulators of oxidative stress under different conditions will be reviewed, emphasizing the case of adipocyte dysfunction, obesity-related vascular alterations, and NAFLD (Figs. 2.3 and 2.4).

5.1 MicroRNAs in Adipose Tissue

As we already know, obese adipose tissue is characterized by adipocyte hypertrophy and hyperplasia, which highly contribute to the increased adipose tissue mass in obesity. In obese subjects, impairment of adipocyte function is associated with endoplasmic reticulum and mitochondrial oxidative stress, which further aggravates adipose tissue dysfunction. Moreover, dysfunctional adipocytes exhibit an inflammatory phenotype, with increased production of proinflammatory adipocytokines and decreased production of antiinflammatory adipocytokines. Which are the roles of miRs within this vicious cycle?

Regarding adipogenesis and differentiation, **miR-103** and **miR-143**, which have been identified as upregulators of these processes, are suppressed in obese subjects while **miR-27a** and **miR-27b**, which have been identified as inhibitors, see their function enhanced. As a result of this, adipocytes experience hyperplasia, hypertrophy, macrophage infiltration, and increased adipokine production. Other miRs have also been proven to impair adipocyte function. Specifically and in relation to oxidative stress, **miR-155**, **miR-183**, and **miR-872** have been associated with increased oxidative damage,

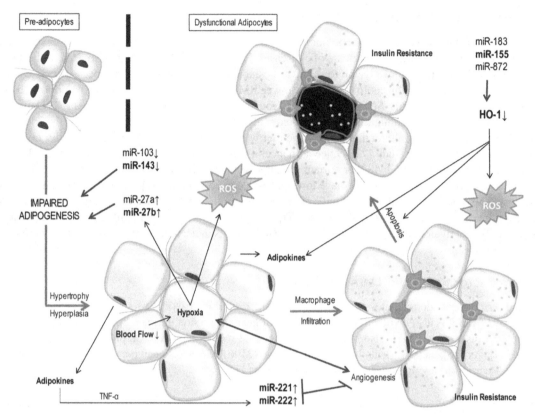

FIGURE 2.3   **MiRs control adipocyte differentiation and promote oxidative damage in adipose tissue of obese subjects.** *Black arrows* between miR and mechanisms indicate stimulation of the process by the corresponding miR. *Blunted arrows* indicate inhibition. miRs in bold have similar expression profiles in adipose and vascular tissues. *HO-1*, heme oxygenase-1; *miRs*, microRNAs; *TNF-α*, tumor necrosis factor alpha.

production of proinflammatory adipocytokines, and apoptosis in adipose tissue [77]. The proposed mechanism underlying this association is the repression of antiinflammatory, antioxidant, and antiapoptotic effects of the **HO-1** [78]. In addition, other miRs such as **miR-221** and **miR-222** have also been associated with adipose tissue dysfunction in obese subjects. Particularly, they both have been reported to be upregulated in obesity and to inhibit endothelial cell (EC) migration, proliferation, and angiogenesis [79]. Thus, they might contribute to hypoxia and consequent oxidative stress in adipose tissue. Interestingly, miR-221/222-induced hypoxia has been reported to be responsible for further inducing inflammatory adipocytokines production and for increasing **miR-27** levels [80], an miR already mentioned to be associated with impaired adipogenesis. Several other miRs have been directly associated with insulin resistance, increased IL-6 production, and other features of adipocyte dysfunction.

Taking all these findings into account, it is clear that dysregulation of certain miRs in obesity leads to increased oxidative stress and oxidative damage in adipose tissue. Indeed, the aforementioned miRs effects on oxidative damage are not isolated alterations but part of a bigger and concerted mechanism by which adipose tissue in obese subjects fails to expand and meet energy storage demands, resulting in lipid spillage from adipocytes to macrophages and the formation of foam cells, which are not able to scavenge apoptotic adipocytes, thereby increasing insulin resistance (Fig. 2.3).

5.2 MicroRNAs in Atherosclerosis

Atherosclerosis is the process of vascular wall thickening and hardening, and it is the primary cause of coronary heart disease, ischemic stroke, and peripheral arterial disease. Given obesity is regarded as an independent risk factor for atherosclerosis-related diseases and that oxidative damage is a key event for endothelial dysfunction, here we summarize the relationship between miRs, oxidative stress, and the atherosclerotic process (Fig. 2.4).

Atherosclerotic lesions preferentially develop on sites with disturbed flow dynamics where the endothelium has become dysfunctional at the cellular and molecular levels. Activated by the disturbed flow, the endothelium supports enhanced adhesion and infiltration of circulating monocytes into vascular intima. While miRs such as **miR-125b** and **miR-146a** have been shown to contribute to this inflammatory process, others such as **miR-10a**, **miR-124a**, **miR-126**, **miR-132**, and **miR-221/222**

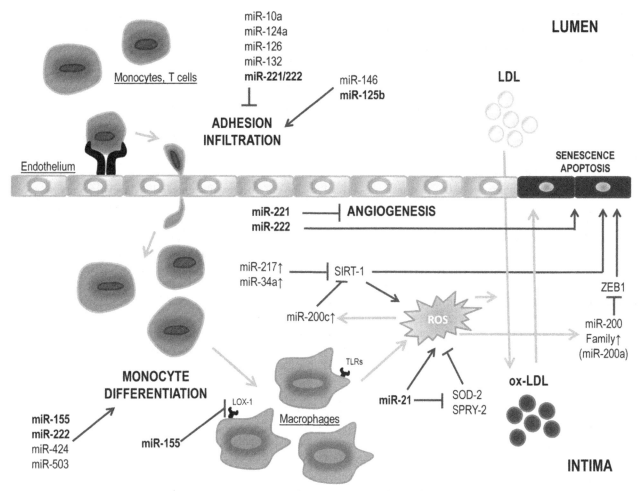

FIGURE 2.4   MiRs control inflammation, oxidative stress, apoptosis, and angiogenesis in atherosclerotic plaques. *Black arrows* between miR and a mechanistic process indicate stimulation of the process by the corresponding miR. *Blunted arrows* indicate inhibition. miRs in bold are miRs deregulated in both adipose and vascular tissues, reflecting common molecular mechanisms. *LDL*, low-density lipoprotein; *miRs*, microRNAs; *ox-LDL*, oxidized-LDL; *TLRs*, toll-like receptors; *ZEB1*, zinc finger e-box binding homeobox 1.

have been reported to elicit antiinflammatory and opposite effects [77,81–85]. Once infiltrated, monocytes differentiate into macrophages and again, several miRs participate in the process, as is the case of **miR-155**, **miR-222**, **miR-424**, and **miR-503**, which synergistically promote monocyte differentiation. MiR-155 and miR-222 also induce apoptosis. Then, activated macrophages express different enzymes, which generate a range of ROS, including superoxide, hydrogen peroxide, and hypochlorous acid. Produced ROS will cause damage to host molecules such as circulating LDL through the oxidation of their phospholipids and this will further induce the formation and accumulation of oxidized-LDL (ox-LDL) into the injured vessel wall. Interestingly and in relation to this, miR-155 significantly reduces ox-LDL-induced lipid uptake by downregulating the expression of scavenger receptors lectin-like oxidized LDL receptor-1, cluster of differentiation (CD) 36, and CD68 in macrophages, and inhibits the release of several proinflammatory cytokines, including IL-6, IL-8, and TNF-α. All these miRs, therefore, indirectly participate inducing or inhibiting oxidative damage in endothelial tissue and thereby accelerating/braking the atherosclerotic process.

Among the aforementioned miRs, several had already been cited in the previous section and identified as key regulators of oxidative stress in adipose tissue of obese subjects—**miR-221** and **miR-222**. Notwithstanding, these two miRs not only induce oxidative stress and dysfunction in adipose tissue of obese rats as we previously remarked. Additionally, both small-RNAs seem to be highly expressed in rat vascular smooth cells (VSMCs) and ECs, where their roles have been extensively studied. In particular, they have been shown to have proliferative, promigratory and antiapoptotic effects in VSMCs; and in contrast, antiproliferative, antimigratory and proapoptotic roles in ECs [86]. These opposite effects might be related to the existence of different expression profiles of their target genes in each of these cell types. Impaired or delayed growth of ECs and enhanced growth of VSMCs are crucial cellular events in atherosclerosis, therefore the miR-

221/222 dysregulation represents a critical event in vascular disease pathogenesis. On the other hand, it has been reported that miR-221 and miR-222 overexpression downregulates eNOS expression in Dicer small interfering RNA-transfected human ECs [87]. This downregulation reduces NO bioavailability, a hallmark of patients with atherosclerosis and cardiovascular diseases, which further induces endothelial dysfunction, in part, by leading to higher oxidative stress.

These mechanisms are only a few of many through which miRs produce oxidative damage and promote atherosclerosis in ECs. Additionally, there are miRs that directly act on key players of the antioxidant defense system, regulating their functionality and switching on/off the ROS production/scavenging. One example is **miR-21**, which has been identified as an inhibitor of both *SOD2*, involved in the mitochondrial oxidative defense, and the sprouty RTK signaling antagonist 2 (*SPRY-2*) protein, which normally leads to extracellular signal—regulated/mitogen-activated protein kinase activation (ERK/MAP) kinase activation. Consequently, both of these repressive effects result in an increased ROS formation and angiogenic progenitor cell migratory defects in vascular tissues [88].

On the other hand, there are miRs that increase oxidative stress by decreasing expression levels of important cell regulatory proteins such as sirtuin 1 (*SIRT1*), a molecule with profound antioxidative and antiinflammatory effects and whose overexpression in endothelium has reported to prevent cellular senescence, to enhance vasodilatory responses, and to attenuate vascular damages [89]. In this line, a link between oxidative stress, miRs, and the SIRT1 pathway in vascular diseases has been extensively described. Some examples are **miR-217 and miR-34a**, which have been reported to be upregulated in vascular diseases and to induce loss of *SIRT1* function, thereby increasing oxidative stress and cell death [90,91]. Other miRs have also been reported to target *SIRT1*, and thus, to affect oxidative stress in a similar way. The case of **miR-199** has also been identified as a downregulator of *SIRT1*. Specifically, reported data have shown this miR is downregulated during hypoxia and that its reduction is required for the rapid upregulation of *SIRT1*, leading to decreased apoptosis in cardiomyocytes [92]. By means of both in silico and experimental validation approaches, aside from these three *SIRT1* target-miRs, many additional miRs have also been identified to target *SIRT1* mRNA and reportedly have a plausible role in the development of atherosclerosis via oxidative damage (miR-520c, miR-373, miR-92a, miR-132, and miR-181) [89].

As we can see, all these processes lead to oxidative stress production. Nevertheless, is there an additional role for miRs when oxidative stress is produced? Do they also act as oxidative damage mediators? Interestingly, once oxidative stress is produced, miRs induction or repression has also been reported to happen. In relation to this, the **miR-200 family** has been shown to be upregulated upon an oxidative stress increase in ECs; this is important since **miR-200c** is likely the main effector of oxidative stress-induced biological responses in ECs. Its overexpression in human umbilical endothelial cells seems to induce cell growth arrest, apoptosis, and cellular senescence. These effects might be mediated, at least in part, by the inhibition of its target the zinc finger e-box binding homeobox 1 (*ZEB1*). These findings underline the importance of miR-200 family upregulation, and in particular of miR-200c, in EC response to oxidative stress, further demonstrating the key role of ZEB1 in ROS-induced apoptosis and senescence [93]. Interestingly, another miR-200 family member, **miR-200a**, which is also induced by oxidative stress, has been identified as a *SIRT1* target-miR [94], further supporting the idea of a prominent role of miR-200 family members in ROS-induced endothelial dysfunction.

Taking all these facts into account, we can see how, in a similar way as it occurs in dysfunctional adipose tissue, miRs also participate in increasing oxidative stress and oxidative damage in the atherosclerotic vessel wall, a common obesity-related alteration. Indeed, some of these identified aberrant miRs share dysfunctional profiles in both vascular and adipose tissues, suggesting that oxidative stress induction mechanisms could be systemic alterations in the context of obesity. Since aberrant miR profiles are potentially modifiable, the downregulation/upregulation of these targets could be a useful therapeutic strategy against the obesity oxidative stress imbalance.

5.3 MicroRNAs in Nonalcoholic Fatty Liver Disease

NAFLD can be defined as a pathologic accumulation of TG within hepatocytes in the absence of significant alcohol consumption. NAFLD shares, in part, the common pathogenesis of metabolic syndrome including obesity, hyperlipidemia, insulin resistance, mitochondrial damage, oxidative stress response, and the release of inflammatory cytokines.

The potential roles of miRs in both physiological health and pathogenesis have been investigated in the liver, and it has been shown that their dysregulation may also contribute to the development and progression of NAFLD as it occurs in obesity [95]. Given NAFLD, as obesity, presents a strong oxidative stress component as hallmark, in this section we focus on the aberrant miR profiles that have been involved to date in the NAFLD etiopathogenesis and check if some of them are shared with previously mentioned alterations in adipose tissue or endothelium.

Among available data we highlight a role of **miR-122** and **miR-33a/b** in the regulation of cholesterol and fatty acid biosynthesis. Specifically, both miRs have been extensively identified as potential molecular targets in the management of metabolic syndrome and NAFLD [96,97]. Notwithstanding and considering the present subject matter, there are even more interesting miRs like those involved in the induction of oxidative liver damage. An example is the **miR-34a**, which has been reported to be highly expressed in patients with NAFLD and T2D, as well as identified as one of the most lipid-responsive hepatic miRs [98]. Intriguingly, it seems this miR mediates its effects through the inhibition of *SIRT1* expression and the blockade of PPARα and liver X receptor, key regulators of energy homeostasis [95]. According to previous sections where the miR-34a has been shown to play exactly the same *SIRT1*-effects in vascular tissues, and keeping in mind oxidative stress is a key feature of NAFLD, this mechanism is very attractive and presumes a plausible role for this small-RNA as an oxidative damage inducer also in NAFLD. Altogether, these data suggest downregulation of miR-34a could be a potential therapeutic strategy not only against atherosclerosis-related diseases but also against NAFLD.

In conclusion, although there are only few available findings pointing to miRs as oxidative damage inducers in NAFLD, it is interesting to see how some of these identified NAFLD-associated aberrant miRs are also key players in other obesity comorbidities such as atherosclerosis and vascular alterations.

Taken together, all these data support the hypothesis that obesity-associated systemic oxidative stress is mediated in large part by the dysregulation of miRs and that consequent oxidative damage plays key roles in the development of severe obesity-related alterations such as atherosclerosis, insulin resistance, or NAFLD.

6. OXIDATIVE STRESS AND EPIGENETIC CHANGES IN OBESITY-RELATED DISEASES

6.1 DNA Methylation and Oxidative Stress

DNA methylation is an epigenetic postreplication modification of DNA carried out by DNA methyltransferases (DNMTs) and consisting of the methylation of CpG dinucleotide cytosines across the whole genome. This methylation process on cytosine bases leads to the generation of 5-methylcytosines, and it is implicated in controlling tissue-specific gene expression patterns and genomic imprinting in humans. The DNA methylation process can be modulated by environmental factors, especially nutrition. Furthermore, modified DNA methylation patterns contribute to susceptibility to a range of complex diseases, cancer being the most studied.

According to this chapter's subject matter, it seems that altered DNA methylation patterns are also involved in the production of ROS as well as in mediating oxidative stress—induced cell responses in humans [99]. Many examples of this have been reported in cancer where numerous studies have been conducted. Such is the case of *SOD2* enzyme, whose transcriptional activity is controlled, in part, by DNA hypermethylation mechanisms at different stages of human cancer development [100]. Specifically, this *SOD* epigenetic impairment has been described to occur in the human KAS6 cell line of multiple myeloma [101], in A549 human lung epithelial cells, and in peripheral blood mononuclear cells [102]. Additionally, it has been shown how the loss of SOD activity may next contribute to changes in epigenetic regulation, thereby establishing a vicious cycle that further drives epigenetic instability in humans [100]. On its side, *CAT*, *GPX3*, and *GPX7* have also been shown to exhibit hypermethylation in different cancers [103,104].

6.2 DNA Methylation, Oxidative Stress, and Metabolic Syndrome

Taking all previous findings into account and given obesity is highly associated with an antioxidant defense imbalance as we already know, we aimed to answer if the same causative relationship observed in cancer (modified DNA methylation patterns induce ROS production in carcinogenesis) also occurs in obesity and metabolic syndrome.

In the context of obesity, DNA methylation has closely been implicated in the emergence of metabolic syndrome components through the epigenetic regulation of numerous candidate genes. In relation to this, while hypomethylation has been reported to happen in the promoter region of neuropeptide Y gene and other sensitive genes implicated in appetite regulation (e.g., leptin and proopiomelanocortin), numerous diabetes-related genes, instead, have been shown to be hypermethylated (the insulin promoter factor 1 [*Pdx-1*] implicated in the pancreatic development and maturation of β cells; the hepatic promoter methylation of PGC1-α implicated in energy metabolism; the unc-13 homolog B [*UNC13B*] implicated in carbohydrate metabolism; and the hepatocyte nuclear factor 4 alpha [*HNF4A*] implicated in the development of the liver, kidneys, and intestine).

Among the aforementioned hypermethylated genes, the *PGC1-α* gene, a key transcriptional regulator of mitochondrial fatty acid oxidation, has been correlated not only with the status of peripheral insulin resistance, but also with the fasting insulin levels of NAFLD patients [105]. In a whole-genome promoter DNA methylation analysis of skeletal muscle, *PGC1-α* hypermethylation was also found in diabetic subjects [106]. In this analysis, methylation levels negatively correlated with the expression of *PGC1-α* and mitochondrial density. Since previously in this chapter *PGC1-α* was identified as a relevant molecule in the regulation of redox state in obesity, these correlations support a prominent role for this gene in obesity-associated oxidative stress induction.

Another interesting study is one conducted in hypertensive rats [107], in which hypermethylation of the *SOD2* gene promoter was reported to happen in the hypertensive group. This hypermethylation could be prevented by the administration of 5-aza-2′-deoxycytidine, a chemical agent and nucleotide analogue that inhibits the methylation of new DNA synthesis, favors the proteasomal degradation of DNMT1, and is associated with a lower level of DNMT1 and DNMT3a protein expression. This last result is very important since it shows how alterations in DNA methylation have the ability to impair the expression of antioxidant genes such as *SOD* not only in cancer but also in a metabolic syndrome disease model. Taking all these data into account and given the fact that oxidative stress and inflammation are major processes in obesity and metabolic syndrome, we conclude that oxidative stress in obesity might also be related to epigenetic modifications (DNA hyper/hypomethylation patterns in key genes) as it has broadly been demonstrated for many cancers. In any case, further investigations are needed to better understand this issue.

6.3 Histone Acetylation, Oxidative Stress, and Metabolic Syndrome

Besides DNA methylation, another important epigenetic modification is histone acetylation, which consists of the introduction of acetyl functional groups into lysine residues. On the contrary, deacetylation is the removal of these acetyl groups. Interestingly, de/acetylation reactions have been reported to play central roles in many types of epigenetic inheritance and diseases.

In relation to oxidative stress, SIRT proteins, which have already been introduced in this chapter as important mediators of oxidative damage in vascular tissues, have also been shown to mediate deacetylation reactions that target histones as part of adaptive responses to metabolic stress by regulating lipid homeostasis and insulin secretion [108]. Although only the SIRT1 isoform has been mentioned before, humans possess seven different sirtuins (SIRT1-7), which localize to several subcellular compartments such as the nucleus (SIRT1, 2, 3, 6, and 7), cytoplasm (SIRT1 and 2), and mitochondria (SIRT3, 4, and 5). Regarding deacetylation reactions, SIRT3 is the primary mitochondrial protein deacetylase that maintains mitochondrial integrity and metabolism during oxidative stress [109]. In this line, SIRT3 deficient mice, fed with a HFD, showed accelerated obesity, insulin resistance, hyperlipidemia, and steatohepatitis compared to wild-type mice [110].

In the context of NAFLD, not only SIRT3 but also SIRT1 isoforms have been found to be activated during redox stress, which means they might modulate crucial responses including adaptation to hypoxia and amelioration of ROS-induced pathologies [111], thus providing a link between histone deacetylation and the cell redox state. In this line and according to reported data, SIRT1 and SIRT3 have been regarded as the crucial gatekeepers of redox status, epigenetic landscape, and lipid homeostasis in hepatocytes.

Taking all this information into account, it is clear how epigenetic modifications including DNA methylation, histone acetylation, and aberrant miRs patterns play an important role in the development of oxidative damage in obesity and metabolic syndrome. Moreover, it seems that these disturbances are not only general inducers of ROS production but also mediators of ROS-induced damage in key metabolic tissues (adipose, vascular, and hepatic tissues). Thus, epigenetic modifications and aberrant miRs profiles could be useful and effective therapeutic targets in the fight against obesity-associated oxidative stress and its comorbidities.

7. OXIDATIVE STRESS, METABOLIC DISEASES, AND CANCER

At this point of the book there is no doubt that genomic and epigenomic aberrancies may induce an exacerbated ROS production in human tissues and that resulting oxidative stress is a major mechanism in the initiation and progression of obesity-associated alterations such as insulin resistance, atherosclerosis, or NAFLD.

However, these alterations may go a step further. In the last years, a relationship between obesity and cancer incidence and mortality has been extensively postulated based on large cohort studies and the evidence of a biological link between both diseases that includes common metabolic, endocrine, and inflammatory processes [112,113]. In this regard, it has been observed that overweight and obese patients present an increased incidence of tumor development.

Given the previously listed evidence of how epigenetic aberrancies induce ROS-production in obesity and metabolic syndrome and the fact that ROS interact with different macromolecules including nucleic acids that become structurally modified by the process of oxidation, could oxidative stress be the link between metabolic disorders and their associated increased incidence of tumor development?

In this regard, the role of ROS as DNA damage inducers cannot be discarded as a plausible explanation. Oxidative stress renders different by-products with an important mutagenic potential. One of these by-products is the damaged base 8-OHdG, a molecule broadly related with tumor development [114]. Based on its ability to induce mismatch incorporation of nucleotides during DNA replication by DNA polymerase, the increased levels of this mutagenic base in obese patients might accelerate the mutational rate of cells and/or interfere with DNA repair mechanisms leading to an increase and accumulation of genetic events that characterize tumor development [115,116]. Thus, 8-OHdG could represent a critical step in obesity-associated carcinogenesis.

Another issue in favor of the hypothesis of oxidative stress being responsible for the higher cancer incidence and mortality in obese subjects is the fact that restriction of caloric intake has been reported to reduce the formation of intracellular ROS and therefore to prevent the oxidative damage to DNA and consequent cancer induction and progression [117].

On the other hand, and in line with the content of the present chapter, epigenetic alterations are common aberrancies in obesity-related cancers. One example is its relation to FoxO proteins and, in particular, to FoxO1, which have beneficial effects with respect to diabetes, as FoxO-dependent transcription of antioxidant enzymes may counteract oxidative stress—induced cellular damage. Interestingly, several studies have shown that miRs modulate *FoxO* levels [25]. In this regard, numerous miRs have been demonstrated to target *FoxO* transcripts in tumor cells; some of them are (miR-137, miR-223, miR-370) and (miR-96, miR-155), which are upregulated in cancer cells where they target *FoxO1a* and *FoxO3a* transcripts, respectively, thereby promoting uncontrolled cell proliferation [25,118]. This fact has been replicated in several cancers including gastric cancer and bladder cancer. Since *FoxO* proteins, and in particular FoxO1, are highly expressed in the major insulin target tissues as well as in the insulin-producing β-cells, these data could be an example of how epigenetic/miRs aberrancies might be indeed the primary alteration leading to oxidative stress, DNA damage, and, at the end, cancer induction in obesity and metabolic disorders.

In any case, although ROS-induced oxidative stress is a promising theory, other traditional metabolic and hormonal alterations associated with obesity have been more extensively studied to date and are still postulated as the main cause for this association. Thus further efforts of the scientific community are required to better understand the proposed cancer—obesity relationship.

8. CONCLUSION

In the present chapter it is made clear that genetic mechanisms are tightly involved in redox regulation in the context of obesity and its associated metabolic abnormalities.

As expected, either an excess or defect in oxidative stress has deleterious consequences for health. Thus an adequate balance between the ROS producing systems and ROS degrading enzymes is needed, together with an appropriate regulation at the cellular and organism level. However, the solution does not rely on a higher activation of antioxidant enzyme's expression, or on the indiscriminate use of antioxidants, but on the avoidance of individual disturbances that affect cellular homeostatic balance through an appropriate regulation.

Interestingly, individual genetic variations, such as SNPs in genes coding enzymes involved in this regulation, are able to affect functionality in such a way as to be associated with the disease or its comorbidities. This way, the identification of variants that confer a higher risk of the disease may be important for the establishment of individualized prevention strategies.

In addition, miRs dysregulation as well as other epigenetic modifications including DNA methylation or histone acetylation reactions also occur in people with obesity. Since many of these disturbances are potentially modifiable either by environmental factors, especially nutrition, or by using synthetic agents such as anti-miR oligonucleotides, many listed alterations in this chapter, therefore, are promising therapeutic targets or useful biomarkers for the fight against obesity-associated oxidative stress and its consequences.

Until now, most studies have been focused on identifying the genetic variants, altered miRs, or hyper/hypomethylated genes associated with oxidative stress in obesity. Nevertheless, although many promising results have been shown to date, additional studies are needed to replicate actual findings as well as to confirm whether the proposed markers could be indeed adequate therapeutic targets for ameliorating the characterized systemic oxidative stress status of obesity and metabolic syndrome.

GLOSSARY

5-aza-2′-deoxycytidine A chemical agent and nucleotide analogue that inhibits the methylation of new DNA synthesis, favors the proteasomal degradation of DNMT1, and is associated with a lower level of DNMT1 and DNMT3a protein expression.

Anti-miRs oligonucleotides (AMOs) Synthetically designed molecules that are used to neutralize microRNA function in cells for desired responses.

Antioxidant response element (ARE) Conserved short sequence present in the promoter of multiple antioxidant genes with the consensus sequence of $TA^{/C}nnA^{/G}TGAC^{/T}nnnGCA^{/G}A^{/T}A^{/T}A^{/T}$.

Atherosclerosis The process of vascular wall thickening and hardening, and the primary cause of coronary heart disease, ischemic stroke, and peripheral arterial disease.

Copy number variant (CNV) Genetic variants characterized by a varying number of repeated contiguous short sequences.

DNA methylation The methylation of CpG dinucleotide cytosines across the whole genome. This methylation process on cytosine bases leads to the generation of 5-methylcytosines instead, and it is implicated in controlling tissue-specific gene expression patterns and genomic imprinting in humans.

DNA methyltransferases (DNMTs) Enzymes that catalyze the transfer of a methyl group to DNA.

Foam cells Fat-laden M2 macrophages seen in atherosclerosis. They are an indication of plaque build-up, or atherosclerosis, which is commonly associated with increased risk of heart attack and stroke.

Functional variant Genetic variant with a direct impact on measurable or observable outcomes in the cell or organism, either through regulatory mechanisms or altered protein codification.

Gene expression Process in which a gene coded in the genome becomes transcribed into messenger RNA, later to be translated into the resulting protein product.

Genetic association study Investigation based on the identification of genomic regions associated with a disease or phenotypic outcome through the analysis of the correlation between the presence of disease and genetic variants.

Genetic variant Change of nucleotide types, length, or number of short sequences in the genome.

Histone acetylation A biochemical reaction that consists of the introduction of acetyl functional groups into lysine residuals of histone proteins. Histone acetylation and deacetylation are essential parts of gene regulation. These reactions are typically catalyzed by enzymes with histone acetyltransferase (HAT) or histone deacetylase (HDAC) activity.

Indel Change in the sequence of the genome in which extra nucleotides are present, or where certain nucleotides are missing.

Linkage disequilibrium The link between two alleles at different loci, observed by a higher frequency in the association of the two variants, which is higher than it would be expected if they were not associated or frequently inherited together.

MicroRNAs (miRs) Highly conserved small noncoding RNAs ranging from 18 to 24 ribonucleotides in length, which act as key post-transcriptional regulators of gene expression. By inducing mRNA degradation or blocking translation, miRs are involved in important cell processes such as cell growth, cell differentiation, and apoptosis, and their dysregulation has been proposed as one of the main triggers of carcinogenesis.

Missense variant Single nucleotide genetic variant that has a functional consequence by also changing the sequence of the coded protein.

Nonalcoholic fatty liver disease (NAFLD) A pathologic accumulation of triglycerides within hepatocytes in the absence of significant alcohol consumption. NAFLD shares, in part, the common pathogenesis of metabolic syndrome including obesity, hyperlipidemia, insulin resistance, mitochondrial damage, oxidative stress response, and the release of inflammatory cytokines.

Promoter Genomic sequence of variable length located prior to the start of the coding sequence of a gene, which often contains conserved and short sequences that can be recognized by the appropriate transcription factors to start gene transcription.

Small interfering RNAs (siRNAs) A class of double-stranded RNA molecules, ranging from 20 to 25 base pairs in length, similar to miRs, which operate within the RNA interference (RNAi) pathway. They interfere with the expression of specific genes with complementary nucleotide sequences by degrading mRNA after transcription resulting in no translation.

Single nucleotide polymorphism (SNP) Change of a single nucleotide for another in one position of the genome.

Thermogenesis Process of heat generation in animal cells, here specifically referred to as nonshivering thermogenesis, which occurs in mitochondria from brown adipose tissue by the uncoupling of oxidative phosphorylation, which generates heat from the unused released energy.

Transcription factor Protein involved in the activation of gene transcription through its direct or indirect binding to the promoter sequence of a target gene.

Upregulation Response of a cellular component to a signal in which the gene expression of a target gene is increased.

LIST OF ACRONYMS AND ABBREVIATIONS

8-OHdG 8-hydroxy-2′-deoxyguanosine
A-FABP Adipocyte fatty acid-binding protein
AMO Anti-miR oligonucleotide
ARE Antioxidant response element
ATP Adenosine triphosphate
BMI Body mass index
CAT Catalase
CD Cluster of differentiation
CEBPβ CCAAT/enhancer-binding protein beta
CNV Copy number variant
DNMT DNA methyltransferase
EC Endothelial cell
EC-SOD Extracellular SOD
eNOS Endothelial nitric oxide synthase

FoxO Forkhead box O
GPX Glutathione peroxidase
GSTA2 Glutathione S-transferase
HDL High-density lipoprotein
HFD High-fat diet
HNF4A Hepatocyte nuclear factor 4 alpha
HO-1 Heme oxygenase-1
HOMA-IR Homeostasis model assessment of insulin resistance
HOMA-β Homeostasis model assessment of β-cell function
HUVEC Human umbilical endothelial cell
IFN-γ Interferon gamma
IGF1 Insulin-like growth factor 1
IL Interleukin
IMT Intima media thickness
indel Deletion or insertion
IRE Insulin responsive element
KEAP1 Kelch-like ECH-associated protein 1
LD Linkage disequilibrium
LDL Low-density lipoprotein
LOX-1 Lectin-like oxidized LDL receptor-1
LXR Liver X receptor
MDA Malondialdehyde
miR MicroRNA
MPO Myeloperoxidase
MsrA Methionine sulphoxide reductase A
NADPH Reduced nicotinamide adenine dinucleotide phosphate
NAFLD Nonalcoholic fatty liver disease
NFκB Nuclear factor kappa-light-chain-enhancer of activated B cells
NO Nitric oxide
NQO1 NADPH quinone oxidoreductase
Nrf2 Nuclear factor (erythroid-derived 2)-like 2
ox-LDL Oxidized-LDL
p22phox Human neutrophil cytochrome b light chain
Pdx-1 Insulin promoter factor 1
PGC1-α Peroxisome proliferative activated receptor (PPAR)-gamma coactivator 1 alpha
POMC Proopiomelanocortin
PON Paraoxonase
PPARγ Peroxisome proliferator-activated receptor gamma
PPRE Peroxisome proliferator response element
PRDX Peroxiredoxin
ROS Reactive oxygen species
siRNA Small interfering RNA
SIRT Sirtuin
SNP Single nucleotide polymorphism
SOD Superoxide dismutase
SPRY-2 Sprouty RTK signaling antagonist 2
T2D Type 2 diabetes
TBARS Thiobarbituric acid reactive substances
TG Triglycerides
TLR Toll-like receptor
TNF-α Tumor necrosis factor alpha
Trx2 Thioredoxin
TrxR2 Thioredoxin reductase
UCP Uncoupling protein
UNC13B unc-13 homolog B
VLDL Very low-density lipoprotein
VSMC Vascular smooth cell
ZEB1 Zinc finger E-box binding homeobox 1

REFERENCES

[1] Lee YS, Kim AY, Choi JW, Kim M, Yasue S, Son HJ, et al. Dysregulation of adipose glutathione peroxidase 3 in obesity contributes to local and systemic oxidative stress. Mol Endocrinol September 2008;22(9):2176−89.

[2] Lijnen HR, Van Hul M, Hemmeryckx B. Caloric restriction improves coagulation and inflammation profile in obese mice. Thromb Res January 2012;129(1):74−9.

[3] Merry TL, Tran M, Stathopoulos M, Wiede F, Fam BC, Dodd GT, et al. High-fat-fed obese glutathione peroxidase 1-deficient mice exhibit defective insulin secretion but protection from hepatic steatosis and liver damage. Antioxid Redox Signal May 10, 2014;20(14):2114−29.

[4] Wei P-C, Hsieh Y-H, Su M-I, Jiang X, Hsu P-H, Lo W-T, et al. Loss of the oxidative stress sensor NPGPx compromises GRP78 chaperone activity and induces systemic disease. Mol Cell December 14, 2012;48(5):747−59.

[5] Chang Y-C, Yu Y-H, Shew J-Y, Lee W-J, Hwang J-J, Chen Y-H, et al. Deficiency of NPGPx, an oxidative stress sensor, leads to obesity in mice and human. EMBO Mol Med August 2013;5(8):1165−79.

[6] Rupérez AI, Olza J, Gil-Campos M, Leis R, Mesa MD, Tojo R, et al. Are catalase -844A/G polymorphism and activity associated with childhood obesity? Antioxid Redox Signal December 1, 2013;19(16):1970−5.

[7] Shin M-J, Park E. Contribution of insulin resistance to reduced antioxidant enzymes and vitamins in nonobese Korean children. Clin Chim Acta March 2006;365(1−2):200−5.

[8] Rindler PM, Plafker SM, Szweda LI, Kinter M. High dietary fat selectively increases catalase expression within cardiac mitochondria. J Biol Chem January 18, 2013;288(3):1979−90.

[9] Huh JY, Kim Y, Jeong J, Park J, Kim I, Huh KH, et al. Peroxiredoxin 3 is a key molecule regulating adipocyte oxidative stress, mitochondrial biogenesis, and adipokine expression. Antioxid Redox Signal February 1, 2012;16(3):229−43.

[10] Nakao C, Ookawara T, Sato Y, Kizaki T, Imazeki N, Matsubara O, et al. Extracellular superoxide dismutase in tissues from obese (ob/ob) mice. Free Radic Res September 2000;33(3):229−41.

[11] Adachi T, Inoue M, Hara H, Maehata E, Suzuki S. Relationship of plasma extracellular-superoxide dismutase level with insulin resistance in type 2 diabetic patients. J Endocrinol June 2004;181(3):413−7.

[12] Liu Y, Qi W, Richardson A, Van Remmen H, Ikeno Y, Salmon AB. Oxidative damage associated with obesity is prevented by overexpression of CuZn- or Mn-superoxide dismutase. Biochem Biophys Res Commun August 16, 2013;438(1):78−83.

[13] Tirosh A, Potashnik R, Bashan N, Rudich A. Oxidative stress disrupts insulin-induced cellular redistribution of insulin receptor substrate-1 and phosphatidylinositol 3-kinase in 3T3-L1 adipocytes. A putative cellular mechanism for impaired protein kinase B activation and GLUT4 translocation. J Biol Chem April 9, 1999;274(15):10595−602.

[14] Styskal J, Nwagwu FA, Watkins YN, Liang H, Richardson A, Musi N, et al. Methionine sulfoxide reductase A affects insulin resistance by protecting insulin receptor function. Free Radic Biol Med March 2013;56:123−32.

[15] Uthus EO, Picklo MJ. Obesity reduces methionine sulphoxide reductase activity in visceral adipose tissue. Free Radic Res September 5, 2011;45(9):1052−60.

[16] Zieleniak A, Wójcik M, Woźniak LA. Structure and physiological functions of the human peroxisome proliferator-activated receptor γ. Arch Immunol Ther Exp (Warsz) October 6, 2008;56(5):331−45.

[17] Vidal-Puig AJ, Considine RV, Jimenez-Liñan M, Werman A, Pories WJ, Caro JF, et al. Peroxisome proliferator-activated receptor gene expression in human tissues. Effects of obesity, weight loss, and regulation by insulin and glucocorticoids. J Clin Invest May 15, 1997;99(10):2416−22.

[18] Luo W, Cao J, Li J, He W. Adipose tissue-specific PPARgamma deficiency increases resistance to oxidative stress. Exp Gerontol March 2008;43(3):154−63.

[19] Houstis N, Rosen ED, Lander ES. Reactive oxygen species have a causal role in multiple forms of insulin resistance. Nature April 13, 2006;440(7086):944−8.

[20] Kadlec AO, Chabowski DS, Ait-Aissa K, Gutterman DD. Role of PGC-1α in vascular regulation: implications for atherosclerosis. Arterioscler Thromb Vasc Biol August 2016;36(8):1467−74.

[21] Singh SP, Schragenheim J, Cao J, Falck JR, Abraham NG, Bellner L. PGC-1 alpha regulates HO-1 expression, mitochondrial dynamics and biogenesis: role of epoxyeicosatrienoic acid. Prostaglandins Other Lipid Mediat September 2016;125:8−18.

[22] Holmström KM, Kostov RV, Dinkova-Kostova AT. The multifaceted role of Nrf2 in mitochondrial function. Curr Opin Toxicol December 2016;1:80−91.

[23] Das SK, Sharma NK, Hasstedt SJ, Mondal AK, Ma L, Langberg KA, et al. An integrative genomics approach identifies activation of thioredoxin/thioredoxin reductase-1-mediated oxidative stress defense pathway and inhibition of angiogenesis in obese nondiabetic human subjects. J Clin Endocrinol Metab August 2011;96(8):E1308−13.

[24] Pi J, Leung L, Xue P, Wang W, Hou Y, Liu D, et al. Deficiency in the nuclear factor E2-related factor-2 transcription factor results in impaired adipogenesis and protects against diet-induced obesity. J Biol Chem March 19, 2010;285(12):9292−300.

[25] Klotz LO, Sánchez-Ramos C, Prieto-Arroyo I, Urbánek P, Steinbrenner H, Monsalve M. Redox regulation of FoxO transcription factors. Redox Biol 2015;6:51−72. Elsevier.

[26] Kim DH, Zhang T, Lee S, Calabuig-Navarro V, Yamauchi J, Piccirillo A, et al. FoxO6 integrates insulin signaling with MTP for regulating VLDL production in the liver. Endocrinology April 2014;155(4):1255−67.

[27] Rupérez AI, Gil A, Aguilera CM. Genetics of oxidative stress in obesity. Int J Mol Sci February 20, 2014;15(2):3118−44. Multidisciplinary Digital Publishing Institute (MDPI).

[28] Kuzuya M, Ando F, Iguchi A, Shimokata H. Glutathione peroxidase 1 Pro198Leu variant contributes to the metabolic syndrome in men in a large Japanese cohort. Am J Clin Nutr June 2008;87(6):1939—44.

[29] Hernández Guerrero C, Hernández Chávez P, Martínez Castro N, Parra Carriedo A, García Del Rio S, Pérez Lizaur A. Glutathione peroxidase-1 PRO200LEU polymorphism (RS1050450) is associated with morbid obesity independently of the presence of prediabetes or diabetes in women from central Mexico. Nutr Hosp October 1, 2015;32(4):1516—25.

[30] Hamanishi T, Furuta H, Kato H, Doi A, Tamai M, Shimomura H, et al. Functional variants in the glutathione peroxidase-1 (GPx-1) gene are associated with increased intima-media thickness of carotid arteries and risk of macrovascular diseases in Japanese type 2 diabetic patients. Diabetes September 2004;53(9):2455—60.

[31] Shuvalova YA, Kaminnyi AI, Meshkov AN, Kukharchuk VV. Pro198Leu polymorphism of GPx-1 gene and activity of erythrocytic glutathione peroxidase and lipid peroxidation products. Bull Exp Biol Med November 2010;149(6):743—5.

[32] Chen Y-I, Wei P-C, Hsu J-L, Su F-Y, Lee W-H. NPGPx (GPx7): a novel oxidative stress sensor/transmitter with multiple roles in redox homeostasis. Am J Transl Res 2016;8(4):1626—40.

[33] Wang Z, Li Y, Wang B, He Y, Wang Y, Xi H, et al. A haplotype of the catalase gene confers an increased risk of essential hypertension in Chinese Han. Hum Mutat March 2010;31(3):272—8.

[34] Adkins S, Gan KN, Mody M, La Du BN. Molecular basis for the polymorphic forms of human serum paraoxonase/arylesterase: glutamine or arginine at position 191, for the respective A or B allozymes. Am J Hum Genet March 1993;52(3):598—608.

[35] Garin MC, James RW, Dussoix P, Blanché H, Passa P, Froguel P, et al. Paraoxonase polymorphism Met-Leu54 is associated with modified serum concentrations of the enzyme. A possible link between the paraoxonase gene and increased risk of cardiovascular disease in diabetes. J Clin Invest January 1, 1997;99(1):62—6.

[36] Rupérez AI, López-Guarnido O, Gil F, Olza J, Gil-Campos M, Leis R, et al. Paraoxonase 1 activities and genetic variation in childhood obesity. Br J Nutr November 21, 2013;110(9):1639—47.

[37] Hiroi M, Nagahara Y, Miyauchi R, Misaki Y, Goda T, Kasezawa N, et al. The combination of genetic variations in the PRDX3 gene and dietary fat intake contribute to obesity risk. Obesity April 2, 2011;19(4):882—7.

[38] Sutton A, Khoury H, Prip-Buus C, Cepanec C, Pessayre D, Degoul F. The Ala16Val genetic dimorphism modulates the import of human manganese superoxide dismutase into rat liver mitochondria. Pharmacogenetics March 2003;13(3):145—57.

[39] Montano MAE, Barrio Lera JP, Gottlieb MGV, Schwanke CHA, da Rocha MIUM, Manica-Cattani MF, et al. Association between manganese superoxide dismutase (MnSOD) gene polymorphism and elderly obesity. Mol Cell Biochem August 5, 2009;328(1—2):33—40.

[40] Pourvali K, Abbasi M, Mottaghi A. Role of superoxide dismutase 2 gene Ala16Val polymorphism and total antioxidant capacity in diabetes and its complications. Avicenna J Med Biotechnol 2016;8(2):48—56.

[41] Tibaut M, Petrovič D. Oxidative stress genes, antioxidants and coronary artery disease in type 2 diabetes mellitus. Cardiovasc Hematol Agents Med Chem 2016;14(1):23—38.

[42] El-Koofy N, El-Karaksy H, Mandour I, Anwar G, El-Raziky M, El-Hennawy A. Genetic polymorphisms in non-alcoholic fatty liver disease in obese Egyptian children. Saudi J Gastroenterol 2011;17(4):265.

[43] Montano MAE, da Cruz IBM, Duarte MMMF, da Costa Krewer C, de Ugalde Marques da Rocha MI, Mânica-Cattani MF, et al. Inflammatory cytokines in vitro production are associated with Ala16Val superoxide dismutase gene polymorphism of peripheral blood mononuclear cells. Cytokine October 2012;60(1):30—3.

[44] Caple F, Williams EA, Spiers A, Tyson J, Burtle B, Daly AK, et al. Inter-individual variation in DNA damage and base excision repair in young, healthy non-smokers: effects of dietary supplementation and genotype. Br J Nutr June 19, 2010;103(11):1585—93.

[45] Bille DS, Banasik K, Justesen JM, Sandholt CH, Sandbæk A, Lauritzen T, et al. Implications of central obesity-related variants in LYPLAL1, NRXN3, MSRA, and TFAP2B on quantitative metabolic traits in adult DanesMailund T, editor. PLoS One June 2, 2011;6(6):e20640.

[46] Yeung E, Qi L, Hu FB, Zhang C. Novel abdominal adiposity genes and the risk of type 2 diabetes: findings from two prospective cohorts. Int J Mol Epidemiol Genet 2011;2(2):138—44.

[47] Hotta K, Nakamura M, Nakamura T, Matsuo T, Nakata Y, Kamohara S, et al. Polymorphisms in NRXN3, TFAP2B, MSRA, LYPLAL1, FTO and MC4R and their effect on visceral fat area in the Japanese population. J Hum Genet November 12, 2010;55(11):738—42.

[48] Scherag A, Dina C, Hinney A, Vatin V, Scherag S, Vogel CIG, et al. Two new loci for body-weight regulation identified in a joint analysis of genome-wide association studies for early-onset extreme obesity in French and German study groupsDermitzakis ET, editor. PLoS Genet April 22, 2010;6(4):e1000916.

[49] Dorajoo R, Blakemore AIF, Sim X, Ong RT-H, Ng DPK, Seielstad M, et al. Replication of 13 obesity loci among Singaporean Chinese, Malay and Asian-Indian populations. Int J Obes January 19, 2012;36(1):159—63.

[50] Nedergaard J, Cannon B. The "novel" "uncoupling" proteins UCP2 and UCP3: what do they really do? Pros and cons for suggested functions. Exp Physiol January 2003;88(1):65—84.

[51] Fisler JS, Warden CH. Uncoupling proteins, dietary fat and the metabolic syndrome. Nutr Metab (Lond) September 12, 2006;3(1):38.

[52] Qian L, Xu K, Xu X, Gu R, Liu X, Shan S, et al. UCP2 -866G/A, Ala55Val and UCP3 -55C/T polymorphisms in association with obesity susceptibility — a meta-analysis studyBuzzetti R, editor. PLoS One April 1, 2013;8(4):e58939. Public Library of Science.

[53] Salopuro T, Pulkkinen L, Lindström J, Kolehmainen M, Tolppanen A-M, Eriksson JG, et al. Variation in the UCP2 and UCP3genes associates with abdominal obesity and serum lipids: the Finnish Diabetes Prevention Study. BMC Med Genet December 21, 2009;10(1):94.

[54] San José G, Moreno MU, Oliván S, Beloqui O, Fortuño A, Díez J, et al. Functional effect of the p22phox -930A/G polymorphism on p22phox expression and NADPH oxidase activity in hypertension. Hypertension 2004;44(2):163—9.

[55] Ochoa MC, Razquin C, Zalba G, Martínez-González MA, Martínez JA, Marti A. G allele of the -930A>G polymorphism of the CYBA gene is associated with insulin resistance in obese subjects. J Physiol Biochem June 2008;64(2):127−33.

[56] Hayaishi-Okano R, Yamasaki Y, Kajimoto Y, Sakamoto K, Ohtoshi K, Katakami N, et al. Association of NAD(P)H oxidase p22 phox gene variation with advanced carotid atherosclerosis in Japanese type 2 diabetes. Diabetes Care February 2003;26(2):458−63.

[57] Schreiber R, Ferreira-Sae MC, Tucunduva AC, Mill JG, Costa FO, Krieger JE, et al. CYBA C242T polymorphism is associated with obesity and diabetes mellitus in Brazilian hypertensive patients. Diabet Med July 2012;29(7):e55−61.

[58] Kim C, Zheng T, Lan Q, Chen Y, Foss F, Chen X, et al. Genetic polymorphisms in oxidative stress pathway genes and modification of BMI and risk of non-Hodgkin lymphoma. Cancer Epidemiol Biomarkers Prev May 1, 2012;21(5):866−8.

[59] van der Veen BS, de Winther MPJ, Heeringa P. Myeloperoxidase: molecular mechanisms of action and their relevance to human health and disease. Antioxid Redox Signal November 2009;11(11):2899−937.

[60] Ergen A, Karagedik H, Karali ZE, Isbir T. An association between MPO -463 G/A polymorphism and type 2 diabetes. Folia Biol (Czech Republic) 2014;60(3):108−12.

[61] Galbete C, Toledo E, Martínez-González MA, Martínez JA, Guillén-Grima F, Marti A. Pro12Ala variant of the *PPARG2* gene increases body mass index: an updated meta-analysis encompassing 49,092 subjects. Obesity July 2013;21(7):1486−95.

[62] Lindi VI, Uusitupa MIJ, Lindström J, Louheranta A, Eriksson JG, Valle TT, et al. Association of the Pro12Ala polymorphism in the PPAR-gamma2 gene with 3-year incidence of type 2 diabetes and body weight change in the Finnish Diabetes Prevention Study. Diabetes August 2002;51(8):2581−6.

[63] Ghoussaini M, Meyre D, Lobbens S, Charpentier G, Clément K, Charles M-A, et al. Implication of the Pro12Ala polymorphism of the PPAR-gamma 2 gene in type 2 diabetes and obesity in the French population. BMC Med Genet March 22, 2005;6(1):11.

[64] Ostgren CJ, Lindblad U, Melander O, Melander A, Groop L, Råstam L. Peroxisome proliferator-activated receptor-gammaPro12Ala polymorphism and the association with blood pressure in type 2 diabetes: skaraborg hypertension and diabetes project. J Hypertens September 2003;21(9):1657−62.

[65] Yang Z, Wen J, Li Q, Tao X, Ye Z, He M, et al. PPARG gene Pro12Ala variant contributes to the development of non-alcoholic fatty liver in middle-aged and older Chinese population. Mol Cell Endocrinol January 2, 2012;348(1):255−9.

[66] Thamer C, Haap M, Volk A, Maerker E, Becker R, Bachmann O, et al. Evidence for greater oxidative substrate flexibility in male carriers of the pro 12 Ala polymorphism in PPARγ2. Horm Metab Res March 26, 2002;34(3):132−6.

[67] Berhouma R, Kouidhi S, Ammar M, Abid H, Ennafaa H, Benammar-Elgaaied A. Correlation of peroxisome proliferator-activated receptor (PPAR-γ) mRNA expression with Pro12Ala polymorphism in obesity. Biochem Genet April 13, 2013;51(3−4):256−63.

[68] O'Rahilly S, Barroso I, Gurnell M, Crowley VEF, Agostini M, Schwabe JW, et al. Dominant negative mutations in human PPARgamma associated with severe insulin resistance, diabetes mellitus and hypertension. Nature 1999;402(6764):880−3.

[69] Fanelli M, Filippi E, Sentinelli F, Romeo S, Fallarino M, Buzzetti R, et al. The Gly482Ser missense mutation of the peroxisome proliferator-activated receptor gamma coactivator-1 alpha (PGC-1 alpha) gene associates with reduced insulin sensitivity in normal and glucose-intolerant obese subjects. Dis Markers 2005;21(4):175−80.

[70] Esterbauer H, Oberkofler H, Linnemayr V, Iglseder B, Hedegger M, Wolfsgruber P, et al. Peroxisome proliferator-activated receptor-gamma coactivator-1 gene locus: associations with obesity indices in middle-aged women. Diabetes April 2002;51(4):1281−6.

[71] Weng S-W, Lin T-K, Wang P-W, Chen I-Y, Lee H-C, Chen S-D, et al. Gly482Ser polymorphism in the peroxisome proliferator-activated receptor gamma coactivator-1alpha gene is associated with oxidative stress and abdominal obesity. Metabolism April 2010;59(4):581−6.

[72] Goyenechea E, Crujeiras AB, Abete I, Parra D, Martínez JA. Enhanced short-term improvement of insulin response to a low-caloric diet in obese carriers the Gly482Ser variant of the PGC-1alpha gene. Diabetes Res Clin Pract November 2008;82(2):190−6.

[73] Okauchi Y, Iwahashi H, Okita K, Yuan M, Matsuda M, Tanaka T, et al. PGC-1alpha Gly482Ser polymorphism is associated with the plasma adiponectin level in type 2 diabetic men. Endocr J December 2008;55(6):991−7.

[74] Nitz I, Ewert A, Klapper M, Döring F. Analysis of PGC-1α variants Gly482Ser and Thr612Met concerning their PPARγ2-coactivation function. Biochem Biophys Res Commun February 9, 2007;353(2):481−6.

[75] Jiménez-Osorio AS, González-Reyes S, García-Niño WR, Moreno-Macías H, Rodríguez-Arellano ME, Vargas-Alarcón G, et al. Association of nuclear factor-erythroid 2-related factor 2, thioredoxin interacting protein, and heme oxygenase-1 gene polymorphisms with diabetes and obesity in Mexican patients. Oxid Med Cell Longev Hindawi 2016 May;4:1−8.

[76] Kim J-R, Jung HS, Bae S-W, Kim JH, Park BL, Choi YH, et al. Polymorphisms in FOXO gene family and association analysis with BMI. Obesity February 2006;14(2):188−93.

[77] Hulsmans M, De Keyzer D, Holvoet P. MicroRNAs regulating oxidative stress and inflammation in relation to obesity and atherosclerosis. FASEB J August 1, 2011;25(8):2515−27.

[78] Chang C-L, Au L-C, Huang S-W, Fai Kwok C, Ho L-T, Juan C-C. Insulin up-regulates heme oxygenase-1 expression in 3T3-L1 adipocytes via PI3-kinase- and PKC-dependent pathways and heme oxygenase-1−associated microRNA downregulation. Endocrinology February 2011;152(2):384−93.

[79] Ortega FJ, Moreno-Navarrete JM, Pardo G, Sabater M, Hummel M, Ferrer A, et al. MiRNA expression profile of human subcutaneous adipose and during adipocyte differentiationWang Y, editor. PLoS One February 2, 2010;5(2):e9022. Public Library of Science.

[80] Lin Q, Gao Z, Alarcon RM, Ye J, Yun Z. A role of miR-27 in the regulation of adipogenesis. FEBS J April 2009;276(8):2348−58. NIH Public Access.

[81] Zhu N, Zhang D, Chen S, Liu X, Lin L, Huang X, et al. Endothelial enriched microRNAs regulate angiotensin II-induced endothelial inflammation and migration. Atherosclerosis April 2011;215(2):286−93.

[82] Fang Y, Shi C, Manduchi E, Civelek M, Davies PF. MicroRNA-10a regulation of proinflammatory phenotype in athero-susceptible endothelium in vivo and in vitro. Proc Natl Acad Sci July 27, 2010;107(30):13450−5.

[83] Guo M, Mao X, Ji Q, Lang M, Li S, Peng Y, et al. miR-146a in PBMCs modulates Th1 function in patients with acute coronary syndrome. Immunol Cell Biol July 2, 2010;88(5):555−64.

[84] Harris TA, Yamakuchi M, Ferlito M, Mendell JT, Lowenstein CJ. MicroRNA-126 regulates endothelial expression of vascular cell adhesion molecule 1. Proc Natl Acad Sci February 5, 2008;105(5):1516−21.

[85] Nakamachi Y, Kawano S, Takenokuchi M, Nishimura K, Sakai Y, Chin T, et al. MicroRNA-124a is a key regulator of proliferation and monocyte chemoattractant protein 1 secretion in fibroblast-like synoviocytes from patients with rheumatoid arthritis. Arthritis Rheum May 2009;60(5):1294−304.

[86] Liu X, Cheng Y, Yang J, Xu L, Zhang C. Cell-specific effects of miR-221/222 in vessels: molecular mechanism and therapeutic application. J Mol Cell Cardiol January 2012;52(1):245−55. NIH Public Access.

[87] Suarez Y, Fernandez-Hernando C, Pober JS, Sessa WC. Dicer dependent microRNAs regulate gene expression and functions in human endothelial cells. Circ Res April 27, 2007;100(8):1164−73.

[88] Fleissner F, Jazbutyte V, Fiedler J, Gupta SK, Yin X, Xu Q, et al. Short communication: asymmetric dimethylarginine impairs angiogenic progenitor cell function in patients with coronary artery disease through a microRNA-21−dependent mechanism. Circ Res 2010;107(1).

[89] Chen Z, Shentu T-P, Wen L, Johnson DA, Shyy JY-J. Regulation of SIRT1 by oxidative stress-responsive miRNAs and a systematic approach to identify its role in the endothelium. Antioxid Redox Signal November 1, 2013;19(13):1522−38. Mary Ann Liebert, Inc.

[90] Menghini R, Casagrande V, Cardellini M, Martelli E, Terrinoni A, Amati F, et al. MicroRNA 217 modulates endothelial cell senescence via silent information regulator 1. Circulation October 13, 2009;120(15):1524−32.

[91] Xu Q, Seeger FH, Castillo J, Iekushi K, Boon RA, Farcas R, et al. Micro-RNA-34a contributes to the impaired function of bone marrow-derived mononuclear cells from patients with cardiovascular disease. J Am Coll Cardiol June 5, 2012;59(23):2107−17.

[92] Rane S, He M, Sayed D, Vashistha H, Malhotra A, Sadoshima J, et al. Downregulation of MiR-199a derepresses hypoxia-inducible factor-1 and sirtuin 1 and recapitulates hypoxia preconditioning in cardiac myocytes. Circ Res April 10, 2009;104(7):879−86.

[93] Magenta A, Cencioni C, Fasanaro P, Zaccagnini G, Greco S, Sarra-Ferraris G, et al. miR-200c is upregulated by oxidative stress and induces endothelial cell apoptosis and senescence via ZEB1 inhibition. Cell Death Differ October 29, 2011;18(10):1628−39.

[94] Eades G, Yao Y, Yang M, Zhang Y, Chumsri S, Zhou Q. miR-200a regulates SIRT1 expression and epithelial to mesenchymal transition (EMT)-like transformation in mammary epithelial cells. J Biol Chem July 22, 2011;286(29):25992−6002.

[95] Panera N, Gnani D, Crudele A, Ceccarelli S, Nobili V, Alisi A. MicroRNAs as controlled systems and controllers in non-alcoholic fatty liver disease. World J Gastroenterol November 7, 2014;20(41):15079−86. Baishideng Publishing Group Inc.

[96] Baffy G. MicroRNAs in nonalcoholic fatty liver disease. J Clin Med December 4, 2015;4(12):1977−88. Multidisciplinary Digital Publishing Institute (MDPI).

[97] Gori M, Arciello M, Balsano C. MicroRNAs in nonalcoholic fatty liver disease: novel biomarkers and prognostic tools during the transition from steatosis to hepatocarcinoma. BioMed Res Int 2014;2014:1−14.

[98] Kong L, Zhu J, Han W, Jiang X, Xu M, Zhao Y, et al. Significance of serum microRNAs in pre-diabetes and newly diagnosed type 2 diabetes: a clinical study. Acta Diabetol March 21, 2011;48(1):61−9.

[99] Hayes P, Knaus UG. Balancing reactive oxygen species in the epigenome: NADPH oxidases as target and perpetrator. Antioxid Redox Signal May 20, 2013;18(15):1937−45.

[100] Cyr AR, Hitchler MJ, Domann FE. Regulation of SOD2 in cancer by histone modifications and CpG methylation: closing the loop between redox biology and epigenetics. Antioxid Redox Signal May 20, 2013;18(15):1946−55.

[101] Hodge DR, Peng B, Pompeia C, Thomas S, Cho E, Clausen PA, et al. Epigenetic silencing of manganese superoxide dismutase (SOD-2) in KAS 6/1 human multiple myeloma cells increases cell proliferation. Cancer Biol Ther May 2005;4(5):585−92.

[102] Kamiya T, Machiura M, Makino J, Hara H, Hozumi I, Adachi T. Epigenetic regulation of extracellular-superoxide dismutase in human monocytes. Free Radic Biol Med August 2013;61:197−205.

[103] Zelko IN, Mueller MR, Folz RJ. CpG methylation attenuates Sp1 and Sp3 binding to the human extracellular superoxide dismutase promoter and regulates its cell-specific expression. Free Radic Biol Med April 1, 2010;48(7):895−904. NIH Public Access.

[104] Peng DF, Razvi M, Chen H, Washington K, Roessner A, Schneider-Stock R, et al. DNA hypermethylation regulates the expression of members of the Mu-class glutathione S-transferases and glutathione peroxidases in Barrett's adenocarcinoma. Gut January 1, 2009;58(1):5−15.

[105] Sookoian S, Rosselli MS, Gemma C, Burgueño AL, Fernández Gianotti T, Castaño GO, et al. Epigenetic regulation of insulin resistance in nonalcoholic fatty liver disease: impact of liver methylation of the peroxisome proliferator-activated receptor γ coactivator 1α promoter. Hepatology December 2010;52(6):1992−2000.

[106] Barrès R, Osler ME, Yan J, Rune A, Fritz T, Caidahl K, et al. Non-CpG methylation of the PGC-1α promoter through DNMT3B controls mitochondrial density. Cell Metab September 2009;10(3):189−98.

[107] Archer SL, Marsboom G, Kim GH, Zhang HJ, Toth PT, Svensson EC, et al. Epigenetic attenuation of mitochondrial superoxide dismutase 2 in pulmonary arterial hypertension: a basis for excessive cell proliferation and a new therapeutic target. Circulation June 22, 2010;121(24):2661−71.

[108] Lee J, Friso S, Choi S-W. Epigenetic mechanisms underlying the link between non-alcoholic fatty liver diseases and nutrition. Nutrients August 21, 2014;6(8):3303−25.

[109] Kim H-S, Patel K, Muldoon-Jacobs K, Bisht KS, Aykin-Burns N, Pennington JD, et al. SIRT3 is a mitochondria-localized tumor suppressor required for maintenance of mitochondrial integrity and metabolism during stress. Cancer Cell January 19, 2010;17(1):41−52.

[110] Hirschey MD, Shimazu T, Jing E, Grueter CA, Collins AM, Aouizerat B, et al. SIRT3 deficiency and mitochondrial protein hyperacetylation accelerate the development of the metabolic syndrome. Mol Cell October 21, 2011;44(2):177−90.

[111] Lee J, Kim Y, Friso S, Choi S-W. Epigenetics in non-alcoholic fatty liver disease. Mol Aspects Med April 2017;54:78−88.

[112] Renehan AG, Tyson M, Egger M, Heller RF, Zwahlen M. Body-mass index and incidence of cancer: a systematic review and meta-analysis of prospective observational studies. Lancet February 16, 2008;371(9612):569−78.

[113] Roberts DL, Dive C, Renehan AG. Biological mechanisms linking obesity and cancer risk: new perspectives. Annu Rev Med February 2010;61(1):301−16.

[114] Collado R, Oliver I, Tormos C, Egea M, Miguel A, Cerdá C, et al. Early ROS-mediated DNA damage and oxidative stress biomarkers in monoclonal B lymphocytosis. Cancer Lett April 28, 2012;317(2):144−9.

[115] Kuchino Y, Mori F, Kasai H, Inoue H, Iwai S, Miura K, et al. Misreading of DNA templates containing 8-hydroxydeoxyguanosine at the modified base and at adjacent residues. Nature May 7, 1987;327(6117):77−9.

[116] Shibutani S, Takeshita M, Grollman AP. Insertion of specific bases during DNA synthesis past the oxidation-damaged base 8-oxodG. Nature January 31, 1991;349(6308):431−4.

[117] Heydari AR, Unnikrishnan A, Lucente LV, Richardson A. Caloric restriction and genomic stability. Nucleic Acids Res 2007;35(22):7485−96. Oxford University Press.

[118] Tan C, Liu S, Tan S, Zeng X, Yu H, Li A, et al. Polymorphisms in microRNA target sites of forkhead box O genes are associated with hepatocellular carcinomaMittal B, editor. PLoS One March 4, 2015;10(3):e0119210. Public Library of Science.

Chapter 3

Molecular Basis of Oxidative Stress and Inflammation

Maria D. Mesa-Garcia, Julio Plaza-Diaz and Carolina Gomez-Llorente
University of Granada, Granada, Spain

1. INTRODUCTION

An increase in oxidative stress—derived inflammation has been hypothesized to be a major mechanism in the pathogenesis and progression of many diseases, specifically in obesity-related disorders [1]. Oxidative stress is caused by an imbalance between the release of oxidative molecules and the antioxidant defenses. When the balance moves toward the formation of free radicals and therefore the organism is not able to eliminate them, they attack other adjacent molecules and tissues. This oxidative stress—derived tissue damage leads to an inflammatory response that tries to eliminate the harmful agents. Additionally, a rise in inflammatory cytokine levels drives a further increase in oxidative stress. The complex and intimate association between both increased oxidative stress and increased inflammation makes it difficult to establish the temporal sequence of this relationship [2] (Fig. 3.1). Oxidative stress machinery and inflammatory signaling not only are interrelated, but their impairment also can lead to the development of a number of noncommunicable diseases.

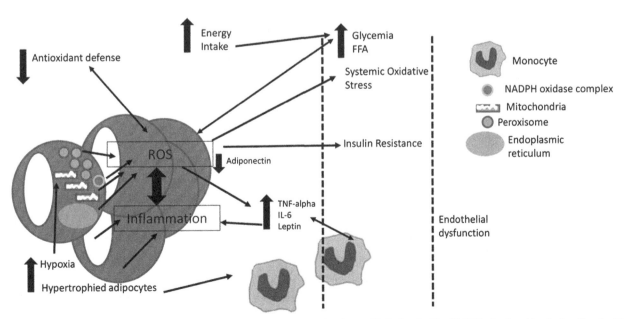

FIGURE 3.1 Relationship between oxidative stress and inflammation. *FFA*, free fatty-acid; *IL*, interleukin; *NADPH*, nicotinamide adenine dinucleotide phosphate; *TNF*, tumor necrosis factor; *ROS*, reactive oxygen species.

Obesity. https://doi.org/10.1016/B978-0-12-812504-5.00003-9

Both oxidative and inflammatory responses share the ability to activate signaling pathways underlying obesity [2]. The present chapter aims at summarizing the main molecular mechanisms of oxidative stress and inflammation.

2. MOLECULAR BASIS OF OXIDATIVE STRESS

2.1 Free Radicals and Reactive Oxygen Species

Free radicals are molecules with an unpaired valence electron, which makes them highly reactive toward other substances, or even toward themselves. Free radicals include reactive oxygen species (ROS) containing oxygen, reactive nitrogen species (RNS) (nitric oxide $-NO-$, peroxynitrite $-ONOO^-$, and related compounds), and other reactive molecules containing carbonyl species (glyoxal, methylglyoxal), carbon, sulfur, halogens, among others. Within ROS, we can find superoxide anion (O_2^-), hydroxyl radical ($HO^\bullet$), hydrogen peroxide (H_2O_2), singlet oxygen ($O_2^\bullet$), and peroxides (Table 3.1). Generally, the terms ROS and free radicals are used interchangeably, although this is not always correct.

In the mid 20th century, free radicals were physically found in biological systems [3] and immediately were suggested to be involved in diverse pathological and physiological processes, including aging. Since then, the understanding of the role of free radicals in living processes has grown enormously. However, free radicals have been considered mainly as damaging species that play deleterious effects on biological organisms. This point of view was strengthened by the discovery of the first protective enzyme against free radicals named superoxide dismutase (SOD) by McCord and Fridovich [4] (Fig. 3.2). Free radicals have been found to be involved in the immune system defense against infection agents [5]. In addition, vascular endothelial cells produce nitric oxide (NO), a molecule acting as an endothelium-derived relaxing factor. That discovery opened the second avenue for nitrogen-derived free radical research [6].

2.2 Generation and Reactivity of Reactive Oxygen Species

Living organisms under aerobic conditions consume oxygen. Into the mitochondria, more than 90% of the consumed oxygen is reduced directly to water by the cytochrome oxidase C in the electron transport chain (ETC), via a four-electron mechanism. This process does not release ROS. The ETC is coupled with oxidative phosphorylation to produce energy as ATP. Less than 10% of the consumed oxygen is reduced via successive one-electron reactions, resulting in the conversion of molecular oxygen to superoxide anion, followed by one-electron reduction with concomitant acceptance of two protons to form hydrogen peroxide. This dismutation of the superoxide anion can be spontaneous or catalyzed by the SOD. Phagocytic cells are also prominent sources of superoxide anion. In the presence of invading pathogens like bacteria, phagocytic cells become activated, and at that state, they generate superoxide radical anions, which may attack the invading pathogens as part of the inflammatory defense response. In this case, superoxide anion is produced from xanthine by the xanthine oxidase enzyme, along with uric acid as a waste product of the purine metabolism.

Although hydrogen peroxide is not a free radical, it is chemically more active than molecular oxygen, and is considered an ROS. The hydrogen peroxide molecule accepts one electron, split into one hydroxyl radical and one hydroxyl anion (OH^-). The hydroxyl radical interacts with another electron and a proton forming a water molecule. In the case of biological systems, the abstraction of the hydrogen atom is mainly carried out from many compounds, such as proteins and

TABLE 3.1 Characteristics of Most Common Free Radicals

	Major Biological Sources	Characteristics
Singlet oxygen ($^1O_2$)	Photo sensibilization reactions	Transfer excitation energy
Superoxide (O_2^-)	Endoplasmic reticulum, mitochondria	Reducing agent, weak oxidizing
Hydroperoxyl ($HO_2^\bullet$)	Protonation of $O_2^\bullet$	Highly reactive
Hydrogen peroxide (H_2O_2)	Distribution of O_2^-	Weak oxidizing agent
Hydroxyl radical ($OH^\bullet$)	Direct, high energy radiation	Highly reactive with most biomolecules
Peroxide ($ROO^\bullet$)	Oxidation of lipids, proteins, DNA	Medium reactivity, highly diffusible
Nitric oxide ($NO^\bullet$)	Macrophages, endothelial cells, neurons	Lipophilic with physiological functions
Hypochlorous acid (HOCl)	Phagocytic cells	Thiol oxidation

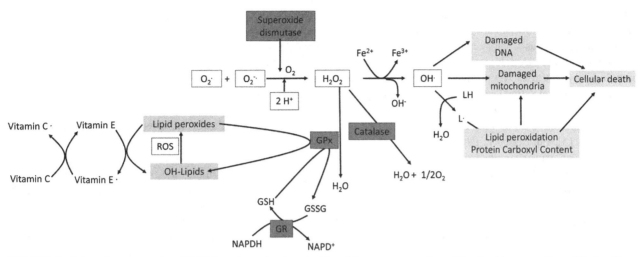

FIGURE 3.2 Schematic representation of ROS formation and main antioxidant defense system reactions. *GPx*, glutathione peroxidase; *GR*, glutathione reductase; *GSH*, reduced glutathione; *GSSG*, oxidized glutathione; *H₂O₂*, hydrogen peroxide; *NADPH*, nicotinamide adenine dinucleotide phosphate; *O₂•*, superoxide anion radical; *OH*, hydroxide; *ROS*, reactive oxygen species.

lipids, resulting in the initiation of the oxidative chain process. In addition, hydrogen peroxide undergoes the Fenton reactions with metal ions like ferrous (Fe^{2+}) or cuprous (Cu^{2+}) to form ferric (Fe^{3+}) or cupric ions (Cu^{3+}), respectively, and hydroxyl ions. Indeed, because of its nonionized and low charged state, hydrogen peroxide has a long diffusion distance, and it can diffuse through hydrophobic membranes, for example from mitochondria. Furthermore, hydrogen peroxide is broken down to O_2 and water by the antioxidant enzyme catalase. In addition to catalase, glutathione peroxidase (GPx) can also reduce hydrogen peroxide and lipid peroxides using reduced glutathione (GSH) to yield water and oxidized glutathione (GSSG) (Fig. 3.2).

The hydroxyl radical is formed not only by the interaction between hydrogen peroxide and the reduced forms of metal ions (i.e., Cu^{2+} and Fe^{2+}), but also by its reduction or after interaction with the superoxide anion [7]. It is particularly unstable and is the most reactive of the free radical molecules. In addition, it is capable of reacting rapidly in a nonspecific fashion with most biological molecules. Despite having a very short half-life (nanoseconds), hydroxyl radicals can provoke severe damage to cells and other intracellular structures by inducing covalent cross-linking of a variety of biological molecules.

Other cellular free radical generation sites besides mitochondrial ETC are endoplasmic reticulum, peroxisomes, and dual oxidase (Duox) 1 and 2 complexes. In addition, a molecular species with a chemical signature similar to that of ozone can be produced by antibodies from singlet oxygen ($^{1}O_2•$) and water, leading to an additional highly efficient unspecific destruction of bacteria, regardless of the antigen specificity of the antibody [8]. Finally, the reaction of hydrogen peroxide with hypochlorite (HOCl) can produce singlet oxygen, a more energetic form of oxygen that can attack double bonds. Cytochrome P450 enzymes, peroxisomal oxidases, and nicotinamide adenine dinucleotide phosphate (NADPH) oxidases are other intracellular sources of ROS [9].

2.3 Generation and Reactivity of Nitrogen-Derived Reactive Species

NO, a potent endothelium-derived relaxing factor, is synthesized through the enzymatic oxidation of L-arginine in a two-step process mediated by nitric oxide synthase (NOS). This metabolic process generates *N*-hydroxyl L-arginine and finally L-citrulline [10]. NOS is an enzyme that exists in three known isoforms: endothelial NOS (eNOS), inducible NOS (iNOS), and neuronal NOS (nNOS). Specifically, eNOS is localized primarily in endothelial cells, closely associated with caveolae/lipid rafts. This isoenzyme is responsible for the physiological endothelial-derived NO production [11]. NO exerts many of its physiological functions by targeting hemoproteins, besides reacting with thiols and superoxide anions. It directly nitrosylates the thiol (SH) groups of protein cysteine residues, to activate signaling molecules, such as the nuclear factor κ-light-chain-enhancer of activated B cell (NF-κB) and the activator protein 1 (AP-1), and to inhibit Ca^{2+}-mediated vasoconstriction [12,13]. At physiological concentrations, NO inhibits mitochondrial respiration. NO competes with oxygen for binding to ETC cytochrome C oxidase (Complex IV), which is the terminal enzyme of the mitochondrial respiratory chain, and thus regulates mitochondrial respiration [14]. In addition, NO diffuses locally within endothelial cells to the luminal surface of the endothelium and into the smooth muscle cells in the vascular wall, where it signals through numerous downstream pathways via guanylate cyclase to regulate the vascular tone. Thus NO, produced from eNOS, has potent vasodilatory and antiinflammatory and antithrombotic properties [6].

Under multiple physiological conditions, eNOS can be upregulated to maintain NO production. On the other hand, in pathological conditions NO production is reduced, even though eNOS protein levels may be normal or even increased, causing an imbalance that leads to endothelial dysfunction. This inconsistency between eNOS protein and NO levels may be due to an increased NO consumption by ROS and by a switch in the enzymatic activity of eNOS to generate the injurious superoxide anion rather than the protective NO. This process, known as eNOS uncoupling, has been studied in vitro [13,15]. Furthermore, iNOS is upregulated by oxidative stress, producing a burst of NO that far exceeds basal levels and can cause significant cellular injury via different mechanisms. For example, NO may directly promote excessive peripheral vasodilation, resulting in vascular decomposition. NO upregulates the transcription of NF-κB, and thus initiates an inflammatory signaling pathway that, in turn, triggers numerous inflammatory cytokines. In addition, NO can react with different ROS, generating other harmful free radical–derived products. Peroxynitrite, obtained from the reaction of the superoxide anion and NO, has been reported to modify proteins with thiol groups, resulting in the generation of nitrosothiols, which can disrupt metal–protein interactions and lead to the generation of other metal-derived free radicals [16].

NO can also react with other oxygen-derived radical and nonradical species generating dangerous RNS (e.g., peroxynitrite, $ONOO^-$), which target proteins and irreversibly affect their structure and function, a phenomenon commonly known as nitrosative stress. Indeed, all mitochondrial ETC complexes are prone to nitrosylation at Fe-hemo-containing centers [17].

2.4 Molecular Cytotoxicity of Reactive Oxygen Species

A delicate balance exists between ROS production and the antioxidant defenses that protect cells. Hyperoxia, inflammation, or ischemia-reperfusion may disturb the homeostasis through an excessive generation of ROS, or in the presence of limited or impaired antioxidant defenses.

Multiple pathways involved in ROS-induced cell death have been proposed. ROS can cause direct injury to proteins, lipids, and nucleic acids, leading to cell death. Protein oxidation and nitrosylation (carbonyl, nitration, and nitrotyrosine formation) can impair a variety of enzymatic processes and growth factors that can result in a marked cellular dysfunction [18]. Phospholipid peroxidation has been associated with cell death, by activation of sphingomyelinase and release of ceramide, which activates apoptosis [19]. Nucleic acid oxidation has been linked to physiologic and premature aging as well as DNA strand breaks, which leads to necrosis and/or maladaptive apoptosis [20]. The magnitude of these changes and the cell's ability to repair this damage determines whether the effects are adaptive or maladaptive.

The brain and the lung are target organ systems prone to be damaged by ROS. In premature and full-term newborns, the control of cerebral perfusion is less tightly regulated, increasing vulnerability to reperfusion-type injury and oxidative stress. For example, the microglial activation causes accumulation of oxidative markers (e.g., nitrotyrosine and carbonyls protein) in oligodendrocytes, leading to the expansion of periventricular leukomalacia [21].

2.5 Reactive Oxygen Species Functions in Cell Signaling

ROS generated during respiration are not always deleterious and have other important functions. The superoxide anion and hydrogen peroxide are examples of signaling molecules inducing the expression of antioxidant enzymes such as SOD and catalase [22]. Redox homeostasis guarantees adequate cell responses to endogenous and exogenous stimuli, mainly by maintaining a relatively reduced intracellular environment that ensures the correct protein structures and functions. However, when redox homeostasis is disturbed, oxidative stress-derived upregulated ROS might lead to aberrant cell dysfunction and death, and further development of disease [22].

Most of the effects driven by ROS are executed by the covalent modification of specific redox-sensitive sulfhydryl residues found in cysteines of target proteins. Oxidation of these specific cysteine residues, in turn, can lead to the reversible modification of their enzymatic activities; for example, those occurring through redox-sensitive cysteine residues of protein tyrosine phosphatases (PTPs) [23]. These PTPs control the phosphorylation state of numerous signal-transducing proteins, and therefore regulating cell functions such as proliferation, differentiation, survival, metabolism, and motility. The catalytic region of PTPs includes cysteine residues, which are susceptible to oxidative inactivation. Thus, ROS decrease phosphatase activity and enhance protein tyrosine phosphorylation levels, thereby influencing signal transduction. ROS can activate kinases like p38 mitogen-activated protein (MAP) kinase and extracellular-related kinases [24].

On the other hand, adequate amounts of ROS can acts as second messengers, activating multiple signal transduction pathways within the cell that facilitate the actions of growth factors, cytokines, and calcium signaling. In this regard, ROS can activate c-Jun N-terminal kinase (possibly through production of lipid peroxide intermediates), which then phosphorylates and releases two Bcl-2—related proteins. These two proteins are normally sequestered within the cell and consequently activate Bax by dissociation from its cytoplasmic anchor. Free Bax translocates to the mitochondria, where it undergoes oligomerization and initiates the release of cytochrome c and other proapoptotic mediators into the cytosol [25].

ROS enhance the signal transduction pathways that affect NF-κB activation and translocation into the nucleus. The DNA-binding potential of oxidized NF-κB is significantly reduced, but it can be reestablished by reductive enzymes, such as redox factor 1 [26]. Hence, NF-κB-dependent inflammatory signals are strongly affected by ROS and RNS levels. Accordingly, the antiinflammatory cyclopentenone prostaglandins, which are strong electrophiles, promptly conjugate with reactive thiols present in cysteine residues of ROS-altered proteins and peptides and consequently dampen ROS-mediated NF-κB signaling [27].

In addition, transcription factors of the forkhead box class O (FoxO) family are important regulators of the cellular stress response and promote the cellular antioxidant defense. FoxO stimulates the transcription of genes encoding for antioxidant proteins present in different subcellular compartments, such as in the mitochondria (e.g., manganese-dependent SOD [MnSOD] and peroxiredoxins [Prxs] 3 and 5) as well as antioxidant proteins found extracellularly in plasma (e.g., selenoprotein P and ceruloplasmin). ROS and other stressful stimuli that elicit their formation may modulate FoxO activity at multiple levels, including posttranslational modifications (such as phosphorylation and acetylation) and interaction with coregulators, thus altering FoxO subcellular localization, protein synthesis, and stability [28].

ROS species can modulate gene expression. This modulation has been found for genes from organisms ranging from bacteria and yeast to humans, and in response to a wide range of oxidant stress agents, such as superoxide, hydrogen peroxide, NO, redox-active quinones, glutathione depletion, and others. Most of those genes have been primarily identified in bacteria and encode for antioxidant enzymes. First studies were stated at the protein level, where it was reported that oxidative stress induces the expression of the antioxidant enzymes SOD and catalase [22]. Further studies demonstrated that, besides these two, dozens of proteins are induced by hydrogen peroxide and superoxide in bacteria, including the expression of genes coding antioxidant enzyme such as alkyl hydroperoxide reductase and glutathione reductase (GR), among others [29].

Reports on the modulation of gene expression by oxidative stress in mammalian cells have lagged behind those in bacteria, perhaps reflecting the surprising lack of a strong modulation of mammalian antioxidant gene expression by ROS (Table 3.2) [30]. It is now known that as with nuclear genes, the expression of mitochondrial genes is modulated by ROS [31,32].

2.6 Beneficial Effects of Reactive Oxygen Species

The presence of ROS has an important role on cell proliferation, immune response, cellular differentiation, development, circadian rhythms, and cell death regulation, which highlight a new view of ROS as being beneficial for life [33]. As previously mentioned, ROS act as signaling molecules to regulate and maintain normal physiological functions, mostly by interacting with cysteine residues of proteins. For example, hydrogen peroxide interacts with these cysteine thiolate anion (Cys—S) residues at physiological pH, and oxidizes them to their sulfenic form (Cys—SOH), changing their structures and functions. Hence, transcription, phosphorylation, and other important signaling events can be affected [34]. The innate immune response has a crucial role for ROS-driven redox signaling. The activation ROS production required for the release of proinflammatory cytokines such as interleukin (IL)-1β, tumor necrosis factor-α (TNF-α), and interferon-γ (IFN-γ), which are required for orchestrating an appropriate immune response. Here we found two scenarios: low ROS levels prevent the activation of the immune response, whereas high ROS levels cause autoimmunity by increasing the release of the aforementioned proinflammatory cytokines [35].

ROS-mediated redox signaling also plays a key role in the emerging field of stem cell research [34]. Consequently, the generation of low levels of ROS by NOX/mitochondria was found to be necessary for the activation of proliferative pathways, supporting stem cell renewal and differentiation. On the other hand, the accumulation of high levels of ROS activates signaling pathways that limit self-renewal in a pathway that involves the DNA-damage checkpoint kinase ataxia-telangiectasia mutated [34]. Finally, recent studies have shown that proliferating cancer cells are susceptible to perturbations in their iron homeostasis. Maintaining levels of cellular iron under control is therefore paramount for keeping ROS within the redox biology range [34,36].

TABLE 3.2 Mammalian Genes Modulated by Reactive Oxygen Species

Genes	Modulating Agent
c-fos, c-myc	Xanthine/xanthine oxidase
c-fos, c-jun, egr-1, JE	Hydrogen peroxide
c-fos	t-Butylhydroperoxide
heme oxygenase	Multiple oxidants
gadd45, gadd153	Hydrogen peroxide
CL100	Hydrogen peroxide
interleukin 8	Hydrogen peroxide
γ-glutamyl transpeptidase	Menadione
Vimentin, cytochrome IV, RP-L4	Diethylmaleate
c-fos, c-jun, c-myc, HSP	Xanthine/xanthine oxidase
glucose-regulated proteins	Singlet oxygen, other oxidants
c-fos and zif/268	Nitric oxide
Adapts	Hydrogen peroxide
catalase, MnSOD, GPx	Hydrogen peroxide
MnSOD	Xanthine/xanthine oxidase
	Hyperbaric oxygen
	Multiple oxidants

GPx, glutathione peroxidase; HSP, heat shock protein; MAPK, mitogen-activated protein kinase; MnSOD, manganese-superoxide dismutase; ROS, reactive oxygen species; RP-L4, ribosomal protein-L4.

2.7 Antioxidant Cellular Defenses

The human body is equipped with a wide variety of antioxidant molecules counteracting and neutralizing the effect of ROS and other oxidants to ensure the homeostasis. Antioxidant defense systems can be divided into two categories: enzymatic and nonenzymatic defenses. They also may be classified as endogenous-produced or exogenous dietary-derived antioxidants [37].

The enzymatic antioxidant defense system includes SOD, catalase, GPx, GR, and thioredoxin system. On the other hand, the nonenzymatic antioxidant system consists of a wide number of molecules of different natures exerting antioxidant effects. This group includes antioxidant vitamins (vitamin A, vitamin E, and vitamin C), carotenes, coenzyme Q (CoQ), uric acid, dietary-derived phenolic compounds, triterpenic acids, and others (Fig. 3.3).

2.7.1 Enzymatic Antioxidant Defenses

Antioxidant enzymes have more effective protective effects against active and massive oxidative attack than nonspecific, nonenzymatic antioxidants due to their ability to decompose ROS [38]. Since superoxide is the primary ROS produced from a variety of sources, its dismutation to oxygen and hydrogen peroxide by SOD is of primary importance for cell defense, while catalase neutralizes the hydrogen peroxide formed after that dismutation, through its degradation into molecular oxygen and water. Therefore, SOD and catalase are the best antioxidants in vivo [38]. Human SOD is present under three isoforms bound to different cofactors: mitochondrial MnSOD, cytosolic copper/zinc (CuZn)-SOD, and extracellular SOD (EC-SOD) especially present in areas containing high amounts of type I collagen fibers and around pulmonary and systemic vessels. EC-SOD has also been found in the bronchial epithelium, alveolar epithelium, and alveolar macrophages, where it represents a fundamental component of lung matrix protection [38]. Overall, CuZn-SOD and MnSOD are generally thought to act as bulk scavengers of superoxide radicals.

Mitochondria are the major producer and target of ROS, where these molecules alter membrane stability and permeability [39]. Disruption of mitochondrial outer membrane will cause the release of cytochrome c and other

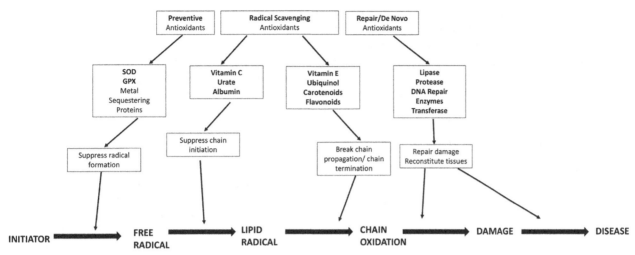

FIGURE 3.3 Oxidative stress mediated disease development and enzymatic and nonenzymatic antioxidant defense roles. *GPx*, glutathione peroxidase; *SOD*, superoxide dismutase.

proapoptotic factors, ultimately triggering caspase activation and cell death [40]. SOD seems to be the first line of defense against oxygen-derived free radicals and can be rapidly induced in some oxidative-stress exposed conditions [41]. In fact, the increased expression of Mn-SOD in response to the inhibition of oxidative stress is due to a massive accumulation of ROS and free radicals in mitochondria. Preliminary studies in patients undergoing a kidney transplant suggest roles of SOD in protecting the allograft from ischemia-reperfusion injury [42].

The hydrogen peroxide that is produced by the action of SODs or other oxidases, such as xanthine oxidase, is reduced to water by the catalase and GPx (Fig. 3.2). Catalase is a tetrameric hemperoxidase enzyme. Degradation of hydrogen peroxide is accomplished via the conversion between two conformations of catalase-ferricatalase (iron coordinated to water) and compound I (iron complexed with an oxygen atom). Catalase also binds NADPH as a reducing equivalent to prevent oxidative inactivation of the enzyme (formation of compound II) by hydrogen peroxide as it is reduced to water [22].

GPx is responsible for the reduction of hydrogen peroxide and lipid hydroperoxides. They are important for the protection of cell membrane from lipid peroxidation; GSH donates protons to membrane lipids and protects them from oxidant attacks [22]. Besides, GPx is a selenium-containing tetrameric enzyme that reduces hydrogen peroxide, lipoperoxides, and other organic hydroperoxides to their corresponding hydroxylated compounds using glutathione as hydrogen donor. It is a family of tetrameric enzymes that contain the unique amino acid selenocysteine within the active sites and use low-molecular-weight thiols, such as GSH, to reduce hydrogen peroxide and lipid peroxides into water or their corresponding alcohols, respectively [43]. Members of GPxs have antioxidant function at different cellular components: (1) GPx1 is present ubiquitously in the cytosol and mitochondria and reduces hydrogen peroxide and fatty acid peroxides, but not esterified peroxyl lipids; (2) GPx2 is found in the cytosol and nucleus, and is localized in gastrointestinal epithelial cells where it reduces dietary peroxides; (3) GPx3 is the only member of the GPx family that resides in the extracellular compartment and plasma, and is believed to be one of the most important extracellular antioxidant enzymes in mammals; whereas (4) GPx4 is a membrane-associated enzyme and appears to protect membranes from oxidative challenge by reducing esterified phospholipid hydroperoxides [38]. It has been described that GPx can regulate the concentration of hydroperoxide mediators, therefore affecting a number of physiological pathways, for example insulin signaling by GPx1 and cell survival/proliferation by GPx4 [38].

GR converts GSSG to GSH, a tripeptide (L-g-glutamyl-L-cysteinyl-L-glycine) that has a thiol (sulfhydryl) group. GSH is a cosubstrate for the GPxs (Fig. 3.2) [22]. NADPH is used as a cofactor by GR and thioredoxins, and maintains catalase in the active form. This NADPH is reduced from NADP by glucose-6-phosphate dehydrogenase. Hence, this enzyme from the pentose phosphate pathway is a critical determinant of cytosolic GSH buffering capacity (GSH/GSSG) and, therefore, can be considered an essential, regulatory antioxidant enzyme [44].

Thiol-containing enzymes, namely thioredoxins, thioredoxin reductases, pyridoxine, and glutaredoxins, are also important against oxidative stress as an endogenous antioxidant system. Thioredoxin antioxidants can use the thiol and selenol groups to repair DNA and proteins by reducing ribonucleotide reductase as well as methionine sulfoxide reductases, and have been involved in the immune response defense [45]. In addition, thioredoxin seems to control apoptosis or metabolic states such as carbohydrate and lipid metabolism [46]. Cytosolic thioredoxin-1 and mitochondrial thioredoxin-2 are the major disulfide reductases that affect cell proliferation and viability by inhibiting apoptosis [45].

Another antioxidant enzyme family is glutathione S-transferase (GST), which regulates the inactivation of secondary metabolites such as unsaturated aldehydes, epoxides, and hydroperoxides. There are three families of GST: cytosolic, mitochondrial, and membrane-associated microsomal GST that has a role in eicosanoid and GSH metabolism [22]. In mammalian, there are seven classes of cytosolic GST designated as alpha (α), mu (μ), pi (π), sigma (σ), theta (θ), omega (ω), and zeta (ζ). During nonstressed conditions, class μ and π GSTs inhibit kinases Ask1 and JNK, respectively [22].

2.7.2 Nonenzymatic Antioxidant Defenses

Nonenzymatic antioxidants include low-molecular-weight compounds, such as GSH, vitamins C, E, and A, or beta-carotene, CoQ, uric acid, bilirubin, and melatonin. In general, nonenzymatic antioxidants mostly help regenerate GSSG back to GSH. Antioxidant vitamins such as A, C, and E and alpha-lipoic acid are among this mechanism (Fig. 3.3). Although all these antioxidant defenses work together to eliminate hydrogen peroxide (and thus superoxide) from the cell, in the presence of reduced transition metals (Cu, Fe) this molecule can be transformed by the Fenton reaction into a hydroxyl radical, which is a highly reactive ROS [22].

GSH is highly abundant in all cell compartments and is the major soluble antioxidant. It is a cofactor for several detoxifying enzymes such as GPx and transferase. Thus GSH/GSSG ratio is a major determinant of oxidative stress [22]. GSH exerts its antioxidant effects in several ways: (1) it reduces and detoxifies hydrogen peroxide and lipid peroxides via action of GPx, and is again reduced into GSH by GR, which uses NADPH as the electron donor as mentioned earlier; (2) it has a role in converting vitamins C and E back to their active forms; (3) it protects cells against apoptosis by interacting with proapoptotic and antiapoptotic signaling pathways; and (4) it also regulates and activates several transcription factors such as AP-1, NF-kB, and Sp-1 [22].

Vitamin C (ascorbic acid) provides intracellular and extracellular aqueous-phase antioxidant capacity primarily by scavenging the superoxide radical anion, hydrogen peroxide, hydroxyl radical, singlet oxygen, and RNS. Vitamin C converts vitamin E free radicals back to vitamin E to sustain its antioxidant potential. Its plasma levels have been shown to decrease with age. Vitamin E, mainly α-tocopherol as the most active form, is concentrated in the hydrophobic interior site of cell membrane and acts as the principal defense against oxidant-induced membrane injury. Vitamin E donates an electron to the peroxyl radical, which is produced during lipid peroxidation, forming tocopheroxyl radicals that are unreactive and unable to continue the oxidative chain reaction, and thus stops lipid peroxidation [47]. Vitamin E triggers apoptosis of cancer cells and inhibits free radical formations. Vitamin A, or retinol, is a carotenoid produced in the liver and resulted from the breakdown of dietary β-carotene. Vitamin A can directly bind and eliminate peroxyl radicals, stopping lipid peroxidation [48]. CoQ can neutralize the oxidative effect of lipid peroxyl radicals and regenerate vitamin E [49].

Furthermore, many metabolites, such as uric acid, bilirubin, and melatonin, exert antioxidant effects. Uric acid is the most potent antioxidant, and hence protects the central nervous system [50]. It can prevent peroxynitrite-induced protein nitrosylation, lipid and protein peroxidation, and the inactivation of tetrahydrobiopterin, which results in scavenging free radical and chelating transitional metal ions [51].

The most important dietary antioxidant minerals are selenium and zinc. They are cofactors of antioxidant enzymes, necessary for maintaining their activity. Zinc may act through different mechanisms: (1) by inhibiting NADPH oxidases that catalyze the production of the singlet oxygen radical from oxygen by using NADPH as an electron donor; (2) as a component of the SOD enzyme; (3) by inducing the production of metallothionein, a scavenger of the hydroxyl radical; and (4) by acting as an effective antiinflammatory agent that inhibits TNF-α-induced NF-κB activation [52].

Other dietary antioxidants may also boost protection against oxidative stress by eliminating free radicals. Carotenoids, apart from the vitamin A precursor activity of β-carotene, are a group of natural pigments derived from plants that present conjugated double bound and capacity to quench radical species. Carotenoids show their antioxidant effects in low oxygen partial pressure, but may have prooxidant effects at higher oxygen concentrations [53]. In addition, carotenoids also affect apoptosis of cells. Both carotenoids and retinoic acids are capable of regulating transcription factors. β-carotene has been found to react with peroxyl, hydroxyl, and superoxide radicals. Moreover, β-carotene is capable of inhibiting the oxidant-induced NF-kB activation and IL-6 and TNF-α production [54]. Retinoic acid has an antiproliferative effect mediated mainly by retinoic acid receptors, which varies among cell types. In mammary carcinoma cells, retinoic acid receptor was shown to trigger growth inhibition by inducing cell cycle arrest, apoptosis, or both [55].

Plant phenolic compounds include phenolic alcohols and acids, cinnamic acids, coumarins, flavonoids (flavones and isoflavones, flavonols, flavanones), and other phenolic compounds exerting antioxidant activity as chelators or free radical scavengers, with special impact over hydroxyl and peroxyl radicals, and superoxide anions. Their antioxidant activity depends on the configuration and total number of hydroxyl functional groups [56].

2.7.3 Molecular Mechanism of Action of Antioxidants

Oxidative stress can block general life cycle programs, such as reproduction or extensive biosynthesis in living organisms, and induce responses to prevent or neutralize negative ROS effects. These ROS protective mechanisms of action are mainly based on upregulation of antioxidant molecules and enzymes.

Animals have multiple systems responsible for adaptive response to oxidative stress. They activate several pathways responding to oxidative stress at different intensities. For example, a low-mild intensity of oxidative stress is sensed by the NF-E2-related factor 2 (Nrf2)/Kelch-like ECH-associated Protein 1 (Keap1) system. Here, the Nrf2 is a transcription factor of the leucine zipper family that operates in concert with Keap1. Under normal conditions, Nrf2 protein interacts with Keap1, on the ligase (E3) complex (Keap1-Cul3-Rbx1) responsible for ubiquitination of Nrf2 prior to proteasomal degradation [57]. ROS and some antioxidants modulate the activity of three separate substrates of the Keap1-Cul3-Rbx1 ubiquitin ligase, preventing Nrf2 for degradation by the proteasome [58]. In response to increased ROS levels, thiol groups of protein Keap1 are oxidized, making it impossible to reach Nrf2. Free Nrf2 moves into the nucleus where it is transiently accumulated and interacts with the so-called antioxidant response element (ARE) in promoters of target genes encoding defense proteins [57]. Recent evidence suggests that some antioxidants act through the Keap1-ARE pathway via the upregulation of Nrf2. Among other functions, antioxidants suppress the degradation of Nrf2 and also enhance its nuclear translocation and expression of target antioxidant enzymes and detoxification genes, and thus regulate the cellular response to oxidants and electrophilic xenobiotics as well as dithiolethiones, isothiocyanates, and triterpenoids [59]. The upregulated genes include those encoding either antioxidant enzymes (SOD, catalase, peroxidases, GST-transferases) or enzymes involved in biosynthesis of antioxidants (such as gamma-glutamylcysteine synthetase, a key enzyme in glutathione biosynthesis), production of reducing equivalents, proteasome function, and others.

Animal responses to intermediate intensity oxidative stress are coordinated by at least three regulatory systems: NF-kB, AP-1 (animal homologue of yeast YAP1), and MAP kinases. These systems upregulate the expression of antioxidant enzymes, but in addition, they also stimulate the expression of certain genes of inflammation and general cellular reprogramming functions [57].

3. MOLECULAR BASIS OF INFLAMMATION

The immune system can be defined as an organization of cells and molecules with specialized roles against infection or any condition in which the organism results altered. To establish an infection, first of all, the pathogen or the infectious agent has to overcome numerous surface barriers, such as enzymes and mucus. Any organism that breaks through this first barrier encounters the immune response. Classically, it has been divided into two main types of response: the innate (natural) and the acquired (adaptive) responses, although both of them are related and connected (Fig. 3.4) [60].

The innate immune response is the first line of defense and it occurs immediately after pathogen exposure. The cells involved in this response are phagocytic cells (neutrophils, monocytes, and macrophages), cells that release inflammatory mediators (basophils, mast cells, and eosinophils), natural killer (NK) cells, and other innate lymphoid cells (Fig. 3.4) (ILCs). The molecular components include the complement, acute-phase proteins and cytokines (e.g., IFNs and ILs) (Fig. 3.5) [60].

The adaptive immune response is generated in the lymph nodes, spleen, and mucosa-associated lymphoid tissue. It is characterized by two classes of lymphocytes, T and B cells, which clonally express different antigen receptors that are produced by somatic site-specific recombination: T cell receptor (TCR) and antibody B cell receptor (BCR). B cells reach maturity within the bone marrow, but T cells need to reach the thymus to completely develop. Naïve T and B cells encounter antigens in specialized lymphoid organs and experience a process of cell division and maturation before exerting their effector functions [61]. Specialized antigen-presenting cells (APCs), such as monocyte/macrophages and dendritic cells expressing both major histocompatibility complex (MHC) class I and II, present the antigen to lymphocytes and collaborate with them in the response against that antigenic agent. B cells secrete immunoglobulins (Igs), also called antibodies, whereas T cells help B cells produce those antibodies, and can eradicate intracellular pathogens by activating macrophages and by killing virally infected cells [60].

Based on the current knowledge about the different T cell and ILC lineages, it has been described that the innate and adaptive immune systems converge into three main types of cell-mediated immunity, which have been classified as type 1,

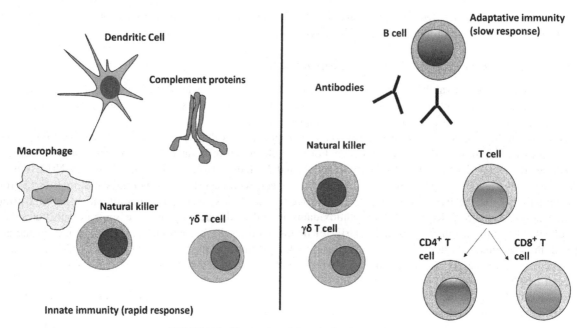

FIGURE 3.4 The innate and the adaptive immune system.

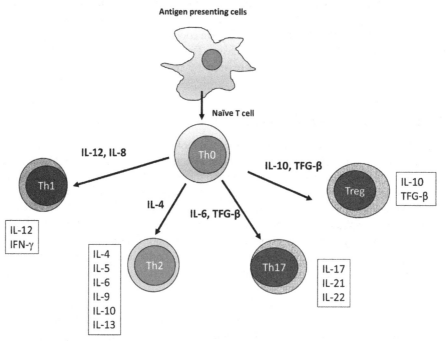

FIGURE 3.5 Th cell differentiation. *IFN-γ*, interferon-gamma; *IL*, interleukin; *TFG-β*, transforming growth factor-beta; *Th0*, naïve T cells; *Th*, helper T cells; *TNF-α*, tumor necrosis factor-alpha; *Treg*, regulatory T cells.

2, and 3 (Fig. 3.5). Type 1 response is determined by cells that secrete IFN-γ, such as T helper (Th) 1 and NK cells. Type 2 immunity consists of cells producing IL-4, IL-5, and IL-13, for example, Th2 cells that activate mast cells, basophils, and eosinophils, as well as Ig E antibody production. Type 3 immunity is characterized by cells (e.g., Th17 cells) that produce IL-17 and IL-22, or both, which activate mononuclear phagocytes but also induce the recruitment of neutrophils and the epithelial antimicrobial response. Type 1 and 3 responses mediate autoimmune diseases, whereas type 2 response causes allergic disease [62].

3.1 The Innate Immune System

When a pathogen reaches an organism it activates a primary, rapid, unspecific immune response driven by phagocytic cells that try to eliminate the foreign body. The innate immune response developed earlier in evolution and consists of all the immune defenses lacking immunologic memory [60]. The innate immune system responds to common structures called pathogen-associated molecular patterns (PAMP), which are shared by the vast majority of pathogens. The primary response to pathogens is triggered by pattern recognition receptors (PRRs), which bind PAMP. PRR are also important in the detection of endogenous damage-associated molecular patterns (DAMPs). Among others, PRR comprise toll-like receptors (TLRs), nucleotide-binding oligomerization domains, adhesion molecules, and lectins [63]. The best studied PRR are TLR, which are transmembrane proteins expressed on various immune and nonimmune cells (Table 3.3). Upon microbial activation, TLR lead to the formation of a large cytoplasmic supramolecular organizing center (SMOC) called myddosome, whose main function is to promote the activation of proinflammatory NF-κB and AP-1 family transcription factors, among others [64]. Therefore, the interaction between PAMP and PRR results in the induction of a signaling cascade against the detected pathogen; this response can include the release of immunomodulatory cytokines, chemokines, or costimulatory molecules [65]. It is worth mentioning that DAMP-triggered inflammation is called sterile inflammation when it occurs in the absence of any foreign pathogens [66].

3.1.1 Soluble Factors of the Innate Immune System

The innate immune response commonly requires the activation of the complement, acute-phase proteins, and cytokines. The complement system is an important part of the innate immune defense. It was named based on its ability to complement the antibody-mediated and cell-mediated immune responses against pathogens. This system functions as a cascade of proteases that activate each other in an enzymatic way. Currently, our understanding about the complement has changed, and we know that it plays an undisputed pivotal role in the regulation of both innate and adaptive immunity. The complement system comprises a large number of distinct blood circulating, cell-surface, and intracellular proteins. It is decisive in the recognition and elimination of pathogens and in the removal of self-derived danger such as apoptotic cells. In addition, it supports innate immune response and the initiation of the inflammatory reactions. Recent experimental and clinical data have revealed that local tissue and intracellular complement (called the complosome) activation impacts normal cell physiology [67]. The complement system has close interactions with macrophages, which are tissue-resident phagocytes differentiated from monocyte precursors. A wide array of complement receptors has been detected on the

TABLE 3.3 Expression Pattern of Toll-Like Receptors in Immune Cells and Their Main Pathogen Derived Activators

Immune Cells	PAMP	TLR
Most immune cells	Triacyl lipopeptides	TLR1/TLR2
Peripheral mononuclear leukocytes, dendritic, monocytes, and T cells	Lipoprotein, peptidoglycans, zymosan, lipoarabinomannan, porins	TLR2
NK, dendritic, and T cells	Double-strand DNA	TLR3
Macrophages, dendritic, and T cells	Lipoopysaccaharide, HSP70	TLR4
Natural killer, monocytes, dendritic, and T cells	Flagellin	TLR5
B and dendritic cells	Diacyl lipopeptides	TLR6/TLR2
Dendritic, monocytes, A and T cells	Single-strand RNA	TLR7
Monocytes, dendritic, NK and T cells	Single-strand RNA	TLR8
Peripheral mononuclear leukocytes, macrophages, NK, dendritic, and B cells	Unmethylated CpG DNA sequences	TLR9
Monocytes, dendritic, B and T cells	Unknown	TLR10

HSP, heat shock protein; NK, natural killer; PAMP, pathogen-associated molecular patterns; TLR, toll-like receptor.

surface of macrophages. To what extent different macrophage subsets, proinflammatory (M1 subclass) versus antiin-flammatory (M2 subclass) differs in their capacity to produce and secrete specific complement proteins remains to be established [67].

Cytokines are other important soluble mediators. They act as messengers both within the immune system and between the immune system and other systems of the body, creating an integrated network involved in the regulation of the immune response. The presence of a cytokine is determined by another cell through specific cytokine receptors. Nevertheless, the distinction between cytokines and their receptors is sometimes confusing, because there are soluble forms of cytokine receptors and membrane-anchored forms of some cytokines [60]. Cytokines are produced transiently and locally con-trolling the duration and the amplitude of the immune response. An excessive or insufficient production of them may significantly contribute to the pathophysiology of a range of diseases.

In response to injury, local inflammatory cells (neutrophil granulocytes and macrophages) secrete a number of cyto-kines, such as TNFα, IL-6, IL-1, and IL-8, into the bloodstream. These molecules activate the liver, which responds by producing a large number of acute-phase proteins or reactants, while reducing the secretion of others, called negative acute-phase reactants. Hence, plasma levels of the acute-phase proteins are modified rapidly in response to infection, inflam-mation, or tissue injury. These acute-phase proteins are responsible for the resolution of the inflammatory response, enhance resistance to infection, and promote the repair of damaged tissue. They include C-reactive protein, serum amyloid A proteins, proteinase inhibitors, and coagulation proteins [60].

3.1.2 Macrophages

Macrophages, together with dendritic cells, are the frontline cells of the innate immunity. Macrophages comprise a highly diverse cell population indispensable for host defense, acting directly as effectors, or indirectly by engaging elements of the innate and adaptive immune systems. Macrophages and their precursors' monocytes reside in every tissue of the body where they phagocyte pathogens and apoptotic cells and produce immune effector molecules. Upon tissue damage or infection, monocytes are rapidly recruited to the tissue driven by different soluble mediators, such as IL-4, where they differentiate to tissue macrophages [60]. Macrophages are singularly plastic and can change their functional phenotype based on the environmental signals they receive. Macrophages are capable of identify invading pathogens thorough the PRR localized on their surface, and activate intracellular signaling cascades leading to the in-duction of a general proinflammatory response trying to eliminate the harmful agent. This response includes the release of antimicrobial mediators, chemokines, and proinflammatory cytokines, which trigger further inflammation, and induce a T and B lymphocyte-mediated adaptive immune response. This adaptive response is more specific than the innate response for a particular invading pathogen [68]. Macrophages and other cells such as neutrophils have receptors for antibodies and complement, so the coating of microorganisms with those antibodies, complement, or both enhances the phagocytosis [60].

Macrophages can arise from multiple sites, namely the bone marrow or yolk sac, adding to the complexity of macrophage biology during health and disease. Bone marrow—derived populations are biologically different from tissue-resident subsets, each playing unique roles in the host defense, maintenance, preservation, and organ integrity. None-theless, this diversity is indispensable for macrophages to respond effectively to different pathologic insults [69]. Macrophages can be classified into two major functional subsets. The classically activated proinflammatory M1 macro-phages are characterized by the production of proinflammatory cytokines (IL-12, IL-23, and IL-1) and by the ability to initiate antimicrobial and tumoricidal programs, at least in part, through the production of RNS and ROS. Classically, active macrophages arise in response to IFN-γ produced by Th1 cells, macrophages, and NK cells. The antiinflammatory activated M2 macrophage phenotypes are induced by signals such as IL-4, IL-10, or IL-13 produced by a different subtype of T lymphocytes, Th2 cells, macrophages, or basophils. M2 macrophages are capable of producing antiinflammatory cytokines such as IL-10 and transforming growth factor (TGF)-β [69].

3.1.3 Dendritic Cells

Dendritic cells are a key cellular component of innate immunity. Human dendritic cells are identified by the high expression of MHC class II and the lack of typical lymphoid lineage markers (CD3, CD19/20, and CD56). Different subsets of dendritic cells have been described based on their markers and location: myeloid, plasmacytoid, Langerhans cells, and monocyte-derived dendritic cells. Myeloid dendritic cells and plasmacytoid dendritic cells are located in circulating blood and in lymphoid and nonlymphoid organs. Myeloid dendritic cells play a major role in the polarization of Th cells (Th1 and Th2 cells), whereas plasmacytoid dendritic cells are the major source of IFN-γ secreted during viral stimulation. Langerhans cells are dendritic cells residing in the epidermis and other stratified squamous epithelia that monitor and capture antigens. Finally monocyte-derived dendritic cells arise from monocytes during the inflammatory response [70].

Dendritic cells are present in various tissues where they reside as immature cells with a high phagocytic capacity. In the immature state, dendritic cells are able to produce functionally active C1q, which is the recognition molecule for the classical pathway of the complement system. However, upon stimulation they lose their ability to produce this molecule [71]. To become activated, the PRRs at the dendritic cell membranes recognize distinctive PAMP on the surface of microorganisms and then act as APC. Endogenous danger signals and heat-shock proteins can also activate dendritic cells. Besides PRR-mediated activation, dendritic cells can indirectly be activated by the capture of apoptotic/necrotic products of other cells, and by pathogen-induced cytokines derived from a wide repertoire of cells, for example, enterocyte, fibroblasts, and innate immune system cells [63]. Mature dendritic cells experience morphological changes by developing extensions that increase cellular surface to improve interaction with T cells [70]. Under maturation signals, mature dendritic cells migrate to the draining lymph node where they are capable of activating T cells. Cytokines and other factors secreted by dendritic cells and other innate immune cells program the differentiation of naïve T cells into Th1, Th2, or Th17 effector cells or T regulatory (Treg) cells (see later) [63].

3.1.4 Innate Lymphoid Cells

ILCs are a type of innate immune cells that play an important role in the modulation of inflammation. These cells exert different functions in the initial stages of immunity in response to microbes, tissue repair, anatomical containment of microbiome, and epithelial barrier function. Modification of the number and function of ILC, and hence their dysregulation, can affect a number of pathologies such as allergies, autoimmunity, and inflammation-based diseases [72].

ILCs are derived from hematopoietic lymphoid precursors. ILCs are characterized by the lack of recombination activating genes and by the absence of lymphoid differentiation lineage markers or antigen receptors, which allow them to discriminate from T and B cells. Recently, it has been demonstrated that all innate lymphocytes might have been developed from a common precursor. The first ILCs identified were NKs and lymphoid tissue inducers [72].

Other ILCs have been recognized and can be divided into three main subsets according to their cytokine release profile, transcription factors, and surface markers: ILC1, ILC2, and ILC3 [72]. ILC2 have been identified in gut mucosa and fat-associated lymphoid cluster and play a key role in metabolic homeostasis of lean healthy adipose tissue. In addition, it has been described that ILCs can switch between different subsets controlled by the local cytokine milieu [73]. For example, ILC1 in the presence of IL-2, IL-23, and IL-1β can be differentiated into ILC3. Furthermore, ILC2 can rise to ILC1-like IFN-γ producer in the presence of IL1, IL-12, and IL18 [73].

ILC2, also called natural helper cells, nuocytes, and innate helper2 cells, are found in the peripheral blood, lung, fetal gut, skin, tonsils, and adipose tissue of humans. ILC2 express GATA-binding protein 3 and secrete characteristic cytokines of type 2 immune response (Th2 immune response), such as IL-13, IL-5, IL-25, IL-33, and thymic stromal lymphopoietin (TSLP). Dysregulation of ILC2 response contributes to inflammatory processes, such as airway hyperreactivity, allergen-induced lung inflammation, and atopic dermatitis [72,74]. Different studies have revealed that ILC2 cells can influence T cell response in a reciprocal fashion, either directly by cell—cell contact or indirectly through cytokine effects on accessory cells, thus activating the adaptive immune system. In addition, ILC2 can also contribute to the support of eosinophils and affect the cell function of basophils, macrophages, dendritic cells, and mast cells, which otherwise can activate ILC2 or suppress their activity [74]. Finally, ILC1 produce IFN-γ, the effector cytokine associated with Th1 response and ILC3 secrete IL-17 and IL-22, cytokines associated with a Th17 response [72].

3.1.5 Natural Killer Cells

NK cells have been classified as lymphocytes on the basis of their morphology, their expression of lymphoid markers, and their origin from common lymphoid progenitor cell in the bone marrow. However, NK cells are considered components of the innate immune defense because of the lack of an antigen-specific receptor on their cell surface. Moreover, NK cells participate in the early control against virus infection. It is worth noting that NK cell biology has attributes of both innate and adaptive immunity that may not be unique to these cells [61].

NK cells are the main producers of IFN-γ, but can also produce other proinflammatory (i.e., TNF-α) and antiinflammatory cytokines (i.e., IL-10), different growth factors, and chemokines [61]. The secretion of chemokines is important for the NK colocalization with other hematopoietic cells such as dendritic cells. Furthermore, the release of IFN-γ by NK cells helps to shape T-cell response in lymph nodes, possible by a direct interaction between naïve T cells and NK cells migrating to secondary lymphoid compartments from inflamed peripheral tissues and by an indirect effect on dendritic cells. Killing target cells by NK can also impact T-cell response, probably by decreasing the antigenic load and because target cell debris could promote antigen cross-presentation to $CD8^+$ cytotoxic T cells [61].

Cytotoxicity and cytokine production mediated by NK cells impact dendritic cells, macrophages, and neutrophils and endow NK cells with regulatory functions affecting subsequent antigen-specific T- and B-cell responses. NK cells need to be priming by various factors, such as IL-15 presented by dendritic cells or macrophages, IL-12 or IL-18 cytokines to reach their full effector potential. This fact highlights the intimate regulatory interactions between NK cells and other components of the immune response [61].

3.1.6 The Inflammasome

Another key feature of the innate immune system is the activation of the inflammasome, a multiprotein complex responsible for caspase-1 activation, caspase-1-dependent proteolytic maturation, and secretion of IL-1β. Several components of the inflammasome, including the nucleotide-binding domain (NOD)-like receptors (NLRs), the leucine-rich repeat containing proteins, the absent in melanoma 2 (AIM)-like receptors (ALRs), and the protein pyrin have been described. Although there are some differences between inflammasomes dependent upon stimuli, in general, a canonical inflammasome serves as a scaffold to recruit the inactive procaspase-1 zymogen. As a consequence of its activation, the relevant NLR or AIM2 can oligomerize to be a caspase-1-activating scaffold. Subsequently, active caspase-1 cleaves the proinflammatory IL-1 family of cytokines into their bioactive forms, IL-1β and IL-18. The inflammasome also can provoke pyroptosis, a type of inflammatory-induced cell death. Inflammasomes have been linked to different autoinflammatory and autoimmune diseases (multiple sclerosis, Alzheimer's and Parkinson's diseases) and metabolic disorders such as atherosclerosis, type 2 diabetes, and obesity [75]. The role of inflammasome-associated IL-1 family of cytokines in shaping adaptive immune responses is well established in regard to the differentiation of Th17 cells and development of the effector functions of Th1 and $CD8^+$ T cells [64].

There is a growing interest in the noncanonical inflammasome, which refers to a complex of procapase-11 and lipopolysaccharide (LPS) activated in mouse macrophages. In humans, caspase-4 and caspase-5 were found to interact directly with the intracellular LPS and activate the noncanonical inflammasome of myeloid cells. These procaspase bindings with intracellular lipid A of LPS oligomerize, and in turn, induce not only pyroptosis but also maturation and secretion of IL-1β and IL-18 [76].

3.2 Adaptive Immune System

The adaptive immunity is activated by the exposure to pathogens, inducing an immunological memory that allows learning how to deal against those threats, and inducing a specific immune response accordingly. Therefore, this immune response requires more time to be effective against threats and infections than the innate immune response, which is primed and ready to fight at all times, but results are more effective than the innate immune response. A characteristic of the adaptive immune system is its ability to remember a previous encounter with an antigen and mount a stronger response. This immunological memory is considered to be a crucial feature of the adaptive immunity. After an initial exposure to an antigen, antigen-specific T and B cells undergo clonal expansion. After antigen clearance, clonal T and B cells are eliminated by apoptosis during the contraction phase. However, some of the T and B cells can survive and progressively be differentiated into long-lived memory cells. These resistant cells can mediate a faster and more robust antigen-specific response than naïve cells [77].

Several studies have noted that the innate immune system also displays adaptive properties. NK cells can retain memory of past antigen confrontation in an autonomously fashion, and consequently they can mediate a more robust secondary response. In the same way, monocytes exposed to pathogens can also exhibit protective recall response to reinfection, suggesting that these cells derived from the myeloid lineage in mammals may have characteristics of the adaptive immunity. This phenomenon involves metabolic reprogramming, leading to epigenetic rewiring. The term *trained immunity* has been proposed for the persistent enhanced state of the innate immune response following the exposure to some infection agents that may result in increased resistance to related or unrelated pathogens [78].

3.2.1 B Lymphocytes

Lymphocytes are the cells responsible for the induction and expression of adaptive immunity. Two major classes of lymphocytes, B and T cells, are found. All the lymphocytes are obtained from a precursor stem cell in the bone marrow. B lymphocytes migrate directly to lymphoid tissues, while progenitor T cells migrate from the bone marrow to the thymus where they undergo maturation.

B cells produce antibody molecules that bind epitopes or individual immune determinants on foreign antigens. Antibodies possess single antigen specificity, therefore, they recognize only a single portion, called epitote or antigenic determinant, of the multitude of determinants on foreign proteins [79]. Antigens recognized by B cells are mainly proteins, but also carbohydrates or nucleic acids, among others. This portion of the foreign antigen binds to a specific antigen receptor on the surface of a B cell and thus stimulates an immune response. When the receptor and epitope are complementary they fit together like two pieces of a puzzle. This event is necessary to activate B cell production of antibodies. The antibodies produced by B cells are targeted specifically to the epitopes that bind to the cells' antigen receptors. Thus the epitope is also the region of the antigen that is recognized by specific antibodies, which bind to and remove the antigen from the body [79].

An antigen may have a variety of distinct epitopes on its structure, reacting with different B cell antigen receptors. Indeed, the blood serum antibodies of an immunized organism are capable of binding, with different affinity, to a variety of surface epitopes of the same antigen. In addition, it is possible for two or more different antigens to have an epitope in common. In these cases, antibodies targeted to one antigen are able to react with all antigens carrying the same epitope. Such antigens are known as cross-reacting antigens [79]. Binding between the antibody and the epitope occurs at the antigen binding site, which is called a paratope and is located at the tip of the variable region on the antibody. This paratope is capable of binding with only one unique epitope. B cells are capable of pinocytosis of soluble protein antigens, but this form of antigen uptake is probably not very efficient [79].

3.2.2 T Lymphocytes

T cells migrate from the bone marrow to the thymus where they undergo maturation. Then mature T lymphocytes emerge from the thymus as naïve T cells that migrate mainly to the spleen and lymph nodes (Fig. 3.5). These T cells are a subset of lymphocytes that play a large role in the immune response. Mature peripheral T lymphocytes generally express either CD4 or CD8. These cell surface structures belong to the immunoglobulin superfamily of molecules. Expression of CD4 or CD8 develops during T cell maturation in the thymus. In general, T cells, which express CD4, usually have helper cell functions, while T cells that express CD8 usually have cytolytic activity, although some CD4$^+$ T cells can be cytolytic, and some CD8$^+$ T cells can carry out some helper functions [80]. The expression of these cell surface structures correlates better with the MHC molecule expressed on their surface, which serves as the restriction element for antigen recognition: CD4$^+$ T cells usually react with antigenic peptides associated with MHC class II molecules, whereas CD8$^+$ T cells are generally restricted to reaction with antigenic peptides associated with MHC class I molecules. The TCR is a complex of integral membrane proteins participating in the activation of T cells in response to an antigen. Stimulation of TCR is triggered by the MHC molecules expressed on cells containing the antigen. Engagement of the TCR initiates positive and negative cascades that ultimately result in cellular proliferation, differentiation, cytokine production, and/or activation-induced cell death, thus regulating T cell development, homeostasis, activation, acquisition of effector's functions, and apoptosis [81].

TCR is composed of six different chains forming the TCR heterodimer responsible for ligand recognition. These chains have a structure similar to the antibody molecule and complementary to the antigen. These receptors recognize amino acids within a peptide bound to a specialized groove on the surface of one of the two MHC class proteins. Peptide fragments that associate with class II molecules are produced through a phagocytic endosomal pathway; those antigens include soluble proteins, bacteria, and killed viruses. Peptide fragments associating with class I molecules are usually synthesized by the APC. Such antigens include newly synthesized viral proteins and tumor and other cellular antigens that are degraded through a cytoplasmic pathway involving proteasomes [80]. Both classes of MHC molecules play essential roles in the initiation (MHC class II) or effector phase (MHC class I) of the immune response by means of their ability to present peptide antigens to CD4$^+$ or CD8$^+$ T lymphocytes, respectively [82]. Activated T cells from many species, with the exception of mice, synthesize and express MHC class II molecules at their cell surface [82].

CD4$^+$ T cells, named Th, act as helper cells supplying antigen-driven signals that induce B or CD8$^+$ cytotoxic T cells, and macrophages proliferation in response to an antigen. CD4$^+$ T cells differentiate into effector subsets in response to environmental signals including cytokines and ligand−receptor interactions from cell−cell contact. These environmental signals promote the development of Th subsets that secrete specific cytokines and perform distinct functions in regulating immunity and inflammation [83]. CD4$^+$ T cells can be classified into several subtypes based on the specific cytokines produced and functions performed; covering Th1, Th2, Th9, Th17, and Treg cells. Each effector Th cell produces cytokines without antigenic stimulation in response to the appropriate stimuli, implying an innate mechanism through which memory CD4$^+$ T cells are recruited by an induced cytokine environment [84]. Indeed, the development of different subtypes of Th cells requires the integration of multiple signals, and clearly a complex cytokine milieu is required for optimal IL production [83].

Th1 cells secrete IFN-γ, IL-2, and TNF-α/β in response to IL-18 and a STAT4 inducer [84], which activates macrophages. They are also responsible for cell-mediated immunity and phagocyte-dependent protective responses [85]. Th1 immune responses critically depend on the ability of dendritic cells to produce IL-12. Th1 cells produce IFNγ and mainly develop following infections by intracellular bacteria and some viruses. Indeed, Th1 cells are involved in the pathogenesis of organ-specific autoimmune disorders, Crohn's disease, *Helicobacter pylori*-induced peptic ulcer, acute kidney allograft rejection, and unexplained recurrent abortions [85].

Th2 cells produce IL-4, IL-5, IL-10, and IL-13, which are responsible for strong antibody production dealing with humoral immunity, eosinophil activation, and inhibition of several macrophage functions, thus providing phagocyte-independent protective responses [85]. IL-4 signaling alone leads to Th2 differentiation. Th2 cells produce IL-13, but not IL-4, in response to IL-33, a member of the IL-1 family, playing an important role in allergic/parasite-induced inflammatory responses [84]. Allergen-specific Th2 responses are responsible for atopic disorders in genetically susceptible individuals. Moreover, Th2 responses against still-unknown antigens predominate in Omenn's syndrome, idiopathic pulmonary fibrosis, and progressive systemic sclerosis. Finally, the prevalence of Th2 responses may play some role in a more rapid evolution of human immunodeficiency virus infection to the full-blown disease [85].

Th9 cells develop from naïve T cells in the presence of TGFβ and IL-4, although TGFβ can be replaced by activin A as a Th9-inducing factor. Importantly, the development of Th9 cells requires a balance of signals from cytokines that would otherwise generate distinct T-helper subsets [83]. Th9 cells produce IL-9, IL-10, and IL-21, and seem to be closely related to Th2 cells [83]. Various cytokines may impact T cell IL-9 production apart from IL-4 and TGFβ. IL-1 family members, such as IL-1 and IL-33, may induce IL-9 secretion under some conditions [86]. IL-2 and presumably the downstream factor STAT5 promote T cell IL-9 production [87], whereas IL-25 plays a critical role in promoting IL-9-dependent immune responses [88]. Furthermore, IFNγ and IL-23 inhibit IL-9 production from T cells [87]. Th9 cells are found in the peripheral blood of allergic patients and in both normal and inflamed skin. In addition, IL-9 responses can also be observed in response to specific antigen stimulation [83].

Th17 cells are induced by IL-6 plus TGFβ and secrete mainly large amounts of IL-17, and also IL-21, and IL-22, and help the B cell expansion, differentiation, and antibody production. Th17 cells produce IL-17A in response to IL-1β and a STAT3 activator [84]. The IL-23 promotes and/or maintains Th17 development and specifically induces IL-22 production. Th17 cells, through the production of both IL-22 and IL-17, might have essential functions in host defense and in the pathogenesis of autoimmune diseases such as psoriasis [89]. In addition, IL-22, as an effector cytokine produced by T cells, mediates the cross-talk between the immune system and epithelial cells [90]. Functionally, Th17 cells play a role in host defense against extracellular pathogens by mediating the recruitment of neutrophils and macrophages to infected tissues. Moreover, it has become evident that aberrant regulation of Th17 cells may play a significant role in the pathogenesis of multiple inflammatory and autoimmune disorders. IL-21 acts in an autocrine manner, whereas IL-22 binds to its receptor on target cells to induce the expression of antimicrobial peptides beta-defensin-2 and beta-defensin-3. In addition, the IL-22 ability to protect hosts against bacterial infections of the lungs and gut has been demonstrated [91].

Treg cells originating from the thymus have a pivotal role in maintaining immunological self-tolerance [63]. These Treg cells express CD25, cytotoxic T lymphocyte-associated antigen 4 (CTLA-4), glucocorticoid-induced TNF receptor family-related gene, lymphocyte activation gene-3, CD127, and the forkhead/winged-helix transcription factor box P3 (FoxP3). FoxP3, a key transcription factor involved in Treg development and function, is considered the most reliable marker for these cells. This observation strongly suggests that T-cell activation is required for T-cell mediated suppression [92]. One important mechanism for the induction of Treg cells by dendritic cells is the release of IL-10 or TGF-β, in the absence of IL-4. This induction results in Th1- and Th3- Treg cells, which in turn also secrete IL-10 and TGF-β, respectively. The IL-10 cytokine has the ability to suppress the Th1 and Th2 immune response, whereas TGF-β antagonizes Th1- and Th2-type inflammatory responses [63].

Suggested functions for Treg cells include (1) prevention of autoimmune diseases by maintaining self-tolerance; (2) suppression of allergy and asthma; (3) induction of tolerance against dietary antigens (i.e., oral tolerance); (4) induction of feto-maternal tolerance; (5) suppression of pathogen-induced immunopathology; (6) regulation of the effector class of the immune response; (7) suppression of T cell activation triggered by weak stimuli; (8) feedback control of the magnitude of the immune response by effector Th cells; (9) protection of commensal bacteria from elimination by the immune system; and (10) prevention of T cells that have been stimulated by their true high-affinity agonist ligand from killing cells that only express low-affinity TCR ligands such as the self-peptide-MHC molecule that positively selected the T cell [92]. In addition, suppression mediated by Treg cells is triggered in an antigen-specific fashion. Concerning the target cell, there are evidences that Treg cells may suppress Th cells with different antigen specificities. However, it is possible that suppression is more effective, and thereby physiologically more relevant, when the Treg cell and the suppressed Th cell have the same antigen specificity [92].

On the other hand, **CD8$^+$ T cells** (cytotoxic T lymphocytes) are generated in the thymus, and once activated can express the TCR. These cells express a dimeric (CD8α/CD8β) coreceptor that recognizes peptides presented by MHC class I molecules. Cytotoxic T lymphocytes are responsible from the local expression of molecules that includes the lytic attack and the production of cytokines that can attract inflammatory cells to the local site [79]. Cytotoxic T lymphocytes are very important for immune defense against intracellular pathogens, including viruses and bacteria, for tumor surveillance, and can also contribute to an excessive immune response leading to autoimmunity [93]. When a CD8$^+$ T cell recognizes an antigen and becomes activated, three major mechanisms to kill infected or malignant cells can be described: (1) secretion of cytokines, primarily TNF-α and IFN-γ, which have antitumor and antiviral microbial effects; (2) production and release of cytotoxic granules, similar to those found in NK cells, containing two families of proteins—perforins (which attack the membrane of target cells causing pores) and granzymes (serin proteases entering through those pores into the infected or malignant cell to cleave intracellular proteins), shutting down the production of viral proteins and resulting in apoptosis of the target cell; and (3) expression of FasL on the cell surface, which binds to its receptor, Fas, initiating the activation of the caspase cascade, and thus the apoptosis of the target cell [94].

3.3 Microbiota and the Immune System

The link between diet, nutrients, and immune response comprises a complex network of factors such as microbial composition, genetic background, and lifestyle. A healthy intestinal microbiota keeps a symbiotic relationship within the gut mucosa, offering essential functions in metabolism, immunology, and protection to the host. This microbiota is also essential for eliminating pathogens from the gut. The abundance and diversity of microbial members play a crucial role in the development of their functions (symbiosis, colonization resistance, clearance of pathogens, etc.) [95]. The intestinal microbiota can influence the adaptive and the innate immune systems; indeed, germ-free mice have poorly developed lymphoid tissues and show perturbations in the development of T and B cells [63]. An alteration of the intestinal composition (dysbiosis) has been related to the development of obesity, type 2 diabetes, and cardiovascular diseases.

Intestinal bacteria can interact directly with host cells through PRR. Particularly diet-induced obesity and genetic obesity were associated with the increase of plasma LPS, called metabolic endotoxemia. An altered intestinal microbiota composition and an increased intestinal permeability contribute to the development of this metabolic endotoxemia [96]. As aforementioned, TLR4 signaling is activated by LPS. First, LPS binds to LPS-binding protein, which transfers an LPS monomer to CD-14 protein. The CD14-LPS complex activates TLR4 and myeloid differentiation protein 2 (MD2) complex. Ligand recognition by TLR4 can trigger two distinct signal transduction pathways, referred to as myeloid differentiation primary response gene 88 (MyD88)-dependent and MyD88-independent. Upon activation, the cytoplasmatic Toll-interleukin receptor homology (TIR) domain of TLR4 associates with TIR-domain containing adaptor molecules such as MyD88, MyD88 adapter-like protein (MAL), TIR-domain-containing adapter inducing IF-β (TRIF), and TRIF-related adapter molecule (TRAM). These interactions result in the recruitment of the IL receptor associated kinase (IRAK) family and TNF receptor associated factor 6 (TRAF6), which in turn lead to the activation of MAP kinases and transcription factors such as NF-κB, which are necessary for the induction of inflammatory and antiinflammatory cytokines [63,97].

One of the functions of the intestinal microbiota is the fermentation of the dietary fiber. As a result of this process, short-chain fatty acids (SCFA), mainly butyrate, acetate, and propionate, are produced in the colon. These SCFA can mediate the communication between the commensal microbiota and the immune system. For example, butyrate, the main energy source for colonocytes, and to a lesser extent acetate and propionate, can facilitate the generation of extrathymic Foxp3$^+$ Tregs, which are crucial for limiting the intestinal inflammation. Moreover, the presence of butyrate during the maturation of human dendritic cells results in a tolerogenic phenotype, with an increased expression of IL-10. SCFA can interact with specific G-protein coupled receptors (GPR41, GPR43y, GPR109), which are particularly expressed in immune cells. GPR43 is also expressed in the colonic epithelium where it can mediate SCFA-regulated effects on epithelial barrier and proliferation. In addition, butyrate has been described as a natural ligand for the transcription factor PPARγ. In addition, butyrate inhibits histone deacetylases and the activation of NF-κB [95]. Interestingly, reduced dietary intake of carbohydrates resulted in decreased butyrate levels in the human feces and correlated with a reduced abundance of butyrate-producing bacteria. In addition, levels of propionate correlated with the amount of *Bacteroidetes* in the gut [98]. Furthermore, in the obese condition, T cells are increased whereas the Treg population is decreased. SCFA promote antiinflammatory response in mucosal and systemic tissues through Treg cells; therefore, it is possible that the intestinal microbiota may control obesity through the generation of Treg cells [98].

The intestinal microbiota is also responsible for the formation of bile acids, which are synthesized in the liver from cholesterol and metabolized in the intestine by its own microbiota. These bile acids act as signaling molecules that regulate intestinal homeostasis through G protein couple bile acid receptor (TGR5) and farnesoid X receptor (FXR) by inhibiting inflammation, preventing pathogen invasion, and maintaining cell integrity. Therefore, the intestinal microbiota, bile acids, and health status are closely related. Whether intestinal dysbiosis and modified bile acid pool are a cause or a consequence of disease is difficult to determine. TGR5 is mainly activated by secondary bile acids; this receptor decreases the production of IL-1α, IL-2β, IL-6, and TNF-α stimulated by LPS in macrophages and Kupffer cells through the inhibition of NF-κB. The activation of the receptor FXR protects against bacterial overgrowth and translocation in the distal small intestine. Uncontrolled increased levels of hydrophobic secondary bile acids are cytotoxic, causing DNA and cell damage possible through the induction of oxidative stress and ROS [99].

Currently, intestinal microbiota can be considered as a new organ able to module the immune system. However, the underlying molecular mechanisms of the intestinal microbiota are not yet fully understood.

GLOSSARY

Adaptive immune response The acquired immune response that depends on the specific recognition of antigens by T and B lymphocytes.
Antioxidant A molecule that inhibits the oxidation of other molecules.
Cytotoxicity The quality of being toxic to cells. Toxic agents are an immune cell or some types of venom.
Gut microbiota Microorganisms that inhabit in the gastrointestinal tract.
Inflammasome A multiprotein complex responsible for the secretion and maturation of interleukin-1 β. It is part of the innate immune system.
Innate immune response First line of defense that occurs immediately after pathogen exposure.
Oxidation A chemical reaction that can produce free radicals, leading to chain reactions that may damage cells.
Reactive oxygen species Chemically reactive chemical species containing oxygen, including peroxides, superoxide, hydroxyl radical, and singlet oxygen.

LIST OF ACRONYMS AND ABBREVIATIONS

ALR Absent in melanoma (AIM)-like receptors
AP-1 Activator protein 1
APC Antigen presenting cells
ARE Antioxidant response element
BCR Antibody B cell receptor
CD Cluster of differentiation
CoQ Coenzyme Q
Cys-OH Cysteine thiolate anions
Cys-SOH Sulfenic form
DAMP Danger-associated molecular pattern
Duox Dual oxidase
eNOS Endothelial NOS
ETC Electron-transport chain
FoxO Forkhead box class O
FXR Farnesoid X receptor
GPR G-protein coupled receptor
GPx Glutathione peroxidase
GR Glutathione reductase
GSH Reduced glutathione
GSSG Oxidized glutathione
GST Glutathione S-transferase
H_2O_2 Hydrogen peroxide
HO· Hydroxyl radical
HOCl Hypochlorite
IFN-γ Interferon-γ
Ig Immunoglobulin
IL Interleukin
ILC Innate lymphoid cell
iNOS Inducible NOS
IRAK IL receptor associated kinase
Keap1 Kelch-like ECH-associated protein 1
LPS Lipopolysaccharide
MAL MyD88 adapter-like protein

MHC Major histocompatibility complex
MnSOD Mn-dependent SOD
NF-κB Nuclear factor κ-light-chain-enhancer of activated B cell
NK Natural killer cell
NLR Nucleotide-binding domain (NOD)-like receptor
nNOS Neuronal NOS
NO Nitric oxide
NOS Nitric oxide synthase
Nrf2 NF-E2-related factor 2
$O_2{}^{\bullet}$ Singlet oxygen
$O_2^{\bullet-}$ Superoxide anion
OH− Hydroxyl anion
ONOO− Peroxynitrite
PAMP Pathogen-associated molecular pattern
PRR Pattern recognition receptor
Prx Peroxiredoxin
PTP Protein tyrosine phosphatase
RNS Reactive nitrogen species
ROS Reactive oxygen species
SCFA Short-chain fatty acid
SH Nitrosylates the thiol
SMOC Supramolecular organizing center
SOD Superoxide dismutase
Treg T regulatory cell
TCR T cell receptor
TGF-β Transforming growth factor β
TGR5 G protein coupled bile acid receptor
Th T helper
TIR Toll-interleukin receptor homology domain
TLR Toll-like receptor
TNF-α Tumor necrosis factor-α
TRAF6 TNF receptor associated factor 6
TRAM TRIF-related adapter molecule
TRIF TIR-domain-containing adapter inducing IF-β
TSLP Thymic stromal lymphopoietin

REFERENCES

[1] Elmarakby AA, Sullivan JC. Relationship between oxidative stress and inflammatory cytokines in diabetic nephropathy. Cardiovasc Ther 2012;30(1):49−59.

[2] Bondia-Pons I, Ryan L, Martinez JA. Oxidative stress and inflammation interactions in human obesity. J Physiol Biochem 2012;68(4):701−11.

[3] Shilov AE. N. N. Semenov and the chemistry of the 20th century (to 100th anniversary of his birth). Pure Appl Chem 1997;69(4):857−63.

[4] McCord JM, Fridovich I. Superoxide dismutase. An enzymic function for erythrocuprein (hemocuprein). J Biol Chem 1969;244:6049−55.

[5] Weiss G, Schaible UE. Macrophage defense mechanisms against intracellular bacteria. Immunol Rev 2015;264(1):182−203.

[6] Libby P, Aikawa M, Jain MK. Vascular endothelium and atherosclerosis. Handb Exp Pharmacol 2006;176(Pt 2):285−306.

[7] Turrens JF. Mitochondrial formation of reactive oxygen species. J Physiol 2003;552(Pt 2):335−44.

[8] Panday A, Sahoo MK, Osorio D, Batra S. NADPH oxidases: an overview from structure to innate immunity-associated pathologies. Cell Mol Immunol 2015;12(1):5−23.

[9] Outten FW, Theil EC. Iron-based redox switches in biology. Antioxid Redox Signal 2009;11(5):1029−46.

[10] Furchgott RF, Zawadzki JV. The obligatory role of endothelial cells in the relaxation of arterial smooth muscle by acetylcholine. Nature 1980;288(5789):373−6.

[11] Paimer RM, Ferrige AG, Moncada S. Nitric oxide release accounts for the biological activity of endothelium-derived relaxing factor. Nature 1987;327(6122):524−6.

[12] Braam B, Verhaar MC. Understanding eNOS for pharmacological modulation of endothelial function: a translational view. Curr Pharm Des 2007;13(17):1727−40.

[13] Montezano AC, Rhian MT. Reactive oxygen species and endothelial function − role of nitric oxide synthase uncoupling and nox family nicotinamide adenine dinucleotide phosphate oxidases. Basic Clin Pharmacol Toxicol 2012;110(1):87−94.

[14] Brown GC, Borutaite V. Nitric oxide and mitochondrial respiration in the heart. Cardiovasc Res 2007;75(2):283−90.

[15] Bouloumie A, Bauersachs J, Linz W. Endothelial dysfunction coincides with an enhanced nitric oxide synthase expression and superoxide anion production. Hypertension 1997;30(4):934–41.

[16] Szabo C, Ischiropoulos H, Radi R. Peroxynitrite: biochemistry, pathophysiology and development of therapeutics. Nat Rev Drug Discov 2007;6(8):662–80.

[17] Suryo Rahmanto Y, Kalinowski DS, Lane DJ, Lok HC, Richardson V, Richardson DR. Nitrogen monoxide (NO) storage and transport by dinitrosyl-dithiol-iron complexes: long-lived NO that is trafficked by interacting proteins. J Biol Chem 2012;287(10):6960–8.

[18] Williams JL, Ji P, Ouyang N, Kopelovich L, Rigas B. Protein nitration and nitrosylation by NO-donating aspirin in colon cancer cells: relevance to its mechanism of action. Exp Cell Res 2011;317(10):1359–67.

[19] Mignard V, Lalier L, Paris F, Vallette FM. Bioactive lipids and the control of Bax pro-apoptotic activity. Cell Death Dis 2014;5:e1266.

[20] Yan M, Tang C, Ma Z, Huang S, Dong Z. DNA damage response in nephrotoxic and ischemic kidney injury. Toxicol Appl Pharmacol 2016;313:104–8.

[21] Auten RL, Davis JM. Oxygen toxicity and reactive oxygen species: the devil is in the details. Pediatr Res 2009;66(2):121–7.

[22] Birben E, Sahiner UM, Sackesen C, Erzurum S, Kalayci O. Oxidative stress and antioxidant defense. World Allergy Organ J 2012;5(1):9–19.

[23] Klomsiri C, Karplus PA, Poole LB. Cysteine-based redox switches in enzymes. Antioxid Redox Signal 2011;14(6):1065–77.

[24] Son Y, Kim S, Chung HT, Pae HO. Reactive oxygen species in the activation of MAP kinases. Methods Enzymol 2013;528:27–48.

[25] Martinou JC, Youle RJ. Mitochondria in apoptosis: Bcl-2 family members and mitochondrial dynamics. Dev Cell 2011;21(1):92–101.

[26] Wink DA, Hines HB, Cheng RY, Switzer CH, Flores-Santana W, Vitek MP, Ridnour LA, Colton CA. Nitric oxide and redox mechanisms in the immune response. J Leukoc Biol 2011;89(6):873–91.

[27] Ida T, Sawa T, Ihara H, Tsuchiya Y, Watanabe Y, Kumagai Y, Suematsu M, Motohashi H, Fujii S, Matsunaga T, Yamamoto M, Ono K, Devarie-Baez NO, Xian M, Fukuto JM, Akaike T. Reactive cysteine persulfides and S-polythiolation regulate oxidative stress and redox signaling. Proc Natl Acad Sci USA 2014;111(21):7606–11.

[28] Klotz LO, Sánchez-Ramos C, Prieto-Arroyo I, Urbánek P, Steinbrenner H, Monsalve M. Redox regulation of FoxO transcription factors. Redox Biol 2015;6:51–72.

[29] Rocha ER, Smith CJ. Role of the alkyl hydroperoxide reductase (ahpCF) gene in oxidative stress defense of the obligate Anaerobe bacteroides fragilis. J Bacteriol 1999;181(18):5701–10.

[30] Scandalios JG. Oxidative stress: molecular perception and transduction of signals triggering antioxidant gene defenses. Braz J Med Biol Res 2005;38(7):995–1014.

[31] Shadel GS. Expression and maintenance of mitochondrial DNA: new insights into human disease pathology. Am J Pathol 2008;172(6):1445–56.

[32] Muir R, Diot A, Poulton J. Mitochondrial content is central to nuclear gene expression: profound implications for human health. Bioessays 2016;38(2):150–6.

[33] Wilking M, Ndiaye M, Mukhtar H, Ahmad N. Circadian rhythm connections to oxidative stress: implications for human health. Antioxid Redox Signal 2013;19(2):192–208.

[34] Mittler R. ROS are good. Trends Plant Sci 2017;22(1):11–9.

[35] Padgett LE, Broniowska KA, Hansen PA, Corbett JA, Tse HM. The role of reactive oxygen species and proinflammatory cytokines in type 1 diabetes pathogenesis. Ann NY Acad Sci 2013;1281:16–35.

[36] Magenta A, Greco S, Gaetano C, Martelli F. Oxidative stress and microRNAs in vascular diseases. Int J Mol Sci 2013;14(9):17319–46.

[37] Ratnam DV, Ankola DD, Bhardwaj V, Sahana DK, Kumar MN. Role of antioxidants in prophylaxis and therapy: a pharmaceutical perspective. J Control Release 2006;113(3):189–207.

[38] He L, He T, Farrar S, Ji L, Liu T, Ma X. Antioxidants maintain cellular redox homeostasis by elimination of reactive oxygen species. Cell Physiol Biochem 2017;44(2):532–53.

[39] Zhang M, Shi J, Jiang L. Modulation of mitochondrial membrane integrity and ROS formation by high temperature in *Saccharomyces cerevisiae*. Electron J Biotechnol 2015;18(3):202–9.

[40] Suen DF, Norris KL, Youle RJ. Mitochondrial dynamics and apoptosis. Genes Dev 2008;22(12):1577–90.

[41] Ma X, He P, Sun P, Han P. Lipoic acid: an immunomodulator that attenuates glycinin-induced anaphylactic reactions in a rat model. J Agric Food Chem 2010;58(8):5086–92.

[42] Land W, Schneeberger H, Schleibner S, Illner WD, Abendroth D, Rutili G, Arfors KE, Messmer K. The beneficial effect of human recombinant superoxide dismutase on acute and chronic rejection events in recipients of cadaveric renal transplants. Transplantation 1994;57(2):211–7.

[43] Han P, Ma X, Yin J. The effects of lipoic acid on soybean beta-conglycinin-induced anaphylactic reactions in a rat model. Arch Anim Nutr 2010;64(3):254–64.

[44] Stanton R. Glucose-6-phosphate dehydrogenase, NADPH, and cell survival. IUBMB Life 2012;64(5):362–9.

[45] Lu J, Holmgren A. The thioredoxin antioxidant system. Free Radic Biol Med 2014;66:75–87.

[46] Lillig CH, Holmgren A. Thioredoxin and related molecules–from biology to health and disease. Antioxid Redox Signal 2007;9(1):25–47.

[47] Burton GW, Traber MG. Vitamin-E. Antioxidant activity, biokinetics, and bioavailability. Annu Rev Nutr 1990;10:357–82.

[48] Jee JP, Lim SJ, Park JS, Kim CK. Stabilization of all-trans retinol by loading lipophilic antioxidants in solid lipid nanoparticles. Eur J Pharm Biopharm 2006;63(2):134–9.

[49] Fan P, Tan Y, Jin K, Lin C, Xia S, Han B, et al. Supplemental lipoic acid relieves post-weaning diarrhoea by decreasing intestinal permeability in rats. J Anim Physiol Anim Nutr (Berl) 2017;101(1):136–46.

[50] Bowman GL, Shannon J, Frei B, Kaye JA, Quinn JF. Uric acid as a CNS antioxidant. J Alzheimers Dis 2010;19(4):1331–6.

[51] Waring WS, Webb DJ, Maxwell SRJ. Systemic uric acid administration increases serum antioxidant capacity in healthy volunteers. J Cardiovasc Pharmacol 2001;38(3):365−71.

[52] Prasad AS, Bao B, Beck FWJ, Kucuk O, Sarkar FH. Antioxidant effect of zinc in humans. Free Radic Biol Med 2004;37(8):1182−90.

[53] Rice-Evans CA, Sampson J, Bramley PM, Holloway DE. Why do we expect carotenoids to be antioxidants in vivo? Free Radic Res 1997;26(4):381−98.

[54] Niles RM. Signaling pathways in retinoid chemoprevention and treatment of cancer. Mutat Res 2004;555(1−2):81−96.

[55] Donato LJ, Noy N. Suppression of mammary carcinoma growth by retinoic acid: proapoptotic genes are targets for retinoic acid receptor and cellular retinoic acid-binding protein II signaling. Cancer Res. 2005;65(18):8193−9.

[56] Heim KE, Tagliaferro AR, Bobilya DJ. Flavonoid antioxidants: chemistry, metabolism and structure-activity relationships. J Nutr Biochem 2002;13(10):572−84.

[57] Lushchak VI. Free radicals, reactive oxygen species, oxidative stress and its classification. Chem Biol Interact 2014;224:164−75.

[58] Kansanen E, Kuosmanen SM, Leinonen H, Levonen AL. The Keap1-Nrf2 pathway: mechanisms of activation and dysregulation in cancer. Redox Biol 2013;1:45−9.

[59] Chen QM, Maltagliati AJ. Nrf2 at the heart of oxidative stress and cardiac protection. Physiol Genomics 2018;50(2):77−97.

[60] Delves PJ, Roitt IM. The immune system. N Engl J Med 2000;343(1):37−49.

[61] Vivier E, Raulet DH, Moretta A, Caligiuri MA, Zitvogel L, Lanier LL, Yokoyama WM, Ugolini S. Innate or adaptive immunity? The example of natural killer cells. Science 2011;331(6013):44−9.

[62] Annunziato F, Romagnani C, Romagnani S. The 3 major types of innate and adaptive cell-mediated effector immunity. J Allergy Clin Immunol 2015;135(3):626−35.

[63] Gomez-Llorente C, Muñoz S, Gil A. Role of toll-like receptors in the development of immunotolerance mediated by probiotics. Proc Nutr Soc 2010;69(3):381−9.

[64] Evavold CL, Kagan JC. How inflammasomes inform adaptive immunity. J Mol Biol 2018;430(2):217−37.

[65] Lebeer S, Vanderleyden J, De Keersmaecker SCJ. Host interactions of probiotic bacterial surface molecules: comparison with commensals and pathogens. Nat Rev Microbiol 2010;8(3):171−84.

[66] Chen GY, Nunez G. Sterile inflammation: sensing and reacting to damage. Nat Rev Immunol 2010;10(12):826−37.

[67] Arbore G, Kemper C, Kolev M. Intracellular complement-the complosome-in immune cell regulation. Mol Immunol 2017;89:2−9.

[68] Janeway CA, Medzhitov R. Innate immune recognition. Annu Rev Immunol 2002;20:197−216.

[69] Twum DYF, Burkard-Mandel L, Abrams SI. The Dr. Jekyll and Mr. Hyde complexity of the macrophage response in disease. J Leukoc Biol 2017;102(2):307−15.

[70] Ahmad S, Zamry AA, Tan HTT, Wong KK, Lim J, Mohamud R. Targeting dendritic cells trough gold nanoparticles: a review on the cellular uptake and subsequent immunological properties. Mol Immunol 2017;91:123−33.

[71] Lubbers R, Essen MF, van Kooten C, Trouw LA. Production of complement components by cells of the immune system. Clin Exp Immunol 2017;188(2):183−94.

[72] Mohammadi H, Sharafkandi N, Hemmatzadeh M, Azizi G, Karimi M, Jadidi-Niaragh F, et al. The role of innate lymphoid cells in health and disease. J Cell Physiol 2017. https://doi.org/10.1002/jcp.26250.

[73] Everaere L, Ait Yahia S, Bouté M, Audousset C, Chenivesse C, Tsicopoulos A. Innate lymphoid cells at the interface between obesity and asthma. Immunology 2018;153(1):21−30.

[74] Symowski C, Voehringer D. Interactions between innate lymphoid cells and cells of the innate and adaptive immune system. Front Immunol 2017;30(8):1422.

[75] Guo H, Callaway JR, Ting JP. Inflammasomes: mechanism of action, role in disease, and therapeutics. Nat Med 2015;21(7):677−87.

[76] Yi YS. Caspase-11 non-canonical inflammasome: a critical sensor of intracellular lipopolysaccharide in macrophage-mediated inflammatory responses. Immunology 2017;152(2):207−17.

[77] Peng H, Tian Z. Natural killer cell memory: progress and implications. Front Immunol 2017;8:1143.

[78] Muraille E, Goriely S. The nonspecific face of adaptive immunity. Curr Opin Immunol 2017;48:38−43.

[79] Wherry EJ, Masopust D. Adaptive immunity. In: Viral pathogenesis. 3rd ed. 2016. ISBN: 978-0-12-800964-2.

[80] Fitch FW. Helper T lymphocytes. In: Encyclopedia of immunology. 2nd ed. 1998.

[81] Lin J, Weiss A. T cell receptor signaling. J Cell Sci 2001;114:243−4.

[82] Holling TM, Schooten E, van Den Elsen PJ. Function and regulation of MHC class II molecules in T-lymphocytes: of mice and men. Hum Immunol 2004;65(4):282−90.

[83] Kaplan MH. Th9 cells: differentiation and disease. Immunol Rev 2013;252:104−15.

[84] Guo L, Wei G, Zhu J, Liao W, Leonard WJ, et al. IL-1 family members and STAT activators induce cytokine production by Th2, Th17, and Th1 cells. Proc Natl Acad Sci USA 2009;106(32):13463−8.

[85] Romagnani S. Th1/Th2 cells. Inflamm Bowel Dis 1999;5(4):285−94.

[86] Blom L, Poulsen BC, Jensen BM, Hansen A, Poulsen LK. IL-33 induces IL-9 production in human CD4 + T cells and basophils. PLoS One 2011;6:e21695.

[87] Fung MM, Chu YL, Fink JL, Wallace A, McGuire KL. IL-2- and STAT5-regulated cytokine gene expression in cells expressing the Tax protein of HTLV-1. Oncogene 2005;24:4624−33.

[88] Angkasekwinai P, Chang SH, Thapa M, Watarai H, Dong C. Regulation of IL-9 expression by IL-25 signaling. Nat Immunol 2010;11:250−6.

[89] Cai Y, Fleming C, Yan J. New insights of T cells in the pathogenesis of psoriasis. Cell Mol Immunol 2012;9(4):302−9.

[90] Zheng Y, Danilenko DM, Valdez P, Kasman I, Eastham-Anderson J, Wu J, Ouyang W. Interleukin-22, a Th17 cytokine, mediates IL-23-induced dermal inflammation and acanthosis. Nature 2007;445(7128):648−51.

[91] Dong C. Th17 cells in development: an updated view of their molecular identity and genetic programming. Nat Rev Immunol 2008;8(5):337−48.

[92] Corthay A. How do regulatory T cells work? Scand J Immunol 2009;70(4):326−36.

[93] Korn T, Kallies A. T cell responses in the central nervous system. Nat Rev Immunol 2017;17:179−94.

[94] Chávez-Galán L, Arenas-Del Angel MC, Zenteno E, Chávez R, Lascurain R. Cell death mechanisms induced by cytotoxic lymphocytes. Cell Mol Immunol 2009;6(1):15−25.

[95] Statovci D, Aguilera M, MacSharry J, Melgar S. The impact of western diet and nutrients on the microbiota and immune response at mucosal interfaces. Front Immunol 2017;28(8):838.

[96] Boulangé CL, Neves AL, Chilloux J, Nicholson JK, Dumas ME. Impact of the gut microbiota on inflammation, obesity, and metabolic disease. Genome Med 2016;8(1):42.

[97] Wan Y, Xiao H, Affolter J, Kim TW, Bulek K, Chaudhuri S, Carlson D, Hamilton T, Mazumder B, Stark GR, Thomas J, Li X. Interleukin-1 receptor-associated kinase 2 is critical for lipopolysaccharide-mediated post-transcriptional control. J Biol Chem 2009;284(16):10367−75.

[98] Andoh A. Physiological role of gut microbiota for maintaining human health. Digestion 2016;93(3):176−81.

[99] Sagar NM, Cree IA, Covington JA, Arasaradnam RP. The interplay of the gut microbiome, bile acids and volatile organic compounds. Gastroenterol Res Pract 2015. 398585.

Chapter 4

Inflammation and Oxidative Stress in Adipose Tissue: Nutritional Regulation

Leyre Martínez-Fernández[1], Marta Fernández-Galilea[1,2], Elisa Felix-Soriano[1], Xavier Escoté[1], Pedro González-Muniesa[1,3,4] and María J. Moreno-Aliaga[1,3,4]

[1]Centre for Nutrition Research, University of Navarra, Pamplona, Spain; [2]Center for Applied Medical Research, University of Navarra, Pamplona, Spain; [3]CIBERobn, Institute of Health Carlos III, Madrid, Spain; [4]IdiSNA, Navarra Institute for Health Research, Pamplona, Spain

1. INTRODUCTION

The rising prevalence of obesity (defined as body mass index [BMI] $\geq 30 \text{ kg/m}^2$) in developed and developing countries has been described as a global pandemic, responsible for 2.8 million deaths each year [1]. According to the World Health Organization, its prevalence has almost doubled between 1980 and 2014, with an increase of 27.5% in the worldwide proportion of overweight and obese [1]. Moreover, estimations predict that obesity prevalence will reach greater proportions, with more than 1 billion people being affected by 2030 [1]. Thus development of effective treatments for obesity and comorbidities is needed.

Obesity, characterized by excessive fat accumulation and accompanied by subacute chronic inflammation, is an important risk factor for some comorbidities such as the metabolic syndrome (MetS), insulin resistance (IR), type 2 diabetes mellitus (T2DM), dyslipidemia, fatty liver disease, hypertension, cardiovascular disease, and certain types of cancer [2]. Growing consensus accepts activation of the immune system and chronic low-grade inflammation as links between excess of adiposity and the development of these obesity-related complications [2].

2. WHITE, BROWN, AND BEIGE ADIPOSE TISSUE: PHYSIOLOGICAL ROLES

It is well known that mammals have two types of adipose tissue: the energy-storing white adipose tissue (WAT) and the energy-dissipating brown adipose tissue (BAT) [3]. Moreover, during the last years a third type of adipocytes has been found within some white adipose depots, but showing functional and morphological features of brown adipocytes. Thus these beige or "brite" (brown-in-white) adipocytes have characteristics that make them similar to both types of fat cells [4]. Differences between white, beige, and brown adipocytes are represented in Fig. 4.1.

2.1 White Adipose Tissue

Certainly, WAT is a long-term storage organ that accumulates excess of energy as triglycerides within its lipid droplets, mobilizing them when needed, through the regulation of lipogenesis and lipolysis, respectively [3]. However, WAT is also a real endocrine organ that secretes pro- and antiinflammatory cytokines, hormones, and growth factors, collectively termed adipokines [5]. Indeed, WAT's plasticity and endocrine function has been reviewed in obesity, in which WAT undergoes processes that comprise hyperplasia and/or hypertrophy, recruitment of inflammatory cells, and adaptations in the extracellular matrix in order to accumulate the excess of energy [6]. However, when inflammation and obesity are sustained, these adaptive mechanisms fail and lead to WAT dysfunction, affecting several distant tissues [6] (Fig. 4.2).

Under these circumstances, adipose tissue dysfunction is characterized by hypertrophic adipocytes that, at first, show an impaired adipokine secretion [7]. This spoiled adipokine secretion, mainly orchestrated by reduced adiponectin and

Obesity. https://doi.org/10.1016/B978-0-12-812504-5.00004-0

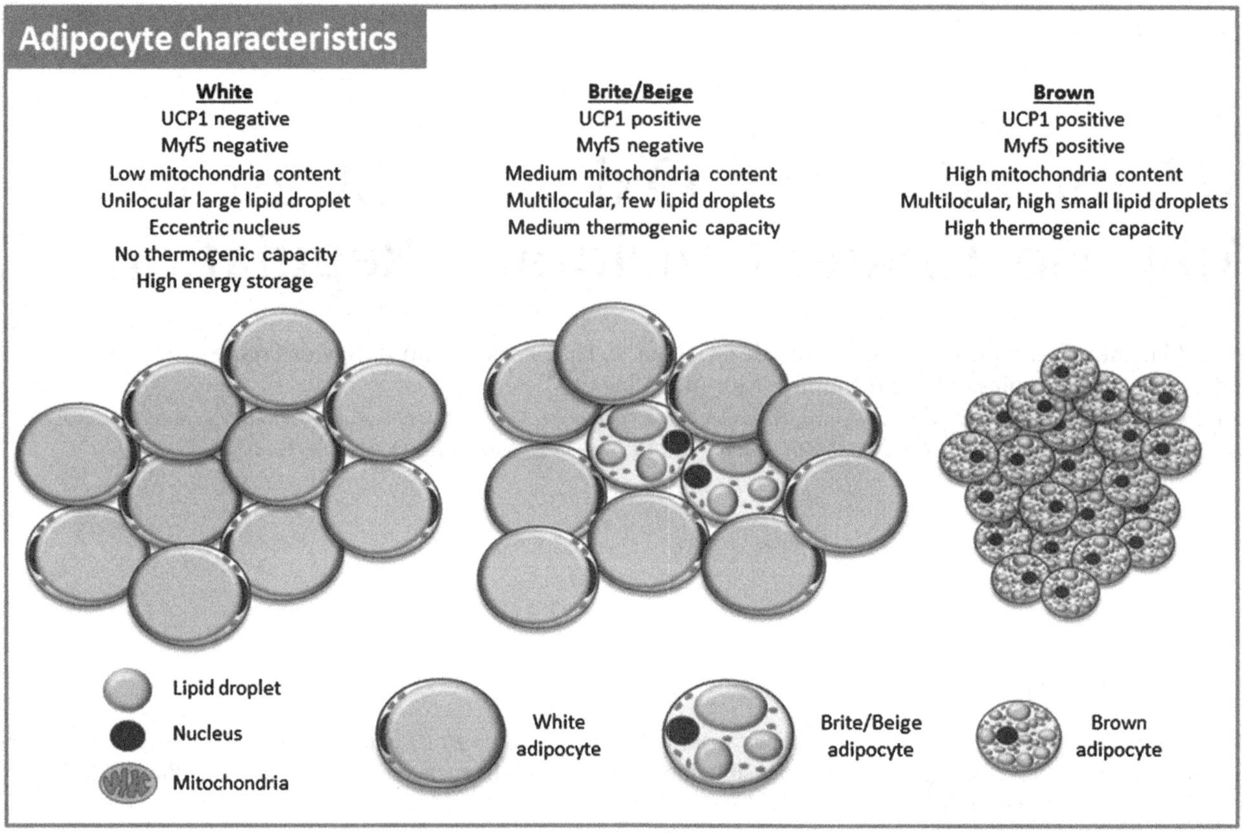

FIGURE 4.1 **Morphological and functional differences between white, brite/beige, and brown adipocytes.** Adipocytes are originated from different precursors that are capable of developing into white, beige, or brown adipocytes. White adipocytes present a unilocular large lipid droplet with an eccentric nucleus. Brown adipocytes are smaller and present multiple small cytoplasmic lipid droplets and a large number of large mitochondria. Brown adipocytes are Myf5-positive cells with a high expression of UCP1. Beige/brite adipocytes are multilocular adipocytes occurring within white fat depots with higher mitochondrial content than white adipocytes and inducible UCP1. *UCP1*, uncoupling protein 1.

increased leptin, resistin, tumor necrosis factor-α (TNF-α), monocyte chemoattractant protein (MCP-1), and interleukins (IL-6, IL-8, IL-1β), attracts and activates immune cells [7]. As a matter of fact, obesity is associated with an increased infiltration of macrophages and a polarization toward their M1 proinflammatory phenotype, instead of the M2 antiinflammatory [8]. M1 macrophages coordinate a significant part of obesity inflammation, as they constitute 50% of immune cells in adipose tissue and secrete proinflammatory cytokines such as IL-6 and MCP-1. M2 macrophages, instead, secrete antiinflammatory cytokines like IL-10 [5]. Not only macrophages, but also many types of immune cells (lymphocytes, eosinophils and killer, mast, dendritic, and foam cells) have been found to appear infiltrated in obese WAT in a higher rate, contributing to the systemic inflammation [5].

WAT dysfunction in obesity is also accompanied by moderate local hypoxia due to enlarged hypertrophic adipocytes. Along with local inflammation, hypoxia causes an increase in adipocyte apoptosis or autophagy. Such necrotic adipocytes appear surrounded by M1 macrophages in a crown-like structure that, together with greater angiogenesis, is believed to represent a compensatory mechanism to facilitate vascularization [5]. However, both angiogenesis and hypoxia-induced fibrosis contribute to the inflammatory state [8].

The whole process leads to high circulating levels of proinflammatory cytokines and free fatty-acids (FFAs), which interfere with insulin actions and signaling in metabolic tissues, causing systemic inflammation and IR [9]. As a consequence, there is a spoiled glucose disposal in muscle and increased lipolysis in adipose tissue. In turn, hyperinsulinemia, hyperglycemia, and hyperlipidemia appear and contribute to the development of obesity associated comorbidities, including T2DM and cardiovascular disease [9].

In summary, adipokines act in an endocrine, paracrine, and autocrine manner, and thus, if their secretion is impaired, the consequences are systemic [10] (Fig. 4.2). In fact, adipose tissue can account for up to 50% of body mass in morbidly obese subjects, representing an important compartment of the immune system capable of influencing systemic inflammation [11]. Noteworthy, a population of metabolically healthy obese subjects has been described as obese people

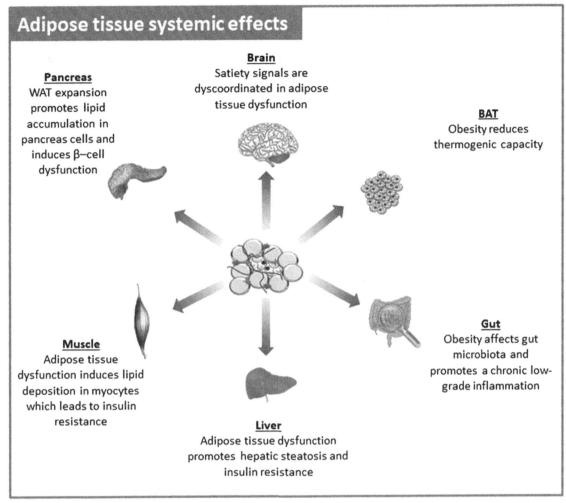

FIGURE 4.2   Adipose tissue dysfunction affects several distant tissues. A long-term positive energy balance, leading to body weight gain, will increase adipocyte size. Adipocyte hypertrophy in obesity is accompanied by disturbances in lipid metabolism and alterations in adipokine secretion, with a shift toward a proinflammatory phenotype. The secretion of proinflammatory factors is further boosted by the infiltration of several immune cells into the adipose tissue. Adipose tissue dysfunction is also accompanied by lipid spillover in the circulation and subsequent ectopic fat storage accumulation (essentially in muscle and liver), contributing to lipotoxicity and systemic low-grade inflammation. *BAT*, brown adipose tissue.

sensitive to insulin with normal plasma glucose, insulin, and lipid levels, together with healthy inflammatory markers and homeostatic model assessment (HOMA)-IR. Among these subjects, adipose tissue appears with lower levels of infiltrated immune cells and smaller adipocytes [2,12].

2.2 Brown Adipose Tissue

BAT, unlike WAT, is a thermogenic tissue whose main function is energy dissipation, with uncoupling protein 1 (UCP1) being a major responsible mechanism. UCP1 is a BAT-specific protein located in the inner mitochondrial membrane, which uncouples the respiratory chain, producing heat instead of energy. This process is known as adaptive thermogenesis, and it is mediated by adrenergic stimulation [13].

In humans, the amount of BAT is relatively abundant at the onset of life, helping to counteract heat loss in neonates, but gradually reduces during aging. Rodents, however, do have BAT depots throughout life, which help them maintain body temperature in response to cold [14]. Recent studies in human adults using ^{18}F-Fluorodeoxyglucose-PET/CT scans have identified active BAT depots mostly in the cervical and supraclavicular regions but also in the axillar, paravertebral, paraaortic, and suprarenal regions [15].

BAT differs from WAT not only in the presence of UCP1, as they arise from different developmental lineages, with Myf5-positive and negative progenitors, respectively [6]. Thus, BAT presents a great number of thermogenic mitochondria and small lipid droplets, which are very accessible for hydrolysis and oxidation of FFAs [16]. Moreover, it is known that BAT relies on glucose and FFAs as metabolic fuels [17], and current investigations have suggested emerging roles of BAT in the physiological regulation of metabolism, such as control of triglyceride [18] and glucose clearance, in both rodents [19] and humans [20]. Although BAT endocrine function is poorly characterized, it has been recently described that BAT produces factors such as fibroblast growth factor 21 and retinol binding protein, which could modulate the function of other metabolic organs [21].

Indeed, BAT mass has been associated with a lean phenotype and lower fasting insulin, as well as reduced IR and inflammatory adipokine secretion in human clinical trials [22]. Upon activation, BAT has been related to weight loss [23] and a decrease in body fat mass [24] both due to an increase in energy expenditure, together with increased local and net glucose disposal [25]. Thus, although BAT represents a small fraction of body mass ($\sim$0.1%), increasing BAT activity is an upcoming promising therapeutic strategy to treat obesity [26].

Interestingly, studies have shown a decreased mass/metabolic activity in BAT among obese subjects associated with increased visceral fat, aging, and hyperglycemia [14,15,27]. In fact, a process of whitening of BAT has been described in animal models of obesity, with enlarged adipocytes showing a loss of response to beta adrenergic stimuli together with mitochondrial dysfunction [28]. Such a process may also take place in humans, given the fact that BAT glucose uptake is impaired among individuals with IR and T2DM [29].

On the other hand, BAT activity among obese individuals is related to a metabolically healthier phenotype [27], and BAT recruitment has been positively associated with weight loss after bariatric surgery [30]. Moreover, BAT transplantation in dietary animal models of obesity improved glucose clearance by increasing insulin sensitivity in heart, muscle, and WAT [19]. Regarding lipid metabolism, there is evidence that BAT activation leads to an improvement in triglyceride and FFA clearance in dyslipidemic humans [31] and in rodent models of obesity [18].

2.3 Beige Adipose Tissue

During the last years a new type of adipose tissue has been found within some white adipose depots, but showing a brown-like adipocytes phenotype. Thus beige or "brite" (brown-in-white) adipocytes are multilocular and have thermogenic properties due to increased mitochondrial function and expression of inducible UCP1 [4] (Fig. 4.1). Such beige cells share Myf5-negative progenitors with WAT [3] but express specific beige genes such as *TBX1*, *TMEM26*, and *CD137* among others. Remarkably, beige adipocytes have been identified in adult humans [4], making this cell type an attractive therapeutic target for obesity and metabolic-related diseases [4].

Although several studies in cultured cells and rodents have suggested that subcutaneous white adipocytes can adopt a BAT-like (beige or brite) phenotype, there is little evidence of browning in human subcutaneous WAT [32]. However, it has been demonstrated that human adult BAT depots consist of a mixed population of brown and beige adipocytes [33], and marker gene studies have recently suggested that supraclavicular and neck BAT actually consist of beige adipocytes [33].

Beige adipocytes have very low UCP1 compared to brown adipocytes, but their UCP1 is highly inducible in response to stimulation. In addition to cold exposure and β-3 adrenergic, these stimuli include other recently found endogenous, pharmacological, and nutritional factors such as natriuretic peptides, irisin, FGF21, cardiotrophin-1, retinoids, and conjugated linoleic acid, among others [34]. Noteworthy, a recent study has also supported the importance of immune-adipose interactions to increase beige fat thermogenesis reliant on eosinophil and macrophage pathways [35].

In mice, browning of WAT due to cold exposure or beta adrenergic stimuli is accompanied by a reduction in diet-induced obesity (DIO), dyslipidemia, and hyperglycemia, along with a macrophage polarization toward M2 antiinflammatory phenotype in BAT and WAT [36]. Interestingly, cold induced an increased gene expression of *UCP1*, *TMEM26*, and *TBX1* in human subcutaneous fat, this process being inhibited by obesity [37].

3. INFLAMMATION AND OXIDATIVE STRESS IN ADIPOSE TISSUE IN OBESITY

Increased fat accumulation is associated with low-grade chronic inflammation, with both hypertrophied adipose tissues and immune cells being contributors to this condition [38]. In lean WAT there is a predominant antiinflammatory environment associated with a Th2-type immune response and a population of M2-like macrophages [39]. In addition, adipocytes and adipose stroma secrete different hormones that contribute to maintain tissue homeostasis, such as adiponectin [39]. In order to accumulate fat excess, adipocytes become hypertrophied and later hyperplastic, leading to an alteration in the secretory pattern of adipose tissue characterized by a decrease of antiinflammatory adipokines, such as adiponectin, and an increase in proinflammatory adipocytokines (i.e., TNF-α, IL-1β, or leptin) and chemokines (i.e., MCP-1) production from adipose tissue. The raised levels of chemokines stimulate macrophage recruitment, which in turn triggers the inflammatory response [38]. In addition, obesity raises B cell number and activates T cells, which promotes the highly proinflammatory M1-like phenotype of macrophages [40].

In addition, obesity involves reactive oxygen species (ROS) overproduction in accumulated adipose tissue accompanied by lower antioxidant defenses, which leads to systemic oxidative stress [41]. There is a strong association between the inflammation triggered in adipose tissue and the increase in oxidative stress. In this sense, local rise of oxidative stress in accumulated fat has been reported to produce a dysregulation in the secretion of adipocytokines [41], which, as stated earlier, plays a pivotal role in the inflammatory response. Moreover, adipose tissue releases adipocytokines including TNF-α, IL-1, and IL-6, which promote increased generation of ROS by immune cells [42], evidencing a strong relationship between both factors.

ROS are highly reactive derivatives of oxygen, including hydrogen peroxide, superoxide radical, and hydroxyl radical, which are found ubiquitously [43]. These molecules are produced by different sources such as peroxisomal fatty acid metabolism, phagocyte cells, cytochrome p450, or the mitochondrial respiratory chain [44]. The organism displays a self-protective antioxidant activity to counteract oxidative damage via endogenously synthesized enzymatic mechanisms (i.e., glutathione peroxidase [GPx], catalase [CAT], superoxide dismutase [SOD]) and nonenzymatic antioxidants (i.e., ascorbic acid, tocopherols, or carotenoids) [45]. In fact, physiological levels of ROS are essential for a number of biological mechanisms, including intracellular messaging and defense against microorganisms among others [43]. However, when ROS production is increased or there is a depression of the antioxidant system, an imbalance between oxidant and antioxidant factors occurs leading to oxidative stress [43]. This oxidative stress is harmful to cellular structures and can also cause an inflammatory response [43].

A number of studies correlate end-products of free radical—mediated oxidative stress with BMI, supporting the idea of obesity-induced oxidative stress [46—48]. In contrast, an inverse association between body fat and antioxidant defense markers in obese subjects has been reported [49]. It should be noted that in chronic obesity, antioxidant sources may be depleted, which is caused by the decreased activity of enzymes including SOD, CAT, and GPx [50]. Furthermore, oxidative stress seems to be an early event in the pathology of metabolic disorders where treatments reducing ROS production ameliorated IR, hyperlipidemia, and hepatic steatosis [41,51]. Moreover, obesity-associated oxidative stress has been found to alter cell and tissue function, such as vascular endothelial cells, pancreatic β cells, or myocytes [46].

There is a strong relationship between oxidative stress and proinflammatory processes. Certain ROS act as second messengers to propagate inflammatory signals and once activated they promote inflammatory status via production of proinflammatory adipocytokines while, as stated earlier, these adipocytokines lead to elevated synthesis of ROS [42].

Concomitant with oxidative stress, there is accumulating evidence highlighting the relevance of the abnormal oxygen tension generated as fat depots expand pathologically [52]. Most authors believe the theory explaining that the tissue enlarges at a higher speed than neovascularization and that the size of hypertrophied adipocytes hinders oxygen diffusion; consequently oxygen tension within the tissue decreases, developing tissue hypoxia [53,54]. On the contrary, other authors believe that oxygen tension increases due to decreased mitochondrial oxygen consumption in the adipocytes from obesity [55].

Whether one option or the other is considered, it seems to be clear that oxygen (low or high) is useful for the treatment of several diseases with inflammatory components [56]. Furthermore, hypoxia has been proposed as a promising therapy for obesity and other related diseases [57], although the results in humans are still not as clear as expected [56].

In this sense, the significance of hypoxia in inflammation is widely accepted for several diseases [58] and for its particular role in obesity and IR among others [59].

In relation with the aforementioned factors, some of the involved adipocytokines that play an important role in the development of a systemic inflammatory state are TNF-α, IL-1β, IL-6, visfatin, resistin, apelin, or adiponectin, to name a few.

TNF-α is a transmembrane protein produced mainly in activated macrophages although it is also released by other cell types such as lymphoid cells, endothelial cells, or cardiac myocytes, among others [60]. TNF-α acts through the activation of two receptors, TNFR1 (TNF type 1 or CD120a) and TNFR2 (TNF type 2 or CD120b) [61], and both TNF-α and its receptors are expressed in WAT [62]. The levels of this cytokine are elevated in obese states [63] and can be reduced by weight loss [64]. TNF-α is implicated in the regulation of processes, including local and systemic inflammation, the immune system as well as apoptosis, and also interferes with the signaling pathway controlling glucose and lipid metabolism [65]. Furthermore, TNF-α signaling leads to ROS production and nuclear factor-κB (NF-κB) activation [66], while hypoxia is also able to activate TNF-α gene promoter and NF-κB in 3T3-L1 adipocytes and NIH3T3 fibroblasts [67].

TNF-α enhances the systemic acute-phase response by increasing IL-6 or plasminogen activator inhibitor-1 (PAI-1) and decreasing the antiinflammatory adiponectin [68].

IL-1β is mostly secreted by monocytes after a tissue injury, immunological challenge, or infection and results in a number of metabolic, inflammatory, immunological, hematological, and physiological effects [69]. Concerning obesity, adipocyte cell death or hypoxia activates the secretion of IL-1α, which initiates the inflammatory cascade, induces IL-1β release that helps maintain the inflammatory process, and downregulates peripheral insulin signaling [70]. IL-1β production is regulated by cytosolic molecular complexes called inflammasomes, which are activated by certain pathogens and diverse stimuli [69]. Interestingly, activation of inflammasome proteins are considerably increased in adipose tissue and liver of obese human and mice and decreased after weight loss in obese T2DM individuals [71,72]. In obesity, the defective autophagy of mitochondria mediated by a decrease of adenosine monophosphate-activated protein kinase (AMPK) activity leads to a higher production of ROS by mitochondria. ROS generation has been suggested to activate nucleotide-binding oligomerization domain, leucine rich repeat and pyrin domain containing 3 (NLRP3) inflammasome leading to an increase in IL-1β release, which, in turn, directly impairs the insulin cascade and promotes production of the proinflammatory response via synthesis of other proinflammatory cytokines including TNF-α or IL-6 and enhanced infiltration of immune cells [72].

Adiponectin, whose reduction plays a key role in obesity-related diseases including IR and cardiovascular disease, is the most abundant protein secreted by adipocytes [73]. It is known to have insulin sensitizing effects and to regulate glucose and lipid metabolism, decreasing lipogenesis and promoting fatty acid oxidation. It exerts potent antiinflammatory and antiatherogenic actions via transformation of macrophages into foam cells, inhibition of adhesion of monocytes to endothelial cells, and reduction of proinflammatory TNF-α and C-reactive protein (CRP) levels as well as elevation of nitric oxide (NO) production in endothelial cells [74]. Some of the molecular mechanisms underlying adiponectin effects on inflammation might be related to direct actions on immune cells that involve a decrease in ROS production, increased expression of the antiinflammatory IL-10, and the suppression of the NF-κB inflammatory signaling pathway [75]. Moreover, adiponectin has been shown to suppress low-density lipoprotein (LDL)-oxidized-induced superoxide generation [76]. It is well documented that adiponectin concentration decreases in obesity and increases after weight loss [77]. This reduction may contribute to the development of IR and cardiovascular disorders [78]. Regarding its regulation, both proinflammatory cytokines, including TNF-α, IL-6, or IL-1β, and high exposition to ROS reduce this adipokine production, being human serum adiponectin levels inversely correlated with systemic oxidative stress [79]. Furthermore, overexpression of adiponectin in obese mice seems to augment angiogenesis and perfusion, within adipose tissue, decreasing tissue hypoxia and increasing the expression of vascular endothelial growth factor-A [80]. This is in line with the fact that adiponectin expression is reduced by hypoxia in murine adipocytes [67].

IL-6 is synthesized by a wide number of cells ranging from adipocytes and macrophages to endothelial cells, immune system cells, fibroblasts, and skeletal muscle cells [44,81] and is highly linked to obesity and IR. This cytokine regulates energy homeostasis and inflammation orchestrating the transition from acute to chronic inflammation by enhancing the production of proinflammatory cytokines and downregulating antiinflammatory mediators [82]. However, it is unclear whether IL-6 plays a harmful or a protective role in this context. Conversely, recent studies have pointed to antiinflammatory effects and even protective actions against IR development. IL-6 levels are directly correlated with the degree of obesity [83] and acute infusion of IL-6 impairs insulin sensitivity in mice [84]. In contrast, deficiency in IL-6 results in adult-onset obesity [85] and hepatic disruption of IL-6 causes resistance to insulin [86]. Moreover, complete blockage of IL-6 may not represent any beneficial effect in mice undergoing a high-fat diet (HFD) feeding [87]. Moreover, inactivation of the IL-6 receptor in myeloid cells results in marked deterioration of diet-induced insulin sensitivity and increased inflammation and macrophage M1 polarization in WAT, BAT, and liver [88]. In addition to this, our group has recently found that those obese people suffering sleep apnea—hypopnea syndrome with a lower oxygen consumption presented a higher secretion and a hypomethylation of IL-6 [89]. Collectively these data may suggest that IL-6 elevated levels in obesity could be the result of a compensatory mechanism.

Inflammation, oxidative stress, and hypoxia in the context of obesity have been hypothesized to play a substantial role in the development and alteration of several highly prevalent diseases including IR/T2DM, cancer, or cardiovascular disease, among others (Fig. 4.3). Obesity is closely associated with the development of IR commonly followed by T2DM. This process implicates several mechanisms including impaired insulin signaling, alterations in glucose transport, pancreatic β cell dysfunction, and increased production of ROS and inflammation [90]. Both IR and T2DM are characterized by hyperglycemia, which leads to an overproduction of ROS [42]. There is evidence indicating that glucose can not only stimulate ROS overproduction but can also activate several enzymatic cascades in mitochondria, such as nicotinamide

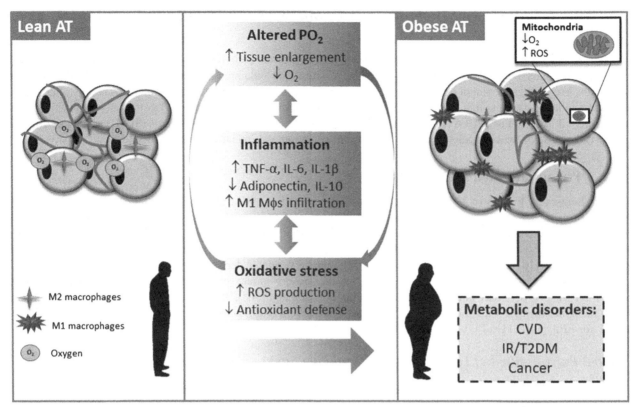

FIGURE 4.3 Inflammation, oxidative stress, and hypoxia occur in adipose tissue during obesity. Oxidative stress, altered PO_2, and inflammation are potential interconnected factors in adipose tissue dysfunction development in obesity, finally leading to associated metabolic disorders. This chronic low-grade inflammation is associated with proinflammatory adipokines release and the concomitant macrophages migration and polarization. Altered PO_2 is related to a tissue enlargement increase at higher speed than neovascularization and to a lower O_2 consumption in mitochondria. Oxidative stress is triggered by an augmented ROS production as well as decreased antioxidant defenses. *CVD*, cardiovascular disease; *IL-1β*, interleukin-1β; *IL-6*, interleukin-6; *IR*, insulin resistance; *Mφs*, macrophages; *O₂*, oxygen; *PO₂*, oxygen tension; *ROS*, reactive oxygen species; *T2DM*, type 2 diabetes mellitus; *TNF-α*, tumor necrosis factor-α.

adenine dinucleotide phosphate (NADPH) oxidase, uncoupling of NO synthases, and stimulation of xanthine oxidase [91]. Oxidative stress may also alter β cell dysfunction by promoting glucolipotoxicity diabetes-associated phenomena [92] and directly impaired insulin signaling in adipocytes [93]. Additionally, the obesity-related chronic inflammation and the altered secretion of key adipocytokines, including TNF-α or adiponectin, contributes to the development of both IR and T2DM [42].

In addition, oxidative stress and a proinflammatory environment are highly implicated in obesity-related conditions that may lead to cardiovascular diseases, including dyslipidemia and hypertension [42]. Dyslipidemia-associated events promote ROS generation including low high-density lipoprotein (HDL) levels as well as elevated triglycerides (TGs) and plasma very low-density lipoprotein (VLDL) [42]. ROS-induced changes in lipid expression may lead to further oxidation-derived products such as oxidative low-density lipoprotein (Ox-LDL), which can play a further critical role in cardio-vascular diseases [94]. There is also an important association between oxidative stress and hypertension. An imbalance in superoxide and NO generation may lead to decreased vasodilation [95]. Other mechanisms involved are the elevated lipid hydroperoxide production [96], the renin-angiotensin-aldosterone system [97], sympathetic nervous system excitation by oxidative stress in the brain [98], and dysfunctional production of adipokines (leptin, adiponectin, ghrelin), cytokines (TNF-α or IL-6), and neuropeptides (α-melanocyte-stimulating hormone and neuropeptide Y) [99].

Furthermore, an association between obesity and both common and less common cancers in many populations worldwide have been described [100]. Particularly rectal and prostate cancers have been associated with BMI in men, and endometrial, gastrointestinal, and postmenopausal breast cancers in women [100]. The suggested mechanisms underlying this association involve genetic factors, insulin/IGF-1 signaling, dysregulated secretion of adipokines and steroid hormones, gut microbiota, IR, hyperinsulinemia, chronic inflammation intimately related to oxidative stress, and altered levels of growth factors [101−103].

4. NUTRITIONAL REGULATION OF INFLAMMATION AND OXIDATIVE STRESS IN OBESITY

It is well documented that high levels of consumption of macronutrients including glucose, saturated fatty acids, or n-6 polyunsaturated fatty acids (n-6 PUFAs) trigger oxidative stress and inflammation through NFκB mediated pathways [104]. Conversely, the selection of other dietary components may simultaneously reduce them. In this context, fatty acids can impact inflammation through a wide range of mechanisms acting from the membrane to the nucleus [105]. In this chapter, we will focus on n-3 PUFAs and their derived specialized proresolving lipid mediators (SPMs) as well as α-lipoic acid (LA), because of their potential to reduce chronic inflammation and oxidative stress associated with obesity.

4.1 n-3 Polyunsaturated Fatty Acids

Omega-3 long-chain PUFAs (n-3 PUFAs) are essential nutrients that can be divided according to their origin, either vegetable or marine. Beneficial effects in several chronic diseases such as cardiovascular disorders or T2DM have been specially attributed to marine origin eicosapentenoic acid (EPA, 20:5) and docosahexaenoic acid (DHA, 22:6) [106], whose main source is fatty fish including salmon, anchovy, sardines, and tuna [21], although they can be also found in krill and marine microalgae [107]. In addition, it has been observed that the vegetable derivative α-linolenic acid (ALA, C18:3) can be converted to EPA and DHA in the organism. However, the conversion rate seems to be poor, so dietary intake of these marine n-3 PUFAs is necessary in order to achieve optimal consumption [108]. This conversion rate depends on gender, in women being between 9.2% and 21% for DHA and EPA, respectively [109], while in men it does not exceed 4% for DHA and 8% for EPA [110,111].

4.1.1 n-3 Polyunsaturated Fatty Acids and Oxidative Stress

As stated earlier, oxidative stress has been identified as a key factor associating obesity with related disorders such as cardiovascular diseases or T2DM. In this sense, the effects of n-3 PUFAs on oxidative stress are still unclear. In spite of the protective effects of these fatty acids on cardiovascular and metabolic diseases, the theoretical concern that the many double bonds of EPA and DHA may lead to an increased unsaturation index once they are incorporated into the membranes and lipoproteins [112] still remains. This could produce higher lipid peroxidation based on the premise that fatty acid oxidizability may be directly associated with the number of double bonds in the fatty acid chain [113]. Even though this could occur in in vitro studies [114], the more complex in vivo systems are influenced by more factors. Indeed, there is substantial evidence that n-3 PUFA effects are more antioxidative than prooxidative either in human trials [115−121] or in animal studies [122,123].

Lipid peroxidation refers to the oxidative degradation of lipids generally located in biological membranes including phospholipids and cholesterol, which propagates free radicals [124]. In order to assess in vivo lipid peroxidation the secondary breakdown products can be quantified. In this sense, F2-isoprostanes have been identified as excellent and highly sensitive biomarkers of in vivo lipid peroxidative damage [124,125]. These compounds are formed in a free radical-dependent manner in cell membranes at the site of free radical attack from arachidonic acid (AA) [125]. Their production has been reported to be altered in many syndromes putatively associated with oxidative stress such as Alzheimer's disease [126].

Some human studies have found no effects on F2-isoprostanes after n-3 PUFA supplementation. In this sense, Petersson et al. [127] reported no effects in urine F2-isoprostanes of individuals suffering from metabolic syndrome after supplementation with 1.24 g/day of n-3 PUFAs for 12 weeks. Similarly, fish oil or krill oil consumption containing either 864 or 543 mg/day of EPA + DHA, respectively, for 7 weeks did not have any effect on urine F2-isoprostanes levels of subjects slightly dyslipidemic [128]. Moreover, some trials administering low doses of EPA + DHA (ranging from 1.24 to 2.4 g/day) described no effects on F2-isoprostanes in human studies [128−131]. However, some investigations have demonstrated that higher doses of n-3 PUFA supplementation reduce plasma and urine F2-isoprostanes in clinical trials [115−121]. For instance, Mori et al. [118,119] indicated that both EPA and DHA at a dose of 4 g/day during 6 weeks equally reduced urine F2-isoprostanes in either overweight, mildly hyperlipidemic men or in treated-hypertensive, T2DM men and women. In fact, the inclusion of one fish meal daily integrated in a low-fat diet for 8 weeks also decreased urine F2-isoprostanes in overweight and dyslipidemic individuals [120]. Furthermore, Barden et al. [115] also showed that fish oil supplementation (4 g/day) during pregnancy resulted in reduced neonates cord plasma F2-isoprostanes.

Some trials observed decreased malondialdehyde (MDA) plasma levels [116,132], increased antioxidative enzymes expression (i.e., CAT, glutathione [GSH], glutathione reductase [GR], GPx, and heme oxygenase 2 [HMOX2]) [133] as well as greater antioxidant capacity [134] after n-3 PUFA supplementation. In contrast, other studies have found no effects of n-3 PUFAs on LDL oxidative susceptibility [135,136] and plasma α-tocopherol concentration [121,128,130,131]. It is difficult to describe the main reason causing discrepant results, given the wide range of doses, differential populations, and duration of treatments as well as the diversity of biomarkers analyzed.

Actually, it remains controversial whether n-3 PUFAs may increase oxidative stress instead of reducing it. Some studies showed even increased lipid peroxidation after n-3 PUFA supplementation [137−143]. Egert et al. [137] reported that fish oil supplementation to male and female led to higher lipid peroxidation by-product thiobarbituric acid reactive substance (TBARS) levels. Nevertheless, it is important to mention that these studies utilized methods that required ex vivo sample preparation (MDA, lipid hydroxides, and oxidation of LDL), which may cause an ex vivo introduction of lipid peroxidation [124].

There are a limited number of studies evaluating the effects of n-3 PUFAs on obesity-induced oxidative stress. As shown in Table 4.1, recent investigations in HFD-induced obese animal models suggest that n-3 PUFA supplementation may increase the activity and levels of antioxidant enzymes [144−146] and decrease ROS production [146]. However, the n-3 PUFA's particular effect on adipose tissue is still unknown. In this context, Molinar-Toribio et al. [122] found that oral administration of n-3 PUFAs at a ratio EPA:DHA 1:1 to spontaneous hypertensive obese rats was able to increase SOD activity in abdominal fat among other tissues as well as decrease urine F2-isoprostanes. In addition, glucose-induced NADPH oxidase activity was inhibited by DHA treatment (250 μM) in 3T3-L1 adipocytes [147].

The mechanism by which oxidative stress is reduced following n-3 PUFA administration is still unresolved, but it is hypothesized that these effects may occur through immunomodulation and decreased leukocyte activation. In this sense, it is known that activated immune cells produce cytokines (i.e., TNF-α or IL-6) that consequently promote ROS generation [42]. Interestingly, numerous studies have demonstrated n-3 PUFA's ability to diminish cytokine production [21]. Moreover, fatty acids may act as antioxidant as a superoxide scavenger in an unsaturation-dependent manner, thus EPA and DHA being more effective given their high unsaturation level [148]. Additionally, EPA and DHA can replace AA into cell membranes decreasing AA concentration [149], which serves as a precursor of F2-isoprostanes. Finally, n-3 PUFAs have been seen to increase cellular concentrations and activity of antioxidant enzymes including CAT, GSH, GR, GPx, and HMOX2 [122,133,145] and to decrease cytochrome p450 enzymes [133].

4.1.2 n-3 Polyunsaturated Fatty Acids and Inflammation

A growing body of evidence has shown that n-3 PUFAs ameliorate adipose tissue inflammation in obese rodents and humans through different mechanisms, including reduction of proinflammatory adipocytokines and increase of antiinflammatory mediators from adipose tissue as well as decrease of M1-macrophage infiltration [21].

Regarding human studies, the literature shows contradictory results. It is clear that n-3 PUFAs generally have no effect on inflammatory markers in healthy subjects [150]. Contrariwise, some reports on individuals with obesity and features of MetS have described that dietary supplementation with n-3 PUFAs with doses ranging from 2 to 7.5 g/day can help to ameliorate the chronic inflammatory state associated with obesity by decreasing serum proinflammatory mediators such as MCP-1, IL-6, or CRP [151−154], as well as increasing adiponectin and IL-10 levels, considered antiinflammatory [155,156]. However, some trials reported no effect on the inflammatory markers evaluated [155,157−161]. Interestingly, Mori et al. [118] showed that after a 6-week intervention in hypertensive and T2DM individuals supplemented with 4 g/day of purified EPA or DHA, inflammatory markers remained unchanged but urine F2-isoprostanes levels were reduced. This may suggest that n-3 PUFA effects may act through a reduction of oxidative stress previous to the antiinflammatory effects.

Additionally, studies in animal models of obesity mostly confirm the downregulatory actions of n-3 PUFAs on proinflammatory adipocytokines, reducing plasma levels and adipose tissue expression of these cytokines either when orally [162] or intraperitoneally injected [163,164] or as a replacement of dietary lipids in the diet [165] (see Table 4.2). In addition, trials in leptin-deficient *ob/ob* and leptin receptor−deficient *db/db* obese mice fed with n-3 PUFA enriched diets found increased serum adiponectin levels [165,166] or adipose tissue mRNA expression [167], although the expression/plasma levels of proinflammatory cytokines, including IL-6 or TNF-α, were not affected. Similar upregulatory effects in serum adiponectin were found in HFD fed mice supplemented with n-3 PUFA concentrate concomitant to a reduction in leptin levels [168].

Furthermore, it has been proposed that n-3 PUFAs may act at the adipose tissue level, reducing the production of chemoattractant proteins and the infiltration of proinflammatory macrophages. Although some human trials have reported no effect on plasma levels of MCP-1, intercellular adhesion molecule (ICAM)-1, vascular cell adhesion molecule (VCAM)-1, and E-selectin [152,157], another trial has shown that supplementation with 4 g/day of fish oil capsules

TABLE 4.1 General Effects of n-3 Polyunsaturated Fatty Acids on Oxidative Stress in Animal Models of Obesity

Study	Model	n-3 PUFA and Dose	Duration (weeks)	Effects on Oxidative Stress Biomarkers
[257]	2-month-old male Ldlr(−/−) mice fed western diet	Replacement of 2% of total energy with either EPA, DHA, or EPA + DHA	16	↓ Hepatic expression of several NADPH oxidase subunits (Nrf2, Hmox1, p22phox, p40phox, p47phox, p67phox)
[146]	8-week-old male apoE-deficient (apoE2/2) mice fed HFD	Replacement of fat with 10% (w/w) fish oil (total EPA and DHA content 64.08 g/kg of diet)	8	↓ ROS production
[122]	11–14-week-old female spontaneously hypertensive (SHR) obese rats	EPA/DHA at rates 1:1; 2:1; 1:2 (0.8 mL/kg BW)	13	*EPA/DHA 1:1* ↑ Plasma LDL-oxidized ↑ SOD activity in erythrocytes, kidneys, abdominal fat, heart, and brain ↑ GR activity in kidney ↑ GPx in kidney *EPA/DHA 2:1* ↑ Plasma LDL-oxidized ↑ SOD activity in kidneys and heart ↑ CAT activity in erythrocytes, kidneys, and heart ↑ GR activity in kidney ↑ GPx in erythrocytes and kidney ↓ Urine 2,3-dinor-15-F2t-IsoP *EPA/DHA 1:2* ↑ Plasma LDL-oxidized ↓ SOD activity in heart ↓ CAT activity in heart ↓ Urine 15-F2t-IsoP, 2,3-dinor-15-F2t-IsoP, 5-F2t-IsoP, 5-F2c-IsoP and 8-F2t-IsoP
[144]	7-week-old male C57BL/6J mice fed HFD	Oral administration of EPA once per day (1 g/kg/day)	12	↑ Hepatic SOD activity ↑ Hepatic GSH content
[258]	13-week-old male C57BL/6J mice fed HFD	Replacement of 5% with EPA or DHA	4	↓ Hepatic HEL, a marker for early stage of lipid oxidation ↓ Hepatic 8-OHdG ↔ SOD expression
[145]	9-week-old female ICR/CD1 mice fed HFD	Diet supplemented with 3 g of EPA and DHA per kg of HFD	6	↑ GSH levels ↑ CAT activity ↓ XO activity

8-OHdG, 8-hydroxy-2′-deoxyguanosine; CAT, catalase; DHA, docosahexenoic acid; EPA, eicosapentenoic acid; GPx, glutathione peroxidase; GR, glutathione reductase; GSH, glutathione; HEL, hexanoyl-lysine; HFD, high-fat diet; ICR, institute of cancer research; IsoP, isoprostane; LDL, low-density lipoprotein; NADPH, nicotinamide adenine dinucleotide phosphate; PUFA, polyunsaturated fatty acid; ROS, reactive oxygen species; SOD, superoxide dismutase; XO, xanthine oxidase.

TABLE 4.2 Effects of n-3 Polyunsaturated Fatty Acids on Adipose Tissue Inflammation in Murine Models of Obesity

Study	Model	n-3 PUFA and Dose	Duration	Effects on Inflammation
[165]	7-week-old male db/db mice fed with HFD	Purified marine n-3 PUFAs (Reesterified to triglycerides) replacing 40% of oil volume	6 weeks	↑ Serum adiponectin ↔ Serum MCP-1 and IL-6 ↓ Serum CRP ↓ Gonadal WAT F4/80 stained macrophage infiltration ↓ Gonadal and subcutaneous WAT expression of MCP-1, CD68, and CD11b
[162]	6-week-old male Wistar rats fed with control or cafeteria diet	EPA ethyl ester (1 g/kg body weight daily; oral gavage)	35 days	↑ Serum leptin in cafeteria-fed rats ↑ Leptin mRNA expression in eWAT ↔ Serum adiponectin ↔ Adiponectin mRNA expression in eWAT ↓ TNF-α mRNA expression in eWAT
[259]				↔ Haptoglobin mRNA expression and serum levels ↓ IL-6 mRNA in eWAT
[166]	6-week-old male C57BL/6J ob/ob mice	Fish meal–free diet supplemented with 5% EPA (wt/wt)	5 weeks	↔ TNF-α and adiponectin mRNA expression in WAT ↑ Serum adiponectin ↑ Epididymal WAT F4/80 stained macrophage infiltration
[171]	3-month-old male C57BL/6N mice fed HFD 4 months prior treatment	DHA (α-ethyl DHA ester) replaced 1.5% of dietary lipids	2 months	↓ Serum leptin and adiponectin ↓MCP-1 mRNA expression in WAT ↓ eWAT MAC-2 immunoreactive macrophages ↓CD68 mRNA expression in WAT
	3-month-old male C57BL/6N and C57BL/6J mice fed HFD	DHA (α-ethyl DHA ester) replaced 1.5% of dietary lipids	4 months	↓ MAC-2 immunoreactive macrophages in eWAT
[167]	Male ob/ob mice	n-3 PUFA-enriched diet (6% of total lipid content)	5 weeks	↑ Adiponectin mRNA expression ↔ Resistin, TNF-α, MCP-1, and IL-6 mRNA expression
[260]	5–6-week-old male C57BL/6J mice fed HFD	EPA ethyl ester (36 g/kg diet [wt/wt])	11 weeks	↓PAI-1, MCP-1 WAT expression ↑ Plasma total adiponectin
	5–6-week-old male C57BL/6J mice fed HFD 6 weeks prior treatment		5 weeks	↓PAI-1 WAT expression ↑ Plasma total adiponectin
[168]	2-month-old male C57BL/6N mice fed HFD	n-3 PUFAs concentrate (46% wt/wt DHA, 14% wt/wt EPA) replacing 15% of dietary lipids	5 weeks	↓ Serum leptin ↑ Serum adiponectin ↔ Serum IL-6 ↔ Macrophage infiltration in eWAT
[164]	7-week-old male C57BL/6J fed HFD for 12 weeks	DHA intraperitoneal injection (4 μg/g body weight)	10 days	↓ MCP-1-α mRNA expression in eWAT ↓ IL-6 and TNF-α mRNA expression in SVC ↔ Macrophages recruitment in eWAT

Continued

TABLE 4.2 Effects of n-3 Polyunsaturated Fatty Acids on Adipose Tissue Inflammation in Murine Models of Obesity—cont'd

Study	Model	n-3 PUFA and Dose	Duration	Effects on Inflammation
[170]	3-month-old male C57BL/6N mice fed HFD with 2 g metformin per kg diet	Supplementation with 30 g DHA/EPA per kg diet	9 weeks	↑ M2 markers Arg1, CD206, Ym1, and IL-10 mRNA expression in eWAT
[261]	6-week-old C57BL/6J mice fed HFD 4 weeks prior treatment	DHA (100 mg/kg) twice a week	6 weeks	↓ MAC-2 immunoreactive macrophages in eWAT ↓ MCP-1 mRNA expression in eWAT ↓ Inflammasome activation in liver and WAT ↓ IL-1β, IL-8, TNF-α, and MCP-1 expression in liver and WAT
[173]	6-week-old male C57BL/6J mice fed HFD	Diet enriched with EPA and DHA (EPAX 1050-TG)	12 weeks	↔ TNF-α, MCP-1 and IL-6 mRNA expression in WAT ↑ Epididymal and mesenchymal WAT F4/80 stained macrophage infiltration ↑ M1 marker CD11c ↑ M2 marker CD206
[169]	Male C57BL/6 fed HFD	15% of fat from the HF diet replaced by EPA ethyl ester	11 weeks	↓ MCP-1 protein in eWAT ↓ Leptin mRNA expression in eWAT ↓ Macrophage infiltration in eWAT
	Male C57BL/6 fed HFD 6 weeks prior treatment		5 weeks	↓ Macrophage infiltration in eWAT
[262]	18- to 24-week-old male or female Elovl2−/− mice	DHA-enriched diet (10% kcal fat, 1% DHA)	3 months	↓ M1 marker CD86 ↑ M2 marker CD206
[163]	7-week-old male C57BL/6J mice fed HFD during 3 months prior treatment	DHA intraperitoneal injection (4 µg/g body weight)	10 days	↔ Serum adiponectin and leptin ↓ F4/80 immunostained macrophages in eWAT ↓ IL-1β and TNF-α mRNA expression in eWAT ↔ MCP-1, IL-6, and adiponectin mRNA expression in eWAT ↓ M1 marker CD11c mRNA expression in eWAT ↔ M2 marker CD163 mRNA expression in eWAT
[172]	3-4 week-old male C57BL/6J mice fed HFD	100 mg/kg n-3 PUFAs from either fish oil, microalgae oil with low DHA purity, or microalgae oil with high DHA purity	16 weeks	↓ eWAT macrophage infiltration

CD, cluster of differentiation; CRP, C-reactive protein; DHA, docosahexenoic acid; EPA, eicosapentenoic acid; eWAT, epididymal white adipose tissue; HFD, high-fat diet; IL, interleukin; MAC-2, macrophage-2 antigen/galectin-3; MCP-1, monocyte chemoattractant protein-1; PPARγ, peroxisome proliferator-activated receptor γ; PUFA, polyunsaturated fatty acid; SVC, stromal vascular cells; TNF-α, tumor necrosis factor-α; WAT, white adipose tissue.

reduced plasma MCP-1 and adipose tissue expression of both MCP-1 and CD68, decreasing the formation of adipose tissue crown-like structures [153]. This is in agreement with a number of animal studies that observed a decrease in adipose tissue macrophage infiltration [163,165,169−172] occasionally accompanied by a decrease in the expression of the chemoattractant protein MCP-1 and CD68 [165,169,171]. In contrast, other studies suggested that n-3 PUFA supplementation had no effects [164,168] or even increased macrophage infiltration [166,173]. It is important to mention that n-3 PUFA antiinflammatory effects have been also attributed to their capacity to polarize to an M2 macrophage antiinflammatory phenotype. In fact, Titos et al. [164] showed that intraperitoneal injection of DHA (4 μg/g, 10 days) in HFD-induced obese mice was able to promote a polarization of macrophages to the antiinflammatory M2 phenotype, although the number of WAT macrophages remained unchanged. This is in accordance with other studies that reported a switch toward an M2 phenotype in murine models of obesity treated with either EPA [169] or DHA [163].

In addition, there is evidence of beneficial effects of n-3 PUFAs on adipose tissue inflammation via regulation of different transcription factors, pattern recognition receptors, and intracellular signaling pathways. NF-κB is a key proinflammatory transcription factor that is involved in the upregulation of proinflammatory cytokines, adhesion molecules, and cyclooxygenase (COX)-2 genes [174,175]. The cytosolic inactive form is activated after inflammatory stimuli through a signaling cascade that involves phosphorylation of an inhibitory subunit IκB. EPA treatment is able to inhibit NF-κB activation in adipocytes [176,177]. Similarly, DHA exerts downregulatory actions on macrophages NF-kB activation [178−180], which leads to reduced expression of different genes including NLRP3, a component of the central regulators of innate immunity inflammasome. Additionally, n-3 PUFAs are naturally occurring ligands of a family of transcription factors called peroxisome proliferator-activated receptors (PPARs) that in conjunction with liver X receptors and sterol regulatory element binding proteins (SREBPs) play a critical role in the regulation of fat metabolism and adipocyte proliferation and differentiation [181] as well as in the release of inflammatory mediators and macrophage infiltration into adipose tissue [182].

Moreover, it has been suggested that n-3 PUFAs decrease the expression of toll-like receptors (TLRs) and nucleotide-binding oligomerization domain proteins (NODs), which may contribute to their antiinflammatory actions. These proteins recognize pathogen-associated molecular patterns activating a downstream signaling cascade that promotes host-defense proinflammatory pathways (i.e., c-Jun N-terminal kinases [JNKs], I kappa B kinase (IKK) as well as transcription factors (i.e., NF-κB) [183]. N-3 PUFAs are known to inhibit SFA and lipopolysaccharide-induced activation of TLR2 and TLR4 [184−186]. These effects may be mediated by the inhibition of the dimerization and recruitment of TLR-4 into lipid drafts, which trigger TLR-4 signaling [186].

Even though a number of studies support the antiinflammatory role of n-3 PUFAs, there are conflicting results that make it complicated to define the efficacy, dose, and type of formula of n-3 PUFA supplementation required to ameliorate the inflammatory response in humans. Further studies are needed to clarify all these issues.

4.1.3 n-3 Polyunsaturated Fatty Acid-Derived Specialized Proresolving Lipid Mediators

Importantly, Serhan and collaborators found that n-3 PUFAs are substrates for the formation of specialized proresolving lipid mediators [187].

Thus n-3 PUFAs can be enzymatically converted into potent antiinflammatory and proresolving lipid mediators that act as braking signals of inflammatory response as well as facilitators of timely resolution of inflammation at nanomolar and even picomolar range [188]. Some of these SPMs include maresins (MaRs), resolvins (RvDs), and protectins (PDs) derived from n-3 PUFAs, or lipoxin (LX) A4, derived from n-6 PUFAs. These SPMs are mainly produced from the release to the cytoplasm of cellular membrane components by phospholipases where COX and lipoxygenase readily converts these free PUFAs into their mediators [188].

Accumulating evidence shows an unbalanced production of some of these n-3 PUFAs-derived lipid mediators including RvD1, PD1, 14-hydroxy-docosahexaenoic acid (HDHA), 17-HDHA and 18-hydroxy-eicosapentaenoic acid in WAT of obese db/db mice and in HFD-induced obese mice [189,190]. In this sense, Titos et al. [191] reported significantly lower levels of the ratios between SPMs (i.e., RvD and E series, PD1, LXs, and MaR1) and AA-derived proinflammatory mediators leukotriene B4 (LTB4) and prostaglandins (PGs) in visceral adipose tissue of obese subjects. This SPM deficit in obesity is not limited to adipose tissue since it has been also observed in muscle, liver, and cutaneous wounds [192,193]. These data suggest that the dysregulated production of SPMs may be associated to an impaired tissue resolution capacity.

In recent years a number of studies have focused on SPM effects on obesity-associated inflammation, which are summarized in Table 4.3. In this sense, RvD1 effects on obesity-related inflammation in vivo were first reported by Hellmann et al. [194], who found that intraperitoneal injection of 2 μg/kg of RvD1 for 8−16 days was able to ameliorate adipose tissue inflammation, decrease macrophage infiltration, and promote a switch toward the antiinflammatory

TABLE 4.3 Specialized Proresolving Lipid Mediator Effects on Inflammatory Markers in Animal Models of Obesity

SPM	Animal Model of Obesity	Treatment (Dose, Administration Method, & Duration)	Inflammatory Outcomes	References
RvE1	Male *ob/ob* mice	1.2 ng/g b.w. (i.p. injection) every 24 h during 4 days	↑ Adiponectin and PPARγ expression in WAT; ↓ F40/80 stained macrophages in liver	[167]
RvD1	8-week-old male *db/db* mice	2 µg/kg b.w. (i.p. injection) for 8–16 days	↑ Adiponectin production in WAT; ↓ IL-6 expression in WAT; ↓ Crown-like structures rich in inflammatory F4/80 + CD11c + macrophages in WAT; ↑ F4/80 + cells expressing MGL-1	[194]
RvD1	6-week-old male C57BL/6J mice HFD for 12 weeks	300 ng (i.p. injection) every 24 h during 3 weeks + calorie restriction	↑ Serum adiponectin; ↑ Hepatic IL-4 and IL-10; ↓ Hepatic JNK phosphorylation; ↓ Hepatic F4/80 + macrophages	[195]
17-HDHA	10-week-old male C57BL/6J mice fed HFD for 17 weeks	50 ng/g b.w. intraperitoneal injection every 12 h during 8 days, or continuous application for 15 days	↓ Expression of MCP-1, TNF-α, IL-6, NF-κB and osteopontin in WAT; ↑ Adiponectin, PPARγ and PPARα expression in WAT; ↓ M1/M2 macrophage phenotype ratio in WAT	[190]
PDX	14-week-old male *db/db* mice	1 µg (i.p. injection) 2.5 h immediately before the 6-h lipid infusion	↑ IL-6 expression in skeletal muscle; ↑ AMPK phosphorylation in skeletal muscle; ↓ CCL-5 and TNF-α in plasma; ↓ Hepatic JNK phosphorylation	[197]
MaR1	8-week-old male *ob/ob* mice	2 µg/kg b.w. (i.p. injection) daily during 20 days	↓ MCP-1, IL-1β, and TNF-α expression in eWAT; ↑ Adiponectin expression in eWAT; ↔ F4/80 + expressing macrophages in eWAT; ↑ M2 phenotype markers CD163 and IL-10 expression in eWAT	[163]
	7-week-old male C57BL/6J mice HFD for 3 months	2 µg/kg b.w. (i.p. injection) daily during 10 days	↓ MCP-1, IL-1β, and TNF-α expression in eWAT; ↑ Adiponectin expression in eWAT; ↑ F4/80 + expressing macrophages in eWAT; ↓ M1 phenotype marker CD11c expression in eWAT	
LXA$_4$	6-week-old C57BL/6J mice fed HFD for 12 weeks	5 ng/g (i.p. injection) three times per week during 7 weeks	↓ CD11c + M1 proinflammatory macrophages in WAT; ↑ CD206 + antiinflammatory macrophages in WAT; ↓ TNF-α expression in WAT; ↔ IL-6 or adiponectin expression in WAT	[196]

17-HDHA, 17-hydroxy docosahexenoic acid; AMPK, AMP-activated protein kinase; b.w., body weight; CCL5, C–C motif chemokine ligand 5; CD, cluster of differentiation; eWAT, epididymal white adipose tissue; HFD, high-fat diet; IL, interleukin; i.p., intraperitoneal; JNK, c-Jun N-terminal kinase; LXA$_4$, lipoxin A4; MaR1, maresin 1; MCP-1, monocyte chemoattractant protein-1; MGL-1, macrophage galactose-type lectin-1; NK-κB, nuclear factor-κB; PDX, protectin DX; PPARγ, peroxisome proliferator-activated receptor γ; RvD1, resolvin D1; RvE1, resolvin E1; SPM, specialized proresolving lipid mediator; TNF-α, tumor necrosis factor-α; WAT, white adipose tissue.

phenotype (M2) in adipose tissue macrophages associated with reduced IL-6 expression and increased adiponectin expression in WAT in *db/db* mice. This was accompanied by an improved glucose tolerance, decreased fasting blood glucose, and increased insulin-stimulated Akt phosphorylation in adipose tissue. Another study also reported that treatment with RvD1 in HFD-induced obese mice in combination with a calorie restricted diet was able to decrease hepatic macrophage infiltration and JNK pathway activation as well as to increase the antiinflammatory IL-10 expression in liver and serum adiponectin levels [195]. Furthermore, the therapeutic potential of RvD1 was corroborated in fat explants from human visceral WAT from obese patients in which RvD1 enhanced inflammatory resolution by blocking STAT1, its target inflammatory genes (i.e., CXCL9), and persistent STAT3 activation as well as promoting the expression of the IL-10 target gene HMOX-1b [191]. In this sense, RvD1 precursor 17-HDHA administration to *db/db* mice also reduce the expression of proinflammatory mediators such as MCP-1, TNF-α, IL-6, and NF-κB and increased adiponectin, PPARγ, and PPARα expression in WAT [190]. Besides, although no effects were reported on the number of crown-like structures in WAT, the ratio between M1/M2 macrophage phenotype was significantly reduced by 17-HDHA treatment supporting the notion that SPMs target tissue macrophages, skewing the phenotype to a proresolutive state [190]. The concept that SPMs exert modulatory actions on macrophage recruitment and phenotype is also supported by a study from our group that found decreased macrophage accumulation and lower M1 markers in WAT of HFD-induced obese mice treated with MaR1 [163]. Interestingly, although MaR1 did not reduce macrophage number in WAT of *ob/ob* mice, M2 markers such as CD163 and IL-10 expression were increased concomitantly with a decrease in the expression of MCP-1, IL-1β, and TNF-α and an increase in adiponectin expression in WAT [163]. These results were in agreement with those reported by Börgeson et al. [196], showing the ability of LXA₄ to promote this switch in WAT macrophages to proresolutive M2 phenotype in parallel with a reduction of TNF-α expression. Given that the majority of macrophages recruited in obese WAT are M1 type, these results strongly support the proresolutive actions of SPMs in obese WAT.

Otherwise, the EPA-derived resolvin E 1 (RvE1) treatment was reported to decrease liver macrophage infiltration in obese *ob/ob* mice, and to increase adiponectin and PPARγ expression in WAT although the proinflammatory adipocytokines TNF-α, IL-6, or MCP-1 remained unchanged [167]. In addition, intravenous PDX administration reduced lipid-induced chemokine (C–C motif) ligand (CCL)-5 and TNF-α plasma levels as well as hepatic JNK pathway activation, although it did not have any impact on adipose tissue inflammation in obese diabetic *db/db* mice [197].

In summary, persistent inflammation in adipose tissue has been suggested to be triggered by an impaired resolution capacity, which, in turn, is likely the consequence of an intrinsic compromised ability to generate the appropriate levels of SPMs in WAT. In this sense, strategies attempt to enhance local SPMs production or exogenous administration of these lipid mediators, which is of great interest in the context of obesity. However, more research will be needed to further elucidate the best approach.

4.2 α-Lipoic Acid: Antioxidant Properties and Beyond

α-LA (thioctic acid, 5-(1,2-dithiolan-3-yl) pentanoic acid; α-LA) is an organosulfur compound, a small molecule (eight carbons; 206.3 g/mol) that contains two oxidized or reduced thiol groups and a single chiral center, an asymmetric carbon, which results in two possible optical isomers: R-α-LA and S-α-LA. α-LA is found naturally in mitochondria, where it acts as the coenzyme for several bioenergetic enzymes such as pyruvate dehydrogenase and α-ketoglutarate dehydrogenase [198]. Both α-LA and its reduced dithiol form, dihydrolipoic acid (DHLA), are powerful antioxidants. Thus, α-LA scavenges hydrogen peroxide, single oxygen, hydroxyl radical, NO radical, and peroxynitrite, and has the capacity to reduce the oxidized forms of several important antioxidants, including glutathione and vitamins C and E. α-LA may also chelate redox-active metals, such as free iron, copper, manganese, and zinc. Together, these properties make α-LA a potentially highly effective therapeutic antioxidant [199]. α-LA can be found in different food sources such as vegetables (i.e., spinach, tomato, broccoli, Brussels sprouts, and rice bran), red meat, and entrails (e.g., liver and kidney) [199]. However, although this molecule is present in food, the dietary intake is unable to provide substantial amounts of α-LA in the bloodstream (2.6 mg/g dry weight, the highest concentration of lipoyllysine detected in beef kidney). For supplementation therapy, α-LA is normally used as a racemic mixture of the R and S forms synthesized in the laboratory [200].

Interestingly, it has been reported that α-LA can be also synthesized endogenously by the lipoic acid synthase (LASY) in mammals from octanoic acid. This is a mitochondrial enzyme directly responsible for important cellular functions such as the maintenance of the antioxidant defense network and mitochondrial function or of decreasing inflammation. LASY deficiency has been linked to serious conditions such as diabetes, atherosclerosis, and neonatal-onset epilepsy [201].

As a nutraceutical compound, α-LA administration at the regular doses administered (600–1200 g/day) is safe due to its very low toxicity. After its oral administration, α-LA is rapidly absorbed and taken up by cells in a pH-dependent manner mediated by two carrier proteins, the monocarboxylate transporter and the Na^+-dependent multivitamin transporter (SMVT) [202].

In fact, given that α-LA is a safe and effective therapy, it has been successfully used as a therapeutic agent for over 60 years in the treatment of diabetic neuropathy, peripheral artery disease, and various skin and liver diseases [203]. In humans, the greatest dose administered in clinical trials were within the ALADIN (I, II, and III), SYDNEY (I and II), and ORPIL trials that used α-LA supplements up to 2400 mg/day with no reported adverse effects versus placebo [200]. Other studies reported that only in some isolated cases and after a high dose (1200−1800 mg/day), transient gastrointestinal problems and itching sensation appeared after α-LA treatment [204−206].

4.2.1 α−Lipoic Acid and Obesity: Evidence From Animal Studies and Human Trials

In addition to the systemic antioxidant and antiinflammatory properties described for α-LA [207,208], there is large and growing evidence in rodents supporting the beneficial effects of α-LA supplementation in the treatment of obesity [209]. Some trials in humans have also proposed that α-LA could be a promising nutraceutical therapy against obesity and obesity-related disorders [204−206].

In this chapter, we will focus on analyzing studies in animals and humans showing that α-LA targets adipose tissue and the mechanisms through which α-LA could ameliorate adipose tissue dysfunction in obesity.

Several studies have been carried out aiming to demonstrate the putative beneficial effects of α-LA on obese animal models. Although many of them evidenced body weight loss and/or adiposity lowering effects, others reported very mild or even no effects. The antiobesity effects of α-LA were first described in a study involving different experimental models of obesity in rodents [210]. Thus dietary supplementation with α-LA (0.25%, 0.5% and 1% w/w of diet) for 2 weeks caused a dose-dependent reduction on food intake and body weight in rats fed on a standard diet. More importantly, the anorexigenic and body fat lowering actions of α-LA supplementation (0.5% w/w, 14−28 weeks) were also observed in models of genetically obese and diabetic rats such as the Otsuka Long-Evans Tokushima Fatty rats [210,211]. Interestingly, the antiobesity properties of α-LA are independent of leptin or leptin receptor signaling since the reduction in food intake and fat mass was also observed in leptin deficient (*ob/ob*) or leptin receptor−deficient (*db/db*) mice [210], and in the obese Zucker rats, a recessive trait (*fa/fa*) of the leptin receptor [212]. In fact, the anorexigenic effects of α-LA are mediated by direct actions on hypothalamic AMPK, a key enzyme that integrates nutritional and hormonal signals and modulates feeding behavior and energy expenditure. Indeed, the activation of hypothalamic AMPK reverses the effects of α-LA on food intake and energy expenditure in rodents [210]. Other studies have provided evidence that dietary supplementation with α-LA (0.25%−0.5% w/w, 8 weeks) is able to prevent the body weight gain and increased adiposity induced by HFD consumption [209,213]. The inclusion of *pair-fed* groups in some of the previously mentioned studies and the finding that α-LA-treated animals weighed significantly less than the *pair-feds* revealed that α-LA, in addition to reduced energy intake, also promotes energy expenditure [210,213].

α-LA antiobesity effects have been also observed in C57BL/6J nondiabetic mice (300 mg/kg of b.w., 9 weeks; 1% w/w, 10 weeks; and 0.23% w/v in drinking water, 9 weeks), and after streptozotocin/nicotinamide treatment (diabetic-induced mice; 200 mg/kg of b.w., 4 weeks) fed on an HFD [214,215]. Interestingly, α-LA reversed HFD deleterious effects not only in adipose tissue weight, but also in immune system by ameliorating T cell oxidative stress [216] and in the central system improving synaptic connections and brain glucose metabolism [217].

Other studies have revealed the efficacy of α-LA treatment on body weight regulation when administered by injection. Thus intraperitoneal injection of α-LA (30 mg/kg b.w.) during 8 weeks to ALS/Lt mice, a T2D mouse model, inhibited progression of T2D, reducing body weight gain and adiposity [218]. Ovariectomy-induced obese rats mediated by estrogen deficiency also showed a downregulation in body weight gain and adiposity, accompanied by a reduction in food intake, after intraperitoneal treatment with α-LA (200 mg/kg b.w., 7 weeks) [217].

However, there are studies reporting neutral effects on body weight after α-LA administration. In this context, the study of Banday et al. [219] in obese Zucker rats showed no effect on body weight or food intake after dietary supplementation with 0.4% α-LA for 2 weeks, although beneficial effects on parameters associated with obesity onset such as oxidative stress were observed. The study of Cummings et al. [220] in the T2D model UC Davis (UCD)-T2DM rats revealed that dietary α-LA supplementation (80 mg/kg b.w., 8 weeks) delayed diabetes onset in fructose-fed animals, without affecting body weight and fat depot weights, or food intake. Furthermore, no anorexigenic and body lowering effects were found in obese Zucker rats treated i.p. with α-LA (92 or 30 mg/kg b.w. for 22 and 2 weeks, respectively), but a marked downregulation in muscle triglyceride accumulation and oxidative damage was observed [221,222].

Some trials in overweight/obese subjects have also reported antiobesity effects of α-LA supplementation, based on the observations of decreased body weight and/or fat mass, as well as some lipid and glucose metabolism biomarkers.

However, other trials did not observe any significant change on anthropometric parameters [223]. Also, it is important to note that the differential effects of the treatments with α-LA observed in the different trials in humans are possibly affected not only by the baseline metabolic characteristics of the subjects, but also by the route of administration and the diet followed during treatment. Therefore, further clinical trials are needed to better characterize the potential therapeutic efficacy of α-LA as an antiobesity candidate in humans.

4.2.2 α–Lipoic Acid Actions in Adipose Tissue: Mechanisms of Action

4.2.2.1 α–Lipoic Acid, Inflammation, and Oxidative Stress

As previously described, expanded dysfunctional adipose tissue in obesity is associated with increased ROS, which leads to impaired adipogenesis, macrophage recruitment and activation, the secretion of inflammatory adipokines, and the damage of biological structures [224]. Based on its antioxidant properties, several studies have suggested that α–LA could help to alleviate the cross-promotion of oxidative stress and inflammation that occurs in obesity, disrupting the feed-forward cycle that can initiate and advance the pathogenesis and progression of obesity-related disorders [225].

Indeed, alleviation of inflammation and oxidative stress in adipose tissue [226] has been proposed as a mechanism by which α-LA appears to ameliorate obesity and related comorbidities. Thus studies in Zucker diabetic fatty rats proposed that the ability of α-LA in preventing body weight gain is a consequence, at least in part, of the prevention of oxidative stress caused by NADPH oxidase activity in adipose tissue [208]. Moreover, in vitro studies in 3T3-L1 adipocytes also suggested that the protective effects of α-LA against the development of IR might be achieved by decreasing oxidative stress [227,228]. In fact, it was described that the α-LA-mediated amelioration of oxidative stress in these cells would cause an increase in glucose transport and accelerate the decline in immunoreactive insulin (biologically active fraction) during incubation in 3T3-L1 cells [227]. The mechanisms proposed for α-LA protection against oxidative stress—induced IR seem not to be mediated by actions on the insulin receptor substrate 1 (IRS1), a well-known molecule involved in oxidative stress—mediated IR, but on actions on increased protein kinase B/Akt activation and on the insulin-stimulated glucose transporter 4 (GLUT4) translocation to plasma membrane [228,229].

In addition to the reported effects on oxidative stress, α-LA showed beneficial effects in ameliorating adipose tissue inflammation. Thus, α-LA counteracted the effects of LPS injection by downregulating the gene expression of several inflammation markers (TLR2, TLR4, NF-κB p65, TNF-α, IL-1α, IL-1β, and IL-6) in mice visceral adipose tissue [207]. In the same line, α-LA decreased the presence of total and activated macrophages in visceral adipose tissue from obese-insulin resistant mice, as well as the number of crown-like structures, markers of adipose tissue inflammation [230]. These effects suggest that α-LA alleviates not only acute inflammation induced by LPS injection, but also obesity-mediated chronic inflammation state in adipose tissue.

Although in human trials the effects of α-LA in adipose tissue oxidative stress and inflammation have not been extensively reported, a recent transcriptomic analysis of adipose tissue showed that α-LA supplementation decreased the expression of genes related with cell adhesion and inflammation in overweight/obese women following a hypocaloric diet [231].

4.2.2.2 α–Lipoic Acid Actions on Adipocyte Metabolic Pathways

In addition to its antioxidant, antiinflammatory, and central actions, α-LA is also able to regulate adipose tissue metabolic function. Its effects involve not only the adipocyte lipid storing function by actions in both anabolic and catabolic pathways, but also the modulation of adipose tissue endocrine function by changes in adipocytes secretory pattern [232,233].

Several studies revealed the ability of α–LA to reduce lipid accumulation by acting on both preadipocytes and mature adipocytes. Thus treatment with α-LA inhibited adipogenesis through mitogen-activated protein kinase activation, the downregulation of early genes such as c-Fos and c-Jun controlling clonal expansion, and further, the negative regulation of integral members of the adipocyte differentiation program, PPARγ and C/EBPα. Together these lead to impaired adipocyte maturation and decreased expression of adipocyte specific genes [234]. Moreover, the inhibitory actions of α-LA on adipogenesis might be also mediated by AMPK signaling pathway through actions on autophagy, which has been described as an essential process for adipocyte differentiation, by regulating lipid droplets formation [235]. Activation of AMPK (phosphorylation at threonine 172), a positive modulator of autophagy, is significantly inhibited by α-LA at the earlier stage of differentiation. These actions together with mammalian target of rapamycin (mTOR) activation promote an inhibition in LC3 lipidation (inhibition on autophagy activation) and p62 accumulation (impaired autophagy flux), indicating that α-LA might be also inhibiting adipogenesis by disturbing autophagy [236].

Within mature adipocytes, α-LA decreased triglyceride accumulation by inhibiting both de novo lipogenesis and fatty acid esterification in primary cultured adipocytes from overweight/obese subjects [232]. These actions were mediated by the downregulation of key lipogenic enzymes such as fatty acid synthase (FAS), stearoyl-Coenzyme A desaturase 1 (SCD1), and diacylglycerol O-acyltransferase 1 (DGAT1). On the contrary of what was observed in early differentiation stages, the effects of α-LA on inhibiting lipogenesis would be mediated by the activation of AMPK and further acetyl CoA carboxylase (ACC) phosphorylation [232].

In addition to actions on preventing the lipid deposition in adipocytes, α-LA also promoted lipid utilization. In this regard, α-LA has been described as a potent lipolytic agent in 3T3-L1 mature adipocytes [237]. Thus α-LA downregulated the adipose-specific phospholipase A2 (AdPLA) levels and AdPLA-mediated PGE2 production, an antilipolytic agent that decreases cAMP levels. Therefore, increased cAMP levels enhance protein kinase A (PKA)-mediated hormone-sensitive lipase (HSL) and perilipin phosphorylation, and therefore, their activation and the increase of adipocyte lipolytic rate [237]. In support of α-LA lipolytic actions, in vivo studies revealed that α-LA counteracts the inhibitory effects of LPS on HSL gene expression and protein levels [207]. After the lipolytic stimulus, within adipocytes, increased intracellular fatty acids levels have been observed to induce fatty acid clearance by their oxidation in mitochondria [238]. By the use of in vivo models of obesity and inflammation it has been demonstrated that α-LA treatment increases mitochondrial functionality by upregulating the expression of most mitochondrial DNA-encoded genes [207]. In fact, in combination with acetyl-L-carnitine, α-LA increases mitochondrial mass, mitochondrial DNA content, and the expression of mitochondrial complexes as well as oxygen consumption rate and fatty acid oxidation in 3T3L1 adipocytes [239]. Further studies in cultured human adipocytes from overweight/obese subjects revealed that α-LA induces mitochondrial biogenesis and promotes adipocyte beiging, based on the following observations: (1) α-LA increased mitochondrial mass, upregulated SIRT1, and decreased peroxisome proliferator-activated receptor gamma coactivator 1-alpha (PGC-1α) acetylation, in parallel with the upregulation of nuclear respiratory factor 1 (Nrf1) and mitochondrial transcription factor (Tfam); (2) α-LA enhanced oxygen consumption and fatty acid oxidation enzymes, carnitine palmitoyl transferase 1 and acyl-coenzyme A oxidase (CPT-1 and ACOX); (3) α-LA upregulated brown-like adipocyte markers as PR domain containing 16 (Prdm16), cell death-inducing DNA fragmentation factor alpha-like effector a (Cidea), T-box 1 (Tbx1), and UCP1 [240]. In addition, the study from Huerta et al. [231] also showed that α-LA supplementation could modulate adipocyte lipid metabolism by inducing the expression of genes involved in the catabolism of lipids while decreasing the mRNA levels of those related with deposition of lipids, in subcutaneous abdominal adipose tissue from overweight/obese healthy women.

4.2.2.3 α-Lipoic Acid Regulates the Adipocyte's Secretory Pattern

Furthermore, the ability of α-LA to modulate both in vitro and/or in vivo the secretion of some key adipokines involved in inflammation and in the regulation of body weight and glucose and lipid metabolism such as leptin, adiponectin, apelin, chemerin, and irisin has been demonstrated [233,241−244].

Although α-LA anorexigenic effects have been described to be independent of leptin, there is substantial evidence supporting the role of α-LA-mediated leptin regulation. Thus, α-LA reduces circulating leptin levels both in animal models and humans, secondary in part to the fat mass loss [244,245]. In vitro studies revealed that α-LA might directly regulate adipocyte leptin production by actions on Sp1, an ubiquitous transcription factor involved in glucose metabolism-induced transcriptional regulation of leptin promoter region [244,246].

Contrary to leptin, adiponectin levels are dramatically reduced in obesity, contributing to impaired glucose tolerance and the inflammatory state associated with obesity [247]. Some studies have suggested that α-LA supplementation restores adiponectin levels independently of its actions on food intake, and this might be contributing to the insulin sensitizing actions of α-LA [243,248]. Paradoxically, α-LA reduces adiponectin secretion in cultured 3T3-L1 adipocytes, suggesting that an indirect mechanism or some in vivo metabolic processing is involved in the regulation of the production of this adipokine after α-LA dietary supplementation [249].

Apelin is an adipokine related to oxidative stress and inflammation [250] and plays a role in the regulation of energy metabolism and insulin sensitivity in rodents and humans [251]. It has been suggested that the overproduction of apelin in obesity could be one of the last protections before the emergence of the obesity-related disorders such as T2D [251]. It was reported that α-LA induced apelin secretion in 3T3-L1 adipocytes [241]. Interestingly, a recent study of our group has reported that α-LA supplementation attenuates the drop in apelin circulating levels induced by the hypocaloric diet-induced weight loss in moderately obese women [252], which could also contribute to the beneficial effects of α-LA supplementation [252].

Chemerin is a proinflammatory adipokine that plays a key role in the pathological process of IR during obesity [253]. Chemerin levels positively correlate with BMI, TNF-α, HOMA-IR, and 8-iso-PGF2α in T2D patients [253], and weight loss promotes a reduction in circulating chemerin concentrations in overweight/obese patients [252]. According to this, α-LA-mediated body weight lowering effects are also accompanied by a fall in chemerin circulating levels [252]. Moreover, studies in cultured adipocytes showed that α-LA lowers chemerin production both in human (subcutaneous and omental adipocytes from overweight and obese subjects) and murine 3T3-L1 adipocytes. Interestingly, α-LA even reversed the TNF-α-induced chemerin production [233]. AMPK activation, as well as AKT inhibition, have been suggested to play a role in α-LA actions on chemerin secretion [233].

Irisin is a myokine/adipokine whose physiological role and regulatory pathways are still unclear. Irisin seems to be induced by exercise in mice and humans and to promote adipose tissue browning [254]. The study of Huerta et al. [242] showed that α-LA upregulates *Fndc5* (irisin) mRNA and irisin secretion in human cultured adipocytes. However, α-LA supplementation to overweight/obese women did not have any additional effects on irisin circulating levels to those caused by the hypocaloric diet-induced weight loss, suggesting than higher doses or longer periods of α-LA supplementation could be required to observe effects on irisin production.

Fig. 4.4 summarizes the described actions of α-LA on adipose tissue metabolism and secretory function.

In summary, α-LA is an important mitochondrial cofactor and antioxidant with potential antiobesity properties. These actions are mediated in part by its ability to modulate adipogenesis as well as oxidative stress and glucose and lipid metabolism in adipose tissue. Moreover, the capability of α-LA to induce mitochondrial biogenesis and brown-like remodeling in white subcutaneous adipocytes suggests that these mechanisms might also contribute to the antiobesity properties of α-LA.

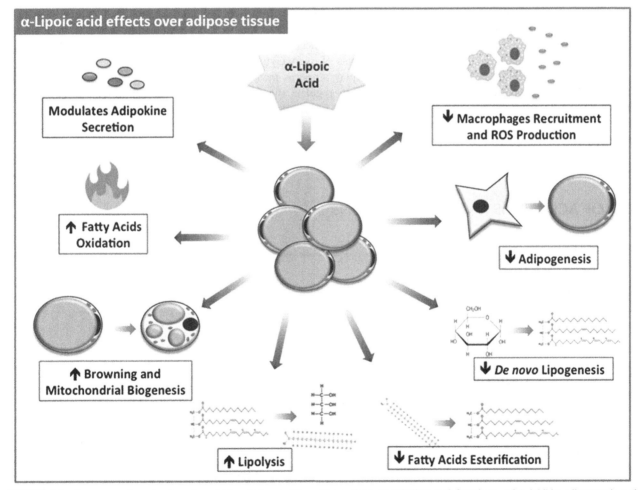

FIGURE 4.4 Summary of mechanisms by which α-LA regulates adipose tissue metabolism and functions. α-LA inhibits adipogenesis and downregulates pathways involved in adipocyte triglyceride accumulation, while upregulates lipid catabolic pathways (lipolysis and fatty acid oxidation). α-LA promotes mitochondrial biogenesis and adipocyte browning, reduces macrophage infiltration and ROS production. α-LA also regulates the secretion of adipokines involved in energy homeostasis, intermediate metabolism, and inflammation, which could also contribute to the beneficial effects of α-LA on glucose and lipid metabolism. *LA*, lipoic acid; *ROS*, reactive oxygen species.

5. CONCLUSIONS AND FUTURE PERSPECTIVES

Dysfunctional adipose tissue plays a key role in the development of obesity and associated comorbidities, with WAT acting as the main energy reservoir and BAT as a major energy dissipating organ. Increased adiposity is accompanied by a low-grade chronic inflammatory state. The hypertrophied adipocytes exhibit an altered secretory pattern characterized by increased secretion of proinflammatory adipokines, cytokines, and chemokines, and reduced production of antiinflammatory adipokines. Progressive infiltration and activation of macrophages and T/B cells also occurs within hypertrophied adipose tissue. There is a strong association between the inflammation triggered in adipose tissue and the increase in oxidative stress. Indeed, dysfunctional adipose tissue has been considered as an independent factor for the generation of systemic inflammation and oxidative stress. Although initially all these inflammatory processes and metabolic disturbances start within the adipose tissue, they can finally derive in a chronic systemic inflammation, affecting the physiology and metabolism of different tissues such as skeletal muscle, liver, and brain, among others. Therefore promoting the resolution of adipose tissue chronic inflammation and oxidative stress could be a key strategy to tackle obesity-associated comorbidities.

Resolution of inflammation is an active process that involves production of several series of SPMs such as LXs, RvDs (series E and D), PDs, and MaRs, biosynthesized within the resolution phase of inflammation. Indeed, obesity is sometimes accompanied by an impaired production of these SPMs, mainly in adipose tissue. Several preclinical studies have unraveled the therapeutic potential of some of these SPMs for reversing adipose tissue inflammation and IR in obese rodents. Because n-3 PUFAs serve as substrates for the formation of these SPMs and can regulate gene transcription in inflammation and nutrient metabolism, they can also constitute a good dietary/therapeutic strategy to promote the resolution of local and systemic inflammation and the subsequent metabolic disorders associated with obesity. Based on its antioxidant properties, but also in its ability to regulate mitochondrial function and adipocyte metabolism and secretory function, α-LA has been also considered as a promising candidate for reducing the inflammation and oxidative stress associated with obesity. Further clinical trials in humans are needed to better characterize their effectiveness to resolve inflammation and oxidative stress in adipose tissue depots of overweight/obese subjects.

Adipose tissue miRNAs have been also shown to play a role as mediators of inflammation associated with obesity. Indeed, it has been reported that specific miRNAs can regulate the production of inflammation-related adipokines. Moreover, adipose-derived circulating miRNAs can regulate gene expression in other tissues [255]. Indeed, exosomes have been recently identified as a new intercellular communication system for transporting proteins and RNAs. Adipocyte exosomes have been involved in metabolism regulation and obesity-related IR [256]. Therefore, modulation of miRNA levels to regulate adipose inflammation and adipose tissue exosomes could also constitute a promising approach to prevent obesity-associated diseases such as IR and T2D.

LIST OF ACRONYMS AND ABBREVIATIONS

AA Arachidonic acid
ACC Acetyl CoA carboxylase
ACOX Acyl-coenzyme A oxidase
AdPLA Adipose-specific phospholipase A2
AMPK AMP-activated protein kinase
BAT Brown adipose tissue
BMI Body mass index
CAT Catalase
CCL-5 Chemokine (C−C motif) ligand 5
CD68 Cluster of differentiation 68
CIDEA Cell death−inducing DFFA-like effector
COX-2 Cyclooxygenase-2
CPT-1 Carnitine palmitoyl transferase 1
CRP C-reactive protein
DGAT1 Diacylglycerol O-acyltransferase
DHA Docosahexenoic acid
DHLA Dihydrolipoic acid
EPA Eicosapentanoic acid
FAS fatty acid synthase
FDG fluorodeoxyglucose
FFA Free fatty-acid

GPx Glutathione peroxidase
GR Glutathione reductase
GSH Glutathione
HDHA Hydroxy-docosahexenoic acid
HDL High-density lipoprotein
HFD High-fat diet
HMOX2 Heme oxygenase 2
HOMA Homeostatic model assessment
HSL Hormone-sensitive lipase
ICAM-1 Intercellular adhesion molecule-1
IKK I kappa B kinase
IL Interleukin
IR Insulin resistance
JNK c-Jun N-terminal kinases
LA Lipoic acid
LASY Lipoic acid synthase
LDL Low-density lipoprotein
LTB4 Leukotriene B4
LX Lipoxin
MAC-2 macrophage-2 antigen/ galectin-3
MaR Maresin
MCP-1 Monocyte chemoattractant protein-1
MDA Malondialdehyde
MetS Metabolic syndrome
mTOR mammalian target of rapamycin
NF-κB Nuclear factor-κB
NLRP3 nucleotide-binding oligomerization domain, leucine rich repeat and pyrin domain containing
NO Nitric oxide
NOD Nucleotide-binding oligomerization domain protein
Nrf1 Nuclear respiratory factor 1
Ox-LDL Oxidative low-density lipoprotein
PD Protectin
PG Prostaglandin
PGC-1α peroxisome proliferator-activated receptor gamma coactivator 1-alpha
PKA Protein kinase A
PPAR Peroxisome proliferator-activated receptor
Prdm16 PR domain containing 16
PUFA Polyunsaturated fatty acid
ROS Reactive oxygen species
RvD Resolvin
SCD1 Stearoyl-coenzyme A desaturase 1
SOD Superoxide dismutase
SPM Specialized proresolving lipid mediator
SREBP Sterol regulatory element binding protein
SVC Stromal vascular cell
T2DM Type 2 diabetes mellitus
TBARS Thiobarbituric acid reactive substance
TBX1 T-box transcription factor
Tfam Mitochondrial transcription factor
TG Triglyceride
TLR Toll-like receptor
TMEM26 Transmembrane protein 26
TNF-α Tumor necrosis factor-α
UCP1 Uncoupling protein 1
VCAM-1 Vascular cell adhesion molecule-1
VLDL Very low-density lipoprotein
WAT White adipose tissue

ACKNOWLEDGMENTS

We thank the Ministry of Economy and Competitiveness from the Government of Spain (ref BFU2015-65937-R, BFU2012-36089, AGL2009-10873/ALI), Government of Navarra (Department of Health ref. 67/2015), and CIBERobn for the grants received. L.M.-F. is supported by a Formación de Personal Investigador predoctoral fellowship and E.F-S. is supported by a predoctoral fellowship from the Centre for Nutrition Research (Universidad de Navarra).

REFERENCES

[1] World Health Organization (WHO). Global status report on noncommunicable diseases. 2014.

[2] Klöting N, Blüher M. Adipocyte dysfunction, inflammation and metabolic syndrome. Rev Endocr Metab Disord 2014;15(4):277−87.

[3] Peirce V, Carobbio S, Vidal-Puig A. The different shades of fat. Nature 2014;510(7503):76−83.

[4] Wu J, Bostrom P, Sparks LM, Ye L, Choi JH, Giang AH, et al. Beige adipocytes are a distinct type of thermogenic fat cell in mouse and human. Cell 2012;150(2):366−76.

[5] Rodríguez A, Ezquerro S, Méndez-Giménez L, Becerril S, Frühbeck G. Revisiting the adipocyte: a model for integration of cytokine signaling in the regulation of energy metabolism. Am J Physiol Endocrinol Metab 2015;309(8):E691−714.

[6] Pellegrinelli V, Carobbio S, Vidal-Puig A. Adipose tissue plasticity: how fat depots respond differently to pathophysiological cues. Diabetologia 2016:1−14.

[7] Pereira SS, Alvarez-Leite JI. Low-grade inflammation, obesity, and diabetes. Curr Obes Rep 2014;3(4):422−31.

[8] Choe SS, Huh JY, Hwang IJ, Kim JI, Kim JB. Adipose tissue remodeling: its role in energy metabolism and metabolic disorders. Front Endocrinol 2016;7:1−16.

[9] Guo S. Insulin signaling, resistance, and the metabolic syndrome: insights from mouse models to disease mechanisms. J Endocrinol 2014;220(2):1−36.

[10] Ouchi N, Parker JL, Lugus JJ, Walsh K. Adipokines in inflammation and metabolic disease. Nat Rev Immunol 2011;11(2):85−97.

[11] Grant RW, Dixit VD. Adipose tissue as an immunological organ. Obesity 2015;23(3):512−8.

[12] Primeau V, Coderre L, Karelis AD, Brochu M, Lavoie ME, Messier V, et al. Characterizing the profile of obese patients who are metabolically healthy. Int J Obes (2005) 2011;35(7):971−81.

[13] Giralt M, Villarroya F. White, brown, beige/brite: different adipose cells for different functions? Endocrinology 2013;154(9):2992−3000.

[14] Virtanen KA, Lidell ME, Orava J, Heglind M, Westergren R, Niemi T, et al. Functional brown adipose tissue in healthy adults. N Engl J Med 2009;360:1518−25.

[15] Cypess AM, Lehman S, Williams G, Tal I, Rodman D, Goldfine AB, et al. Identification and importance of brown adipose tissue in adult humans. N Engl J Med 2009;360(15):1509−17.

[16] Jeremic N, Chatuverdi P, Tyagi SC. Browning of white fat: novel insight into factors, mechanisms and therapeutics. J Cell Physiol 2016;232(1):61−8.

[17] Bolsoni-Lopes A, Deshaies Y, Festuccia WT. Regulation of brown adipose tissue recruitment, metabolism and thermogenic function by peroxisome proliferator-activated receptor γ. Temperature 2015;8940:1−7.

[18] Bartelt A, Bruns OT, Reimer R, Hohenberg H, Ittrich H, Peldschus K, et al. Brown adipose tissue activity controls triglyceride clearance. Nat Med 2011;17(2):200−5.

[19] Stanford KI, Middelbeek RJ, Townsend KL, An D, Nygaard EB, Hitchcox KM, et al. Brown adipose tissue regulates glucose homeostasis and insulin sensitivity. J Clin Invest 2013;123(1):215−23.

[20] Hanssen MJW, Hoeks J, Brans B, van der Lans AA, Schaart G, van den Driessche JJ, et al. Short-term cold acclimation improves insulin sensitivity in patients with type 2 diabetes mellitus. Nat Med 2015;21(8):863−5.

[21] Martínez-Fernández L, Laiglesia LM, Huerta AE, Martínez JA, Moreno-Aliaga MJ. Omega-3 fatty acids and adipose tissue function in obesity and metabolic syndrome. Prostaglandins Other Lipid Mediat 2015;121(Pt A):24−41.

[22] Zhang Q, Ye H, Miao Q, Zhang Z, Wang Y, Zhu X, et al. Differences in the metabolic status of healthy adults with and without active brown adipose tissue. Wien Klin Wochenschr 2013;125(21−22):687−95.

[23] Peterson CM, Lecoultre V, Frost EA, Simmons J, Redman LM, Ravussin E. The thermogenic responses to overfeeding and cold are differentially regulated. Obesity (Silver Spring) 2015;24(1):37−54.

[24] Yoneshiro T, Aita S, Matsushita M, Kayahara T, Kameya T, Kawai Y, et al. Recruited brown adipose tissue as an antiobesity agent in humans. J Clin Invest 2013;123(8):3404−8.

[25] Blondin DP, Labbé SM, Tingelstad HC, Noll C, Kunach M, Phoenix S, et al. Increased brown adipose tissue oxidative capacity in cold-acclimated humans. J Clin Endocrinol Metab 2014;99(3):438−46.

[26] Nedergaard J, Bengtsson T, Cannon B. New powers of brown fat: fighting the metabolic syndrome. Cell Metab 2011;13(3):238−40.

[27] Orava J, Nuutila P, Noponen T, Parkkola R, Viljanen T, Enerbäck S, et al. Blunted metabolic responses to cold and insulin stimulation in brown adipose tissue of obese humans. Obesity 2013;21(11):2279−87.

[28] Xu F, Zheng X, Lin B, Liang H, Cai M, Cao H, et al. Diet-induced obesity and insulin resistance are associated with brown fat degeneration in SIRT1-deficient mice. Obesity 2016;24(3):634−42.

[29] Blondin DP, Labbé SM, Noll C, Kunach M, Phoenix S, Guérin B, et al. Selective impairment of glucose but not fatty acid or oxidative metabolism in brown adipose tissue of subjects with type 2 diabetes. Diabetes 2015;64(7):2388−97.

[30] Vijgen GH, Bouvy ND, Teule GJ, Brans B, Hoeks J, Schrauwen P, et al. Increase in brown adipose tissue activity after weight loss in morbidly obese subjects. J Clin Endocrinol Metab 2012;97(7):E1229−33.

[31] Hoeke G, Kooijman S, Boon MR, Rensen PC, Berbeé JF. Role of brown fat in lipoprotein metabolism and atherosclerosis. Circ Res 2016;118(1):173−82.

[32] Sidossis LS, Porter C, Saraf MK, Børsheim E, Radhakrishnan RS, Chao T, et al. Browning of subcutaneous white adipose tissue in humans after severe adrenergic stress. Cell Metab 2015;22(2):219−27.

[33] Cypess AM, White AP, Vernochet C, Schulz TJ, Xue R, Sass C a, et al. Anatomical localization, gene expression profiling, and functional characterization of adult human neck brown fat. Nat Med 2013;19(5):635−9.

[34] Villarroya F, Vidal-Puig A. Beyond the sympathetic tone: the new brown fatactivators. Cell Metab 2013;17(5):638−43.

[35] Qiu Y, Dguyen KD, Odergaar JI, Cui X, Tian X, Locksley RM, et al. Eosinophils and type 2 cytokine signaling in macrophages orchestrate development of functional beige fat. Cell 2014;72(2):181−204.

[36] Preite NZ, Nascimento BP, Muller CR, Américo AL, Higa TS, Evangelista FS, et al. Disruption of beta3 adrenergic receptor increases susceptibility to DIO in mouse. Endocrinol 2016;231(3):259−69.

[37] Kern PA, Finlin BS, Zhu B, Rasouli N, McGehee RE, Westgate PM, et al. The effects of temperature and seasons on subcutaneous white adipose tissue in humans: evidence for thermogenic gene induction. J Clin Endocrinol Metab 2014;99(12):E2772−9.

[38] Asghar A, Sheikh N. Role of immune cells in obesity induced low grade inflammation and insulin resistance. Cell Immunol 2017;315:18−26.

[39] Wensveen FM, Valentić S, Šestan M, Turk Wensveen T, Polić B. The "Big Bang" in obese fat: events initiating obesity-induced adipose tissue inflammation. Eur J Immunol 2015;45(9):2446−56.

[40] Ray I, Mahata SK, De RK. Obesity: an immunometabolic perspective. Front Endocrinol 2016;7:157.

[41] Furukawa S, Fujita T, Shimabukuro M, Iwaki M, Yamada Y, Nakajima Y, et al. Increased oxidative stress in obesity and its impact on metabolic syndrome. J Clin Invest 2004;114(12):1752−61.

[42] Marseglia L, Manti S, D'Angelo G, Nicotera A, Parisi E, Di Rosa G, et al. Oxidative stress in obesity: a critical component in human diseases. Int J Mol Sci 2014;16(1):378−400.

[43] Roberts CK, Sindhu KK. Oxidative stress and metabolic syndrome. Life Sci 2009;84(21−22):705−12.

[44] Fernández-Sánchez A, Madrigal-Santillán E, Bautista M, Esquivel-Soto J, Morales-González Á, Esquivel-Chirino C, et al. Inflammation, oxidative stress, and obesity. Int J Mol Sci 2011;12(5):3117−32.

[45] Poprac P, Jomova K, Simunkova M, Kollar V, Rhodes CJ, Valko M. Targeting free radicals in oxidative stress-related human diseases. Trends Pharmacol Sci 2017;38(7):592−607.

[46] Le Lay S, Simard G, Martinez MC, Andriantsitohaina R. Oxidative stress and metabolic pathologies: from an adipocentric point of view. Oxid Med Cell Longev 2014;2014:908539.

[47] Sankhla M, Sharma TK, Mathur K, Rathor JS, Butolia V, Gadhok AK, et al. Relationship of oxidative stress with obesity and its role in obesity induced metabolic syndrome. Clin Lab 2012;58(5−6):385−92.

[48] Vincent HK, Taylor AG. Biomarkers and potential mechanisms of obesity-induced oxidant stress in humans. Int J Obes 2006;30(3):400−18.

[49] Chrysohoou C, Panagiotakos DB, Pitsavos C, Skoumas I, Papademetriou L, Economou M, et al. The implication of obesity on total antioxidant capacity in apparently healthy men and women: the ATTICA study. Nutr Metab Cardiovasc Dis 2007;17(8):590−7.

[50] Amirkhizi F, Siassi F, Minaie S, Djalali M, Rahimi A, Chamari M. Is obesity associated with increased plasma lipid peroxidation and oxidative stress in women? ARYA Atheroscler 2007;2(4):189−92.

[51] Houstis N, Rosen ED, Lander ES. Reactive oxygen species have a causal role in multiple forms of insulin resistance. Nature 2006;440(7086):944−8.

[52] González-Muniesa P, Mártinez-González MA, Hu FB, Després JP, Matsuzawa Y, Loos RJF, et al. Obesity. Nat Rev Dis Primer 2017;15(3):17034.

[53] Trayhurn P. Hypoxia and adipose tissue function and dysfunction in obesity. Physiol Rev 2013;93(1):1−21.

[54] Trayhurn P, Wood IS. Adipokines: inflammation and the pleiotropic role of white adipose tissue. Br J Nutr 2004;92(3):347−55.

[55] Goossens GH, Blaak EE. Adipose tissue dysfunction and impaired metabolic health in human obesity: a matter of oxygen? Front Endocrinol 2015;6:55.

[56] González-Muniesa P, Lopez-Pascual A, de Andrés J, Lasa A, Portillo MP, Arós F, et al. Impact of intermittent hypoxia and exercise on blood pressure and metabolic features from obese subjects suffering sleep apnea-hypopnea syndrome. J Physiol Biochem 2015;71(3):589−99.

[57] Urdampilleta A, González-Muniesa P, Portillo MP, Martínez JA. Usefulness of combining intermittent hypoxia and physical exercise in the treatment of obesity. J Physiol Biochem 2012;68(2):289−304.

[58] Biddlestone J, Bandarra D, Rocha S. The role of hypoxia in inflammatory disease (review). Int J Mol Med 2015;35(4):859−69.

[59] Norouzirad R, González-Muniesa P, Ghasemi A. Hypoxia in obesity and diabetes: potential therapeutic effects of hyperoxia and nitrate. Oxid Med Cell Longev 2017;2017:5350267.

[60] Locksley RM, Killeen N, Lenardo MJ. The TNF and TNF receptor superfamilies: integrating mammalian biology. Cell 2001;104(4):487−501.

[61] Chen G, Goeddel DV. TNF-R1 signaling: a beautiful pathway. Science 2002;296(5573):1634−5.

[62] Fain JN, Madan AK, Hiler ML, Cheema P, Bahouth SW. Comparison of the release of adipokines by adipose tissue, adipose tissue matrix, and adipocytes from visceral and subcutaneous abdominal adipose tissues of obese humans. Endocrinology 2004;145(5):2273−82.

[63] Hotamisligil GS, Arner P, Caro JF, Atkinson RL, Spiegelman BM. Increased adipose tissue expression of tumor necrosis factor-alpha in human obesity and insulin resistance. J Clin Invest 1995;95(5):2409−15.

[64] Chou CY, Lang HF, Sheu WH, Lin JY. Weight loss improves serum mediators and metabolic syndrome features in android obese subjects. Obes Res Clin Pract 2013;7(1):e81−8.

[65] Tzanavari T, Giannogonas P, Karalis KP. TNF-alpha and obesity. Curr Dir Autoimmun 2010;11:145−56.

[66] Chandel NS, Schumacker PT, Arch RH. Reactive oxygen species are downstream products of TRAF-mediated signal transduction. J Biol Chem 2001;276(46):42728−36.

[67] Ye J, Gao Z, Yin J, He Q. Hypoxia is a potential risk factor for chronic inflammation and adiponectin reduction in adipose tissue of ob/ob and dietary obese mice. Am J Physiol Endocrinol Metab 2007;293(4):E1118−28.

[68] Wang B, Trayhurn P. Acute and prolonged effects of TNF-alpha on the expression and secretion of inflammation-related adipokines by human adipocytes differentiated in culture. Pflugers Arch 2006;452(4):418−27.

[69] Abderrazak A, Syrovets T, Couchie D, El Hadri K, Friguet B, Simmet T, et al. NLRP3 inflammasome: from a danger signal sensor to a regulatory node of oxidative stress and inflammatory diseases. Redox Biol 2015;4:296−307.

[70] Ballak DB, Stienstra R, Tack CJ, Dinarello CA, van Diepen JA. IL-1 family members in the pathogenesis and treatment of metabolic disease: focus on adipose tissue inflammation and insulin resistance. Cytokine 2015;75(2):280−90.

[71] Stienstra R, Joosten LAB, Koenen T, van Tits B, van Diepen JA, van den Berg SA, et al. The inflammasome-mediated caspase-1 activation controls adipocyte differentiation and insulin sensitivity. Cell Metab 2010;12(6):593−605.

[72] Vandanmagsar B, Youm YH, Ravussin A, Galgani JE, Stadler K, Mynatt RL, et al. The NLRP3 inflammasome instigates obesity-induced inflammation and insulin resistance. Nat Med 2011;17(2):179−88.

[73] Achari AE, Jain SK. Adiponectin, a therapeutic target for obesity, diabetes, and endothelial dysfunction. Int J Mol Sci 2017;18(6).

[74] Ouedraogo R, Gong Y, Berzins B, Wu X, Mahadev K, Hough K, et al. Adiponectin deficiency increases leukocyte-endothelium interactions via upregulation of endothelial cell adhesion molecules in vivo. J Clin Invest 2007;117(6):1718−26.

[75] Ouchi N, Walsh K. Adiponectin as an anti-inflammatory factor. Clin Chim Acta 2007;380(1−2):24−30.

[76] Motoshima H, Wu X, Mahadev K, Goldstein BJ. Adiponectin suppresses proliferation and superoxide generation and enhances eNOS activity in endothelial cells treated with oxidized LDL. Biochem Biophys Res Commun 2004;315(2):264−71.

[77] Kaser S, Tatarczyk T, Stadlmayr A, Ciardi C, Ress C, Tschoner A, et al. Effect of obesity and insulin sensitivity on adiponectin isoform distribution. Eur J Clin Invest 2008;38(11):827−34.

[78] Turer AT, Scherer PE. Adiponectin: mechanistic insights and clinical implications. Diabetologia 2012;55(9):2319−26.

[79] Deng Y, Scherer PE. Adipokines as novel biomarkers and regulators of the metabolic syndrome. Ann NY Acad Sci 2010;1212:E1−19.

[80] Aprahamian TR. Elevated adiponectin expression promotes adipose tissue vascularity under conditions of diet-induced obesity. Metabolism 2013;62(12):1730−8.

[81] Sánchez-Muñoz F, García-Macedo R, Alarcón-Aguilar F, Cruz M. Adipocitokines, adipose tissue and its relationship with immune system cells. Gac Med Mex 2005;141(6):505−12.

[82] Naugler WE, Karin M. The wolf in sheep's clothing: the role of interleukin-6 in immunity, inflammation and cancer. Trends Mol Med 2008;14(3):109−19.

[83] Weiss R, Dziura J, Burgert TS, Tamborlane WV, Taksali SE, Yeckel CW, et al. Obesity and the metabolic syndrome in children and adolescents. N Engl J Med 2004;350(23):2362−74.

[84] Kim H-J, Higashimori T, Park S-Y, Choi H, Dong J, Kim Y-J, et al. Differential effects of interleukin-6 and -10 on skeletal muscle and liver insulin action in vivo. Diabetes 2004;53(4):1060−7.

[85] Wallenius V, Wallenius K, Ahrén B, Rudling M, Carlsten H, Dickson SL, et al. Interleukin-6-deficient mice develop mature-onset obesity. Nat Med 2002;8(1):75−9.

[86] Wunderlich FT, Ströhle P, Könner AC, Gruber S, Tovar S, Brönneke HS, et al. Interleukin-6 signaling in liver-parenchymal cells suppresses hepatic inflammation and improves systemic insulin action. Cell Metab 2010;12(3):237−49.

[87] Chen X, Gong Q, Wang CY, Zhang K, Ji X, Chen Y-X, et al. High-fat diet induces distinct metabolic response in interleukin-6 and tumor necrosis factor-α knockout mice. J Interferon Cytokine Res 2016;36(10):580−8.

[88] Mauer J, Chaurasia B, Goldau J, Vogt MC, Ruud J, Nguyen KD, et al. Signaling by IL-6 promotes alternative activation of macrophages to limit endotoxemia and obesity-associated resistance to insulin. Nat Immunol 2014;15(5):423−30.

[89] Lopez-Pascual A, Lasa A, Portillo MP, Arós F, Mansego ML, González-Muniesa P, et al. Low oxygen consumption is related to a hypomethylation and an increased secretion of IL-6 in obese subjects with sleep apnea-hypopnea syndrome. Ann Nutr Metab 2017;71(1−2):16−25.

[90] Paneni F, Costantino S, Cosentino F. Insulin resistance, diabetes, and cardiovascular risk. Curr Atheroscler Rep 2014;16(7):419.

[91] Pitocco D, Tesauro M, Alessandro R, Ghirlanda G, Cardillo C. Oxidative stress in diabetes: implications for vascular and other complications. Int J Mol Sci 2013;14(11):21525−50.

[92] Poitout V, Robertson RP. Glucolipotoxicity: fuel excess and beta-cell dysfunction. Endocr Rev 2008;29(3):351−66.

[93] Wang CH, Wang CC, Huang HC, Wei YH. Mitochondrial dysfunction leads to impairment of insulin sensitivity and adiponectin secretion in adipocytes. FEBS J 2013;280(4):1039−50.

[94] Parthasarathy S, Raghavamenon A, Garelnabi MO, Santanam N. Oxidized low-density lipoprotein. Methods Mol Biol 2010;610:403−17.

[95] Touyz RM. Reactive oxygen species, vascular oxidative stress, and redox signaling in hypertension: what is the clinical significance? Hypertension 2004;44(3):248−52.

[96] Lacy F, Kailasam MT, O'Connor DT, Schmid-Schönbein GW, Parmer RJ. Plasma hydrogen peroxide production in human essential hypertension: role of heredity, gender, and ethnicity. Hypertension 2000;36(5):878−84.

[97] Landsberg L, Aronne LJ, Beilin LJ, Burke V, Igel LI, Lloyd-Jones D, et al. Obesity-related hypertension: pathogenesis, cardiovascular risk, and treatment—a position paper of the The Obesity Society and The American Society of Hypertension. Obesity (Silver Spring) 2013;21(1):8−24.

[98] Nagae A, Fujita M, Kawarazaki H, Matsui H, Ando K, Fujita T. Sympathoexcitation by oxidative stress in the brain mediates arterial pressure elevation in obesity-induced hypertension. Circulation 2009;119(7):978−86.

[99] Ferrante AW. Obesity-induced inflammation: a metabolic dialogue in the language of inflammation. J Intern Med 2007;262(4):408−14.

[100] Renehan AG, Tyson M, Egger M, Heller RF, Zwahlen M. Body-mass index and incidence of cancer: a systematic review and meta-analysis of prospective observational studies. Lancet 2008;371(9612):569−78.

[101] Jochem C, Leitzmann M. Obesity and colorectal cancer. Recent Results Cancer Res 2016;208:17−41.

[102] Laiyemo AO. The risk of colonic adenomas and colonic cancer in obesity. Best Pract Res Clin Gastroenterol 2014;28(4):655−63.

[103] Prieto-Hontoria PL, Perez-Matute P, Fernandez-Galilea M, Bustos M, Martinez JA, Moreno-Aliaga MJ. Role of obesity-associated dysfunctional adipose tissue in cancer: a molecular nutrition approach. Biochim Biophys Acta 2011;1807(6):664−78.

[104] Muñoz A, Costa M. Nutritionally mediated oxidative stress and inflammation. Oxid Med Cell Longev 2013;2013:610950.

[105] Calder PC. Long-chain fatty acids and inflammation. Proc Nutr Soc 2012;71(2):284−9.

[106] Calder PC. Marine omega-3 fatty acids and inflammatory processes: effects, mechanisms and clinical relevance. Biochim Biophys Acta 2015;1851(4):469−84.

[107] Martins DA, Custódio L, Barreira L, Pereira H, Ben-Hamadou R, Varela J, et al. Alternative sources of n-3 long-chain polyunsaturated fatty acids in marine microalgae. Mar Drugs 2013;11(7):2259−81.

[108] Calder PC. Functional roles of fatty acids and their effects on human health. J Parenter Enteral Nutr 2015;39(1 Suppl.):18S−32S.

[109] Burdge GC, Wootton SA. Conversion of α-linolenic acid to eicosapentaenoic, docosapentaenoic and docosahexaenoic acids in young women. Br J Nutr 2002;88(4):411−20.

[110] Burdge GC, Jones AE, Wootton SA. Eicosapentaenoic and docosapentaenoic acids are the principal products of alpha-linolenic acid metabolism in young men. Br J Nutr 2002;88(4):355−63.

[111] Emken EA, Adlof RO, Gulley RM. Dietary linoleic acid influences desaturation and acylation of deuterium-labeled linoleic and linolenic acids in young adult males. Biochim Biophys Acta 1994;1213(3):277−88.

[112] Nenseter MS, Drevon CA. Dietary polyunsaturates and peroxidation of low density lipoprotein. Curr Opin Lipidol 1996;7(1):8−13.

[113] Liu J, Yeo HC, Doniger SJ, Ames BN. Assay of aldehydes from lipid peroxidation: gas chromatography-mass spectrometry compared to thiobarbituric acid. Anal Biochem 1997;245(2):161−6.

[114] Crnkovic S, Riederer M, Lechleitner M, Hallström S, Malli R, Graier WF, et al. Docosahexaenoic acid-induced unfolded protein response, cell cycle arrest, and apoptosis in vascular smooth muscle cells are triggered by Ca^{2+}-dependent induction of oxidative stress. Free Radic Biol Med 2012;52(9):1786−95.

[115] Barden AE, Mori TA, Dunstan JA, Taylor AL, Thornton CA, Croft KD, et al. Fish oil supplementation in pregnancy lowers F2-isoprostanes in neonates at high risk of atopy. Free Radic Res 2004;38(3):233−9.

[116] Higdon JV, Liu J, Du SH, Morrow JD, Ames BN, Wander RC. Supplementation of postmenopausal women with fish oil rich in eicosapentaenoic acid and docosahexaenoic acid is not associated with greater in vivo lipid peroxidation compared with oils rich in oleate and linoleate as assessed by plasma malondialdehyde and F2-isoprostanes. Am J Clin Nutr 2000;72(3):714−22.

[117] Kiecolt-Glaser JK, Epel ES, Belury MA, Andridge R, Lin J, Glaser R, et al. Omega-3 fatty acids, oxidative stress, and leukocyte telomere length: a randomized controlled trial. Brain Behav Immun 2013;28:16−24.

[118] Mori TA, Woodman RJ, Burke V, Puddey IB, Croft KD, Beilin LJ. Effect of eicosapentaenoic acid and docosahexaenoic acid on oxidative stress and inflammatory markers in treated-hypertensive type 2 diabetic subjects. Free Radic Biol Med 2003;35(7):772−81.

[119] Mori TA, Puddey IB, Burke V, Croft KD, Dunstan DW, Rivera JH, et al. Effect of omega 3 fatty acids on oxidative stress in humans: GC-MS measurement of urinary F2-isoprostane excretion. Redox Rep 2000;5(1):45−6.

[120] Mori TA, Dunstan DW, Burke V, Croft KD, Rivera JH, Beilin LJ, et al. Effect of dietary fish and exercise training on urinary F2-isoprostane excretion in non-insulin-dependent diabetic patients. Metabolism 1999;48(11):1402−8.

[121] Nälsén C, Vessby B, Berglund L, Uusitupa M, Hermansen K, Riccardi G, et al. Dietary (n-3) fatty acids reduce plasma F2-isoprostanes but not prostaglandin F2alpha in healthy humans. J Nutr 2006;136(5):1222−8.

[122] Molinar-Toribio E, Pérez-Jiménez J, Ramos-Romero S, Romeu M, Giralt M, Taltavull N, et al. Effect of n-3 PUFA supplementation at different EPA: DHA ratios on the spontaneously hypertensive obese rat model of the metabolic syndrome. Br J Nutr 2015;113(6):878−87.

[123] Quaggiotto P, Leitch JW, Falconer J, Murdoch RN, Garg ML. Plasma F2α-isoprostane levels are lowered in pigs fed an (n-3) polyunsaturated fatty acid supplemented diet following occlusion of the left anterior descending coronary artery. Nutr Res May 1, 2000;20(5):675−84.

[124] Kelley NS, Yoshida Y, Erickson KL. Do n-3 polyunsaturated fatty acids increase or decrease lipid peroxidation in humans? Metab Syndr Relat Disord October 2014;12(8):403−15.

[125] Lawson JA, Rokach J, FitzGerald GA. Isoprostanes: formation, analysis and use as indices of lipid peroxidation in vivo. J Biol Chem 1999;274(35):24441−4.

[126] Praticò D, Lee VMY, Trojanowski JQ, Rokach J, Fitzgerald GA. Increased F2-isoprostanes in Alzheimer's disease: evidence for enhanced lipid peroxidation in vivo. FASEB J 1998;12(15):1777−83.

[127] Petersson H, Risérus U, McMonagle J, Gulseth HL, Tierney AC, Morange S, et al. Effects of dietary fat modification on oxidative stress and inflammatory markers in the LIPGENE study. Br J Nutr 2010;104(9):1357−62.

[128] Ulven SM, Kirkhus B, Lamglait A, Basu S, Elind E, Haider T, et al. Metabolic effects of krill oil are essentially similar to those of fish oil but at lower dose of EPA and DHA, in healthy volunteers. Lipids 2011;46(1):37−46.

[129] Kirkhus B, Lamglait A, Eilertsen KE, Falch E, Haider T, Vik H, et al. Effects of similar intakes of marine n-3 fatty acids from enriched food products and fish oil on cardiovascular risk markers in healthy human subjects. Br J Nutr 2012;107(9):1339−49.

[130] Ottestad I, Vogt G, Retterstøl K, Myhrstad MC, Haugen JE, Nilsson A, et al. Oxidised fish oil does not influence established markers of oxidative stress in healthy human subjects: a randomised controlled trial. Br J Nutr 2012;108(2):315−26.

[131] Wu WH, Lu SC, Wang TF, Jou HJ, Wang TA. Effects of docosahexaenoic acid supplementation on blood lipids, estrogen metabolism, and in vivo oxidative stress in postmenopausal vegetarian women. Eur J Clin Nutr 2006;60(3):386−92.

[132] Parra D, Bandarra NM, Kiely M, Thorsdottir I, Martínez JA. Impact of fish intake on oxidative stress when included into a moderate energy-restricted program to treat obesity. Eur J Nutr 2007;46(8):460−7.

[133] Schmidt S, Stahl F, Mutz KO, Scheper T, Hahn A, Schuchardt JP. Transcriptome-based identification of antioxidative gene expression after fish oil supplementation in normo- and dyslipidemic men. Nutr Metab 2012;9(1):45.

[134] Hajianfar H, Paknahad Z, Bahonar A. The effect of omega-3 supplements on antioxidant capacity in patients with type 2 diabetes. Int J Prev Med 2013;4(Suppl. 2):S234−8.

[135] Brude IR, Drevon CA, Hjermann I, Seljeflot I, Lund-Katz S, Saarem K, et al. Peroxidation of LDL from combined-hyperlipidemic male smokers supplied with omega-3 fatty acids and antioxidants. Arterioscler Thromb Vasc Biol 1997;17(11):2576−88.

[136] Frankel EN, Parks EJ, Xu R, Schneeman BO, Davis PA, German JB. Effect of n-3 fatty acid-rich fish oil supplementation on the oxidation of low density lipoproteins. Lipids 1994;29(4):233−6.

[137] Egert S, Lindenmeier M, Harnack K, Krome K, Erbersdobler HF, Wahrburg U, et al. Margarines fortified with α-linolenic acid, eicosapentaenoic acid, or docosahexaenoic acid alter the fatty acid composition of erythrocytes but do not affect the antioxidant status of healthy adults. J Nutr 2012;142(9):1638−44.

[138] Egert S, Somoza V, Kannenberg F, Fobker M, Krome K, Erbersdobler HF, et al. Influence of three rapeseed oil-rich diets, fortified with alpha-linolenic acid, eicosapentaenoic acid or docosahexaenoic acid on the composition and oxidizability of low-density lipoproteins: results of a controlled study in healthy volunteers. Eur J Clin Nutr 2007;61(3):314−25.

[139] Filaire E, Massart A, Rouveix M, Portier H, Rosado F, Durand D. Effects of 6 weeks of n-3 fatty acids and antioxidant mixture on lipid per-oxidation at rest and postexercise. Eur J Appl Physiol 2011;111(8):1829−39.

[140] Harats D, Dabach Y, Hollander G, Ben-Naim M, Schwartz R, Berry EM, et al. Fish oil ingestion in smokers and nonsmokers enhances perox-idation of plasma lipoproteins. Atherosclerosis 1991;90(2−3):127−39.

[141] Meydani M, Natiello F, Goldin B, Free N, Woods M, Schaefer E, et al. Effect of long-term fish oil supplementation on vitamin E status and lipid peroxidation in women. J Nutr 1991;121(4):484−91.

[142] Palozza P, Sgarlata E, Luberto C, Piccioni E, Anti M, Marra G, et al. n-3 fatty acids induce oxidative modifications in human erythrocytes depending on dose and duration of dietary supplementation. Am J Clin Nutr 1996;64(3):297−304.

[143] Suzukawa M, Abbey M, Howe PR, Nestel PJ. Effects of fish oil fatty acids on low density lipoprotein size, oxidizability, and uptake by mac-rophages. J Lipid Res 1995;36(3):473−84.

[144] Hirotani Y, Ozaki N, Tsuji Y, Urashima Y, Myotoku M. Effects of eicosapentaenoic acid on hepatic dyslipidemia and oxidative stress in high fat diet-induced steatosis. Int J Food Sci Nutr 2015;66(5):569−73.

[145] Hunsche C, Hernandez O, Gheorghe A, Díaz LE, Marcos A, De la Fuente M. Immune dysfunction and increased oxidative stress state in diet-induced obese mice are reverted by nutritional supplementation with monounsaturated and n-3 polyunsaturated fatty acids. Eur J Nutr 2017. https://doi.org/10.1007/s00394-017-1395-1.

[146] Sun R, Wang X, Liu Y, Xia M. Dietary supplementation with fish oil alters the expression levels of proteins governing mitochondrial dynamics and prevents high-fat diet-induced endothelial dysfunction. Br J Nutr 2014;112(2):145−53.

[147] Han CY, Umemoto T, Omer M, Hartigh LJD, Chiba T, LeBoeuf R, et al. NADPH oxidase-derived reactive oxygen species increases expression of monocyte chemotactic factor genes in cultured adipocytes. J Biol Chem 2012;287(13):10379−93.

[148] Richard D, Kefi K, Barbe U, Bausero P, Visioli F. Polyunsaturated fatty acids as antioxidants. Pharmacol Res 2008;57(6):451−5.

[149] Adkins Y, Kelley DS. Mechanisms underlying the cardioprotective effects of omega-3 polyunsaturated fatty acids. J Nutr Biochem 2010;21(9):781−92.

[150] Rangel-Huerta OD, Aguilera CM, Mesa MD, Gil A. Omega-3 long-chain polyunsaturated fatty acids supplementation on inflammatory biomakers: a systematic review of randomised clinical trials. Br J Nutr 2012;107(Suppl. 2):S159−70.

[151] Browning LM, Krebs JD, Moore CS, Mishra GD, O'Connell MA, Jebb SA. The impact of long chain n-3 polyunsaturated fatty acid supple-mentation on inflammation, insulin sensitivity and CVD risk in a group of overweight women with an inflammatory phenotype. Diabetes Obes Metab 2007;9(1):70−80.

[152] Kelley DS, Siegel D, Fedor DM, Adkins Y, Mackey BE. DHA supplementation decreases serum C-reactive protein and other markers of inflammation in hypertriglyceridemic men. J Nutr 2009;139(3):495−501.

[153] Spencer M, Finlin BS, Unal R, Zhu B, Morris AJ, Shipp LR, et al. Omega-3 fatty acids reduce adipose tissue macrophages in human subjects with insulin resistance. Diabetes 2013;62(5):1709−17.

[154] Tousoulis D, Plastiras A, Siasos G, Oikonomou E, Verveniotis A, Kokkou E, et al. Omega-3 PUFAs improved endothelial function and arterial stiffness with a parallel antiinflammatory effect in adults with metabolic syndrome. Atherosclerosis 2014;232(1):10−6.

[155] Krebs JD, Browning LM, McLean NK, Rothwell JL, Mishra GD, Moore CS, et al. Additive benefits of long-chain n-3 polyunsaturated fatty acids and weight-loss in the management of cardiovascular disease risk in overweight hyperinsulinaemic women. Int J Obes 2006;30(10):1535–44.

[156] Neff LM, Culiner J, Cunningham-Rundles S, Seidman C, Meehan D, Maturi J, et al. Algal docosahexaenoic acid affects plasma lipoprotein particle size distribution in overweight and obese adults. J Nutr 2011;141(2):207–13.

[157] Bragt MCE, Mensink RP. Comparison of the effects of n-3 long chain polyunsaturated fatty acids and fenofibrate on markers of inflammation and vascular function, and on the serum lipoprotein profile in overweight and obese subjects. Nutr Metab Cardiovasc Dis 2012;22(11):966–73.

[158] Dewell A, Marvasti FF, Harris WS, Tsao P, Gardner CD. Low- and high-dose plant and marine (n-3) fatty acids do not affect plasma inflammatory markers in adults with metabolic syndrome. J Nutr 2011;141(12):2166–71.

[159] Skulas-Ray AC, Kris-Etherton PM, Harris WS, Heuvel JP, Wagner PR, West SG. Dose-response effects of omega-3 fatty acids on triglycerides, inflammation, and endothelial function in healthy persons with moderate hypertriglyceridemia. Am J Clin Nutr 2011;93(2):243–52.

[160] Su HY, Lee HC, Cheng WY, Huang SY. A calorie-restriction diet supplemented with fish oil and high-protein powder is associated with reduced severity of metabolic syndrome in obese women. Eur J Clin Nutr 2015;69(3):322–8.

[161] Wong AT, Chan DC, Barrett PH, Adams LA, Watts GF. Supplementation with n3 fatty acid ethyl esters increases large and small artery elasticity in obese adults on a weight loss diet. J Nutr 2013;143(4):437–41.

[162] Pérez-Matute P, Pérez-Echarri N, Martínez JA, Marti A, Moreno-Aliaga MJ. Eicosapentaenoic acid actions on adiposity and insulin resistance in control and high-fat-fed rats: role of apoptosis, adiponectin and tumour necrosis factor-alpha. Br J Nutr 2007;97(2):389–98.

[163] Martínez-Fernández L, González-Muniesa P, Laiglesia LM, Sáinz N, Prieto-Hontoria PL, Escoté X, et al. Maresin 1 improves insulin sensitivity and attenuates adipose tissue inflammation in ob/ob and diet-induced obese mice. FASEB J 2017;31(5):2135–45.

[164] Titos E, Rius B, González-Périz A, López-Vicario C, Morán-Salvador E, Martínez-Clemente M, et al. Resolvin D1 and its precursor docosa-hexaenoic acid promote resolution of adipose tissue inflammation by eliciting macrophage polarization toward an M2-like phenotype. J Immunol 2011;187(10):5408–18.

[165] Todoric J, Löffler M, Huber J, Bilban M, Reimers M, Kadl A, et al. Adipose tissue inflammation induced by high-fat diet in obese diabetic mice is prevented by n-3 polyunsaturated fatty acids. Diabetologia 2006;49(9):2109–19.

[166] Itoh M, Suganami T, Satoh N, Tanimoto-Koyama K, Yuan X, Tanaka M, et al. Increased adiponectin secretion by highly purified eicosapentaenoic acid in rodent models of obesity and human obese subjects. Arterioscler Thromb Vasc Biol 2007;27(9):1918–25.

[167] González-Périz A, Horrillo R, Ferré N, Gronert K, Dong B, Morán-Salvador E, et al. Obesity-induced insulin resistance and hepatic steatosis are alleviated by omega-3 fatty acids: a role for resolvins and protectins. FASEB J 2009;23(6):1946–57.

[168] Flachs P, Ruhl R, Hensler M, Janovska P, Zouhar P, Kus V, et al. Synergistic induction of lipid catabolism and anti-inflammatory lipids in white fat of dietary obese mice in response to calorie restriction and n-3 fatty acids. Diabetologia 2011;54(10):2626–38.

[169] LeMieux MJ, Kalupahana NS, Scoggin S, Moustaid-Moussa N. Eicosapentaenoic acid reduces adipocyte hypertrophy and inflammation in diet-induced obese mice in an adiposity-independent manner. J Nutr 2015;145(3):411–7.

[170] Rossmeisl M, Jilkova ZM, Kuda O, Jelenik T, Medrikova D, Stankova B, et al. Metabolic effects of n-3 PUFA as phospholipids are superior to triglycerides in mice fed a high-fat diet: possible role of endocannabinoids. PLoS One 2012;7(6):e38834.

[171] Rossmeisl M, Jelenik T, Jilkova Z, Slamova K, Kus V, Hensler M, et al. Prevention and reversal of obesity and glucose intolerance in mice by DHA derivatives. Obesity (Silver Spring) 2009;17(5):1023–31.

[172] Yu J, Ma Y, Sun J, Ran L, Li Y, Wang N, et al. Microalgal oil from *Schizochytrium* sp. prevents HFD-induced abdominal fat accumulation in mice. J Am Coll Nutr 2017;36(5):347–56.

[173] Ludwig T, Worsch S, Heikenwalder M, Daniel H, Hauner H, Bader BL. Metabolic and immunomodulatory effects of n-3 fatty acids are different in mesenteric and epididymal adipose tissue of diet-induced obese mice. Am J Physiol Endocrinol Metab 2013;304(11):E1140–56.

[174] Kumar A, Takada Y, Boriek AM, Aggarwal BB. Nuclear factor-kappaB: its role in health and disease. J Mol Med (Berl Ger) 2004;82(7):434–48.

[175] Sigal LH. Basic science for the clinician 39: NF-kappaB-function, activation, control, and consequences. J Clin Rheumatol 2006;12(4):207–11.

[176] Lorente-Cebrián S, Bustos M, Marti A, Fernández-Galilea M, Martinez JA, Moreno-Aliaga MJ. Eicosapentaenoic acid inhibits tumour necrosis factor-α-induced lipolysis in murine cultured adipocytes. J Nutr Biochem 2012;23(3):218–27.

[177] Siriwardhana N, Kalupahana NS, Fletcher S, Xin W, Claycombe KJ, Quignard-Boulange A, et al. n-3 and n-6 polyunsaturated fatty acids differentially regulate adipose angiotensinogen and other inflammatory adipokines in part via NF-κB-dependent mechanisms. J Nutr Biochem 2012;23(12):1661–7.

[178] Martinez-Micaelo N, González-Abuín N, Terra X, Richart C, Ardèvol A, Pinent M, et al. Omega-3 docosahexaenoic acid and procyanidins inhibit cyclo-oxygenase activity and attenuate NF-κB activation through a p105/p50 regulatory mechanism in macrophage inflammation. Biochem J 2012;441(2):653–63.

[179] Oliver E, McGillicuddy FC, Harford KA, Reynolds CM, Phillips CM, Ferguson JF, et al. Docosahexaenoic acid attenuates macrophage-induced inflammation and improves insulin sensitivity in adipocytes-specific differential effects between LC n-3 PUFA. J Nutr Biochem 2011;23(9):1192–200.

[180] Williams-Bey Y, Boularan C, Vural A, Huang NN, Hwang IY, Shan-Shi C, et al. Omega-3 free fatty acids suppress macrophage inflammasome activation by inhibiting NF-κB activation and enhancing autophagy. PLoS One 2014;9(6):e97957.

[181] Ferre P. The biology of peroxisome proliferator-activated receptors: relationship with lipid metabolism and insulin sensitivity. Diabetes 2004;53(Suppl. 1):S43–50.

[182] Odegaard JI, Ricardo-Gonzalez RR, Goforth MH, Morel CR, Subramanian V, Mukundan L, et al. Macrophage-specific PPARgamma controls alternative activation and improves insulin resistance. Nature 2007;447(7148):1116–20.

[183] Lee JY, Zhao L, Hwang DH. Modulation of pattern recognition receptor-mediated inflammation and risk of chronic diseases by dietary fatty acids. Nutr Rev 2010;68(1):38–61.

[184] Lee JY, Zhao L, Youn HS, Weatherill AR, Tapping R, Feng L, et al. Saturated fatty acid activates but polyunsaturated fatty acid inhibits toll-like receptor 2 dimerized with toll-like receptor 6 or 1. J Biol Chem 2004;279(17):16971–9.

[185] Lee JY, Sohn KH, Rhee SH, Hwang D. Saturated fatty acids, but not unsaturated fatty acids, induce the expression of cyclooxygenase-2 mediated through toll-like receptor 4. J Biol Chem 2001;276(20):16683–9.

[186] Wong SW, Kwon M-J, Choi AMK, Kim H-P, Nakahira K, Hwang DH. Fatty acids modulate toll-like receptor 4 activation through regulation of receptor dimerization and recruitment into lipid rafts in a reactive oxygen species-dependent manner. J Biol Chem 2009;284(40):27384–92.

[187] Serhan CN. Systems approach to inflammation resolution: identification of novel anti-inflammatory and pro-resolving mediators. J Thromb Haemost 2009;7(Suppl. 1):44–8.

[188] Clària J, López-Vicario C, Rius B, Titos E. Pro-resolving actions of SPM in adipose tissue biology. Mol Aspects Med 2017;58:83–92.

[189] Claria J, Dalli J, Yacoubian S, Gao F, Serhan CN. Resolvin D1 and resolvin D2 govern local inflammatory tone in obese fat. J Immunol 2012;189(5):2597–605.

[190] Neuhofer A, Zeyda M, Mascher D, Itariu BK, Murano I, Leitner L, et al. Impaired local production of proresolving lipid mediators in obesity and 17-HDHA as a potential treatment for obesity-associated inflammation. Diabetes 2013;62(6):1945–56.

[191] Titos E, Rius B, López-Vicario C, Alcaraz-Quiles J, García-Alonso V, Lopategi A, et al. Signaling and immunoresolving actions of resolvin D1 in inflamed human visceral adipose tissue. J Immunol 2016;197(8):3360–70.

[192] Tang Y, Zhang MJ, Hellmann J, Kosuri M, Bhatnagar A, Spite M. Proresolution therapy for the treatment of delayed healing of diabetic wounds. Diabetes 2013;62(2):618–27.

[193] White PJ, Arita M, Taguchi R, Kang JX, Marette A. Transgenic restoration of long-chain n-3 fatty acids in insulin target tissues improves resolution capacity and alleviates obesity-linked inflammation and insulin resistance in high-fat-fed mice. Diabetes 2010;59(12):3066–73.

[194] Hellmann J, Tang Y, Kosuri M, Bhatnagar A, Spite M. Resolvin D1 decreases adipose tissue macrophage accumulation and improves insulin sensitivity in obese-diabetic mice. FASEB J 2011;25(7):2399–407.

[195] Rius B, Titos E, Moran-Salvador E, Lopez-Vicario C, Garcia-Alonso V, Gonzalez-Periz A, et al. Resolvin D1 primes the resolution process initiated by calorie restriction in obesity-induced steatohepatitis. FASEB J 2014;28(2):836–48.

[196] Börgeson E, Johnson AMF, Lee YS, Till A, Syed GH, Ali-Shah ST, et al. Lipoxin A4 attenuates obesity-induced adipose inflammation and associated liver and kidney disease. Cell Metab 2015;22(1):125–37.

[197] White PJ, St-Pierre P, Charbonneau A, Mitchell PL, St-Amand E, Marcotte B, et al. Protectin DX alleviates insulin resistance by activating a myokine-liver glucoregulatory axis. Nat Med 2014;20(6):664–9.

[198] Packer L, Witt EH, Tritschler HJ. alpha-Lipoic acid as a biological antioxidant. Free Radic Biol Med 1995;19(2):227–50.

[199] Packer L, Kraemer K, Rimbach G. Molecular aspects of lipoic acid in the prevention of diabetes complications. Nutrition 2001;17(10):888–95.

[200] Shay KP, Moreau RF, Smith EJ, Smith AR, Hagen TM. Alpha-lipoic acid as a dietary supplement: molecular mechanisms and therapeutic potential. Biochim Biophys Acta 2009;1790(10):1149–60.

[201] Padmalayam I, Hasham S, Saxena U, Pillarisetti S. Lipoic acid synthase (LASY): a novel role in inflammation, mitochondrial function, and insulin resistance. Diabetes 2009;58(3):600–8.

[202] Dörsam B, Fahrer J. The disulfide compound α-lipoic acid and its derivatives: a novel class of anticancer agents targeting mitochondria. Cancer Lett 2016;371(1):12–9.

[203] Foster TS. Efficacy and safety of alpha-lipoic acid supplementation in the treatment of symptomatic diabetic neuropathy. Diabetes Educ 2007;33(1):111–7.

[204] Kim NW, Song YM, Kim E, Cho HS, Cheon KA, Kim SJ, et al. Adjunctive α-lipoic acid reduces weight gain compared with placebo at 12 weeks in schizophrenic patients treated with atypical antipsychotics: a double-blind randomized placebo-controlled study. Int Clin Psychopharmacol 2016;31(5):265–74.

[205] Koh EH, Lee WJ, Lee SA, Kim EH, Cho EH, Jeong E, et al. Effects of alpha-lipoic acid on body weight in obese subjects. Am J Med 2011;124(1):85.e1–8.

[206] Ziegler D, Ametov A, Barinov A, Dyck PJ, Gurieva I, Low PA, et al. Oral treatment with alpha-lipoic acid improves symptomatic diabetic polyneuropathy: the SYDNEY 2 trial. Diabetes Care 2006;29(11):2365–70.

[207] Guo J, Gao S, Liu Z, Zhao R, Yang X. Alpha-lipoic acid alleviates acute inflammation and promotes lipid mobilization during the inflammatory response in white adipose tissue of mice. Lipids 2016;51(10):1145–52.

[208] Midaoui AE, Talbot S, Lahjouji K, Dias JP, Fantus IG, Couture R. Effects of alpha-lipoic acid on oxidative stress and kinin receptor expression in obese Zucker diabetic fatty rats. J Diabetes Metab 2015;6(6):1–7.

[209] Prieto-Hontoria PL, Perez-Matute P, Fernandez-Galilea M, Barber A, Martinez JA, Moreno-Aliaga MJ. Lipoic acid prevents body weight gain induced by a high fat diet in rats: effects on intestinal sugar transport. J Physiol Biochem 2009;65(1):43–50.

[210] Kim MS, Park JY, Namkoong C, Jang PG, Ryu JW, Song HS, et al. Anti-obesity effects of alpha-lipoic acid mediated by suppression of hypothalamic AMP-activated protein kinase. Nat Med 2004;10(7):727–33.

[211] Song KH, Lee WJ, Koh JM, Kim HS, Youn JY, Park HS, et al. alpha-Lipoic acid prevents diabetes mellitus in diabetes-prone obese rats. Biochem Biophys Res Commun 2005;326(1):197–202.

[212] Butler JA, Hagen TM, Moreau R. Lipoic acid improves hypertriglyceridemia by stimulating triacylglycerol clearance and downregulating liver triacylglycerol secretion. Arch Biochem Biophys 2009;485(1):63–71.

[213] Timmers S, de Vogel-van den Bosch J, Towler MC, Schaart G, Moonen-Kornips E, Mensink RP, et al. Prevention of high-fat diet-induced muscular lipid accumulation in rats by alpha lipoic acid is not mediated by AMPK activation. J Lipid Res 2010;51(2):352—9.

[214] Chen WL, Kang CH, Wang SG, Lee HM. α-Lipoic acid regulates lipid metabolism through induction of sirtuin 1 (SIRT1) and activation of AMP-activated protein kinase. Diabetologia 2012;55(6):1824—35.

[215] Jang A, Kim D, Sung KS, Jung S, Kim HJ, Jo C. The effect of dietary α-lipoic acid, betaine, l-carnitine, and swimming on the obesity of mice induced by a high-fat diet. Food Funct 2014;5(8):1966—74.

[216] Cui J, Huang D, Zheng Y. Ameliorative effects of α-lipoic acid on high-fat diet-induced oxidative stress and glucose uptake impairment of T cells. Free Radic Res 2016;50(10):1106—15.

[217] Liu Z, Patil I, Sancheti H, Yin F, Cadenas E. Effects of lipoic acid on high-fat diet-induced alteration of synaptic plasticity and brain glucose metabolism: a PET/CT and (13)C-NMR study. Sci Rep 2017;7(1):5391.

[218] Mathews CE, Bagley R, Leiter EH. ALS/Lt: a new type 2 diabetes mouse model associated with low free radical scavenging potential. Diabetes 2004;53(Suppl. 1):S125—9.

[219] Banday AA, Fazili FR, Marwaha A, Lokhandwala MF. Mitogen-activated protein kinase upregulation reduces renal D1 receptor affinity and G-protein coupling in obese rats. Kidney Int 2007;71(5):397—406.

[220] Cummings BP, Stanhope KL, Graham JL, Evans JL, Baskin DG, Griffen SC, et al. Dietary fructose accelerates the development of diabetes in UCD-T2DM rats: amelioration by the antioxidant, alpha-lipoic acid. Am J Physiol Integr Comp Physiol 2010;298(5):R1343—50.

[221] Muellenbach EM, Diehl CJ, Teachey MK, Lindborg KA, Hasselwander O, Matuschek M, et al. Metabolic interactions of AGE inhibitor pyridoxamine and antioxidant alpha-lipoic acid following 22 weeks of treatment in obese Zucker rats. Life Sci 2009;84(15—16):563—8.

[222] Saengsirisuwan V, Kinnick TR, Schmit MB, Henriksen EJ. Interactions of exercise training and lipoic acid on skeletal muscle glucose transport in obese Zucker rats. J Appl Physiol (Bethesda Md 1985) 2001;91(1):145—53.

[223] Fernández-Galilea M, Prieto-Hontoria PL, Martínez JA, Moreno-Aliaga MJ. Antiobesity effects of α-lipoic acid supplementation. Clin Lipidol 2013;8(3):371—83.

[224] Picklo M, Claycombe KJ, Meydani M. Adipose dysfunction, interaction of reactive oxygen species, and inflammation. Adv Nutr (Bethesda Md) 2012;3(5):734—5.

[225] Bryan S, Baregzay B, Spicer D, Singal PK, Khaper N. Redox-inflammatory synergy in the metabolic syndrome. Can J Physiol Pharmacol 2013;91(1):22—30.

[226] Kathirvel E, Morgan K, French SW, Morgan TR. Acetyl-L-carnitine and lipoic acid improve mitochondrial abnormalities and serum levels of liver enzymes in a mouse model of nonalcoholic fatty liver disease. Nutr Res (NY) 2013;33(11):932—41.

[227] Greene EL, Nelson BA, Robinson KA, Buse MG. alpha-Lipoic acid prevents the development of glucose-induced insulin resistance in 3T3-L1 adipocytes and accelerates the decline in immunoreactive insulin during cell incubation. Metabolism 2001;50(9):1063—9.

[228] Rudich A, Tirosh A, Potashnik R, Khamaisi M, Bashan N. Lipoic acid protects against oxidative stress induced impairment in insulin stimulation of protein kinase B and glucose transport in 3T3-L1 adipocytes. Diabetologia 1999;42(8):949—57.

[229] Potashnik R, Bloch-Damti A, Bashan N, Rudich A. IRS1 degradation and increased serine phosphorylation cannot predict the degree of metabolic insulin resistance induced by oxidative stress. Diabetologia 2003;46(5):639—48.

[230] Deiuliis JA, Kampfrath T, Ying Z, Maiseyeu A, Rajagopalan S. Lipoic acid attenuates innate immune infiltration and activation in the visceral adipose tissue of obese insulin resistant mice. Lipids 2011;46(11):1021—32.

[231] Huerta AE, Prieto-Hontoria PL, Fernández-Galilea M, Escoté X, Martínez JA, Moreno-Aliaga MJ. Effects of dietary supplementation with EPA and/or α-lipoic acid on adipose tissue transcriptomic profile of healthy overweight/obese women following a hypocaloric diet. BioFactors (Oxf Engl) 2017;43(1):117—31.

[232] Fernández-Galilea M, Pérez-Matute P, Prieto-Hontoria PL, Sáinz N, López-Yoldi M, Houssier M, et al. α-Lipoic acid reduces fatty acid esterification and lipogenesis in adipocytes from overweight/obese subjects. Obesity (Silver Spring Md) 2014;22:2210—5.

[233] Prieto-Hontoria PL, Pérez-Matute P, Fernández-Galilea M, López-Yoldi M, Sinal CJ, Martínez JA, et al. Effects of alpha-lipoic acid on chemerin secretion in 3T3-L1 and human adipocytes. Biochim Biophys Acta 2016;1861(3):260—8.

[234] Cho KJ, Moon HE, Moini H, Packer L, Yoon DY, Chung AS. Alpha-lipoic acid inhibits adipocyte differentiation by regulating pro-adipogenic transcription factors via mitogen-activated protein kinase pathways. J Biol Chem 2003;278(37):34823—33.

[235] Salle-Teyssières L, Auclair M, Terro F, Nemani M, Elsayed SM, Elsobky E, et al. Maladaptive autophagy impairs adipose function in congenital generalized lipodystrophy due to cavin-1 deficiency. J Clin Endocrinol Metab 2016;101(7):2892—904.

[236] Hahm JR, Noh HS, Ha JH, Roh GS, Kim DR. Alpha-lipoic acid attenuates adipocyte differentiation and lipid accumulation in 3T3-L1 cells via AMPK-dependent autophagy. Life Sci 2014;100(2):125—32.

[237] Fernández-Galilea M, Pérez-Matute P, Prieto-Hontoria PL, Martinez JA, Moreno-Aliaga MJ. Effects of lipoic acid on lipolysis in 3T3-L1 adipocytes. J Lipid Res 2012;53(11):2296—306.

[238] Kim SJ, Tang T, Abbott M, Viscarra JA, Wang Y, Sul HS. AMPK phosphorylates desnutrin/ATGL and hormone-sensitive lipase to regulate lipolysis and fatty acid oxidation within adipose tissue. Mol Cell Biol 2016;36(14):1961—76.

[239] Shen W, Liu K, Tian C, Yang L, Li X, Ren J, et al. R-alpha-lipoic acid and acetyl-L-carnitine complementarily promote mitochondrial biogenesis in murine 3T3-L1 adipocytes. Diabetologia 2008;51(1):165—74.

[240] Fernández-Galilea M, Pérez-Matute P, Prieto-Hontoria PL, Houssier M, Burrell MA, Langin D, et al. α-Lipoic acid treatment increases mitochondrial biogenesis and promotes beige adipose features in subcutaneous adipocytes from overweight/obese subjects. Biochim Biophys Acta 2015;1851(3):273—81.

[241] Fernández-Galilea M, Perez-Matute P, Prieto-Hontoria P, Martinez JA, Moreno-Aliaga MJ. Effects of lipoic acid on apelin in 3T3-L1 adipocytes and in high-fat fed rats. J Physiol Biochem 2011;67(3):479–86.

[242] Huerta AE, Prieto-Hontoria PL, Fernández-Galilea M, Sáinz N, Cuervo M, Martínez JA, et al. Circulating irisin and glucose metabolism in overweight/obese women: effects of á-lipoic acid and eicosapentaenoic acid. J Physiol Biochem 2015;71(3):547–58.

[243] Prieto-Hontoria PL, Perez-Matute P, Fernandez-Galilea M, Martinez JA, Moreno-Aliaga MJ. Effects of lipoic acid on AMPK and adiponectin in adipose tissue of low- and high-fat-fed rats. Eur J Nutr 2012;52(2):779–87.

[244] Prieto-Hontoria PL, Perez-Matute P, Fernandez-Galilea M, Martinez JA, Moreno-Aliaga MJ. Lipoic acid inhibits leptin secretion and Sp1 activity in adipocytes. Mol Nutr Food Res 2011;55(7):1059–69.

[245] Huerta AE, Navas-Carretero S, Prieto-Hontoria PL, Martínez JA, Moreno-Aliaga MJ. Effects of α-lipoic acid and eicosapentaenoic acid in overweight and obese women during weight loss. Obesity 2015;23(2):313–21.

[246] Moreno-Aliaga MJ, Swarbrick MM, Lorente-Cebrián S, Stanhope KL, Havel PJ, Martínez JA. Sp1-mediated transcription is involved in the induction of leptin by insulin-stimulated glucose metabolism. J Mol Endocrinol 2007;38(5):537–46.

[247] Tishinsky JM, Robinson LE, Dyck DJ. Insulin-sensitizing properties of adiponectin. Biochimie 2012;94(10):2131–6.

[248] Vidović B, Milovanović S, Stefanović A, Kotur-Stevuljević J, Takić M, Debeljak-Martačić J, et al. Effects of alpha-lipoic acid supplementation on plasma adiponectin levels and some metabolic risk factors in patients with schizophrenia. J Med Food 2017;20(1):79–85.

[249] Prieto-Hontoria PL, Fernández-Galilea M, Pérez-Matute P, Martínez JA, Moreno-Aliaga MJ. Lipoic acid inhibits adiponectin production in 3T3-L1 adipocytes. J Physiol Biochem September 2013;69(3):595–600.

[250] Zhou Q, Cao J, Chen L. Apelin/APJ system: a novel therapeutic target for oxidative stress-related inflammatory diseases (review). Int J Mol Med 2016;37(5):1159–69.

[251] Bertrand C, Valet P, Castan-Laurell I. Apelin and energy metabolism. Front Physiol 2015;6:115.

[252] Huerta AE, Prieto-Hontoria PL, Sáinz N, Martínez JA, Moreno-Aliaga MJ. Supplementation with α-lipoic acid alone or in combination with eicosapentaenoic acid modulates the inflammatory status of healthy overweight or obese women consuming an energy-restricted diet. J Nutr 2016;146(4):889S–96S.

[253] Yu S, Zhang Y, Li MZ, Xu H, Wang Q, Song J, et al. Chemerin and apelin are positively correlated with inflammation in obese type 2 diabetic patients. Chin Med J (Engl) 2012;125(19):3440–4.

[254] Boström P, Wu J, Jedrychowski MP, Korde A, Ye L, Lo JC, et al. A PGC1-α-dependent myokine that drives brown-fat-like development of white fat and thermogenesis. Nature 2012;481(7382):463–8.

[255] Thomou T, Mori MA, Dreyfuss JM, Konishi M, Sakaguchi M, Wolfrum C, et al. Adipose-derived circulating miRNAs regulate gene expression in other tissues. Nature 2017;542(7642):450–5.

[256] Zhang Y, Yu M, Tian W. Physiological and pathological impact of exosomes of adipose tissue. Cell Prolif 2016;49(1):3–13.

[257] Depner CM, Philbrick KA, Jump DB. Docosahexaenoic acid attenuates hepatic inflammation, oxidative stress, and fibrosis without decreasing hepatosteatosis in a Ldlr(−/−) mouse model of western diet-induced nonalcoholic steatohepatitis. J Nutr 2013;143(3):315–23.

[258] Suzuki-Kemuriyama N, Matsuzaka T, Kuba M, Ohno H, Han S-I, Takeuchi Y, et al. Different effects of eicosapentaenoic and docosahexaenoic acids on atherogenic high-fat diet-induced non-alcoholic fatty liver disease in mice. PLoS One 2016;11(6):e0157580.

[259] Pérez-Echarri N, Pérez-Matute P, Marcos-Gómez B, Baena MJ, Marti A, Martínez JA, et al. Differential inflammatory status in rats susceptible or resistant to diet-induced obesity: effects of EPA ethyl ester treatment. Eur J Nutr 2008;47(7):380–6.

[260] Kalupahana NS, Claycombe K, Newman SJ, Stewart T, Siriwardhana N, Matthan N, et al. Eicosapentaenoic acid prevents and reverses insulin resistance in high-fat diet-induced obese mice via modulation of adipose tissue inflammation. J Nutr 2010;140(11):1915–22.

[261] Yan Y, Jiang W, Spinetti T, Tardivel A, Castillo R, Bourquin C, et al. Omega-3 fatty acids prevent inflammation and metabolic disorder through inhibition of NLRP3 inflammasome activation. Immunity 2013;38(6):1154–63.

[262] Talamonti E, Pauter AM, Asadi A, Fischer AW, Chiurchiù V, Jacobsson A. Impairment of systemic DHA synthesis affects macrophage plasticity and polarization: implications for DHA supplementation during inflammation. Cell Mol Life Sci 2017;74(15):2815–26.

Chapter 5

Vascular Damage in Metabolic Disorders: Role of Oxidative Stress

Álvaro Pejenaute[1] and Guillermo Zalba Goñi[1,2]

[1]University of Navarra, Pamplona, Spain; [2]IdiSNA, Navarra Institute for Health Research, Pamplona, Spain

1. METABOLIC SYNDROME

1.1 Definition and Classification

The metabolic syndrome is a major public-health problem in the developed world whose prevalence has been increasing in the last years. It is defined as a clustering of several clinical risk factors such as elevated plasma glucose (hyperglycemia), insulin resistance, central obesity, atherogenic dyslipidemia (high triglycerides and low high-density lipoprotein levels), and elevated blood pressure (hypertension) in the same individual [1].

Although the term "metabolic syndrome" was first used in 1975 by Hermann Haller, it has its origins in 1923, when Kylin described an aggrupation of three metabolic alterations: hypertension, hyperglycemia, and gout in patients. In 1988, Reaven introduced the designation of syndrome X as a constellation of metabolic alterations, which included insulin resistance, glucose intolerance, hyperinsulinemia, dyslipidemia, and hypertension but missed obesity in the definition [2]. In 1989, the metabolic syndrome was called The Deadly Quartet, referring to the combination of obesity, hypertension, glucose intolerance, and hypertriglyceridemia; later in 1992 it was renamed The Insulin Resistance Syndrome [3]. Since 1988 several international organizations have established the clinical factors that are implicated in the metabolic syndrome and define the criteria for metabolic syndrome diagnosis (Table 5.1).

The first diagnosis definition was developed by the World Health Organization (WHO) in 1998, in which insulin resistance, obesity, dyslipidemia, and arterial hypertension were the main characteristics that describes the metabolic syndrome. One year later, in 1999, the European Group for the study of Insulin Resistance modified the WHO definition by excluding type 2 diabetes mellitus and including the waist circumference as a parameter to classify obesity. In 2001 the National Cholesterol Education Program Adult Treatment Panel III (NCEP-ATPIII) proposed a new definition for the metabolic syndrome as a constellation of metabolic alterations including dyslipidemia, hyperglycemia, and hypertension but excluded insulin resistance as a clinical criterion for its diagnosis [4]. Two years later, the American Association of Clinical Endocrinologists reintroduced insulin resistance in the metabolic syndrome definition. In 2005, two new definitions were proposed, one by the International Diabetes Federation (IDF) and the other by the American Heart Association (AHA) and the National Heart, Lung, and Blood Institute (NHLBI) [5]; both of them were based on the NCEP-ATPIII definition with minor modifications (Table 5.1).

Due to the variety of definitions, a precise diagnosis of metabolic syndrome could be challenging. For this reason a joint statement of the IDF Task Force on Epidemiology and Prevention, NHLBI, AHA, World Heart Federation, International Atherosclerosis Society, and International Association for the Study of Obesity was published [6] in order to set a single definitive definition of the metabolic syndrome. According to this last definition, insulin resistance and obesity are not prerequisites for metabolic syndrome diagnosis; it requires the presence of three of the five metabolic alterations described in Table 5.2.

Obesity. https://doi.org/10.1016/B978-0-12-812504-5.00005-2

TABLE 5.1 Metabolic Syndrome Definition and Clinical Diagnosis Criteria by Different International Associations

Criterion	WHO	EGIR	NCEP-ATPIII	AACE	IDF	AHA/NHLBI
Obesity	Waist to hip ratio >0.90 (men)/0.85 (women) BMI > 30 kg/m²	WC > 94 cm (men)/80 cm (women)	WC > 102 cm (men)/88 cm (women)	BMI > 25 kg/m²	Increased WC (ethnicity and gender specific)	WC > 102 cm (men)/88 cm (women)
Lipids	Triglycerides ≥ 150 mg/dL and/or HDLc < 35 mg/dL (men)/39 mg/dL (women)	Triglycerides ≥ 177 mg/dL or HDLc < 39 mg/dL	Triglycerides ≥ 150 mg/dL and/or HDLc < 40 mg/dL (men)/50 mg/dL (women)	Triglycerides ≥ 150 mg/dL and/or HDLc < 40 mg/dL (men)/50 mg/dL (women)	Triglycerides ≥ 150 mg/dL and/or HDLc < 40 mg/dL (men)/50 mg/dL (women) or receiving treatment	Triglycerides ≥ 150 mg/dL and/or HDLc < 40 mg/dL (men)/50 mg/dL (women) or receiving treatment
Blood pressure (systolic/diastolic)	≥140/90 mmHg	≥140/90 mmHg or receiving treatment	≥135/85 mmHg	≥135/85 mmHg	≥135/85 mmHg or receiving treatment	≥135/85 mmHg or receiving treatment
Glucose	Impaired fasting glucose, impaired glucose tolerance, or type 2 diabetes	Impaired fasting glucose or impaired glucose tolerance	≥110 mg/dL	Impaired fasting glucose or impaired glucose tolerance	≥110 mg/dL or type 2 diabetes	≥110 mg/dL or receiving treatment
Insulin resistance	Yes	Hyperinsulinemia	No	Impaired fasting glucose or impaired glucose tolerance	No	No
Other factors	Microalbuminuria					
Required criteria	Impaired glucose tolerance or type 2 diabetes + 2 factors	Insulin resistance + 2 factors	At least 3 of 5 factors	At least 2 of 4 factors	Impaired fasting glucose or impaired glucose tolerance + 2 factors	At least 3 of 5 factors

AACE, American Association of Clinical Endocrinologists; *AHA*, American Heart Association; *BMI*, body mass index; *EGIR*, European Group for the Study of Insulin Resistance; *HDLc*, high-density lipoprotein cholesterol; *IDF*, International Diabetes Federation; *NCEP-ATPIII*, National Cholesterol Education Program Adult Treatment Panel III; *NHLBI*, National Heart, Lung, and Blood Institute; *WC*, waist circumference; *WHO*, World Health Organization.

TABLE 5.2 Metabolic Syndrome Definition and Clinical Diagnosis Criteria by the International Diabetes Federation Task Force on Epidemiology and Prevention; National Heart, Lung, and Blood Institute; American Heart Association; World Heart Federation; International Atherosclerosis Society; and International Association for the Study of Obesity

Criterion	Threshold
Obesity	Elevated waist circumference (population and country specific)
Triglycerides	$\geq$150 mg/dL or receiving treatment
HDLc	<40 mg/dL (men)/50 mg/dL (women) or receiving treatment
Blood pressure (systolic/diastolic)	$\geq$135/85 mmHg or receiving treatment
Glucose	Elevated fasting glucose ($\geq$110 mg/dL) or receiving treatment

HDLc, high-density lipoprotein cholesterol.

1.2 Epidemiology and Clinical Repercussion

Early identification of patients with metabolic syndrome is critical, since several studies have associated the presence of metabolic syndrome with a twofold increase in the risk of developing cardiovascular disease and a fivefold increase in the risk of type 2 diabetes mellitus. Taking into account that the prevalence of metabolic syndrome is increasing worldwide, to a great extent due to the rise of sedentary lifestyle and obesity, metabolic syndrome can be considered a major public-health concern. In fact, a study performed with the offspring from the participants of the Framingham Heart Study revealed that in 10 years the prevalence of metabolic syndrome has increased from 23.5% to 40.6% [7].

Cardiovascular diseases, such as type 2 diabetes mellitus and coronary artery disease, are chronic diseases whose prevalence is rising and that increase morbidity and mortality of patients. For this reason, mortality of patients with metabolic syndrome is increased when compared with subjects without metabolic syndrome, and the risk is even greater if the patients with metabolic syndrome have diabetes. It has been shown that in subjects with metabolic syndrome the risk of stroke is 2—4 times higher and the risk of myocardial infarction is 3—4 times higher. In both cases the risk of dying is twofold increased in patients with metabolic syndrome [3].

Recently, other risk factors have been identified to be associated with metabolic syndrome, such as nonalcoholic fatty liver disease, atherosclerosis, the proinflammatory state, and oxidative stress [8].

2. OXIDATIVE STRESS

2.1 Introduction

Reactive oxygen species (ROS) are a family of molecules derived from molecular oxygen produced by the uncompleted reduction of oxygen to water in all mammalian cells. The most representative molecules of the ROS family are superoxide radical anion ($\cdot O_2^-$), hydroxyl radical ($\cdot OH$), hydrogen peroxide (H_2O_2), radical nitric oxide ($\cdot NO$), peroxynitrites ($ONOO^-$), and hypochlorous acid (HOCl).

The majority of ROS are produced from molecular oxygen, which can suffer a series of sequential reactions that originate the rest of ROS (Fig. 5.1) [9]. Molecular oxygen is in a triplet state and is relatively inert, despite the fact that it is a free biradical due to the parallel electron spins. For this reason the first reactions have to be catalyzed by enzymes. Molecular oxygen can be reduced by different oxidase enzymes to superoxide anions or react with L-arginine catalyzed nitric oxide synthase to form nitric oxide, which can be oxidized to nitrites (NO_2^-) or nitrates (NO_3^-). Nitric oxide half-life is short (around 3—5 s) and can easily react with superoxide anion to form peroxynitrites, which can be protonated in acid medium to peroxynitrous acid, which ultimately can be decomposed into hydroxyl radical and dioxide of nitrogen (NO_2). Superoxide anion can be dismutated into H_2O_2 by superoxide dismutase enzymes (SODs) and can be further transformed into hydroxyl radical, converted into water by enzymes (catalase or glutathione peroxidase) or transformed into hypochlorous acid by myeloperoxidase [10]. ROS can be generated intracellularly, extracellularly, or inside specific intracellular compartments.

ROS play an important role as second messengers in redox signaling, controlling growth, cellular adhesion, apoptosis, and cellular survival. This variety of actions of ROS is possible thanks to the diversity of ROS molecules and their finely

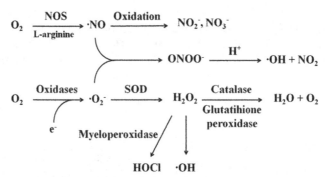

FIGURE 5.1   Scheme of reactive oxygen species metabolism. e^-, electron; H^+, proton; H_2O, water; H_2O_2, hydrogen peroxide; *HOCl*, hypochlorous acid; •*NO*, nitric oxide; NO_2, dioxide of nitrogen; NO_2^-, nitrites; NO_3^-, nitrates; *NOS*, nitric oxide synthase; O_2, molecular oxygen; •O_2^-, superoxide anion; •*OH*, hydroxyl radical; *ONOO*$^-$, peroxynitrites; *ROS*, reactive oxygen species; *SOD*, superoxide dismutase.

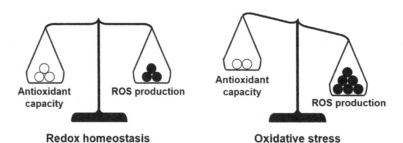

FIGURE 5.2   Schematic representation of a situation of redox homeostasis and oxidative stress. *ROS*, reactive oxygen species.

controlled production in a precise localization and right kinetic [11]. ROS are highly reactive and can oxidize biologic macromolecules like proteins, DNA, lipids, and carbohydrates; for this reason they have to be in balance with the antioxidant defenses (redox homeostasis) and their production has to be perfectly regulated.

Oxidative stress is a pathological situation in which there is an imbalance in redox homeostasis (Fig. 5.2). This takes place when there is an excessive production of ROS and/or when the antioxidant capacity is compromised. In this situation ROS can participate in the development of cardiovascular pathology through the activation of hypertrophic signaling, induction of apoptosis, inflammation, fibrosis, and macromolecular damage (proteins, lipids, and DNA) [12].

2.2 Cellular Consequences of Pathological Reactive Oxygen Species Production

In physiological conditions ROS play a key role in redox signaling cascades (through redox regulation of protein phosphorylation, ion channels, and transcription factors); they also take part in host defense since they are used to destroy bacteria and are required for synthetic reactions (like thyroid hormone production and cross-linking of extracellular matrix) [9]. In pathological conditions, ROS production can be diminished, leading to decreased antimicrobial defense (for example in chronic granulomatous disease) and lack of redox signaling, which can cause hypothyroidosis and low blood pressure. On the other hand excessive ROS production will lead to oxidative stress, with exacerbated redox signaling and tissue damage [9]. The two main pathological effects of oxidative stress at a cellular level are the reduction of nitric oxide bioavailability and the production of peroxynitrites.

2.2.1 Nitric Oxide Bioavailability

Nitric oxide was first denominated as the endothelium-derived relaxing factor in 1980 for its vasodilator effects to induce vasorelaxation, but the molecule responsible for that activity was unknown. In 1987 it was identified as nitric oxide, and the work of Robert F. Furchgott, Louis J. Ignarro, and Ferid Murad about nitric oxide signaling in the cardiovascular system was awarded the Nobel Prize in Physiology or Medicine in 1998.

The reaction between superoxide anion and nitric oxide is around three times faster than the dismutation of superoxide anion catalyzed by SOD. In physiological conditions superoxide dismutation is sufficient and SOD can keep superoxide anion concentration under control and consequently nitric oxide levels are not compromised. However, in a pathological situation ROS production is exacerbated and/or the antioxidant systems are not able to control the concentration of superoxide, which reacts with nitric oxide, decreasing its bioavailability [13].

Since nitric oxide is one of the main vasodilator agents, its depletion has an enormous impact on the regulation of the vascular tone, leading to endothelial dysfunction.

2.2.2 Peroxynitrites Production

The reaction between superoxide anion and nitric oxide results in the production of peroxynitrites. However, this does not reduce the potential oxidative stress created by superoxide anion, since peroxynitrites are strong oxidant molecules and more stable than superoxide anion and nitric oxide. In physiological conditions, peroxynitrite half-life is about one second, which limits its diffusion and prevents its accumulation and interaction with other biological molecules. Peroxynitrite detoxification is performed by reaction with thiol-rich molecules to generate nitrosothiols and the regeneration of nitric oxide.

However, in pathological situations peroxynitrite formation is increased. Peroxynitrites are powerful oxidant and nitrating agents, able produce DNA fragmentation [14], depletion of antioxidant substances (like glutathione), lipid peroxidation, and oxidative damage to proteins. Peroxynitrites can interact with proteins by reaction with transition metal centers (heme group, iron-sulfur clusters, or Zn^{2+} sulfur motifs) or by reacting with specific amino acids (tyrosine nitration or by cysteine, tryptophan, methionine, and histidine oxidation) [15]. These alterations in proteins can lead to loss of their activity, gain altered function, or be tagged to degradation, which affects cellular modulation of signaling cascades, resulting in cellular and organic dysfunction. It should be noted that endothelial nitric oxide 3 (NOS3) cofactor tetrahydrobiopterin can be oxidized by peroxynitrites, leading to the uncoupling of the enzyme by inducing the production of superoxide anion instead of nitric oxide.

Peroxynitrites can attack target molecules through two different mechanisms:

- Peroxynitrite is protonated to peroxynitrous acid (ONOOH) and induces oxidative reaction by one- or two-electron transfer.
- Peroxynitrite is transformed into hydroxyl radical and nitrogen dioxide radical ($\cdot NO_2$) by homolytic decomposition of peroxynitrous acid.

2.3 Oxidative Stress and Cardiovascular and Metabolic Disease

Oxidative stress plays a key role in several pathological situations like hypertension, obesity, and/or hypertriglyceridemia, which are part of the factors that define the metabolic syndrome [16].

The relationship between oxidative stress and hypertension has been shown in several animal models like spontaneously hypertensive rat (SHR), angiotensin II infused rat, and deoxycorticosterone acetate (DOCA) salt hypertensive rat [17]. An increased production of ROS, especially superoxide anion, accompanied by reduced nitric oxide bioavailability and H_2O_2 in the vasculature and kidney, promotes a chain of physiological modifications that lead to functional and structural alterations in the vascular wall, increasing peripheral resistances and raising blood pressure.

In human and mice models of obesity, oxidative stress is associated with a reduction of antioxidant systems, thus promoting the development of the metabolic syndrome by an alteration in adipokines production. Increased ROS levels from adipose tissue in peripheral blood in obese subjects are associated with the development of insulin resistance in skeletal muscle and adipose tissue and in insulin secretion [18].

Oxidative stress is involved in the pathogenesis of atherosclerosis. ROS promotes the activation of extracellular matrix metalloproteinases, low-density lipoprotein (LDL) oxidation, endothelial dysfunction, vascular smooth muscle cell growth, migration, and apoptosis, so ROS participates in the initial step, the progression, and the end event of the atherosclerotic process [19].

2.4 Enzymatic Sources of Superoxide Anion

Several enzymatic sources can produce ROS in the vascular wall, such as cyclooxygenases (COXs), lipoxygenase, uncoupled nitric oxide synthases [20], the mitochondrial electron transport chain, xanthine oxidase, cytochrome P450, and nicotinamide adenine dinucleotide phosphate (NADPH) oxidase (NOX).

Xanthine oxidase is an enzyme that has two interconvertible forms, xanthine oxidase and xanthine reductase. Xanthine oxidase catalyzes the oxidation of hypoxanthine and xanthine, the last two steps of purine metabolism, in which molecular oxygen is reduced to superoxide anion. It has been shown that SHR has elevated levels of endothelial xanthine oxidase with enhanced ROS production accompanied by increased arteriolar tone, and in hypertensive rats induced by DOCA and salt, xanthine oxidase promotes superoxide anion production [21]. In human subjects xanthine oxidase has been implicated in the development of hypertension, since its inhibition with allopurinol is associated with lower blood pressure.

Endothelial nitric oxide synthase is the main source of nitric oxide in the vascular wall. In pathological conditions of oxidative stress, deficiency of the substrate L-arginine and/or the deficiency or oxidation of tetrahydrobiopterin leads to uncoupling of nitric oxide synthase, which starts to produce superoxide anion instead of nitric oxide [22], contributing to the development of hypertension. In the SHR and DOCA animal models, treatment with tetrahydrobiopterin reduced blood pressure values. Clinical studies in patients also support the role of decreased tetrahydrobiopterin availability and reduced nitric oxide production, opening the possibility of using tetrahydrobiopterin treatment as a therapeutic approach in endothelial dysfunction.

Numerous studies have demonstrated that NOXs are the main source of superoxide anion in the vascular wall (in endothelial cells, vascular smooth muscle cells, and fibroblasts) and that plays a critical role in the development of cardiovascular diseases.

3. NICOTINAMIDE ADENINE DINUCLEOTIDE PHOSPHATE OXIDASES

The NOX family is one of the main producers of ROS in cardiovascular context. NOXs catalyze the transfer of an electron from NADPH cofactor to reduce molecular oxygen, generating superoxide anion and/or H_2O_2 outside the cells or inside different intracellular components (phagosomes, endosomes, the endoplasmic reticulum, or perinuclear compartment) [23]. However, unlike other enzymatic systems, ROS production for NOXs is its primary catalytic function instead of a side product of their activity or the result of an aberrant function in a pathological situation. For this reason NOXs are defined as professional ROS producers [24].

NOXs were first discovered in phagocytes (macrophages/monocytes, neutrophils), which produce great amounts of superoxide anion to generate a respiratory burst used in defense against bacterial and fungal infection. Since then, NOXs were also identified in endothelial cells, vascular smooth muscle cells [25], fibroblasts, cardiomyocytes, platelets, and others. NOXs are expressed in most mammalian cells. Nonphagocytic NOXs act as an oxygen sensor and modulate redox signaling pathways that control key cellular functions like contraction, growth, differentiation, migration, proliferation, and cellular death [26].

The NADPH family is composed of five homologs (Nox 1−5) and the dual oxidases (DUOXs 1 and 2) in mammals [27], but they are also expressed in plants and lower organisms. Each homolog is encoded by its own respective gene and it is formed by a core catalytic transmembrane subunit and up to five regulatory subunits (Fig. 5.3).

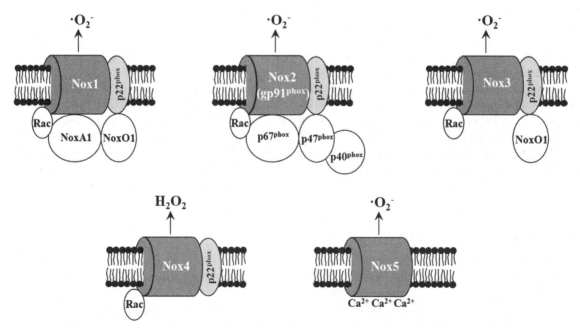

FIGURE 5.3 NADPH oxidase structure and subunits. Transmembrane catalytic units (Nox 1 to 5) and regulatory units (p22phox) are shown as *dark gray*; cytosolic regulatory units are presented as *light gray* (RAC, NOXA1, NOXO1, p47phox, p40phox, and p67phox); EF-hand motifs that bind to Ca^{2+} are shown as Ca^{2+}. *NADPH*, nicotinamide adenine dinucleotide phosphate; *Nox*, NADPH oxidase; *RAC*, Rac family small GTPase.

The catalytic subunit of each NOX homolog is composed by a long C-terminal reductase domain, with conserved flavin adenine dinucleotide (FAD) and NADPH binding sites followed by six transmembrane α-helical segments [28]. The transmembrane domains posses two heme groups (in NOX proteins, but not in the DUOX; helix 3 and 5 contains four conserved histidine residues near the membrane interface where the heme groups are anchored). Finally, there is a cytoplasmic N-terminal domain, and in the DUOX this N-terminal domain has a large extracellular peroxidase-like domain and an additional transmembrane segment [23].

The regulatory subunits play important roles in the expression (p22phox, and DUOX activators—DUOXA1 and DUOXA2-), activation (p67phox and NOX activator—NOXA1) and spatial organization (p47phox, p40phox, and NOX organizer—NOXO1) of the enzyme complex [23]. p22phox is a regulatory transmembrane subunit whose main function is to serve as a connector between the catalytic subunit and the other cytosolic regulatory subunits (p47phox and p67phox), taking part in enzyme assembly; it is present in Nox 1, 2, 3, and 4. Nox 1, 2, and 3 also requires the guanosine trisphosphate (GTP)ase Rac family small GTPase (RAC)1 or RAC2 for their activation. Nox 5 and the DUOX do not require cytosolic regulatory nor p22phox to be activated; instead they are regulated by Ca^{2+} due to the presence of EF-hand motifs.

When NOXs are activated, electrons are transferred from the NADPH cofactor, transported across the electron transport chain of catalytic subunit, and used to reduce molecular oxygen. In Nox 1, 2, and 5 this reduction results in the release of superoxide anion, but Nox 4 and the DUOX generate hydrogen peroxide directly. It has been suggested that the extracytosolic E-loop of Nox 4 delays the release of superoxide anion, so it is still linked to the enzyme when a second molecule of superoxide anion is produced and both react producing dismutation and release of H_2O_2 [29]. In the DUOX the peroxidase-like domain is responsible for superoxide conversion into H_2O_2 [23].

3.1 Nicotinamide Adenine Dinucleotide Phosphate Oxidases Localization

NOXs are present in most cell types in mammalian organisms; however, not all the NOX homologs are expressed in the same tissues/cells with the same level of expression or at the same time. In fact, different homologs can be expressed in parallel in the same cell, but in different subcellular organelles or localizations. This is an indicator that shows the complexity of this enzyme family, the specialization and different function of each homolog [30].

Nox 1 (originally named Mox1) is expressed mainly in the colon and vessel wall, but also in the heart and brain. Nox 2 (also named gp91phox) is the homolog identified as the phagocytic NOX, so its highest levels of expression are found in phagocytes, but can be also found in the vessel wall, heart, brain, and lungs [31]. Nox 3 is expressed in the inner ear and fetal kidney. Nox 4 homolog is highly expressed in the kidney and also found in the vessel, heart, liver, lungs, and prostate. Nox 5 was found in the vessel, spleen, heart, lymph nodes, ovaries, sperm, and testes. Finally both DUOX are mainly expressed in the thyroid gland; DUOX1 is also found in cerebellum and lung (bronchi) and DUOX2 in lung (bronchi), prostate, uterus, and pancreatic islets (Table 5.3).

Focusing in the vasculature, NOX homologs Nox 1, 2, 4, and 5 have been identified in the vascular wall [28]. Nox 1 is expressed in endothelial cells [32] and vascular smooth muscle cells. Nox 2 is found in circulating white blood cells, in endothelial cells [31], and in adventitial fibroblasts [33]. Nox 4 appears ubiquitously in all cell types of the vascular wall (in

TABLE 5.3 NADPH Oxidase and DUOX Homolog Regulatory Subunits and Tissue Localization

NADPH Oxidase	Regulatory Subunits	Tissue Localization
Nox 1	p22phox, p47phox/NOXO1, NOXA1, RAC1	Colon, vessel, heart, brain
Nox 2	p22phox, p47phox, p67phox, p40phox, RAC1/RAC2	Phagocytes, vessel, heart, brain, lungs
Nox 3	p22phox, NOXO1, NOXA1, RAC1	Inner ear, fetal kidney
Nox 4	p22phox, POLDIP2	Kidney, vessel, heart, liver, lungs, prostate
Nox 5	EF-hand motifs	Vessel, spleen, heart, lymph nodes, ovaries, sperm, testes
DUOX1	DUOXA1, EF-hand motifs	Thyroid gland, bronchi, cerebellum
DUOX2	DUOXA2, EF-hand motifs	Thyroid gland, bronchi, prostate, uterus, pancreatic islets

DUOX, dual oxidase; *DUOXA1*, DUOX activator 1; *DUOXA2*, DUOX activator 2; *NADPH*, nicotinamide adenine dinucleotide phosphate; *Nox*, NADPH oxidase; *NOXA1*, NOX activator 1; *NOXO1*, NOX organizer 1; *POLDIP2*, polymerase δ-interacting protein 2; *RAC1*, Rac family small GTPase 1; *RAC2*, Rac family small GTPase 2.

endothelial cells, vascular smooth muscle cells, and fibroblasts) [34], and compared with the other homologs, is highly expressed. Nox 5 expression is found in endothelial cells [35], vascular smooth muscle cells, and recently it has been shown that Nox 5 is also present in human monocytes and macrophages.

Inside vascular cells, NOX homologs are present in different compartments. Nox 1 has been detected in the plasma membrane, in caveolae and endosomes on the cell surface [34]. Nox 2 is found in the plasma membrane, endosomes, phagosomes, and in intracellular membranes [24]. Nox 4 is expressed in focal adhesions [34], the nucleus, the endoplasmic reticulum, and the mitochondria. Nox 5 in the absence of stimulation is placed in intracellular membranes, but it is transported to the plasma membrane in response to phosphatidylinositol 4,5-biphosphate (PIP2) due the interaction of PIP2 with Nox5 N-terminal polybasic domain.

3.2 Nicotinamide Adenine Dinucleotide Phosphate Oxidase Regulation

NOX activity is regulated by interactions with the regulatory subunits, by humoral factors, by hemodynamic factors, by controlling the expression levels, and by transcriptional regulation.

Nox 1, 2, and 3 are regulated by interacting and binding to regulatory subunits (Table 5.2). First, they need the transmembrane subunit p22phox as a membrane-stabilizing subunit, which is essential to form the core cytochrome [36]. Second, they are under control of the cytosolic regulatory subunits [37], which are classified in three groups [23]:

- The small GTPase Rac bound to GTP RAC1 and RAC2
- The NOX activators: p67phox or NOXA1, the GTP-dependent targets of RAC
- The organizer or adaptor proteins: p40phox and p47phox or NOXO1, which are responsible for the interactions between the NOX activators and the core cytochrome

Nox 1 and 2 are completely inactive in the absence of stimulation so their control is performed by posttranslational modification of the regulatory units, while Nox 3 has constitutive activity [23].

Nox 4 is constitutively active in a high expression level, but also requires p22phox subunit and is regulated by polymerase δ-interacting protein 2 (POLDIP2). Nox 4 activity is determined by controlling its expression level [26] or by direct posttranslational modification [38]. Nox 5 does not require any regulatory subunits for its activation and like DUOX1 and DUOX2 are regulated by Ca^{2+} by the EF-hand motifs [39]. DUOX1 and DUOX2 also bind to the transmembrane DUOX activator DUOXA1 and DUOXA2, respectively.

NOXs can be regulated by hemodynamic factors; they are sensitive to mechanical forces [40]. Laminar shear stress seems to limit NOX expression in cultured endothelial cells while cyclic strain induces ROS production by NOXs and oscillatory shear stress activates Nox 1. Pulsatile stretch enhances superoxide production in smooth muscle cells and flow overload induce Nox 2 and Nox 4 expression.

NOXs can be also activated by humoral stimuli like [41]

- Growth factors whose targets are G-protein-coupled receptors. Their most representative example is angiotensin II [25], which activates NOXs through angiotensin II type 1 receptor leading to protein kinase C (PKC) activation, which phosphorylates p47phox. Thrombin also activates NOX activity by p47phox phosphorylation. Other NOX activating factors are endothelin-1 [20], aldosterone [20], histamine, serotonin, and prostaglandins.
- Growth factors whose targets are tyrosine kinases receptors, like platelet-derived growth factor [42] and transforming growth factor β (TGF-β) [32].
- Cytokines like leptin, interleukin-4, interleukin-1, erythropoietin, and tumor necrosis factor α (TNFα) [43].
- Signaling lipids like lysophosphatidylcholine, lysophosphatidic acid, and oxidized LDL [44].

Elevated glucose concentration activates NOXs by PKC induction [45]. Hypoxia increases ROS production by NOX activation in endothelial cells. Some epigenetic mechanisms have been discovered to modify NOX expression. In vascular endothelial cells senescence miR-146a induces Nox 4 while miR-25 downregulation increases Nox 4 activity in diabetic rats. Acetylation of histones H2BK16 and H3K9 by histone acetyltransferases GCN5 is required for Nox 2 expression in leukocytes.

4. PHAGOCYTIC NICOTINAMIDE ADENINE DINUCLEOTIDE PHOSPHATE OXIDASE AND METABOLIC DISORDERS

NOXs play a central role in cardiovascular diseases such as hypertension, diabetes, atherosclerosis, and cerebrovascular disease [46]. This role has been determined in experimental models of disease as well as in human diseases.

In cardiovascular diseases not only vascular oxidases but also the phagocytic NOX plays an important role in superoxide production, since monocytes and lymphocytes can infiltrate cardiovascular tissues.

NOX is the major inducible source of superoxide in phagocytic cells, including lymphocytes, monocytes, and neutrophils. The phagocytic oxidase is a membrane-bound enzyme that catalyses the single electron reduction of molecular oxygen to form superoxide. It consists of a membrane-associated cytochrome b558, and three cytosolic components p47phox, p67phox, and RAC1/2. Cytochrome b558 comprises a large subunit, gp91phox (Nox 2), and a smaller, p22phox, and functions as the final electron transporter from NADPH to molecular oxygen [47].

Phagocytic NOX activity and expression are enhanced in atherosclerosis and in its vascular and metabolic risk factors. Thus this oxidase might play a key role in the morbidity and mortality in these diseases by favoring deleterious prooxidant processes on cellular macromolecules, after exposition to acute and chronic oxidative stress situations.

4.1 Arterial Hypertension

The potential role of phagocytic NOX in the pathogenesis of hypertension is unclear. The augmented infiltration of monocytes and lymphocytes in the vascular wall in the experimental hypertension associates with enhanced superoxide production that impairs the endothelial function. Clinical data show that peripheral monocytes/macrophages and lymphocytes are activated in human hypertension [48].

Circulating phagocytic cells from hypertensive patients exhibit a state of preactivation, including increased adherence to endothelial cells, enhanced release of cytokines upon stimulation, and alteration in gene expression profile [49,50]. Superoxide generation is also increased in neutrophils from hypertensive patients [51]. Interestingly, NOX-dependent superoxide production is increased in lymphoblasts derived from hypertensive subjects [52]. Accordingly, NOX-dependent superoxide production is increased in mononuclear cells (monocytes and lymphocytes) from hypertensive patients [17].

- NOX-dependent superoxide correlated inversely with nitric oxide metabolites in hypertensive patients. Nitric oxide is oxidized to nitrite and then to nitrate by superoxide, among others, so the major oxidative metabolites are nitrite and nitrate. Nitric oxide is able to react with superoxide to form peroxynitrate, though this compound may lead to nitration of tyrosine or may isomerase to nitrates. Thus measurements of nitric oxide metabolites reflect real changes in nitric oxide generation. Impaired expression/activity of endothelial nitric oxide synthase could cause the diminished production of nitric oxide observed in hypertensive patients. In addition, endothelial nitric oxide synthase-mediated nitric oxide production may be reduced when the enzyme is deprived of its critical cofactor tetrahydrobiopterin or its substrate L-arginine, a phenomenon known as endothelial nitric oxide synthase uncoupling [22]. The association between exaggerated phagocytic NOX-dependent superoxide production and diminished nitric oxide generation in hypertensive patients allows us to speculate that phagocytic NOX might be involved in a diminished nitric oxide availability in essential hypertension.

- Enhanced phagocytic NOX-dependent superoxide production may also be involved in the damage of target organs in hypertension. Thus, left ventricular hypertrophy is an independent marker of mortality in hypertension, and inflammation and oxidative stress may favor its development. In this sense, NOX-dependent superoxide anion production is enhanced in peripheral blood mononuclear cells from hypertensive patients with left ventricular hypertrophy as compared with cells from both hypertensives without left ventricular hypertrophy and normotensive subjects [53]. Interestingly, activation of the NOX in peripheral blood mononuclear cells might promote a systemic and cardiac proinflammatory and prohypertrophic profile, thus supporting that the peripheral blood mononuclear cells NOX overactivity may play a major role in left ventricular hypertrophy in hypertensive patients. Hypertensive heart might produce higher levels of proinflammatory molecules, which can promote white cell infiltration. Such activated, infiltrated white cells thus turn into local sources of oxidative stress, proinflammatory cytokines, and matrix metalloproteinases, contributing to myocardial remodeling. Monocytes and lymphocytes may play a relevant role in the genesis of hypertension, in part attributable to NOX-dependent mechanisms. Local NOXs play a role in the development and outcome of cardiovascular diseases. In addition, the NOX of circulating cells is influenced by a systemic proinflammatory state and contributes to cardiac oxidative stress. Interestingly, in hypertensive patients with left ventricular hypertrophy, the reduction in the left ventricular mass index by treatment with antihypertensive drugs correlated with a reduction in ROS produced by monocytes [54].

4.2 Metabolic Syndrome

Metabolic syndrome associates with elevated systemic oxidative stress [55]. Among other effects, an excess of superoxide may inactivate nitric oxide, thus leading to endothelial dysfunction and, in turn, facilitating vascular abnormalities.

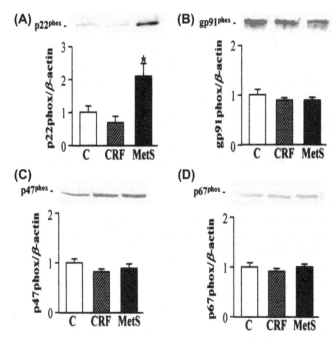

FIGURE 5.4 **Expression of NADPH oxidase subunits in phagocytic cells.** Representative Western blots for (A) p22phox, (B) gp91phox, (C) p47phox, and (D) p67phox. Densitometric analysis revealed increased p22phox in the *MetS* group compared with *C* and *CRF* groups. *C*, control subjects; *CRF*, individuals with one or two cardiovascular risk factors; *MetS*, metabolic syndrome patients; *NADPH*, nicotinamide adenine dinucleotide phosphate. *Adapted from Fortuno A, San Jose G, Moreno MU, Beloqui O, Diez J, Zalba G. Phagocytic NADPH oxidase overactivity underlies oxidative stress in metabolic syndrome. Diabetes 2006;55(1):209−15.*

In addition, an increased production of superoxide may facilitate oxidative modification of proteins by rendering nitro-tyrosine; levels of nitrotyrosine are increased in diabetic patients [56] and constitute a strong and independent predictor of cardiovascular disease [57]. Superoxide is also involved in LDL oxidation, a key step in the initiation and progression of atherosclerosis. LDL is oxidized by myeloperoxidase in the presence of peroxide hydrogen. Because increased NOX-dependent superoxide production associates with increased levels of H_2O_2 [58], it has been suggested that phagocytic NOX overactivity might facilitate the oxidation of LDL.

Phagocytic NOX expression and activity is enhanced in patients with metabolic syndrome [16]. In particular, the enhanced NOX activity associated with upregulated levels of the p22phox subunit, but not with changes in the other NOX subunits (Fig. 5.4). Thus it is likely that p22phox levels constitute a limiting factor capable of regulating NOX activity in metabolic disorders. Interestingly, NOX overactivity is involved in oxidative stress and atherosclerosis in metabolic syndrome patients. Thus patients with metabolic syndrome exhibit features of oxidative stress (i.e., increased levels of oxidized LDL and hydrogen peroxide), which associates with phagocytic NOX activity. Finally, NOX overactivity also associated with enhanced carotid intima-media thickness, an independent risk factor for coronary heart disease events, stroke, and transient cerebral ischemia that provides a useful surrogate marker for atherosclerotic disease.

Obesity, a key component defining metabolic syndrome, also associates with increased production of superoxide via the phagocytic NOX pathway [59]. Because obesity associates with increased ROS generation by mononuclear phagocytic cells, probably in relation to increased macronutrient intake, and a majority of the metabolic syndrome patients are obese, the NOX overactivity in metabolic syndrome patients might be related to obesity.

Metabolic syndrome associates with insulin resistance, thus increasing the cardiovascular risk. NOX-dependent superoxide production is augmented in insulin-resistant metabolic syndrome patients with respect to insulin sensitive patients [60]. Moreover, increased NOX-dependent superoxide production associated with higher p22phox expression in insulin-resistant than in insulin-sensitive patients. This association results in highest cardiovascular risk in metabolic syndrome patients.

4.3 Atherosclerosis

The phagocytic NOX plays a major role in human atherosclerosis. In fact, contribution of NOX to lesion progression is due almost entirely to infiltrated monocytes [61,62]. The severity of atherosclerotic lesion associates with p22phox overexpression in coronary arteries [63]. In addition, gp91phox and p22phox increase considerably along the progression of human atherosclerotic plaques, thus suggesting a causal link between the phagocytic NOX and the development of lesions. Finally, ROS production, mainly generated by infiltrated inflammatory cells, associates with p22phox in atherosclerotic human coronary arteries [64]. In human endarterectomies, upregulated NOX subunits colocalize with higher infiltration of monocytes/macrophages, higher expression of extracellular matrix metalloproteinase 9, and lower amount of collagen [65]. Interestingly, phagocytic NOX activity is already increased in asymptomatic subjects, apparently free of clinical atherosclerosis. In these subjects, NOX activity associates with carotid intima-media thickness [19], a surrogate marker of atherosclerosis, and with systemic levels of extracellular matrix metalloproteinase 9 [65], a surrogate marker of thrombosis.

5. REGULATION OF PHAGOCYTIC NICOTINAMIDE ADENINE DINUCLEOTIDE PHOSPHATE OXIDASE IN METABOLIC DISORDERS

5.1 Humoral Agonists

5.1.1 Angiotensin II and Endothelin-1

In the setting of cardiovascular and metabolic diseases, we can find several potential stimulating factors of the NOX. Humoral factors play a key role in the activation of NOX. Thus, angiotensin II and endothelin-1 enhances NOX activity in several kinds of cells, including smooth muscle cells and monocytes [66]. Interestingly, superoxide production in response to angiotensin II and endothelin-1 is higher in phagocytic cells from hypertensive patients than in cells from normotensive subjects [17].

5.1.2 Cytokines

Cardiotrophin-1 is a member of the interleukin-6 superfamily of cytokines. Although originally characterized as a survival factor, chronically elevated cardiotrophin-1 may contribute to left ventricular growth and dysfunction in hypertension. In fact, cardiotrophin-1 can contribute to systemic oxidative stress by activating the NOX in phagocytic cells, and that consequently, a further proinflammatory and prohypertrophic profile (interleukin-6 secretion) is induced [53]. Interleukin-6 is a pleiotropic cytokine expressed in a multitude of cells, especially in monocytes and macrophages. Interestingly, interleukin-6 infusion induces cardiac hypertrophy and fibrosis in mice, yielding a myocardial phenotype that resembles hypertensive heart disease [67]. Thus phagocytic NOX may play a major role in left ventricular hypertrophy in hypertensive patients. In addition, other proinflammatory cytokines, including TNF-α, may also activate phagocytic NOX [68].

5.2 Metabolic Agonists

5.2.1 Leptin

Oxidative stress is associated with obesity and is a unifying mechanism in the development of obesity-related comorbidities. Among the mechanisms linking obesity to cardiovascular diseases, recent analyses point to the role of mediators secreted by white adipose tissue. Among these leptin seems to play a key role in the pathogenesis of obesity-associated atherosclerosis [69]. Circulating levels of leptin are related with hypertension in clinical obesity. In particular, leptin induces proliferation and matrix metalloproteinase 2 expression in human vascular smooth muscle cells through the activation of NOX [70]. We have found that leptin is also able to activate NOX in human phagocytic cells and in murine macrophages [59]. Moreover, leptin-stimulated superoxide production was associated with the translocation of p47phox from cytosolic to membrane fraction in macrophages, through underlying mechanisms involving PI3K/PKC axis.

5.2.2 Insulin

A number of factors may be related to an increased phagocytic NOX-mediated superoxide production in metabolic syndrome, although growing evidence suggests a determinant role for hyperinsulinemia. Insulin is involved in the activation of the NOX in vascular smooth muscle cells, fibroblasts, and adipocytes [71,72]. Interestingly, insulin also activates NOX in human phagocytic cells [16]. Moreover, in metabolic syndrome patients, insulin-stimulated superoxide production is higher in insulin-resistant subjects than in insulin-sensitive ones [60]. Thus, chronic hyperinsulinemia might favor NOX overactivation in metabolic syndrome.

5.3 Genetics Profile

A great number of studies suggest a significant role of the genetic background in NOX regulation [47]. Among the key subunits involved in NOX activation, we can underline a key role for the p22phox subunit, which is a common regulator component of NOX1 to NOX4-dependent forms of the NOX. Monocytic and/or lymphocytic p22phox levels are increased in human arterial hypertension [17,52], obesity [59], metabolic syndrome [16], and diabetes [73]. Moreover, the enhanced activity of phagocytic NOX described in subclinical and clinical atherosclerosis is associated with upregulation of p22phox subunit [19,62−65]. In the last years, a great number of studies have described a relationship between genetic variability of p22phox and the pathophysiology of metabolic and cardiovascular diseases.

The human gene encoding the p22phox subunit, *CYBA*, is localized on chromosome 16q24. Variants in the gene are numerous, most of them mutations linked to chronic granulomatous disease. Among the huge amount of polymorphisms characterized, there are several single nucleotide polymorphisms (SNPs) with an effect in complex diseases, including arterial hypertension, obesity, metabolic syndrome, diabetes, and atherosclerosis. Four of these are localized in the promoter region of the gene, two nonconservative allelic variants in the coding region and another in the 3′ untranslated region [46].

Functionality of polymorphisms mainly depends on location within the gene [74]. Variants in the 5′ region may affect transcription rate and therefore alter protein quantity. Protein levels may also be affected by variants in the 3′ untranslated region, since they may alter the stability and translation rate of the messenger RNA (mRNA). Such effects are cell- or tissue-specific, as they depend on the mechanisms that regulate transcription and translation within the cell, such as transcription factors and microRNAs. This type of variant may display a molecular functional effect only under specific conditions. Alternatively, variants that affect the coding region are independent of such regulation and therefore not tissue-specific but of systemic effect. They alter protein quality and sometimes quantity, affecting the length of the protein, its structure and stability, how it interacts with other proteins, and, in the case of enzymes, the catalytic capacity. In this regard, polymorphisms affecting the *CYBA* gene will modify p22phox mRNA and/or protein levels or else cytochrome stability and functionality, resulting in altered NOX-dependent release of superoxide and greater oxidative stress.

5.3.1 Polymorphism -930A>G

The -930A>G variant is localized in the promoter of *CYBA* [75] and displays in vitro functional effects in hypertension [76]. The G allele may interact with CCAAT/enhancer binding protein (C/EBP) delta and promote higher transcription levels than the A allele. This is in agreement with clinical data showing that hypertensive patients exhibit a higher prevalence of the GG genotype, which is accompanied with higher levels of p22phox and enhanced NOX-derived oxidative stress.

The diverse ethnicity of the subjects in study, the variable distribution of the polymorphism, and the range of pathologies considered may be taken in mind in order to explain controversial results. Thus in a Brazilian study, the authors did not find association of the -930A>G polymorphism with hypertension [77]. On the other hand, a higher prevalence of the GG genotype in hypertension has been described in Japanese population [78].

In an association study carried out on coronary artery disease, the authors detected no association of the -930A>G polymorphism with ROS production and the disease, which may be explained by their use of lymphoblastoid cells in basal conditions [79]. Nevertheless, in view that C/EBP delta is implicated in the regulation of this variant and given the possible implication of C/EBP delta in hypertension, atherosclerosis, and diabetes, we cannot discard the role of the -930A>G variant in coronary artery disease. In fact, a study has shown that the -930A>G polymorphism is associated with coronary artery disease in the Polish population [80]. Interestingly, the -930G allele carriers were particularly at risk of consequences of obesity and tobacco smoke exposure.

5.3.2 Polymorphism -675T>A

The -675T>A variant was described together with the -852G>C and the -536C>T polymorphisms. Despite the very asymmetric distribution of the -675T>A variant, we detected a significant reduction of the A allele in the hypertensive population [81]. In vitro studies identified the transcription factor hypoxia inducible factor 1-α as one of the mediators of the increased promoter activity derived by the A allele in accordance with evidence related to the existence of the regulation of p22phox and NOX activity by hypoxia. Given the known activation of the factor hypoxia inducible factor 1-α by both the hypoxia associated with the atherosclerotic process and also by cardiovascular agonists such as angiotensin II, it would be of great interest to investigate if patients carrying the A allele may present a higher p22phox transcription rate in cardiovascular tissues, and thus, if they may be under greater risk of coronary artery disease and complications.

5.3.3 Polymorphism 242C>T

The 242C>T is the best known *CYBA* polymorphism. It results in an amino acid change (histidine to tyrosine) in position 72 of the p22phox protein; the Tyrosine residue derived from the T allele may alter p22phox interaction with the heme group, thus diminishing the cytochrome capacity for electron transfer. Functional studies have shown that the T allele was associated with reduced white-cell NOX activity in control subjects and in hypertensive patients as well as in saphenous veins of atherosclerotic patients [82–84]. Lymphoblastoid cells from coronary artery disease patients with the CC genotype for 242C>T exhibited enhanced NOX activity [79]. In contrast, other studies have not detected an effect of the C242T polymorphism on granulocyte NOX activity in healthy subjects.

Despite robust indication of a functional effect of the 242C>T variant, the association of the 242C>T polymorphism with clinical phenotypes has yielded conflicting results. Such controversy is due in part to the low numbers of some studies, the differential genotype frequencies for this variant among different populations, and the diversity of clinical phenotypes assessed. Their relevance in cardiovascular disease has been reviewed elsewhere.

As well as having evidence of the association of the 242C>T with risk factors for coronary artery disease (essential hypertension, diabetes, hypercholesterolemia, smoking) several studies report association of the 242C>T polymorphism with verified coronary artery disease. In a Japanese population, the prevalence of the T allele is reduced in patients. Similarly, in another study performed in Caucasians, the authors reported again a reduced prevalence of the T allele in coronary artery disease and associated the polymorphism [85]. Along similar lines, the T allele associated with reduced systemic oxidative stress markers in patients with coronary stenosis and a possible protective effect against future events [86]. A recent metaanalysis highlights the ethnic heterogeneity of the 242C>T prevalence and a possible protective effect of the T allele only for the Asian population [87].

In summary, current approaches indicate a functionality of the 242C>T, which has not been substantiated by clinical association studies. Discrepancies may be due to the small number of subjects under study and their diverse ethnicity, varied phenotyping methodologies, as well as for being mainly single-gene studies.

5.3.4 Polymorphism 640A>G

The 640A>G variant of the 3′ region of *CYBA* does not have a known mechanism of action yet. It does not seem to have an impact on the ex vivo NOX-dependent superoxide-release from human neutrophils or lymphoblasts [79,82]. However, these studies were carried out in basal conditions, which my lack the molecular environment in which the 640A>G may display functional effects.

Association studies of this variant with cardiovascular disease are somehow conflicting, with both positive and negative results. As in the case of the 242C>T variant, association studies of the 640A>G are somewhat conflicting: some authors did not find an association of the variant with coronary artery disease in a Japanese population [88]; conversely, others have detected a significant reduction of the G allele in patients with coronary artery disease [89].

In this setting, we have recently demonstrated that A640 G polymorphism is associated with diabetes [90]. Subjects with the GG genotype presented higher NOX-dependent superoxide production by their peripheral blood mononuclear cells and subclinical atherosclerosis. Therefore, the A640G polymorphism may identify individuals at greater risk of developing vascular complications in the setting of type 2 diabetes mellitus. It should be noticed that a polymorphism may not be active by itself but rather a marker of risk, maybe due to other genetic causes. In this regard, preliminary linkage disequilibrium studies of the A640G polymorphism with other functional *CYBA* polymorphisms (namely the -930A/G and the C242T) have shown that linkage is low. This suggests that the prooxidant profile associated with the A640G polymorphism is not due to these other polymorphisms. We are aware that a single variant can explain only a reduced part of the phenotypic variability of a complex disease, and that the environmental factors play a significant role as well.

6. CONCLUSIONS

Phagocytic NOX activity and expression are enhanced in traditional vascular and metabolic risk factors, thus promoting the development of pathological processes in diabetes and atherosclerosis. This oxidase might increase the morbidity and mortality in these diseases by favoring deleterious prooxidant processes on cellular macromolecules after exposition to acute and chronic oxidative stress situations (Fig. 5.5).

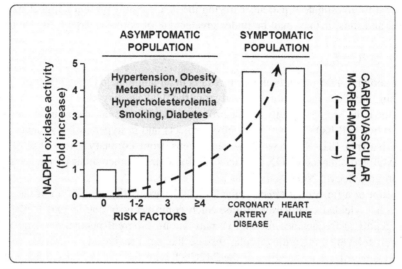

FIGURE 5.5 Phagocytic NADPH oxidase activity, traditional vascular and metabolic risk factors, and morbidity/mortality. *NADPH*, nicotinamide adenine dinucleotide phosphate.

LIST OF ACRONYMS AND ABBREVIATIONS

AACE American Association of Clinical Endocrinologists
AHA American Heart Association
BMI Body mass index
COX Cyclooxygenase
C/EBP CCAAT/enhancer binding protein
DNA Deoxyribonucleic acid
DOCA Deoxycorticosterone acetate
DUOX Dual oxidase
DUOXA DUOX activator
EGIR European Group for the Study of Insulin Resistance
FAD Flavin adenine dinucleotide
GTP Guanosine trisphosphate
HDLc High-density lipoprotein cholesterol
H2O2 Hydrogen peroxide
IDF International Diabetes Federation
LDL Low-density lipoprotein
NADPH Nicotinamide adenine dinucleotide phosphate
NCEP-ATPIII National Cholesterol Education Program Adult Treatment Panel III
NHLBI National Heart, Lung, and Blood Institute
•NO Nitric oxide
NOS Nitric oxide synthase
NOX NADPH oxidase
NOXA NADPH oxidase activator
NOXO NADPH oxidase organizer
•NO2 Nitrogen dioxide radical
•OH Hydroxyl radical
ONOO⁻ Peroxynitrites
•O2⁻ Superoxide anion radical
Phox Phagocyte oxidase
PIP2 Phosphatidylinositol 4,5-biphosphate
PI3K Phosphatidylinositol 3 kinase
PKC Protein kinase C
POLDIP2 Polymerase δ-interacting protein 2
RAC Rac family small GTPase
ROS Reactive oxygen species

SHR Spontaneously hypertensive rat
SOD Superoxide dismutase
TGF-β Transforming growth factor β
WC Waist circumference
WHO World Health Organization

REFERENCES

[1] O'Neill S, O'Driscoll L. Metabolic syndrome: a closer look at the growing epidemic and its associated pathologies. Obes Rev 2015;16(1):1−12.

[2] Reaven GM. Banting lecture 1988. Role of insulin resistance in human disease. Diabetes 1988;37(12):1595−607.

[3] Kaur J. A comprehensive review on metabolic syndrome. Cardiol Res Pract 2014;2014:943162.

[4] Cleeman JI. Executive summary of the third report of The National Cholesterol Education Program (NCEP) Expert Panel on detection, evaluation, and treatment of high blood cholesterol in adults (Adult Treatment Panel III). J Am Med Assoc 2001;285(19):2486−97.

[5] Grundy SM, Cleeman JI, Daniels SR, Donato KA, Eckel RH, Franklin BA, et al. Diagnosis and management of the metabolic syndrome: an American Heart Association/National Heart, Lung, and Blood Institute scientific statement. Circulation 2005;112(17):2735−52.

[6] Alberti KG, Eckel RH, Grundy SM, Zimmet PZ, Cleeman JI, Donato KA, et al. Harmonizing the metabolic syndrome: a joint interim statement of the International Diabetes Federation Task Force on Epidemiology and Prevention; National Heart, Lung, and Blood Institute; American Heart Association; World Heart Federation; International Atherosclerosis Society; and International Association for the Study of Obesity. Circulation 2009;120(16):1640−5.

[7] Franco OH, Massaro JM, Civil J, Cobain MR, O'Malley B, D'Agostino Sr RB. Trajectories of entering the metabolic syndrome: the framingham heart study. Circulation 2009;120(20):1943−50.

[8] Elnakish MT, Hassanain HH, Janssen PM, Angelos MG, Khan M. Emerging role of oxidative stress in metabolic syndrome and cardiovascular diseases: important role of Rac/NADPH oxidase. J Pathol 2013;231(3):290−300.

[9] Brieger K, Schiavone S, Miller Jr FJ, Krause KH. Reactive oxygen species: from health to disease. Swiss Med Wkly 2012;142(w13659):1−14.

[10] Guzik TJ, West NE, Black E, McDonald D, Ratnatunga C, Pillai R, Channon KM. Vascular superoxide production by NAD(P)H oxidase: association with endothelial dysfunction and clinical risk factors. Circ Res 2000;86(9):E85−90.

[11] Droge W. Free radicals in the physiological control of cell function. Physiol Rev 2002;82(1):47−95.

[12] Schulz E, Gori T, Münzel T. Oxidative stress and endothelial dysfunction in hypertension. Hypertens Res 2011;34(6):665−73.

[13] Gryglewski RJ, Palmer RM, Moncada S. Superoxide anion is involved in the breakdown of endothelium-derived vascular relaxing factor. Nature 1986;320(6061):454−6.

[14] Beckman JS, Koppenol WH. Nitric oxide, superoxide, and peroxynitrite: the good, the bad, and ugly. Am J Physiol 1996;271(5):C1424−37.

[15] Pacher P, Beckman JS, Liaudet L. Nitric oxide and peroxynitrite in health and disease. Physiol Rev 2007;87(1):315−424.

[16] Fortuno A, San Jose G, Moreno MU, Beloqui O, Diez J, Zalba G. Phagocytic NADPH oxidase overactivity underlies oxidative stress in metabolic syndrome. Diabetes 2006;55(1):209−15.

[17] Fortuno A, Olivan S, Beloqui O, San Jose G, Moreno MU, Diez J, et al. Association of increased phagocytic NADPH oxidase-dependent superoxide production with diminished nitric oxide generation in essential hypertension. J Hypertens 2004;22(11):2169−75.

[18] Furukawa S, Fujita T, Shimabukuro M, Iwaki M, Yamada Y, Nakajima Y, et al. Increased oxidative stress in obesity and its impact on metabolic syndrome. J Clin Investig 2004;114(12):1752−61.

[19] Zalba G, Beloqui O, San Jose G, Moreno MU, Fortuno A, Diez J. NADPH oxidase-dependent superoxide production is associated with carotid intima-media thickness in subjects free of clinical atherosclerotic disease. Arterioscler Thromb Vasc Biol 2005;25(7):1452−7.

[20] Briones AM, Touyz RM. Oxidative stress and hypertension: current concepts. Curr Hypertens Rep 2010;12(2):135−42.

[21] Viel EC, Benkirane K, Javeshghani D, Touyz RM, Schiffrin EL. Xanthine oxidase and mitochondria contribute to vascular superoxide anion generation in DOCA-salt hypertensive rats. Am J Physiol Heart Circ Physiol 2008;295(1):H281−8.

[22] Vásquez-Vivar J. Tetrahydrobiopterin, superoxide, and vascular dysfunction. Free Radic Biol Med 2009;47(8):1108−19.

[23] Leto TL, Morand S, Hurt D, Ueyama T. Targeting and regulation of reactive oxygen species generation by Nox family NADPH oxidases. Antioxid Redox Signal 2009;11(10):2607−19.

[24] Montezano AC, Touyz RM. Reactive oxygen species and endothelial function−role of nitric oxide synthase uncoupling and Nox family nicotinamide adenine dinucleotide phosphate oxidases. Basic Clin Pharmacol Toxicol 2012;110(1):87−94.

[25] Griendling KK, Minieri CA, Ollerenshaw JD, Alexander RW. Angiotensin II stimulates NADH and NADPH oxidase activity in cultured vascular smooth muscle cells. Circ Res 1994;74(6):1141−8.

[26] Sirker A, Zhang M, Shah AM. NADPH oxidases in cardiovascular disease: insights from in vivo models and clinical studies. Basic Res Cardiol 2011;106(5):735−47.

[27] Drummond GR, Selemidis S, Griendling KK, Sobey CG. Combating oxidative stress in vascular disease: NADPH oxidases as therapeutic targets. Nat Rev Drug Discov 2011;10(6):453−71.

[28] Touyz RM, Briones AM, Sedeek M, Burger D, Montezano AC. NOX isoforms and reactive oxygen species in vascular health. Mol Interv 2011;11(1):27−35.

[29] Takac I, Schröder K, Zhang L, Lardy B, Anilkumar N, Lambeth JD, et al. The E-loop is involved in hydrogen peroxide formation by the NADPH oxidase Nox4. J Biol Chem 2011;286(15):13304−13.

[30] Takac I, Schröder K, Brandes RP. The Nox family of NADPH oxidases: friend or foe of the vascular system? Curr Hypertens Rep 2012;14(1):70–8.

[31] Li JM, Shah AM. Differential NADPH- versus NADH-dependent superoxide production by phagocyte-type endothelial cell NADPH oxidase. Cardiovasc Res 2001;52(3):477–86.

[32] Brown DI, Griendling KK. Nox proteins in signal transduction. Free Radic Biol Med 2009;47(9):1239–53.

[33] Chamseddine AH, Miller Jr FJ. Gp91phox contributes to NADPH oxidase activity in aortic fibroblasts but not smooth muscle cells. Am J Physiol Heart Circ Physiol 2003;285(6):H2284–9.

[34] Hilenski LL, Clempus RE, Quinn MT, Lambeth JD, Griendling KK. Distinct subcellular localizations of Nox1 and Nox4 in vascular smooth muscle cells. Arterioscler Thromb Vasc Biol 2004;24(4):677–83.

[35] BelAiba RS, Djordjevic T, Petry A, Diemer K, Bonello S, Banfi B, et al. NOX5 variants are functionally active in endothelial cells. Free Radic Biol Med 2007;42(4):446–59.

[36] Dahan I, Issaeva I, Gorzalczany Y, Sigal N, Hirshberg M, Pick E. Mapping of functional domains in the p22(phox) subunit of flavocytochrome b(559) participating in the assembly of the NADPH oxidase complex by "peptide walking". J Biol Chem 2002;277(10):8421–32.

[37] Brandes RP, Schröder K. Differential vascular functions of Nox family NADPH oxidases. Curr Opin Lipidol 2008;19(5):513–8.

[38] Lambeth JD. NOX enzymes and the biology of reactive oxygen. Nat Rev Immunol 2004;4(3):181–9.

[39] Bánfi B, Tirone F, Durussel I, Knisz J, Moskwa P, Molnár GZ, et al. Mechanism of Ca^{2+} activation of the NADPH oxidase 5 (NOX5). J Biol Chem 2004;279(18):18583–91.

[40] De Keulenaer GW, Chappell DC, Ishizaka N, Nerem RM, Alexander RW, Griendling KK. Oscillatory and steady laminar shear stress differentially affect human endothelial redox state: role of a superoxide-producing NADH oxidase. Circ Res 1998;82(10):1094–101.

[41] Brandes RP, Weissmann N, Schröder K. Nox family NADPH oxidases: molecular mechanisms of activation. Free Radic Biol Med 2014;76C:208–26.

[42] Marumo T, Schini-Kerth VB, Fisslthaler B, Busse R. Platelet-derived growth factor-stimulated superoxide anion production modulates activation of transcription factor NF-kappaB and expression of monocyte chemoattractant protein 1 in human aortic smooth muscle cells. Circulation 1997;96(7):2361–7.

[43] De Keulenaer GW, Alexander RW, Ushio-Fukai M, Ishizaka N, Griendling KK. Tumour necrosis factor alpha activates a p22phox-based NADH oxidase in vascular smooth muscle. Biochem J 1998;329(Pt 3):653–7.

[44] Kranenburg O, Moolenaar WH. Ras-MAP kinase signaling by lysophosphatidic acid and other G protein-coupled receptor agonists. Oncogene 2001;20(13):1540–6.

[45] Inoguchi T, Li P, Umeda F, Yu HY, Kakimoto M, Imamura M, Aoki T, Etoh T, et al. High glucose level and free fatty acid stimulate reactive oxygen species production through protein kinase C–dependent activation of NAD(P)H oxidase in cultured vascular cells. Diabetes 2000;49(11):1939–45.

[46] Zalba G, San José G, Moreno MU, Fortuño A, Díez J. NADPH oxidase-mediated oxidative stress: genetic studies of the p22(phox) gene in hypertension. Antioxid Redox Signal 2005;7(9–10):1327–36.

[47] San José G, Fortuño A, Beloqui O, Díez J, Zalba G. NADPH oxidase CYBA polymorphisms, oxidative stress and cardiovascular diseases. Clin Sci (Lond) 2008;114(3):173–82.

[48] Hilgers KF. Monocytes/macrophages in hypertension. J Hypertens 2002;20(4):593–6.

[49] Dörffel Y, Lätsch C, Stuhlmüller B, Schreiber S, Scholze S, Burmester GR, Scholze J. Preactivated peripheral blood monocytes in patients with essential hypertension. Hypertension 1999;34(1):113–7.

[50] Chon H, Gaillard CA, van der Meijden BB, Dijstelbloem HM, Kraaijenhagen RJ, van Leenen D, et al. Broadly altered gene expression in blood leukocytes in essential hypertension is absent during treatment. Hypertension 2004;43(5):947–51.

[51] Kristal B, Shurtz-Swirski R, Chezar J, Manaster J, Levy R, Shapiro G, et al. Participation of peripheral polymorphonuclear leukocytes in the oxidative stress and inflammation in patients with essential hypertension. Am J Hypertens 1998;11(8):921–8.

[52] Pettit AI, Wong RKM, Lee V, Jennings S, Quinn PA, Ng LL. Increased free radical production in hypertension due to increased expression of the NADPH oxidase subunit p22phox in lymphoblast cell lines. J Hypertens 2002;20(4):677–83.

[53] Moreno MU, San José G, Pejenaute A, Landecho MF, Díez J, Beloqui O, et al. Association of phagocytic NADPH oxidase activity with hypertensive heart disease: a role for cardiotrophin-1? Hypertension 2014;63(3):468–74.

[54] Yasunari K, Maeda K, Watanabe T, Nakamura M, Yoshikawa J, Asada A. Comparative effects of valsartan versus amlodipine on left ventricular mass and reactive oxygen species formation by monocytes in hypertensive patients with left ventricular hypertrophy. J Am Coll Cardiol 2004;43(11):2116–23.

[55] Holvoet P, Kritchevsky SB, Tracy RP, Mertens A, Rubin SM, Butler J, et al. The metabolic syndrome, circulating oxidized LDL, and risk of myocardial infarction in well-functioning elderly people in the health, aging, and body composition cohort. Diabetes 2004;53(4):068–73.

[56] Ceriello A, Mercuri F, Quagliaro L, Assaloni R, Motz E, Tonutti L, Taboga C. Detection of nitrotyrosine in the diabetic plasma: evidence of oxidative stress. Diabetologia 2001;44(7):834–8.

[57] Shishehbor MH, Aviles RJ, Brennan ML, Fu X, Goormastic M, Pearce GL, et al. Association of nitrotyrosine levels with cardiovascular disease and modulation by statin therapy. JAMA 2003;289(13):1675–80.

[58] Zafari AM, Ushio-Fukai M, Akers M, Yin Q, Shah A, Harrison DG, et al. Role of NADH/NADPH oxidase-derived H_2O_2 in angiotensin II-induced vascular hypertrophy. Hypertension 1998;32(3):488–95.

[59] Fortuño A, Bidegain J, Baltanás A, Moreno MU, Montero L, Landecho MF, et al. Is leptin involved in phagocytic NADPH oxidase overactivity in obesity? Potential clinical implications. J Hypertens 2010;28(9):1944–50.

[60] Fortuño A, Bidegain J, San José G, Robador PA, Landecho MF, Beloqui O, et al. Insulin resistance determines phagocytic nicotinamide adenine dinucleotide phosphate oxidase overactivation in metabolic syndrome patients. J Hypertens 2009;27(7):1420−30.

[61] Kalinina N, Agrotis A, Tararak E, Antropova Y, Kanellakis P, Ilyinskaya O, et al. Cytochrome b558-dependent NAD(P)H oxidase-phox units in smooth muscle and macrophages of atherosclerotic lesions. Arterioscler Thromb Vasc Biol 2002;22(12):2037−43.

[62] Sorescu D, Weiss D, Lassegue B, Clempus RE, Szocs K, Sorescu GP, et al. Superoxide production and expression of nox family proteins in human atherosclerosis. Circulation 2002;105(12):1429−35.

[63] Azumi H, Inoue N, Takeshita S, Rikitake Y, Kawashima S, Hayashi Y, et al. Expression of NADH/NADPH oxidase p22phox in human coronary arteries. Circulation 1999;100(14):1494−8.

[64] Azumi H, Inoue N, Ohashi Y, Terashima M, Mori T, Fujita H, et al. Superoxide generation in directional coronary atherectomy specimens of patients with angina pectoris. Important role of NAD(P)H oxidase. Arterioscler Thromb Vasc Biol 2002;22(11):1838−44.

[65] Zalba G, Fortuño A, Orbe J, San José G, Moreno MU, Belzunce M, et al. Phagocytic NADPH oxidase-dependent superoxide production stimulates matrix metalloproteinase-9: implications for human atherosclerosis. Arterioscler Thromb Vasc Biol 2007;27(3):587−93.

[66] Li L, Fink GD, Watts SW, Northcott CA, Galligan JJ, Pagano PJ, Chen AF. Endothelin-1 increases vascular superoxide via endothelin(A)-NADPH oxidase pathway in low-renin hypertension. Circulation 2003;107(7):1053−8.

[67] Meléndez GC, McLarty JL, Levick SP, Du Y, Janicki JS, Brower GL. Interleukin 6 mediates myocardial fibrosis, concentric hypertrophy, and diastolic dysfunction in rats. Hypertension 2010;56(2):225−31.

[68] Fortuño A, Bidegain J, Robador PA, Hermida J, López-Sagaseta J, Beloqui O, et al. Losartan metabolite EXP3179 blocks NADPH oxidase-mediated superoxide production by inhibiting protein kinase C: potential clinical implications in hypertension. Hypertension 2009;54(4):744−50.

[69] Martin SS, Qasim A, Reilly MP. Leptin resistance: a possible interface of inflammation and metabolism in obesity-related cardiovascular disease. J Am Coll Cardiol 2008;52(15):1201−10.

[70] Li L, Mamputu JC, Wiernsperger N, Renier G. Signaling pathways involved in human vascular smooth muscle cell proliferation and matrix metalloproteinase-2 expression induced by leptin: inhibitory effect of metformin. Diabetes 2005;54(7):2227−34.

[71] Mahadev K, Motoshima H, Wu X, Ruddy JM, Arnold RS, Cheng G, et al. The NAD(P)H oxidase homolog Nox4 modulates insulin-stimulated generation of H_2O_2 and plays an integral role in insulin signal transduction. Mol Cell Biol 2004;24(5):1844−54.

[72] Ceolotto G, Bevilacqua M, Papparella I, Baritono E, Franco L, Corvaja C, et al. Insulin generates free radicals by an NAD(P)H, phosphatidylinositol 3′-kinase-dependent mechanism in human skin fibroblasts ex vivo. Diabetes 2004;53(5):1344−51.

[73] Adaikalakoteswari A, Balasubramanyam M, Rema M, Mohan V. Differential gene expression of NADPH oxidase (p22phox) and hemoxygenase-1 in patients with Type 2 diabetes and microangiopathy. Diabet Med 2006;23(6):666−74.

[74] Moreno MU, Zalba G. CYBA gene variants as biomarkers for coronary artery disease. Drug News Perspect 2010;23(5):316−24.

[75] Moreno MU, San José G, Orbe J, Páramo JA, Beloqui O, Díez J, Zalba G. Preliminary characterisation of the promoter of the human p22(phox) gene: identification of a new polymorphism associated with hypertension. FEBS Lett 2003;542(1−3):27−31.

[76] San José G, Moreno MU, Oliván S, Beloqui O, Fortuño A, Díez J, Zalba G. Functional effect of the p22phox -930A/G polymorphism on p22phox expression and NADPH oxidase activity in hypertension. Hypertension 2004;44(2):163−9.

[77] Sales ML, Ferreira MC, Leme Jr CA, Velloso LA, Gallani MC, Colombo RC, et al. Non-effect of p22-phox -930A/G polymorphism on end-organ damage in Brazilian hypertensive patients. J Hum Hypertens 2007;21(6):504−6.

[78] Doi K, Noiri E, Nakao A, Fujita T, Kobayashi S, Tokunaga K. Haplotype analysis of NAD(P)H oxidase p22 phox polymorphisms in end-stage renal disease. J Hum Genet 2005;50(12):641−7.

[79] Mehranpour P, Wang SS, Blanco RR, Li W, Song Q, Lassègue B, et al. The C242T CYBA polymorphism as a major determinant of NADPH oxidase activity in patients with cardiovascular disease. Cardiovasc Hematol Agents Med Chem 2009;7(3):251−9.

[80] Niemiec P, Nowak T, Iwanicki T, Krauze J, Gorczynska-Kosiorz S, Grzeszczak W, Ochalska-Tyka A, Zak I. The -930A>G polymorphism of the CYBA gene is associated with premature coronary artery disease. A case-control study and gene-risk factors interactions. Mol Biol Rep 2014;41(15):3287−94.

[81] Moreno MU, San José G, Fortuño A, Beloqui O, Redón J, Chaves FJ, et al. A novel CYBA variant, the -675A/T polymorphism, is associated with essential hypertension. J Hypertens 2007;25(8):1620−6.

[82] Wyche KE, Wang SS, Griendling KK, Dikalov SI, Austin H, Rao S, et al. C242T CYBA polymorphism of the NADPH oxidase is associated with reduced respiratory burst in human neutrophils. Hypertension 2004;43(6):1246−51.

[83] Moreno MU, San José G, Fortuño A, Beloqui O, Díez J, Zalba G. The C242T CYBA polymorphism of NADPH oxidase is associated with essential hypertension. J Hypertens 2006;24(7):1299−306.

[84] Guzik TJ, West NE, Black E, McDonald D, Ratnatunga C, Pillai R, Channon KM. Functional effect of the C242T polymorphism in the NAD(P)H oxidase p22phox gene on vascular superoxide production in atherosclerosis. Circulation 2000;102(15):1744−7.

[85] Fan M, Kähönen M, Rontu R, Lehtinen R, Viik J, Niemi M, et al. The p22phox C242T gene polymorphism is associated with a reduced risk of angiographically verified coronary artery disease in a high-risk Finnish Caucasian population. The Finnish Cardiovascular Study. Am Heart J 2006;152(3):538−42.

[86] Ueno T, Watanabe H, Fukuda N, Tsunemi A, Tahira K, Matsumoto T, et al. Influence of genetic polymorphisms in oxidative stress related genes and smoking on plasma MDA-LDL, soluble CD40 ligand, E-selectin and soluble ICAM1 levels in patients with coronary artery disease. Med Sci Mon 2009;15(7):CR341−8.

[87] Di Castelnuovo A, Soccio M, Iacoviello L, Evangelista V, Consoli A, Vanuzzo D, et al. The C242T polymorphism of the p22phox component of NAD(P)H oxidase and vascular risk. Two case-control studies and a meta-analysis. Thromb Haemost 2008;99(3):594−601.

[88] Inoue N, Kawashima S, Kanazawa K, Yamada S, Akita H, Yokoyama M. Polymorphism of the NADH/NADPH oxidase p22 phox gene in patients with coronary artery disease. Circulation 1998;97(2):135−7.

[89] Gardemann A, Mages P, Katz N, Tillmanns H, Haberbosch W. The p22 phox A640G gene polymorphism but not the C242T gene variation is associated with coronary heart disease in younger individuals. Atherosclerosis 1999;145(2):315−23.

[90] Moreno MU, San Jose G, Fortuño A, Miguel-Carrasco JL, Beloqui O, Diez J, Zalba G. The A640G *CYBA* polymorphism associates with subclinical atherosclerosis in diabetes. Front Biosci (Elite Ed) 2011;3:1467−74.

Chapter 6

Obesity and Nonalcoholic Fatty Liver Disease: Role of Oxidative Stress

M. Vanessa Bullón-Vela[1], Itziar Abete[1,2], J. Alfredo Martínez[1,2,3] and M. Angeles Zulet[1,2,3]

[1]Department of Nutrition, Food Science and Physiology, Faculty of Pharmacy and Nutrition, University of Navarra, Pamplona, Spain; [2]Biomedical Research Centre Network in Physiopathology of Obesity and Nutrition (CIBERobn), ISCIII, Madrid, Spain; [3]Navarra Institute for Health Research (IdiSNA), Pamplona, Spain

1. INTRODUCTION

Obesity is a metabolic disorder which is assumed to contribute to a proinflammatory and prooxidant state accompanied by the excessive accumulation of body fat [1]. This state promotes lipotoxicity and alterations in the adipokines production, leading to oxidative stress and overproduction of reactive oxygen species (ROS), inducing liver damage [2,3]. This chronic disease is also associated with a lipid and glucose/carbohydrate-abnormal metabolism, which is closely related to several diseases, such as type 2 diabetes mellitus and cardiovascular disease, among others including metabolic syndrome (MetS) features [4]. In this context, several studies have suggested the emerging role of obesity in the development of nonalcoholic fatty liver disease (NAFLD) [5–7].

This chapter highlights recent scientific evidence about the close relationship between obesity and oxidative stress, which may induce liver damage mediated by several biological pathways involving NAFLD pathogenesis.

2. DEFINITION

NAFLD is characterized by an excessive accumulation of lipid droplets in >5% of hepatocytes by histology [8]. The diagnosis excludes conditions associated with hepatic steatosis and daily alcohol consumption (less than 30 g in men and 20 g in woman) (Table 6.1). In early stages, NAFLD initiates a nonalcoholic fatty liver (NAFL), characterized by the presence of hepatic steatosis without evidence of hepatocytes injury or fibrosis; this can progress to nonalcoholic steatohepatitis (NASH), which includes hepatic steatosis, inflammation, and ballooning hepatocellular injury with or without fibrosis, which can progress to cirrhosis and finally may develop into hepatocellular carcinoma (HCC) [9] (Table 6.2).

The liver structure is organized in acinos that have two portal spaces and two central lobular veins. They are distributed in three acinar zones: zone 1 is close to the portal space; zone 2 is located between zones 1 and 3, and zone 3 is near to the lobular center vein. Zone 1 receives a blood flow with high oxygen concentration, while in zone 3 hepatocytes receive a lower concentration of oxygen; zone 3 is thus more susceptible to hypoxia. Zone 2 shows intermediate characteristics between zones 1 and 3 [10]. The degree of steatosis is determined by considering the amount of hepatocytes compromised by fat vacuoles, predominantly macrovesicular or a combination of small and large vacuoles mainly concentrated in zone 3. Another feature in NASH is the ballooned hepatocytes, characterized by a "balloon" shape with no vacuolar cytoplasm and associated with inflammation and damage. It has been suggested that alterations of intermediate filaments of the cytoskeleton, such as cytokeratin 8 and 18, are related to hepatocyte ballooning, and oxidative stress might induce alterations of these keratin filaments in liver diseases [11]. In fact, ballooning and inflammation are crucial features for the diagnosis of steatohepatitis, but in patients with NASH is not common to find neutrophil leukocytes and polymorphonuclear cells surrounding hepatocytes ballooning, called "satelitosis," in comparison to alcoholic patients [12]. In advanced stages, fibrous septal can be observed as collagen deposits in zone 3 of the hepatic lobule (perivenular or

TABLE 6.1 Conditions Associated With Hepatic Steatosis

Congenital[a,b,c]	Metabolic[b,c]	Nutritional[b,c]	Drugs[a,c]	Others[c]
Abetalipoproteinemia	Diabetes mellitus	Marasmus	Methotrexate	Inflammatory bowel
Hypobetalipoproteinemia	Obesity	Kwashiorkor	azauridine	disease
Familial combined hyperlipidemia	Hyperlipidemias	Starvation	L-asparaginase	HIV infection
Glycogen storage disease		Parenteral nutrition	Bleomycin	Hepatotoxins
Galactosemia			Puromycin	Small intestinal
Hereditary fructose intolerance			Azaserine	bacterial overgrowth
Lipodystrophy			tetracycline	Celiac disease
Tyrosinemia			Amiodarone	Bariatric surgery
Systemic carnitine deficiency			Tamoxifen	Jejunoileal bypass
Homocystinuria			Dichloroethylene	
Weber–Christian disease			Estrogens	
Wilson's disease			Glucocorticoids	
Gaucher's disease				

HIV, human immunodeficiency virus.
[a]Raman, Allard. Can J Gastroenterol 2006;20:345–9.
[b]Kneeman, Misdraji, Corey. Ther Adv Gastroenterol 2012;5(3):199–207.
[c]Feldman M, et al. Gastrointestinal and Liver Disease. 2010. pp. 1401–11.

TABLE 6.2 Spectrum of Nonalcoholic Fatty Liver Disease

Terms	Definition
Nonalcoholic Fatty Liver Disease (NAFLD)	Chronic liver disease not caused by abusive alcohol consumption; it includes several conditions, ranging from steatosis to steatohepatitis and cirrhosis.
Nonalcoholic Fatty Liver (NAFL)	Presence of lipid droplets in hepatocytes (more than 5% macrovesicular steatosis) without hepatocyte damage (ballooning or fibrosis).
Nonalcoholic steatohepatitis (NASH)	Presence of hepatic steatosis (more than 5% macrovesicular steatosis) accompanied by hepatocyte inflammation and ballooning with or without fibrosis.
Cirrhosis[a,b]	Liver disease characterized by hepatocellular damage; liver tissue is replaced by scar tissue, increasing portal hypertension.
Cryptogenic cirrhosis[c]	Last stage of chronic liver disease of unknown etiology; subjects diagnosed with cryptogenic cirrhosis present obesity and several components of MetS that are key factors in developing this condition.

[a]Mercado-Irizarry, Torres. Clin Liver Dis 2016;7(4):69–72.
[b]Schuppan, Afdhal. Lancet 2008;371(9615):838–51.
[c]Desai. J Assoc Physicians India 2009;57(11).

perisinusoidal central region) that extends toward the portal space, replacing it with a fibrosis scar and promoting sclerosing hyaline necrosis. Other findings are that the megamitochondria and eosinophilic bodies measuring between 3 and 10 microns are related to oxidative stress as a result of lipid peroxidation [13].

Another pathological alteration in NASH is the presence of Mallory–Denk bodies, which are irregular eosinophilic aggregates located predominantly in the ballooned hepatocytes of zone 3; they also contain cytokeratin 18 and 8, ubiquitin, and P62. This alteration is linked to the grade of severity in steatohepatitis and fibrosis [14]. However, the presence of these aggregates is not necessarily specific in steatohepatitis, but is associated with alcoholic patients [15]. To evaluate the grade/severity of steatosis, the Kleiner scale takes into account the percentage of macrovesicular and/or microvesicular steatosis. Minimal steatosis (scale 0) involves <5% of hepatocytes containing fat vacuoles, mild steatosis (scale 1) refers to <33% of hepatocytes compromised, moderate steatosis indicates between 34% and 66% (scale 2), and >66% (scale 3) matches with severe steatosis [8]. Thus the score system Brunt proposed as a classification for steatohepatitis considers necroinflammation and the stage of fibrosis (location and extension). Stage 1 indicates zone 3 perisinusoidal fibrosis; stage 2 includes portal fibrosis; stage 3 involves bridging fibrosis; and stage 4 refers to cirrhosis [16].

3. PREVALENCE AND TRENDS

NAFLD is the most common cause of chronic liver disease worldwide [5], and the principal cause of liver-related morbidity and mortality. The incidence of this pathology has grown due to the increasing rates of obesity, diabetes, and MetS [17] and the high prevalence of cardiovascular disease [18]. As previously mentioned, NAFLD includes a wide spectrum of liver damage characterized by an accumulation of intrahepatic fat until it becomes NASH, which can eventually lead to cirrhosis and HCC if it is not detected and treated in the early stages [17]. Liver biopsy is the gold standard to confirm the diagnosis of NASH, but it is an invasive and expensive procedure which involves some clinical risk. Therefore NAFLD prevalence is heterogeneous because studies use different kinds of diagnostic methods, such as noninvasive biomarkers of liver status, image tests, and heterogeneity of population [9]. Several clinical and epidemiological studies indicate that NAFLD prevalence is growing, especially in Western countries [17].

A recent systematic review and metaanalysis using PubMed and MEDLINE sources and considering publications from 1989 to 2015 reported that the prevalence of NAFLD worldwide is 25.2% and NASH prevalence between biopsied NAFLD patients is 59.1%. The highest rate was reported in South America (30.5%), followed by the Middle East (31.8%), Asia (27.4%), Europe (23.7%), and North America (21.1%), and the lowest rate was seen in Africa population (14%) [5]. Also, epidemiological data shows that 30% and 5% of the US population suffer from NAFLD and NASH, respectively [17], whereas in the Asia-Pacific region the prevalence ranges from 30% to 90% in diabetic patients [19].

It is expected that 6%−13% of patients with steatosis can progress to steatohepatitis. Of those, 10%−29% will progress to liver cirrhosis within 10 years and 4%−27% may get HCC [20]. In addition, the presence of NAFLD increases the risk of mortality associated to hepatic disease (13%), cardiovascular diseases (25%), and malign tumors (28%) [21].

At least 90% of patients with NAFLD are diagnosed with MetS and 75% show insulin resistance [22] and impaired fasting glucose status [21], with the presence of dyslipidemias between 20% and 92% [23]. The prevalence of NAFLD in the pediatric population is higher in males and increases with age and body mass index (BMI) [24].

3.1 Ethnicity, Gender, and Age

Ethnicity and gender differences in the spectrum of NAFLD are connected to the interaction between lifestyle, environmental, and genetic factors [25]. Several population-based studies have reported that NAFLD is more prevalent in Hispanics [9,25]. Moreover, Smits et al. [26] examined data from the US National Health and the Nutrition Examination Survey (1988−94) of three ethnic groups using ultrasonography to diagnose NAFLD. Results showed that the prevalence of NAFLD changes between race, and is higher in Mexican Americans (39.4%) than in nonHispanic Whites (29.8%) and nonHispanic Blacks (23.1%) [26]. Similarly, in another study Hispanics exhibited a high prevalence of hepatic steatosis measured by proton magnetic resonance spectroscopy [27]. The findings of these studies reveal racial and genetic disparities in the prevalence of NAFLD. Other literature showed that the incidence and severity of NAFLD differ by gender but increase in the elderly [28]. In relation to gender, several studies reported that the rate of NAFLD is higher in men than in woman [25]; however, in postmenopausal women a higher prevalence than in men has been observed. In this context, Carulli et al. [29] suggested that the circulating levels of estrogens could exert a protective effect on the development of steatosis. These results indicate that a fertile woman has a low risk of developing steatosis, but this protection disappears after menopause. Likewise, in a cohort study involving 351 patients with NAFLD proved by liver biopsy, data showed that NAFLD affects mainly middle-aged (≥50 to <60 years) and old-aged people (≥60 years), and demonstrated increasing risk factors related to NAFLD development, such as obesity, hypertension, diabetes mellitus, and hyperlipidemia [30].

4. RISK FACTORS ASSOCIATED WITH NONALCOHOLIC FATTY LIVER DISEASE

The global prevalence of NAFLD is rising, and this is related to other medical illnesses such as obesity, dyslipidemia, type 2 diabetes mellitus, and MetS complications due mainly to a sedentary lifestyle and unhealthy dietary patterns [31]. Specific conditions such as insulin resistance alter the lipid metabolism, leading to an excess of lipid droplets into the hepatocyte and dysfunctional adipose tissue, and contributing to the activation of several complex mechanisms that induce oxidative stress and inflammation, which are the most important features in NAFLD pathogenesis [3,32,33].

4.1 Obesity

Obesity is a chronic disease characterized by a low-grade inflammation and increased adipose tissue deposition. Adipocytes secret several bioactive molecules, which promote ROS and cause a prooxidative stress balance and disruptions in the mitochondrial metabolism [1]. In this context, a large number of clinical studies have reported that the rate of NAFLD has been increasing in parallel to increases in numbers of overweight and obese people, mainly associated with visceral obesity [3,34]. According to a metaanalysis, the prevalence of obesity in NAFLD subjects is 51.3%, and it is 81.8% in NASH subjects [5]. A later metaanalysis that included 21 cohort studies aimed to evaluate whether obesity or raised BMI increase the risk of NAFLD [6]. The results showed that obese subjects had a 3.5-fold increased risk of developing NAFLD, and there is a direct relationship between higher BMI and NAFLD risk [6]. Pang et al. (2015) [6a] carried out another metaanalysis, reviewing databases to search for studies that estimate the influence of central obesity on NAFLD [7]; 20 studies were analyzed, and the main finding was that the sum of odds ratio (OR) values per unit increased by 1.07 in waist circumference and 1.25 in BMI for NAFLD. In this sense, obesity and central obesity appear as independent factors associated with increased risk of NAFLD [7]. Furthermore, a study evaluated the prevalence of NAFLD in 105 liver biopsies of morbidly obese subjects without MetS according to the International Diabetes Foundation. The findings of this analysis indicated that 73% of the samples has histologically proven NAFLD, 56% had steatosis, and 17% had NASH, suggesting a high prevalence of NAFLD in this population [35]. Taking this evidence together, it might be concluded that the rising prevalence of NAFLD is closely associated with obesity.

On the other hand, obesity is related to hyperglycemia, which increases the levels of free fatty acids (FFAs) to induce lipotoxicity [36]. This state results in an increased ectopic fat accumulation on the pancreatic beta-cells, myocytes, and hepatocytes, inducing apoptosis and cell death, and a disruption in intracellular signals related to energy homeostasis promoting insulin resistance and overproduction of oxygen-derived free radicals [2]. Moreover, a chronic increase in FFA levels and insulin resistance induce hepatic steatosis and mitochondrial dysfunction. Supporting these arguments, a number of studies in humans have investigated the relationship between hepatic steatosis and body adiposity, especially central obesity. A study by Thomas et al. [37] measured fat tissue content, including intrahepatocellular lipids, by magnetic resonance imaging (MRI). The principal finding was that intrahepatocellular lipid levels were significantly higher in overweight (BMI > 25 kg/m^2) compared with lean subjects, and increased by 22% for each 1% increase in total adipose tissue, by 21% for each 1% increase in total subcutaneous adipose tissue, and by 72% for each 1% increase in subcutaneous abdominal adipose tissue [37]. In line with this, another study evaluated liver fat content by MRI in 4949 participants in the UK Biobank [38]. The results showed that subjects with BMI < 25 kg/m^2 presented a lower content of liver fat in comparison to subjects with BMI > 30 kg/m^2 increasing the prevalence of high liver fat around 1 in 3 [38]. As noted previously, obesity is characterized by a chronic proinflammatory state which facilitates liver failure and malignancy by activating carcinogenic mechanisms. Hence obesity plays a crucial role in the progression of steatosis to NASH (inflammation and fibrosis) by activating several inflammatory and oxidative stress networks that can lead to HCC progression [39]. Moreover, several epidemiological studies have suggested that obesity is related to an increased risk of HCC. A systematic metaanalysis has been published which includes 11 cohort studies related to overweight or obesity and risk of liver cancer. Data analysis showed an increased risk factor for the onset of liver cancer in overweight and obese subjects of 17% and 89%, respectively, compared to subjects with normal weight. These results indicate that increased body weight is strongly related to increased risk of liver cancer [40]. Additionally, the European Prospective Investigation into Cancer and Nutrition multicenter cohort study evaluated the association between obesity, abdominal obesity, and the risk of HCC. Results showed that waist to height ratio (related to abdominal obesity) and weight gain had the strongest association with the development of HCC [41]. Clearly, relevant evidence supports the view that obesity should be considered a key risk factor in the onset and progression of HCC; it induces systemic oxidative stress and other damaging metabolic pathways, such as insulin resistance and increased production of inflammatory adipocytokines, leading to activation of hepatic stellate cells (HSCs) and inducing hepatocyte apoptosis and liver damage [3,39].

4.1.1 Adipose Tissue in Nonalcoholic Fatty Liver Disease

Adipose tissue produces several adipokines that have a number of biological activities closely related to hepatic insulin resistance and obesity [36]. However, obesity induces a dysregulated storage production of these molecules and alterations in their endocrine functions, activating the expression of proinflammatory mediators that promote metabolic disorders and MetS. Thus adipose tissue plays a key role in the generation of systemic oxidative stress [42]. In NAFLD pathogenesis an imbalance of proinflammatory mediators is established; these are involved in many biological signaling pathways related to necroinflammation, fibrosis, and cancer, as well as in the regulation of lipid and carbohydrate metabolism [3]. These conditions induce liver failure that leads to an altered metabolic state, systemic inflammation, insulin resistance, mitochondrial dysfunction, and oxidative stress [3,43]. The main adipokines related to hepatic insulin resistance, steatosis, and liver fibrosis are leptin, adiponectin, tumor necrosis factor (TNF-α), plasminogen activator inhibitor 1 (PAI-1) [44].

Leptin is involved in the regulation of food intake, energy balance, and body weight [45]. High serum levels of leptin are found in patients with obesity associated with insulin resistance [46]. In this context, a cross-sectional study

[46a] carried out with 402 nondiabetic adolescents aged between 10 and 19 years old revealed that plasma leptin levels were positively correlated with adiposity, as found in many other investigations. In addition, leptin was associated with insulin resistance independently of age, gender, and BMI [47]. Thus diverse studies suggest that leptin may have a profibrogenic action because of the activation of Kupffer and HSCs that lead to oxidative stress exacerbation [43]. In a study where activated rat HSCs were cultured and treated with leptin, the treatment showed a significant HSC mitogenesis playing a key role in HSC survival in the apoptosis process [48]. However, in human studies the relationship between liver fibrosis and leptin has provided controversial results [43,44]. A cross-sectional study evaluating the association between serum leptin and serum adiponectin levels and the severity of NAFLD in 338 subjects found high levels of leptin and low levels of adiponectin in the early-stage NASH group independent of gender. However, fibrosis was not predicted by these adipokines [49]. Another study evaluated leptin levels in 49 patients with biopsy-proven NASH, 32 patients with chronic hepatitis without cirrhosis diagnosed by biopsy, and 30 healthy adult subjects. Results showed higher levels of leptin in the NASH group than in other groups [50]. In line with this, Chandrashekaran et al. (2016) [50a] showed that in vitro and in vivo increased levels of leptin as a result of oxidative stress caused by cytochrome P450, family 2, subfamily E, polypeptide 1 (CYP2E1) induces high glucose transporter type 4 (GLUT-4) protein levels in HSCs.

Leptin has been suggested to have a profibrogenic effect and to induce oxidative stress. On the other hand, some studies proposed that adiponectin has a protective effect in liver injury. In this regard, Polyzos et al. [52] performed a systematic review and metaanalysis including 27 studies in patients with NAFLD, NASH, and control (n = 2243). Data indicated that the control group had higher levels of adiponectin in comparison to other groups. Moreover, the NASH group presented lower levels of adiponectin than the NAFLD group. Hence hypoadiponectinemia can be implicated in the progression of NAFLD to NASH [52]. In line with these findings, a cross-sectional study showed that hypoadiponectinemia is associated with liver histologic damage (NASH), and specifically lobular inflammation and fibrosis in severely obese subjects [52a]. A study performed using an animal model and primary culture of mouse HSCs to evaluate the role of adiponectin in fibrosis showed that treatment with adiponectin inhibits proliferation and migration of HSCs; hence adiponectin is demonstrated to have an antifibrogenic effect [53]. Moreover, adiponectin has antiinflammatory effects by inhibiting the expression, production, secretion, and actions of TNF-α and interleukin (IL)-6 by the suppression of the nuclear factor κB (NF-κB) [36].

Obesity and insulin resistance facilitate an environment of inflammation; as a consequence, TNF-α is secreted by several types of cells, such as macrophage (adipose tissue), hepatocytes, and Kupffer cells, and contributes to inflammation, necrosis, apoptosis, and finally liver failure [54]. It has been suggested that TNF-α promotes an accumulation of intracellular fat in the liver. Rodents injected with TNF-α showed high serum levels of FFAs and a significant increase of lipids in liver cells. Also, TNF-α affected the expression of sterol regulatory element binding protein-1c (SREBP-1c), which is linked to lipid metabolism and consequently developing hepatic steatosis [55]. A study consisting of a four-year follow-up of 363 healthy subjects showed that NAFLD was present in 29.2% of the population, and the NAFLD group had higher levels of TNF-α compared to the nonNAFLD group. Also, high serum levels of TNF-α increase significantly the risk of developing NAFLD [56].

In relation to PAI-1, a few studies have suggested an important role in NAFLD. PAI-1 is involved in the fibrinolytic system and is linked to insulin resistance [57]. A study by Holzberg et al. [58] suggested that high concentrations of PAI-1 are significantly associated with the degree of hepatic steatosis in overweight children regardless of BMI, insulin resistance, visceral fat, and other inflammatory markers.

4.2 Insulin Resistance

Insulin resistance is defined as a clinical condition where cells fail to respond normally to exogenous or endogenous insulin to increase glucose uptake and utilization as a consequence of impaired sensitivity to insulin mediated by glucose disposal [59]. In the majority of cases this pathophysiological abnormality is related to several abnormalities and clinical syndromes [60]. Nevertheless, it is important to distinguish between the role of insulin resistance versus compensatory hyperinsulinemia, which is a mechanism to maintain normal blood glucose levels as the response of peripheral insulin resistance in muscle and adipose tissue [61]. Hence some subjects with insulin resistance syndrome have more risk of developing diabetes because they lose the capacity to secrete insulin due to the insulin resistance, and if hyperinsulinemia continues, metabolic abnormalities increase the risk of the onset of cardiovascular disease and NAFLD [62]. Insulin resistance can be evaluated using several methods: the euglycemic hyperinsulinemic clamp, which is the gold standard, and alternative methods such as mathematical models, including the homeostasis model assessment of insulin resistance and the Quantitative Insulin Sensitivity Check Index [63].

Scientific evidence points out that oxidative stress influences insulin sensitivity adversely by impairing glucose tolerance or increasing insulin resistance. This state contributes to maintaining an oxidative environment that plays a critical role in the development of hepatic steatosis. Hence low whole-body insulin sensitivity could be involved in the progression from fatty liver (FL) to NASH [64]. The prevalence of diabetes associated with NAFLD is 22.5%, and it is 43.6% in NASH [5]. Generally, subjects with NAFLD are obese and present high abdominal fat, which is characterized by a decrease of insulin sensitivity and high levels of inflammatory and oxidative markers [65]. Moreover, this state is more severe in subjects diagnosed with NASH than in individuals with FL. Supporting this last statement, a study evaluated 32 subjects diagnosed with NAFLD by liver biopsy with insulin resistance (n = 21) and without (n = 11), and showed that subjects with insulin resistance exhibited significantly higher levels of malondialdehyde (MDA) in tissue and an enhanced degree of steatosis and necroinflammatory grades compared to those without insulin resistance. Furthermore, MDA levels increased the risk of developing NASH. In this context, insulin resistance in NAFLD promotes hepatic necroinflammation and disease progression [33]. In line with this, Gholam et al. [66] found that severely obese subjects with NASH presented a serious Insulin resistance in comparison to those only diagnosed with steatosis. Moreover, Videla et al. (2006) [32] indicated the close association between oxidative stress and insulin resistance in NAFLD, showing that dysregulation of the ROS system and FFAs promotes an impairment of tyrosine phosphorylation of insulin receptor substrate (IRS) proteins, leading to a decrease of the insulin signaling pathway and inducing an initial state of insulin resistance in steatosis [32]. The researchers suggested that insulin resistance in NAFLD might be associated with an overwhelmed intrahepatic and intramyocellular lipid content and/or depletion of liver n-3 polyunsaturated fatty acids (PUFAs), which are involved as regulators in lipid metabolism [32]. Meanwhile, the progression of steatosis to steatohepatitis in NAFLD could be related to ROS production that induces an environment of liver oxidative stress joined to lipotoxicity and excess ketones because of the increased activity of CYP2E1 associated with diabetes and obesity [67].

4.3 Dyslipidemias

Dyslipidemia induces an upregulation of transcription factors related to de novo lipogenesis (DNL) that also promotes the inhibition of FFA oxidation triggering a lipid atherogenic lipid profile [68]. The chronic state of hepatic lipid excess due to oxidative stress plays a crucial role in the development of cardiovascular disease in NAFLD subjects [69]. In fact, prevalence of hypertriglyceridemia is 69.2% in NAFLD and 72.1% in NASH [5], and several studies report that NAFLD is an independent risk factor for cardiovascular disease, which is the principal cause of death among patients with NAFLD [18]. In this context, a disrupted serum lipid profile in subjects with NAFLD is characterized by low levels of high-density lipoprotein cholesterol (HDL-c) and high levels of triglycerides, both of which increase the risk of atherosclerosis and induce changes in cardiac structure and function [70].

Evidence suggests that some fatty acids are responsible for hepatocellular damage and death, which induce disease progression to NASH and increase the risk of developing cirrhosis and HCC in the majority of patients with NAFLD [71,72]. Supporting this, Neuschwander-Tetri [71] proposed a lipotoxicity model of NASH where an increased uptake of FFAs and overwhelmed fatty acid oxidation induce liver inflammation, necrosis, and even fibrosis. In addition, triglyceride accumulation in liver, skeletal muscle, and other tissues could have a protective function by preventing the effects of other lipotoxicity mediators such as FFAs, diacylglycerides, ceramides, and free cholesterol, but in NAFLD pathogenesis a chronic lipotoxic condition leads to hepatocyte collapse and developing NASH [71,73].

Ceramides are a group of lipids that exert effects over several biological mechanisms involved in insulin resistance, inflammation, oxidative stress, cell dysfunction, and death [72,74]. They can inhibit insulin pathways, which promotes insulin resistance and production of ROS and oxidative stress, the principal features triggering NASH. Pagadala et al. (2012) suggested a model where ceramides play a key role in NAFLD progression: obesity and insulin resistance increase the level of proinflammatory cytokines, mainly TNF-α, and decrease the levels of adiponectin joined to increased FFA release by adipose tissue. This state promotes ceramide production, inducing hepatic insulin resistance (caused by protein phosphatase 2A and the attenuation of the Akt pathway) and leading to mitochondrial dysfunction and apoptosis [74].

In relation to cholesterol, Musso et al. [69] published a review summarizing the relationship between cholesterol toxicity and steatohepatitis. They concluded that alterations in cholesterol homeostasis induce oxidative stress, mitochondrial dysfunction, and endoplasmic reticulum (ER) stress. Activation of the hepatic Kupffer cells and HSCs that increase inflammation and fibrosis was found [69]. Consequently, free cholesterol might be a key mediator of lipotoxicity and liver injury [69,72].

4.4 Metabolic Syndrome

NAFLD and MetS share common risk factors [26,75,76], and it was suggested that NAFLD is a characteristic hepatic manifestation of MetS. The principal components of MetS, such as high levels of fasting glucose, visceral fat, and dyslipidemias, were associated with the progression of NAFLD to NASH, leading to oxidative stress and lipid peroxidation [75]. The prevalence of MetS is 42.5% in NAFLD and 70.7% in NASH [5].

The main components of MetS are dyslipidemias, characterized by elevated levels of triglycerides and apolipoprotein B (apoB), HDL-c, high blood pressure, and impaired glucose homeostasis as principal pathophysiological alterations. Central obesity and insulin resistance have been considered as other attributes of MetS [77].

A study evaluated the prevalence of MetS in 304 NAFLD patients without diabetes: prevalence increased from 18% in patients with normal BMI to 67% in obese patients, and exhibited a strong association with insulin resistance [78]. Moreover, 88% of NASH patients and 67% of patients with FL had MetS, which also increased the risk of NASH, mainly in severe fibrosis [78]. Supporting this finding, many authors suggest that MetS is strongly related to an increased risk of severe fibrosis mainly associated with a disruption of insulin sensitivity and mitochondrial dysfunction [75,79]. Moreover, Patton et al. [79] suggested that MetS is strongly related to NAFLD in children. In their study they evaluated whether MetS components are associated with histological characteristics and severity in NAFLD in 254 children between 6 and 17 years old with NAFLD. Results indicated that children with severe steatosis had increased risk of MetS. In relation to histological features, hepatocellular ballooning was strongly associated with MetS; in fibrosis, children in stage 3 or 4 showed an OR for MetS of 3.21 in comparison to children in stage 0. Also, children with MetS exhibited significant higher values on the NAFLD activity score than children without MetS [79]. Koehler et al. [76] evaluated 2811 participants from a Rotterdam study; the results reveal that features of MetS are independent factors in NAFLD. The features significantly associated with NAFLD were waist circumference >88 cm for women and >102 cm for men (OR = 4.89), fasting glucose concentration ≥100 mg/dL (OR = 2.11), blood pressure ≥130/85 mmHg (OR = 1.80), and triglycerides ≥150 mg/dL (OR = 1.56) [76].

Obesity mediated by increased production of cytokines and insulin resistance (MetS components) leads to an alteration in the lipid homeostasis and oxidative stress, increasing the risk of developing NASH [3,5,43]. Furthermore, evidence regarding the MetS/NAFLD relationship has shown that the majority of individuals diagnosed with NAFLD present at least one component of MetS and insulin resistance, which is the principal factor to link NAFLD and MetS [26,78−80]. The American Association for the Study of Liver Disease (AASLD) indicated that MetS could predict the existence of steatohepatitis in subjects with NAFLD, which might be used in performing liver biopsies [9].

Despite all this evidence, MetS includes a cluster of risk factors that increase the risk of developing NAFLD. However, it is still not clear whether MetS contributes to NAFLD or vice versay, and the mechanism implicated is not fully understood [80].

5. PATHOGENESIS: THE HITS HYPOTHESIS

An established theory proposes that the development of simple steatosis into NASH follows a two-hit model [81]. The first hit is characterized by an excessive accumulation of lipids in hepatocytes, increasing the risk of developing the second hit, a state of oxidative stress and mitochondrial dysfunction, which leads to increased ROS production. Thus the second hit is a prerequisite to progress from NAFLD to NASH, and eventually to cirrhosis [81].

In this context, several mechanisms are involved in NAFLD pathogenesis (Fig. 6.1), including insulin resistance, a lipodystrophic state that promotes hepatocyte susceptibility to oxidative stress, and the activation of several pathways related to inflammation and apoptosis.

5.1 First Hit: Lipid Accumulation in Hepatocytes

The excessive hepatic fat accumulation is derived from several sources and characterized by an excessive lipid deposition in the liver. Donnelly et al. (2005) [81a] quantified the principal sources of hepatic and plasma triacylglycerol in patients with NAFLD by the method of multiple stable isotopes; they showed that around 60% of triglycerides are derived from nonesterified fatty acids, which are products of lipolysis from adipose tissue, 26% from DNL, and 15% from diet. These findings indicate that a disruption in peripheral fatty acid flux and DNL increases hepatic fat accumulation in NAFLD [81a].

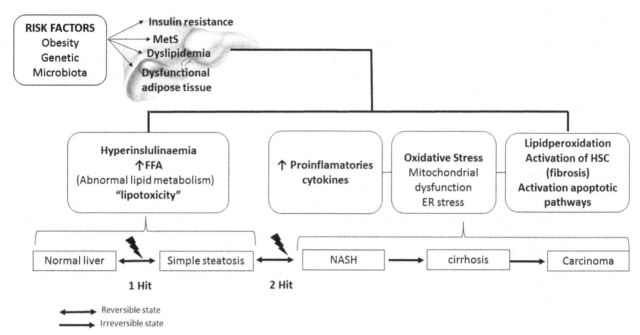

FIGURE 6.1 Pathogenesis of nonalcoholic fatty liver disease. Several risk factors mainly induce insulin resistance and dysfunctional adipose tissue. This state increases production of several proinflammatory mediators and promotes alterations in lipid metabolism, developing a state of lipotoxicity which leads to hepatic steatosis (first hit). This environment of oxidative stress induces increased ROS production, mitochondrial dysfunction, and ER stress, leading to liver damage by activation of HSC and apoptotic pathways (second hit). *ER*, endoplasmic reticulum; *FFA*, free fatty acid; *HSC*, hepatic stellate cell; *MetS*, metabolic syndrome; *NASH*, nonalcoholic steatohepatitis; *ROS*, reactive oxygen species.

Steatosis occurs when there is an imbalance between the rate of lipid input and the rate of lipid output. In addition, there are many pathways which allow an increased influx of triglycerides in the hepatocytes [34], including the hepatic fatty acid uptake (increased synthesis), de novo fatty acid synthesis (increased delivery), the fatty acid oxidation (reduced fatty oxidation), and the fatty acid export (reduced very low-density lipoprotein (VLDL) secretion).

5.1.1 Fatty Acid Uptake

Insulin stimulates the activity of the adipocyte lipoprotein lipase, an enzyme which hydrolyzes triglycerides in lipoproteins to FFAs, so FFAs are delivered into the adipocyte and stored in esterified triglycerides. Thus FFAs are mobilized from the white adipocytes under fasting conditions via lipolysis by the action of the hormone-sensitive lipase to export FFAs into the plasma [83]. In a condition of insulin resistance, these abilities are reduced due to the increased rate of lipolysis and raised FFA plasma levels increasing the risk to develop hepatic steatosis [83]. Furthermore, Nielsen et al. [82] evaluated the contribution of visceral adipose tissue lipolysis to hepatic FFAs delivered to lean and obese subjects by isotope dilution hepatic vein catheterization techniques. This study revealed that levels of FFAs in plasma are 20% greater in obese subjects compared with lean subjects. In subjects with less visceral fat, around 5% of the hepatic FFA is derived from adipose tissue lipolysis [82]. Supporting this finding, Fabbrini et al. (2009) [84] reported FFA kinetics in obese subjects with NAFLD with normal ($\leq$5.5%) or high (>10%) amount of intrahepatic triglyceride content determined by magnetic resonance spectroscopy. The hyperinsulinemic clamp procedure and deuterated palmitate tracer infusion were performed to measure the FFA kinetics. The results showed high adipose tissue lipolysis among obese subjects with high amount of intrahepatic triglyceride content during fasting and feeding conditions. This observation indicates an increase of the FFA flux into plasma during the day [84]. Genes related to lipid metabolism and fatty acid transport are also upregulated in subjects with NAFLD. In this context, a study was conducted to investigate the gene expression on liver samples from individuals diagnosed with NAFLD and with a severe degree of steatosis but no histological signs of inflammation, compared to individuals with low lipid fat accumulation. The expression of fatty-acid-binding protein 4 adipocyte (FABP4) and CD36 molecule (thrombospondin receptor), which are genes related to lipid metabolism, were correlated positively with liver fat content. Taken together this shows a reduced efficacy of lipolysis and an increased fatty acid uptake might be associated with hepatocellular lipid accumulation, and can lead to a progression of liver disease [85].

5.1.2 De Novo Fatty Acid Synthesis

DNL is a process that mainly occurs in the liver and adipose tissue. These metabolic steps take place in the cytoplasm (mitochondria), where excess carbohydrates are converted into fatty acids and esterified into triglyceride. DNL starts with the conversion of acetyl-CoA into malonil-CoA by acetyl-CoA carboxylase, which involves several cycles and reactions [86]. The malonil-CoA is used as a substrate to produce 16-carbon palmitic acyl-CoA by the enzyme fatty acid synthase, which plays a pivotal role in fatty acid synthesis [86]. Thus the contribution of fatty acids via the DNL pathway in NAFLD is important. Indeed, a study has shown that patients with higher FL content have more than threefold rates of fatty acid synthesis via DNL compared to individuals with lower FL amounts [87]. Furthermore, postprandial blood glucose and insulin levels rise and promote hepatic lipogenesis. This state activates the principal pathways involved in the regulation of DNL, which are the SREBP-1 that is stimulated by the effect of glucose and the carbohydrate response element binding protein (ChREBP) activated by insulin. These transcription factors increase the expression of glycolytic and lipogenic genes [88]. SREBPs are responsible for activating almost 30 genes related to lipid metabolism in hepatocyte cells involved in DNL. Three isoforms of SREBPs, SREBP-1a, SREBP-1c, and SREBP-2, are encoded by the human genome. SREBP-1c is responsible for modulating genes related to fatty acid and triglyceride metabolism, while SREBP-2 modulates genes involved in cholesterol metabolism [89].

A review has been published summarizing the evidence from several studies in rodents to determine the action of the transcription factor SREBP-1c in DNL and hepatic steatosis. In the livers of ob/ob or lipodystrophic mice with severe hepatic insulin resistance, hyperglycemia, and steatosis, the hepatic levels of SREBP-1c are disrupted. Authors have also suggested that insulin resistance and especially ER stress induce hyperstimulation in the lipogenic pathway by inducing SREBP-1c, explaining the "paradoxical stimulation of lipogenesis in an insulin-resistant liver" [90]. Thus activation of SREBP-1c increases malonyl-CoA in the mitochondrial membrane by inhibiting β-oxidation of FFAs, and is directed toward the formation of triglycerides. This metabolic situation increases the production and accumulation of lipids at a hepatocellular level, leading to hepatic steatosis [68]. For ChREBP, evidence suggests that this molecule/gene plays a crucial role in the development of steatosis. Dentin et al. [91] showed a higher liver gene expression of ChREBP in leptin-deficient ob/ob mice, and silencing ChREBP expression diminished liver steatosis significantly [91]. Linked to this, visceral adipose tissue promotes the alteration of glucose and lipid metabolism by increasing the production of FFAs in the liver (DNL) by overexpression of these transcription factors [68]. Keeping with the contention that SREBP-1c and ChREBP are involved in the pathogenesis of NAFLD, high levels of postprandial glucose and insulin promote hepatic fat accumulation.

5.1.3 Fatty Acid Oxidation

Fatty acid oxidation is a major source of adenosine triphosphate in tissues such as liver, skeletal muscle, and heart; especially in fasting conditions where glucose availability is limited, fatty acids are used as the main source [92]. Thus fatty acid oxidation can occur in the mitochondria, peroxisomes, and ER. Under an excessive flux of FFAs and elevated insulin resistance, oxidation of long-chain and very-long-chain fatty acids in peroxisomes and ER leads to an over-production of ROS and lipotoxicity [93]. The principal pathway is β-oxidation, which is a cyclic process where fatty acids of short, medium, and long chains are broken down within mitochondria. Acyl-CoA (long chain) is converted to acyl-carnitine by the action of carnitine palmitoyltransferase (CPT) 1, which occurs in the outer mitochondrial membrane, and then shuttled inside by carnitine acylcarnitine translocase. Finally, CPT 2 reconverts the acylcarnitine into acyl-CoA, which is able to enter inside the mitochondria matrix to initiate the β-oxidation. This process is necessary for long-chain fatty acids such as palmitoyl-CoA, oleoyl-CoA, and linoleoyl-CoA, but short- and medium-chain lengths are able to penetrate the mitochondrial membrane by diffusion and may not need the action of carnitine [92]. This process includes several complex cycles of dehydrogenation, hydration, and cleavage reactions that depend on the length of the fatty acid [92]. Each cycle shortens the fatty acyl-CoA by two carbon atoms, an acetyl-CoA, one flavin adenine dinucleotide (FADH$_2$), and one nicotinamide adenine dinucleotide (NADH) that is released as acetyl-CoA [92]. The acetyl-CoA generated enters in the Krebs cycle for oxidation, or is converted to ketone bodies such as acetoacetate, D-β-hydrox-ybutyrate, and acetone, used as energy fuel for several extrahepatic tissues including the brain [94]. Furthermore, the fatty acid oxidation process is regulated by the peroxisome proliferator activated receptor (PPAR)-α; hence a disruption in PPAR-α or fatty acid oxidation leads to a reduced capacity to use FFA energy and the development of steatosis [94]. Moreover, the activation of SREBP-1c increases malonyl CoA in the mitochondrial membrane by the inhibition of FFA β-oxidation, as it is directed toward the formation of triglycerides. The increase in lipid production and accumulation causes hepatic steatosis [68]. However, the precise mechanisms involved in the increase of fatty acid oxidation are not fully elucidated in subjects with NAFLD. Several studies conducted in rodents exposed to high amount of FFAs showed upregulated expression of CPT 1a [93,95], but data from another study suggested that fatty acid oxidation genes are overexpressed while CPT 1a and PPAR-α expressions are decreased by 50% in human livers with NAFLD in comparison to normal livers [96].

5.1.4 Fatty Acid Export

The VLDL assembly is a complex process which has two steps; the principal protein structure is the apoB, and there is also the microsomal triglyceride transfer protein (MTP) located in ER luminal that have an action as lipid transfer between membranes with a several functions such as apo B translocation and folding [97]. Barrows and Parks (2006) [98] evaluated the different sources of FFAs involved in lipoprotein synthesis during the transition from postabsorptive to fed state in healthy men, and found that approximately 77% of the principal substrate during postabsorptive conditions originates from recycled adipose tissue fatty acids and around 4% from lipogenesis. Also, during feeding, the adipose tissue fatty acids give up 44%, lipogenesis more up to 8%, around 15% from the chylomicron-remnant triglyceride, and approximately 10% from dietary [98]. In this context, a chronic hepatic lipid overload coming to DNL or exogenous fatty acids facilitated lipid accumulation and storage into hepatocytes or increased VLDL secretion [97]. Indeed, a state of insulin resistance induces VLDL and apoB secretion due to inhibition of hepatic MTP expression. Hence both conditions develop into hepatic steatosis [99]. In line with these findings, Choi and Ginsberg (2011) reviewed the relationship between insulin resistance and abnormality in VLDL assembly in hepatic steatosis, and suggested that uncoupled protein response (UPR) and ER stress are strongly associated [100]. The mechanism of UPR inhibiting hepatic VLDL output occurs in two ways: increasing cotranslational degradation of apoB by the proteasome, or promoting post-ER degradation of apoB and VLDL by autophagy. In low grades of ER stress, fatty acid overload in the hepatocytes induces VLDL secretion and triglyceride storage. But in severe ER stress the UPR is not able to reestablish the ER protein-folding homeostasis, so it initiates several apoptotic signaling pathways [100]. A study evaluated apoB-100 synthesis in seven subjects with NASH proven by liver biopsy, seven obese subjects without NASH, and seven lean healthy subjects using an isotope ^{13}C-leucine. Data showed that the absolute synthesis and metabolic clearance rates of apoB-100 were significantly lower in subjects with NASH than in only obese and lean subjects. These results indicate that lower synthesis of apoB-100 has contributed to retention of lipids within hepatocytes [101].

The accumulation of lipids at the liver level causes activation of Kupffer cells, factor NFκB, leading to increased expression of inflammatory cytokines such as TNFα, IL-6, and IL-8; a disruption of adiponectin and leptin levels associated with insulin resistance; and mitochondrial dysfunction and ER stress due to excessive FFAs, causing ROS and lipid peroxidation. Hence this chronic lipotoxic state activates several pathways linked to insulin resistance, inflammation, and apoptosis that promote hepatocyte necroinflammation, fibrosis, and the progression of this disease toward liver cancer.

5.2 Second Hit: Oxidative Stress

5.2.1 Oxidative Stress in Nonalcoholic Fatty Liver Disease

The mechanism of NAFLD pathogenesis as previously explained could be defined by the hits hypothesis. In the first hit, several factors such as inadequate dietary patterns, obesity, insulin resistance, and MetS induce an excessive lipid accumulation that promotes an environment of lipotoxicity, triggering a second hit that leads to the activation of inflammatory and oxidative cascades contributing to hepatocellular damage, impaired liver regeneration capacity, and hepatocellular death, which increases the risk of developing HCC.

Oxidative stress is a state of imbalance between the production of reactive nitrogen species (RNS) or ROS and the antioxidant molecules of the organism responsible for the detoxification of these radicals, which leads to cellular injury and damage. ROS includes several molecules, such as superoxide anion radical, hydrogen peroxide, and hydroxyl radical. Moreover, the production of ROS stimulates the enzymes involved in cell protection, such as superoxide dismutase, glutathione peroxidase, and catalase. However, in an environment of oxidative stress, the overproduction of prooxidant species saturates the antioxidant machinery. Furthermore, ROS is closely related to lipid peroxidation, which is relevant in the pathogenesis of NAFLD [102]. In this sense, during oxidative stress the PUFAs are the main substrate for lipid peroxidation by ROS species [103], so this process activates reactive products such as hexanal, 4-hydroxynonenal (4-HNE) derived from omega 6, 4-hydroxy-2-hexenal (4-HHE) from omega 3, and MDA that can diffuse into intracellular or extracellular spaces, affecting other cells linked to pathological conditions, tissue damage, and liver failure by stimulating HSCs [68,104].

5.2.1.1 Mitochondrial Dysfunction

Lipotoxicity induces the progression of simple steatosis to NASH; this leads to oxidative damage promoting the activation of many cell signaling pathways related to proinflammatory cytokines production and activation of HSCs, in which mitochondrial dysfunction leads to ROS and cytokines play a pivotal role in NAFLD pathogenesis [105−107].

Mitochondrial dysfunction and structural changes have been observed in hepatocytes of NASH patients. These mitochondrial changes include a depletion in mitochondrial DNA, decreased activity of the respiratory chain, and impaired mitochondrial β-oxidation [105]. The principal abnormalities of mitochondria morphology in NASH are mega-mitochondria containing linear crystalline inclusions, and loss of cristae and paracrystalline inclusion bodies [108].

Mitochondrial DNA damage has been reported in NASH subjects. Kawahara et al. [106] evaluated mutations in mitochondrial DNA in 24 subjects with alcoholic hepatitis (AL-Hep), NASH, and FL. NASH and AL-Hep groups showed significantly increased mutations in mitochondrial NADH dehydrogenase subunit 1 (ND1) and mitochondrial cytochrome c oxidase subunit II (COII) of the coding region in comparison to the FL group. These results indicate that gene mutations in mitochondrial DNA are observed in AL-Hep and NASH subjects, which could play a key role in liver pathogenesis [106].

Another mitochondrial dysfunction is related to the respiratory chain. Some clinical studies have reported alterations in complexes I, III, IV, and V in NASH subjects [109]. One study directly quantified mitochondrial respiration in liver tissue in obese (OBE) insulin-resistant patients diagnosed with NAFL (OBE NAFL+), without NAFL (OBE NAFL−), with NASH (OBE NASH), and lean without NAFLD (CON). Data showed that obese IR subjects diagnosed with NAFLD or no NAFLD exhibited 4.3- to 5.3-fold higher maximal respiration rates than lean subjects. Moreover, NASH patients had higher mitochondrial mass but lower maximal respiration. Thus OBE NASH showed elevated JNK (c-Jun N-terminal kinase) phosphorylation and a disruption of hepatic catalase activity, important for detoxification of hydrogen peroxide. This metabolic evidence suggests that in initial stages of obesity and insulin resistance the mitochondria suffers an adaptation considered as "hepatic mitochondrial flexibility." However, this capacity is lost in OBE NASH subjects, who present lower mitochondrial respiration and proton leakage with an increase of oxidative stress as a consequence of a reduced antioxidant capacity [109].

As previously mentioned, increased fatty acid β-oxidation in steatosis leading to increased ROS induces dysfunction in the electron transport chain, contributing to an imbalance of NADH/NAD+ and FADH2/FAD (flavin adenine dinucleotide) ratios which affects the oxidative capacity of the mitochondria and overproduction of ROS. This redox disequilibrium increased CYP2E1 activity, which is related to NASH. CYP2E1 is suppressed by insulin, but in a state of insulin resistance is overexpressed and predisposes to oxidative stress in humans and animal models [67]. Abdelmegeed et al. [110] evaluated the CYP2E1 activity in wild-type mice with steatohepatitis induced by a high-fat diet. The mice exhibited insulin resistance, increased CYP2E1 activity and JNK phosphorylation, MDA and hydroxyalkenals, and lipid peroxidation [110].

Wei et al. (2008) proposed a mechanism that can explain mitochondrial abnormalities in NAFLD. This encompasses overproduction of ROS, increased TNF-α expression, and alteration of the transcription coactivator PPAR-γ coactivator-1α (PGC-1) [105]. In this context, TNF-α might promote cell death by activating the caspase cascade (proapoptotic) and NF-κB (antiapoptotic) pathways in hepatocytes [107]. Thus TNF-α cytotoxicity could promote damage in the mitochondrial respiratory chain at complex III, triggering increased production of ROS and RNS [111]. On the other hand, impaired activity of PGC-1 affects mitochondrial biogenesis [105].

5.2.1.2 Endoplasmic Reticulum Stress

The ER is a dynamic organelle involved in fundamental cell processes, including production, secretion, and transport of membrane proteins, lipid biosynthesis, carbohydrate metabolism, and intracellular calcium storage. The ER is a complex system of tubular membranes that includes two continuous membranes: the nuclear envelope and the peripheral ER. An oxidative stress environment can trigger crucial changes in the ER membrane environment which have a negative impact on ER functions and UPR activation. The UPR signaling is mediated by the protein kinase-like ER kinase, inositol-requiring enzyme (IRE) 1α, and activating transcription factor 6α [112,113]. Furthermore, these UPR transmembrane sensors are involved in lipid metabolism [114]. The progression of NAFLD to NASH is thus strongly associated with ER stress and UPR activation.

UPR/ER stress has been linked to activation of inflammatory (NF-κB, JNK, ROS, TNF-α, IL-6) and insulin pathways [115], lipotoxicity, and apoptotic cell death, which are common features in NAFLD and obesity [114]. Pagliassotti et al. [113] published a review evaluating the link between ER stress and UPR and obesity and related chronic disease manifestations, which suggested that ER stress might be activated by three mechanisms: the increased levels of protein synthesis inducing ER stress; a downregulation of the folding capacity leading to ER stress mediated by a disequilibrium of calcium homeostasis between ER lumen and cytosol increasing the production of chaperones; and a reduction in the degradation of misfolded ER proteins [113]. However, the precise mechanism in progression to the pathogenesis of NAFLD is not fully defined.

ER stress might play a crucial role in steatosis by the action of lipid transcription factors [116]. Colgan et al. [116] evaluated the effects of ER stress on lipid metabolism. Cell lines (HeLa and MCF7) treated with ER stress-inducing agents showed that ER stress induces SREBP-2 activation, leading to lipid accumulation. Moreover, cholesterol accumulation and SREBP-2 activation are mediated by site-1 serine protease (S1P) and site-2 zinc metalloproteinase (S2P) proteolytic networks [116].

On the other hand, several studies have documented that FFAs are implicated in the activation of UPR and liver injury [115]. Arruda et al. (2014) studied the impact of saturated fatty acids over the ER in rat hepatoma cell lines (H4IIE liver cells) and primary hepatocytes. Data showed that palmitate promotes the activation of UPR and the markers associated with ER stress and cell death. Saturated fatty acids also induce changes in calcium transport activity that triggers hepatocytes death [117]. Zhang et al. [114] reviewed the role of ER stress in NAFLD, finding that ER stress might induce hepatocyte death throught C/EBP-homologous protein (CHOP) pathway; the induction of the JNK pathway by mediated IRE1 recruitment of protein TNFα receptor-associated factor 2 TRAF2; and a dysregulation of calcium homeostasis signaling pathways [114].

In summary, an increased uptake of FFA induces hepatic lipotoxicity, inflammation, and oxidative stress inducing ER perturbation. This state promotes the activation of many pathways to establish the normal ER homeostasis. However, in a constant lipotoxic environment, ER dysfunction induces steatosis and hepatocyte injure.

6. DIAGNOSIS

6.1 Liver Biopsy

Liver biopsy is currently the reference standard for the diagnosis of patients with NAFLD and the differentiation of steatosis from steatohepatitis. It is an invasive procedure which can lead to several clinical complications. Histological lesions are not equally distributed (sampling variability), while histological sampling error can lead to an inaccurate diagnosis [118]. Moreover, liver biopsy might carry some complications [9], increasing the risk of morbidity between 0.06% and 0.35% and the risk of mortality by 0.1%−0.01% [15].

6.2 Noninvasive Techniques

6.2.1 General Biochemistry

Among the principal routine laboratory tests linked to liver function, the blood chemistry panel includes serum concentrations of aminotransferases, gamma glutamyl transferase (GGT), and alkaline phosphatase. A complete blood count and prothrombin time may also be useful [119]. Serum alanine aminotransferase (ALT) concentration is usually the most evaluated biomarker in patients with liver disease. Commonly, patients with NAFLD exhibited high levels of ALT and aspartate aminotransferase (AST), especially in patients with NASH. High levels of ALT are associated with an increased progression of NAFLD. However, the evaluation of ALT levels in patients with NAFLD reports different results [17,120]. Maximos et al. [121] assessed the role of insulin resistance and intrahepatic fat content over ALT serum levels in overweight or obese subjects with NAFLD or NASH: 440 patients were evaluated and randomly assigned into three groups of no NAFLD, NAFLD/normal ALT levels, and NAFLD/high ALT levels. The authors found that insulin resistance and triglyceride contents were strongly associated with the increase of ALT plasma levels, but no differences in fibrosis, ballooning, or inflammation were found among NASH patients with high or normal ALT plasma levels [121]. In this context, ALT plasma levels are apparently variable among patient groups, which also suggests that other factors such as metabolic status and demographic variables have an impact on ALT concentrations [120], but a consensus criterion of cut-off point has not been established yet. Prati et al.(2017) redefined ALT plasma level limits, undertaking a retrospective cohort study that evaluated ALT plasma levels of blood-donor candidates negative in hepatitis and NAFLD. Results showed that a cut-off of <30 IU/L in men and <19 IU/L in women exhibited higher sensitivity (76.3%) and sensibility (88.5%) than the conventional cut-off of <40 IU/L in men and <30 IU/L in women in patients with hepatitis virus C infection, increasing the possibility of including patients with minimal or mild histological lesions [122].

6.2.2 Markers of Liver Damage

A key feature of the progression of NAFLD to NASH is apoptosis, which correlates with the severity of steatohepatitis and fibrosis [123]. During the apoptosis process, proteolytic enzymes called caspases are activated to degrade several substrates, including cytokeratin 18 fragments (CK18). The CK18 is a type 1 intermediate filament protein and pairs with CK8, a complementary type 2 keratin protein. CK18 and CK8 are indispensable for the development of the keratin filaments that are altered during apoptosis [124]. Furthermore, it has been suggested that CK18 seems to play a role in the development of cancer by the activation of several cell signaling pathways related to carcinogenesis [125]. Nowadays, CK18 is one of the most promising blood biomarkers studied because of it is predictive potential to diagnose NASH and the progression of NAFLD. One systematic review and metaanalysis to evaluate noninvasive biomarkers covered 22 studies; among the principal findings, a cut-off between 261.4 and 670 U/L showed 24%−86% sensitivity and 91%−100% specificity. In general, CK18 exhibited 66% sensitivity and 82% specificity, but the variability of the studies made it difficult to establish proper limits for diagnostic accuracy [126]. Feldstein et al. [123] evaluated CK18 plasma levels in 201 children with NAFLD proven by liver biopsy. Serum CK18 levels were significantly higher in children with NASH compared to no NASH, and it turned out to be a better predictor of NASH than AST and GGT. They found a strong correlation between steatosis, inflammation, ballooning, fibrosis, and portal inflammation as well [123]. Nevertheless, this biomarker still reports contradictory results and needs to be tested in powered studies. Another study evaluated 420 multiethnic subjects whose intrahepatic fat content was measured by MRI, magnetic resonance spectroscopy and liver biopsy. Data showed that CK18 serum levels increased in steatosis and inflammation; nevertheless, no differences were found concerning ballooning features [127].

6.2.3 Imaging Tests

Liver biopsy is the gold standard for the diagnosis of NAFLD to assess fat content and estimate the stage of NASH more accurately, but other tests include ultrasonography, MRI, computed tomography, and elastography [128]. Most imaging tests are inexpensive and could be useful to diagnose NAFLD, although some are not able to distinguish between steatosis or steatohepatitis and the different stages of NASH, showing a high sensitivity only when the liver fat content is higher than 33%; thus they are only useful to diagnose moderate and severe stages of steatohepatitis [128]. Hepatic ultrasonography is the most commonly used imaging technique for the diagnosis of NAFLD [127]. To assess the accuracy of ultrasonography in the diagnosis of steatosis, one systematic review and metaanalysis covered 47 studies with 4720 subjects, and the results were compared to liver histology as the reference. In 34 studies involving 2815 patients, the sensitivity was 84.8% and the specificity was 93.6% to detect moderate−severe FL content. Also, the data analysis showed a significant heterogeneity in the area under the curve. In 29 studies, the sensitivity was 87.2% and the specificity was 79.2% to differentiate steatosis from other histological features. The authors concluded that ultrasonography could be useful to diagnose steatosis. However, additional studies about criteria are needed considering individual parameters [129]. Computed tomography is no more sensitive than ultrasonography in diagnosing FL, although it can determine other liver pathologies more accurately compared to ultrasonography [128]. MRI is one of the most sensitive noninvasive techniques, but the high cost limits its use [127]. In a cohort study, 38 subjects who had undergone a liver biopsy were evaluated by MRI and ultrasonography; the main findings were that MRI exhibits a better correlation than ultrasonography for lipid content, but MRI and ultrasonography show a good correlation in macrovesicular steatosis. Nevertheless, fat content assessed by MRI varied between 19% and 40%. MRI has shown good accuracy in identifying minor degrees of FL compared to ultrasonography [130]. However, both MRI and computed tomography are not feasible for large-scale epidemiological studies due to the high cost involved [128]. Among other techniques, the transient elastography or FibroScan is a rapid and noninvasive procedure. This method measures the propagation speed of elastic waves, measuring the stiffness or elasticity of a tissue through the liver [131]. FibroScan can also measure the elasticity of a cylinder of hepatic parenchyma approximately 1 cm in diameter and 2−4 cm in length, exploring a volume of up to 100 times more compared to liver biopsy [132]. This technique presents several advantages, such as a reduced risk of complications, and it is capable of detecting liver stiffness and steatosis. It has demonstrated good reproducibility and can be used in studies with large populations. However, in morbidly obese subjects it is necessary to use an XL probe [133].

6.2.4 Models to Assess Steatosis

6.2.4.1 Fatty Liver Index

In 2006 the fatty liver index (FLI) was derived from the cohort of DIONYSOS, a study of the prevalence of chronic liver diseases in the general population of two communities in northern Italy; 216 subjects with suspected liver disease and 280 without were evaluated. Ultrasonography was used for the diagnosis of NAFLD. They identified an algorithm to predict hepatic steatosis included in the model, anthropometric variables (BMI and waist circumference), and biochemical variables (triglycerides and GGT). A cut-off value of <30 that can be used to rule out steatosis showed a sensitivity of 87%, and a value of ≥60 exhibited 86% specificity to diagnose steatohepatitis [134].

6.2.4.2 Lipid Accumulation Product

In the cross-sectional DIONYSOS nutrition and liver study a new predictor that considered two variables of the FLI model was assessed. Liver steatosis was diagnosed by ultrasonography, and 588 patients were included, stratified according to the degree of steatosis: 56% normal, 20% intermediate, and 24% severe. Authors evaluated the lipid accumulation product (LAP), which considers waist circumference and triglycerides by sex. Results showed that increased values of LAP are associated with moderate and severe steatosis [135].

6.2.4.3 Hepatic Steatosis Index

The hepatic steatosis index was proposed in 2010 by Lee and colleagues. Investigators performed a cross-sectional case-control study that evaluated a total of 10,724 participants according to age and sex-matched controls; patients were randomly assigned to a derivation cohort (2680 pairs) or a validation cohort (2862 pairs) of patients diagnosed with NAFLD defined by ultrasonography. The formulated index included the ALT/AST ratio and BMI, and added two points for the presence of diabetes mellitus and two points for sex (female). In the derivation cohort it was found that a cut-off of <30 has a sensitivity of 92.5% to exclude NAFLD and a cut-off of >36 could detect NAFLD with a specificity of 92.4%, and 85.6% of subjects were accurately classified. On the other hand, in the validation cohort a cut-off of <30 has a sensitivity of 93.1% to exclude NAFLD and a cut-off of >36 could detect NAFLD with a specificity of 92.4%. Moreover, in the validation cohort showed that a value of <30 could ruled out NAFLD with a sensitivity of 93.1% and a value of >36 could detect NAFLD with a specificity of 93.1% [136].

6.2.4.4 Nonalcoholic Fatty Liver Disease Liver Fat Score

The NAFLD Liver Fat Score (NAFLD-LFS) considers the presence of MetS, diabetes mellitus, insulin levels, AST, and AST/ALT ratio [137]. Cheung et al. [137] evaluated within the third US National Health and Nutrition Examination Survey 5184 subjects between 20 and 74 years old. Hepatic steatosis was determined by ultrasonography. An NAFLD-LFS ≥1.257 cut-off exhibited an area under curve of 0.771. A second study was carried out to establish an association between NAFLD-LFS and mortality (follow-up of 14.7 years). Data showed that high values of NAFLD-LFS are associated with cardiovascular and liver-related mortality [137].

6.2.5 Model to Assess Hepatic Fibrosis

6.2.5.1 BAAT Score

The BAAT score was proposed by Ratziu et al. [138] and includes BMI, age, serum levels of ALT, and triglycerides as variables. They assessed a retrospective study which included 93 subjects with BMI >25 kg/m^2 and abnormal biomarkers related to liver function (AST, ALT, and GGT) who had undergone liver biopsy. Results indicated that four variables are strongly associated to septal fibrosis and represent 30% of the variability. The model awards one point for each parameter (age ≥ 50 years old, BMI ≥ 28 kg/m^2, ALT ≥ 2N, and triglyceride ≥1.7 mmol/L); a score of 0−1 showed 100% sensitivity and 47% specificity for a diagnosis of hepatic septal fibrosis (related with necroinflammatory activity), and a score of 4 exhibited 14% sensitivity and 100% specificity [138].

6.2.5.2 BARD Score

The BARD score system was proposed by Harrison et al. [139]. Researchers evaluated 827 participants with biopsy-proven NAFLD from two care centers (669 subjects had NASH), and found that the principal parameters associated with NASH were BMI ≥ 28, AST/ALT ratio ≥0.8, and presence of diabetes mellitus. These variables increase the risk of fibrosis in NASH by 2.4 times. Moreover, the receiver operator characteristic areas under the curve and a score of 4 could detect advanced liver fibrosis (stages 3−4) with a positive predictive value of 43% and a negative predictive value of 96%, using liver biopsy as a reference standard [139].

7. DIETARY TREATMENT

Emerging clinical studies suggest that diet might improve the principal features related to NAFLD [9] [140—142]. The AASLD recommends a weight loss between 3% and 5% to improve hepatic steatosis, and almost ≥10% may be necessary to improve necroinflammation [9]. As it is overwhelmed FFA-disrupted oxidative capacity that induces oxidative stress, causing hepatocellular injury, healthy eating patterns can not only promote weight loss but also include foods that might improve the antioxidant capacity of the diet. Several intervention studies have reported that dietary components with antioxidant activity are able to reduce oxidative stress and tissue damage [143]. The Mediterranean diet is recognized as a healthy eating pattern which provides bioactive substances with a high antioxidant content and antiinflammatory effects. It is characterized by a high consumption of specific fatty acids such as PUFAs and monounsaturated fatty acids, fruits, vegetables, and legumes; moderate consumption of fish, seafood, fermented dairy products, poultry, and eggs; moderate intake of wine; and low consumption of red and processed meat and sweets [144]. One principal epidemiological study is the Prevención con Dieta Mediterránea (PREDIMED—Prevention with Mediterranean diet), a parallel-group, multicenter, randomized trial with 5 years follow-up involving 7447 subjects with high cardiovascular risk but without cardiovascular disease. Subjects were randomized into three groups: a Mediterranean diet supplemented with extravirgin olive oil, a Mediterranean diet supplemented with mixed nuts (30 g/day), and a control diet (advice to reduce dietary fat). After 3 months of intervention, a Mediterranean diet supplemented with olive oil was associated with a reduction of blood glucose. The two Mediterranean diets improved fasting insulin and insulin resistance in nondiabetic subjects. In relation to the lipoprotein profile, the low-fat diet group did not exhibit any changes, but the Mediterranean diet groups reported a reduction of low-density lipoprotein cholesterol levels and increased levels of HDL-c. Furthermore, the PREDIMED study showed that Mediterranean diets reduce the biomarkers related to inflammation and oxidative stress, such as serum C-reactive protein IL-6, compared to a low-fat diet [145]. Moreover, a high dietary inflammatory score is related to high FLI score (>60) in obese subjects [146]. This evidence suggests that a Mediterranean dietary pattern enhances antioxidant capacity and might improve the principal risk factors related to NAFLD, such as insulin resistance, dyslipidemia, and MetS (Table 6.3). In another randomized cross-sectional study, 12 nondiabetic subjects with NASH confirmed by liver biopsy were enrolled. During the 6 weeks of intervention participants consumed a Mediterranean diet, a control diet, and a low-fat, high-carbohydrate diet (LF/HCD) with a 6-week washout period in between. The results showed a significant reduction of hepatic steatosis after Mediterranean diet consumption compared with the other diets, plus an improvement in insulin sensitivity in comparison to the LF/HCD diet [140]. Trovato et al. [141] reported that Mediterranean diet might improve hepatic fat accumulation in subjects with NAFLD; 90 nondiabetic patients with NAFLD proven by ultrasonography were enrolled in this trial. After 6 months of intervention, subjects adhering to the Mediterranean diet showed a significant decrease in Bright Liver Score [141]. Furthermore, unsaturated fatty acids (one of the principal features of a Mediterranean diet) have been associated with healthy effects in subjects with NAFLD. These effects could be attributed to an improvement in hepatic lipid metabolism, which plays a pivotal role in the oxidative stress mechanism and progression to NASH [142]. The intake of omega-3 PUFA could induce weight loss and reduction of body fat mass in overweight or obese individuals, probably through alteration of gene expression related to fat oxidation upregulation. Thus omega-3 PUFA promotes a reduction of fatty deposition in adipose tissue and modulates food intake [147]. In a systematic review and metaanalysis, authors focused in clinical investigations that used omega-3 PUFA supplementation in NAFLD patients. A total of 355 patients were included in the analysis. The average treatment with omega-3 PUFA lasted 6 months with a dose of 4 g/day. Omega-3 PUFA treatment exerted beneficial effects in the liver related to reduced lipid droplet and AST levels [142]. However, the heterogeneity of the studies and the correct dose have not been determined yet, so clinical studies are required to evaluate its efficacy in patients with NAFLD [142]. The AASLD indicated that the use of omega-3 PUFA in NAFLD or NASH required more studies to establish the dose and its validity to treat this disease [9]. Among the principal components with a high-power antioxidant with antiinflammatory action are the polyphenols, which are bioactive compounds of fruits and vegetables. Polyphenols are shown to have effects on glucose and lipid metabolism. Salomone et al. [148] published a review with experimental and clinical evidence of using polyphenols in NAFLD, suggesting that they might improve liver steatosis and liver damage by several mechanisms [148]. Furthermore, animal and experimental models have reported that polyphenols have beneficial effects on hepatocytes by the suppression of DNL and stimulation of fatty acid oxidation, improving insulin sensitivity, activating the adenosine monophosphate-activated protein kinase pathway, and decreasing the production of inflammatory cytokines in Kuppfer cells. They are also linked to the inhibition of HSC proliferation, and ROS and fibrogenic cascade [148].

Several studies have suggested the beneficial action of vitamin E. In the TONIC study (Treatment of Nonalcoholic Fatty Liver Disease in Children) a randomized, multicenter, double-masked, placebo-controlled trial evaluated the action of vitamin E or metformin in 173 nondiabetic children with NAFLD proven by liver biopsy. Participants were randomized

TABLE 6.3 Interventional Studies on Mediterranean Diet in Nonalcoholic Fatty Liver Disease

Study Design	Patients	Intervention	Follow-up	Results
Random clinical trial[a]	322 obese subjects (male = 277)	Three intervention groups Low-fat (LF) and restricted calorie Mediterranean diet (MD) Low-carbohydrate nonrestrictive calorie (LC)	2 years	Body weight reduction: LF = −3.3 ± 4.1 kg MD = −4.6 ± 6.0 kg LC = −5.5 ± 7.0 kg MD group showed a significant reduction of fasting plasma glucose and insulin levels in diabetic subjects versus others Significant reduction of PCR in MD (21%) and LC (29%) Changes in biomarkers related to liver function (bilirubin, alkaline phosphatase, and ALT) were similar in all groups
Post hoc analysis parallel-design quasirandomized control trial[b]	259 obese subjects with diabetes	Subjects were randomized in three groups: American Diabetes Association diet (ADA) (n = 85) Low glycaemic index diet (LGI) (n = 89) Modified Mediterranean diet (MMD)	12 months	MMD = significant decrease of ALT levels compared to other groups
Prospective study[c]	14 obese men with NAFLD and MetS	Spanish ketogenic Mediterranean diet	12 weeks	Significant reduction of body weight, LDL, ALT, AST, and steatosis
Case-control study[d]	518 cases of HCC and 772 controls of two countries	Evaluated the association between MD (based on 9 dietary components and a scale from 0 (lowest adherence) to 9 (high adherence)) and liver cancer		MD adherence ≥5 reduced around 50% of incidence of HCC

ADA, American Diabetes Association diet; ALT, alanine aminotransferase; AST, aspartate aminotransferase; HCC, hepatocellular carcinoma; LC, low-carbohydrate, nonrestrictive calorie; LDL, low-density lipoprotein; LF, low-fat restricted calorie; LGI, low glycemic index diet; MD, Mediterranean diet; MetS, metabolic syndrome; NAFLD, non-alcoholic fatty liver disease; PCR, C-reactive protein.
[a]Shai et al. N Engl J Med 2008;359(3):229–41.
[b]Fraser et al. Diabetologia 2008;51(9):1616–22.
[c]Pérez-Guisado, Munoz-Serrano. J Med Food 2011;14(7–8):677–80.
[d]Turati et al. J Hepatol 2014;60(3):606–11.

into three groups, metformin oral 500 mg (twice daily), vitamin E oral 400 IU (twice daily), or placebo (twice daily), for 96 weeks of treatment with a 24-week washout period. Results showed a statistical reduction of ALT levels in all groups: vitamin E (-48.3 U/L), metformin (-41.7 U/L), and placebo (-35.2 U/L). The reduction of hepatocellular ballooning score was -0.5 with vitamin E, -0.3 with metformin, and -0.7 with placebo. In relation to the NAFLD activity score, all groups showed a reduction, but only vitamin E exhibited a significant improvement compared to placebo (-1.8 versus -0.7) and a reduction of NASH (58%) versus placebo (28%) [149]. In a pilot study Sanyal et al. [150] evaluated vitamin E and pioglitazone (an insulin sensitizer) in nondiabetic patients with biopsy-proven NASH; 20 patients were randomized to groups of vitamin E (400 IU/day) or vitamin E (400 IU/day) and pioglitazone (30 mg/day). Treatment with vitamin E showed a significant decrease of steatosis, and the therapy combination gave a decrease not only of the steatosis but also in histological parameters such as ballooning, Mallory's hyaline, and pericellular fibrosis. Moreover, this therapy induced a significant decrease of fasting FFAs and insulin [150]. The AASLD indicated that a daily dose of 800 IU might give improvements in liver histology in nondiabetic adults with NASH proved by liver biopsy, and it also has to be considered as a first-line treatment in this population (Strength 1, Quality B) [9].

Taking this evidence together, it appears that systematic oxidative stress plays a crucial role in the progression of liver damage. Increasing evidence suggests that dietary antioxidative therapy might promote hepato-protective effects and improve MetS components through several mechanisms related to glucose and lipid metabolism andinflammatory and fibrogenic networks [141,143,148].

8. CONCLUSIONS

There is much evidence suggesting that obesity and components of MetS are strongly associated, but the mechanism underlying NAFLD is not yet fully understood. Nevertheless, insulin resistance, obesity, and oxidative stress play a pivotal role in NAFLD pathogenesis.

At present there is no specific medical treatment for NAFLD, but several clinical studies report that weight loss and lifestyles changes are cornerstones of its treatment. Emerging data discloses the effectiveness of a Mediterranean diet in controlling steatosis, liver enzymes, and several factors related to insulin resistance, inflammation, and oxidative stress. It is crucial to identify new molecules that can modulate oxidative cascade and regulate the expression of proinflammatory and apoptotic genes. New ways must be opened with the aim of providing new insights to establish optimal strategies and clinical therapies to prevent and manage NAFLD.

GLOSSARY

Cirrhosis Liver disease characterized by fibrosis and hepatocyte injure with an alteration of the liver architecture.
Hepatic stellate cells (HSCs) These type of cells are located within the space of disease and are closely related to the development of liver fibrosis.
Hepatocellular carcinoma (HCC) A type of liver adenocarcinoma.
Nonalcoholic fatty liver (NAFL) Characterized by hepatic triglyceride accumulation (hepatic steatosis), mainly macrovesicular.
Nonalcoholic fatty liver disease (NAFLD) Chronic liver disease not caused for abuse alcohol consumption characterized by increased lipid accumulation into hepatocytes.
Nonalcoholic steatohepatitis (NASH) Presence of hepatic steatosis with hepatocyte damage (inflammation, ballooning with or without fibrosis).

LIST OF ABBREVIATIONS

4-HHE 4-hydroxy-2-hexenal
4-HNE 4-hydroxynonenal
AASLD American Association for the Study of Liver Disease
ALT Alanine aminotransferase
ApoB Apolipoprotein
AST Aspartate aminotransferase
BMI Body mass index
CD36 Cluster of differentiation 36
ChREBP Carbohydrate response element binding protein
CK18 Cytokeratin 18
COII Mitochondrial cytochrome c oxidase subunit II
CPT Carnitine palmitoyltransferase

CYP2E1 Cytochrome P450, family 2, subfamily E, polypeptide 1
DNA Deoxyribonucleic acid
DNL De novo lipogenesis
ER Endoplasmic reticulum
FABP4 Fatty-acid-binding protein 4
FADH$_2$ Flavin adenine dinucleotide
FFA Free fatty acid
FLI Fatty liver index
GGT Glutamyl transferase
GLUT-4 Glucose transporter type 4
HCC Hepatocellular carcinoma
HDL-c High-density lipoprotein cholesterol
HSC Hepatic stellate cell
IL-6 Interleukin 6
IRE Inositol-requiring enzyme
IRS Insulin receptor substrate
JNK c-Jun N-terminal kinase
LAP Lipid accumulation product
LF/HCD Low-fat high-carbohydrate diet
MDA Malondialdehyde
MetS Metabolic syndrome
MRI magnetic resonance imaging
MTP Microsomal triglyceride transfer protein
NADH Nicotinamide adenine dinucleotide
NAFL Nonalcoholic fatty liver
NAFLD-LFS NAFLD Liver Fat Score
NAFLD Nonalcoholic fatty liver disease
NASH Nonalcoholic steatohepatitis
ND1 NADH dehydrogenase subunit 1
NF-κB Nuclear factor κB
PAI-1 Plasminogen activator inhibitor 1
PGC-1 Peroxisome proliferator-activated receptor-γ coactivator-1α
PPAR-α Peroxisome proliferator activated receptor
PREDIMED Prevención con Dieta Mediterránea
PUFA Polyunsaturated fatty acid
RNS Reactive nitrogen species
ROS Reactive oxygen species
S1P Site-1 serine protease
S2P Site-2 zinc metalloprotease
SREBP-1c Sterol regulatory binding protein-1c
TNF-α Tumor necrosis factor
UPR Uncoupled protein response
VLDL Very low-density lipoprotein

REFERENCES

[1] Bondia-Pons I, Ryan L, Martinez JA. Oxidative stress and inflammation interactions in human obesity. J Physiol Biochem 2012;68(4):701–11.

[2] Brookheart RT, Michel CI, Schaffer JE. As a matter of fat. Cell Metab July 2009;10(1):9–12.

[3] Tilg H. Adipocytokines in nonalcoholic fatty liver disease: key players regulating steatosis, inflammation and fibrosis. Curr Pharm Des 2010;16(17):1893–5.

[4] Fernández-Sánchez A, Madrigal-Santillán E, Bautista M, Esquivel-Soto J, Morales-González Á, Esquivel-Chirino C, et al. Inflammation, oxidative stress, and obesity. Int J Mol Sci 2011;12(5):3117–32.

[5] Younossi ZM, Koenig AB, Abdelatif D, Fazel Y, Henry L, Wymer M. Global epidemiology of nonalcoholic fatty liver disease-meta-analytic assessment of prevalence, incidence, and outcomes. Hepatology July 2016;64(1):73–84.

[6] Li L, Liu DW, Yan HY, Wang ZY, Zhao SH, Wang B. Obesity is an independent risk factor for non-alcoholic fatty liver disease: evidence from a meta-analysis of 21 cohort studies. Obes Rev 2016;17(6):510–9.

[6a] Pang Q, Zhang J-Y, Song S-D, Qu K, Xu X-S, Liu S-S, et al. Central obesity and nonalcoholic fatty liver disease risk after adjusting for body mass index, Central obesity and nonalcoholic fatty liver disease risk after adjusting for body mass index. World J Gastroenterol 2015;21(5):1650.

[7] Pang Q. Central obesity and nonalcoholic fatty liver disease risk after adjusting for body mass index. World J Gastroenterol 2015;21(5):1650.

[8] Kleiner DE, Brunt EM, Van Natta M, Behling C, Contos MJ, Cummings OW, et al. Design and validation of a histological scoring system for nonalcoholic fatty liver disease. Hepatology 2005;41(6):1313−21.

[9] Chalasani N, Younossi Z, Lavine JE, Diehl AM, Brunt EM, Cusi K, et al. The diagnosis and management of non-alcoholic fatty liver disease: practice guideline by the American Association for the Study of Liver Diseases, American College of Gastroenterology, and the American Gastroenterological Association. Hepatology 2012;55(6):2005−23.

[10] Ovalle WK, Nahirney PC, Netter FH. Netter's essential histology. Philadelphia: Saunders/Elsevier, Cop; 2008.

[11] Lackner C, Gogg-Kamerer M, Zatloukal K, Stumptner C, Brunt EM, Denk H. Ballooned hepatocytes in steatohepatitis: the value of keratin immunohistochemistry for diagnosis. J Hepatol 2008;48(5):821−8.

[12] Brunt EM. Alcoholic and nonalcoholic steatohepatitis. Clin Liver Dis 2002;6(2):399−420.

[13] Takahashi Y. Histopathology of nonalcoholic fatty liver disease/nonalcoholic steatohepatitis. World J Gastroenterol 2014;20(42):15539.

[14] Zatloukal K, French SW, Stumptner C, Strnad P, Harada M, Toivola DM, et al. From Mallory to Mallory−Denk bodies: what, how and why? Exp Cell Res 2007;313(10):2033−49.

[15] Brunt EM. Pathology of nonalcoholic fatty liver disease. Nat Rev Gastroenterol Hepatol 2010;7(4):195−203. Nature Publishing Group.

[16] Brunt EM, Janney CG, Di Bisceglie AM, Neuschwander-Tetri BA, Bacon BR. Nonalcoholic steatohepatitis: a proposal for grading and staging the histological lesions. Am J Gastroenterol 1999;94(9):2467−74.

[17] Rinella ME. Nonalcoholic fatty liver disease: a systematic review. J Am Med Assoc June 9, 2015;313(22):2263−73.

[18] Francque SM, Van Der Graaff D, Kwanten WJ. Review non-alcoholic fatty liver disease and cardiovascular risk: pathophysiological mechanisms and implications. J Hepatol 2016;65(2):425−43. European Association for the Study of the Liver.

[19] Amarapurkar DN, Hashimoto E, Lesmana LA, Sollano JD, Chen P. How common is non-alcoholic fatty liver disease in the Asia − Pacific region and are there local differences. J Gastroenterol Hepatol 2007;22:788−93.

[20] Hsu C-S, Kao J-H. Non-alcoholic fatty liver disease: an emerging liver disease in Taiwan. J Formos Med Assoc 2012;111(10):527−35. Elsevier Taiwan LLC.

[21] Adams LA, Lymp JF, Sauver JST, Sanderson SO, Lindor KD, Feldstein A, et al. Population-based cohort study. Gastroenterology 2005:113−21.

[22] Abd El-Kader SM, El-Den Ashmawy EMS. Non-alcoholic fatty liver disease: the diagnosis and management. World J Hepatol 2015;7(6):846−58.

[23] Gaggini M, Morelli M, Buzzigoli E, Defronzo RA, Bugianesi E, Gastaldelli A. Non-alcoholic fatty liver disease (NAFLD) and its connection with insulin resistance, dyslipidemia, atherosclerosis and coronary heart disease. Nutrients 2013:1544−60.

[24] Anderson EL, Howe LD, Jones HE, Higgins JPT, Lawlor DA, Fraser A. The prevalence of non-alcoholic fatty liver disease in children and adolescents: a systematic review and meta-analysis. PLoS One 2015;10(10):e0140908.

[25] Pan J-J, Fallon MB. Gender and racial differences in nonalcoholic fatty liver disease. World J Hepatol 2014;6(5):274−83.

[26] Smits MM, Ioannou GN, Boyko EJ, Utzschneider KM. Non-alcoholic fatty liver disease as an independent manifestation of the metabolic syndrome: results of a US national survey in three ethnic groups. J Gastroenterol Hepatol 2013;28(4):664−70.

[27] Browning JD, Szczepaniak LS, Dobbins R, Nuremberg P, Horton JD, Cohen JC, et al. Prevalence of hepatic steatosis in an urban population in the United States: impact of ethnicity. Hepatology 2004;40(6):1387−95.

[28] Suzuki A, Abdelmalek MF. Nonalcoholic fatty liver disease in women. Womens Health (Engl) 2009;5(2):191−203.

[29] Carulli L, Lonardo A, Lombardini S, Marchesini G, Loria P. Gender, fatty liver and GGT. Hepatology 2006;44(1):278−9.

[30] Frith J, Day CP, Henderson E, Burt AD, Newton JL. Non-alcoholic fatty liver disease in older people. Gerontology 2009:607−13.

[31] Fan J-G, Cao H-X. Role of diet and nutritional management in non-alcoholic fatty liver disease. J Gastroenterol Hepatol 2013;28:81−7.

[32] Videla LA, Rodrigo R, Araya J, Poniachik J. Insulin resistance and oxidative stress interdependency in non-alcoholic fatty liver disease. Trends Mol Med 2006;12(12):555−8.

[33] Koroglu E, Canbakan B, Atay K, Hatemi I, Tuncer M, Dobrucali A, et al. Role of oxidative stress and insulin resistance in disease severity of non-alcoholic fatty liver disease. Turk J Gastroenterol 2016;27(4):361−6.

[34] Fabbrini E, Sullivan S, Klein S. Obesity and nonalcoholic fatty liver disease: biochemical, metabolic, and clinical implications. Hepatology 2010:679−89.

[35] Qureshi K, Abrams GA. Prevalence of biopsy-proven non-alcoholic fatty liver disease in severely obese subjects without metabolic syndrome. Clin Obes 2016;6(2):117−23.

[36] Qureshi K, Abrams GA. Metabolic liver disease of obesity and role of adipose tissue in the pathogenesis of nonalcoholic fatty liver disease. World J Gastroenterol 2007;13(26):3540−53.

[37] Thomas EL, Hamilton G, Patel N, O'Dwyer R, Doré CJ, Goldin RD, et al. Hepatic triglyceride content and its relation to body adiposity: a magnetic resonance imaging and proton magnetic resonance spectroscopy study. Gut 2005;54(1):122−7.

[38] Wilman HR, Kelly M, Garratt S, Matthews PM, Milanesi M, Herlihy A, et al. Characterisation of liver fat in the UK Biobank cohort. PLoS One 2017;12(2):e0172921.

[39] Streba LAM, Vere CC, Rogoveanu I, Streba CT. Nonalcoholic fatty liver disease, metabolic risk factors, and hepatocellular carcinoma: an open question. World J Gastroenterol 2015;21(14):4103−10.

[40] Larsson SC, Wolk A. Overweight, obesity and risk of liver cancer: a meta-analysis of cohort studies. Br J Cancer 2007:1005−8.

[41] Schlesinger S, Aleksandrova K, Pischon T, Fedirko V, Jenab M, Trepo E, et al. Abdominal obesity, weight gain during adulthood and risk of liver and biliary tract cancer in a European cohort. Int J Cancer 2013;132(3):645−57.

[42] Moreno MJ, Martínez JA. Adipose tissue: a storage and secretory organ. An Sist Sanit Navar 2002;25(1):29−39.

[43] Schäffler A, Schölmerich J, Büchler C. Mechanisms of disease: adipocytokines and visceral adipose tissue—emerging role in nonalcoholic fatty liver disease. Nat Clin Pract Gastroenterol Hepatol 2005;2(6):273—80.

[44] Wieckowska A, Mccullough AJ, Feldstein AE. Noninvasive diagnosis and monitoring of nonalcoholic steatohepatitis: present and future. Hepatology 2007;46(2):582—9.

[45] Friedman JM, Halaas JL. Leptin and the regulation of body weight in mammals. Nature 1998;395(6704):763—70.

[46] Sáinz N, Barrenetxe J, Moreno-Aliaga MJ, Martínez JA. Leptin resistance and diet-induced obesity: central and peripheral actions of leptin. Metabolism 2015;64(1):35—46.

[46a] Huang K, Lin RCY, Kormas N, Lee L, Chen C, Gill TP, et al. Plasma leptin is associated with insulin resistance independent of age, body mass index, fat mass, lipids, and pubertal development in nondiabetic adolescents. Int J Obes Relat. Metab Disord 2004;28(4):470—5.

[47] Zuo H, Shi Z, Yuan B, Dai Y, Wu G, Hussain A. Association between serum leptin concentrations and insulin resistance: a population-based study from China. PLoS One 2013;8(1):e54615.

[48] Saxena NK. Leptin as a novel profibrogenic cytokine in hepatic stellate cells: mitogenesis and inhibition of apoptosis mediated by extracellular regulated kinase (Erk) and Akt phosphorylation. FASEB J 2004;30(1):1—31.

[49] Zelber-Sagi S, Ratziu V, Zvibel I, Goldiner I, Blendis L, Morali G, et al. The association between adipocytokines and biomarkers for nonalcoholic fatty liver disease-induced liver injury: a study in the general population. Eur J Gastroenterol Hepatol 2012;24(3):262—9.

[50] Uygun A, Kadayifci A, Yesilova Z, Erdil A, Yaman H, Saka M, et al. Serum leptin levels in patients with nonalcoholic steatohepatitis. Am J Gastroenterol 2000;95(12):3584—9.

[50a] Chandrashekara V, Das S, Seth RK, Dattaroy D, Alhasson F, Michelotti G, et al. Purinergic receptor X7 mediates leptin induced GLUT4 function in stellate cells in nonalcoholic steatohepatitis. Biochimica et Biophysica Acta 2016;1862(1):32—45.

[51] Peper JS, Dahl RE. HHS Public Access 2015;22(2):134—9.

[52] Polyzos SA, Toulis KA, Goulis DG, Zavos C, Kountouras J. Serum total adiponectin in nonalcoholic fatty liver disease: a systematic review and meta-analysis. Metabolism 2011;60(3):313—26. Elsevier Inc.

[52a] Machado MV, Coutinho J, Carepa F, Costa A, Proença H, Cortez-Pinto H. How adiponectin, leptin, and ghrelin orchestrate together and correlate with the severity of nonalcoholic fatty liver disease. Eur J Gastroenterol Hepatol 2012;24(10):1166—72.

[53] Kamada Y, Tamura S, Kiso S, Matsumoto H, Saji Y, Yoshida Y, et al. Enhanced carbon tetrachloride-induced liver fibrosis in mice lacking adiponectin. Gastroenterology 2003;125(6):1796—807.

[54] Stojsavljević S, Palčić MG, Jukić LV, Duvnjak LS, Duvnjak M. Adipokines and proinflammatory cytokines, the key mediators in the pathogenesis of nonalcoholic fatty liver disease. World J Gastroenterol 2014;20(48):18070—91.

[55] Endo M, Masaki T, Seike M, Yoshimatsu H. TNF-alpha induces hepatic steatosis in mice by enhancing gene expression of sterol regulatory element binding protein-1c (SREBP-1c). Exp Biol Med 2007;232(5):614—21.

[56] Seo YY, Cho YK, Bae J-C, Seo MH, Park SE, Rhee E-J, et al. Tumor necrosis factor-α as a predictor for the development of nonalcoholic fatty liver disease: a 4-year follow-up study. Endocrinol Metab 2013;28(1):41.

[57] Kershaw EE, Flier JS. Adipose tissue as an endocrine organ. J Clin Endocrinol Metab 2004;89(6):2548—56.

[58] Holzberg JR, Jin R, Le N-A, Ziegler TR, Brunt EM, McClain CJ, et al. Plasminogen activator inhibitor-1 predicts quantity of hepatic steatosis independent of insulin resistance and body weight. J Pediatr Gastroenterol Nutr 2016;62(6):819—23.

[59] Lebovitz HE. Insulin resistance: definition and consequences. Exp Clin Endocrinol Diabetes 2001;109.

[60] Reaven G. The metabolic syndrome or the insulin resistance syndrome? Different names, different concepts, and different goals. Endocrinol Metab Clin North Am 2004;33:283—303.

[61] Wilcox G. Insulin and insulin resistance. Clin Biochem Rev May 2005;26:19—39.

[62] Einhorn D. American College of Endocrinology position statement on the insulin resistance syndrome. Endocr Pract 2003;9(3):240—52.

[63] Trout KK, Homko C, Tkacs NC. Methods of measuring insulin sensitivity. Biol Res Nurs 2007;8(4):305—18.

[64] Bugianesi E, Moscatiello S, Ciaravella MF, Marchesini G. Insulin resistance in nonalcoholic fatty liver disease. Curr Pharm Des 2010;6(17):1941—51.

[65] Kelley DE, McKolanis TM, Hegazi RAF, Kuller LH, Kalhan SC. Fatty liver in type 2 diabetes mellitus: relation to regional adiposity, fatty acids, and insulin resistance. Am J Physiol Endocrinol Metab 2003;285(4):E906—16.

[66] Gholam PM, Flancbaum L, MacHan JT, Charney DA, Kotler DP. Nonalcoholic fatty liver disease in severely obese subjects. Am J Gastroenterol 2007;102(2):399—408.

[67] Lieber CS. CYP2E1: from ASH to NASH. Hepatol Res 2004;28(1):1—11.

[68] Browning JD, Horton JD. Molecular mediators of hepatic steatosis and liver injury. J Clin Invest 2004;114(2):147—52.

[69] Musso G, Gambino R, Cassader M. Cholesterol metabolism and the pathogenesis of non-alcoholic steatohepatitis. Prog Lipid Res 2013;52(1):175—91. Elsevier Ltd.

[70] Chatrath H, Vuppalanchi R, Chalasani N. Dyslipidemia in patients with nonalcoholic fatty liver disease. Semin Liver Dis 2012;32(1):22—9.

[71] Neuschwander-Tetri BA. Hepatic lipotoxicity and the pathogenesis of nonalcoholic steatohepatitis: the central role of nontriglyceride fatty acid metabolites. Hepatology 2010;52(2):774—88.

[72] Ioannou GN. The role of cholesterol in the pathogenesis of NASH. Trends Endocrinol Metab 2016;27(2):84—95. Elsevier Ltd.

[73] Cusi K. Role of insulin resistance and lipotoxity in non-alcoholic steatohepatitis. Clin Liver Dis 2009;13(4):545—63.

[74] Pagadala M, Kasumov T, McCullough AJ, Zein NN, Kirwan JP. Role of ceramides in nonalcoholic fatty liver disease. Trends Endocrinol Metab 2012;23(8):365—71.

[75] Sundaram SS, Zeitler P, Nadeau K. The metabolic syndrome and nonalcoholic fatty liver disease in children. Curr Opin Pediatr 2009;21(4):529−35.

[76] Koehler EM, Schouten JNL, Hansen BE, Van Rooij FJA, Hofman A, Stricker BH, et al. Prevalence and risk factors of non-alcoholic fatty liver disease in the elderly: results from the Rotterdam study. J Hepatol 2012;57(6):1305−11. European Association for the Study of the Liver.

[77] Kassi E, Pervanidou P, Kaltsas G, Chrousos G. Metabolic syndrome: definitions and controversies. BMC Med 2011:1−13. Appendix 1.

[78] Marchesini G, Bugianesi E, Forlani G, Cerrelli F, Lenzi M, Manini R, et al. Nonalcoholic fatty liver, steatohepatitis, and the metabolic syndrome. Hepatology 2003:917−23.

[79] Patton HM, Yates K, Unalp-Arida A, Behling CA, Huang TT-K, Rosenthal P, et al. Association between metabolic syndrome and liver histology among children with nonalcoholic fatty liver disease. Am J Gastroenterol September 6, 2010;105(9):2093−102.

[80] Asrih M, Jornayvaz FR. Metabolic syndrome and nonalcoholic fatty liver disease: is insulin resistance the link? Mol Cell Endocrinol 2015;418:55−65. Elsevier Ireland Ltd.

[81] Day CP, James OFW. Steatohepatitis: a tale of two "hits"? Gastroenterology 1998;114(4):842−5.

[81a] Donnelly KL, Smith CI, Schwarzenberg SJ, Jessurun J, Boldt MD, Parks EJ. Sources of fatty acids stored in liver and secreted via lipoproteins in patients with nonalcoholic fatty liver disease. J Clin Invest 2005;115(5):1343−51.

[82] Nielsen S, Guo Z, Johnson CM, Hensrud DD, Jensen MD. Splanchnic lipolysis in human obesity. J Clin Invest 2004;113(11):1582−8.

[83] Bradbury MW. Lipid metabolism and liver inflammation. I. Hepatic fatty acid uptake: possible role in steatosis. Am J Physiol Gastrointest Liver Physiol 2006;290(12):194−8.

[84] Fabbrini E, deHaseth D, Deivanayagam S, Mohammed BS, Vitola BE, Klein S. Alterations in fatty acid kinetics in obese adolescents with increased intrahepatic triglyceride content. Obesity (Silver Spring) 2009;17(1):25−9.

[85] Greco D, Kotronen A, Westerbacka J, Puig O, Arkkila P, Kiviluoto T, et al. Gene expression in human NAFLD. Am J Physiol Gastrointest Liver Physiol 2008:1281−7.

[86] Paglialunga S, Dehn CA. Clinical assessment of hepatic de novo lipogenesis in non-alcoholic fatty liver disease. Lipids Health Dis 2016;15(1):159.

[87] Lambert JE, Ramos-Roman MA, Browning JD, Parks EJ. Increased de novo lipogenesis is a distinct characteristic of individuals with nonalcoholic fatty liver disease. Gastroenterology 2014;146(3):726−35. Elsevier, Inc.

[88] Ameer F, Scandiuzzi L, Hasnain S, Kalbacher H, Zaidi N. De novo lipogenesis in health and disease. Metabolism 2014;63(7):895−902. Elsevier Inc.

[89] Horton JD, Goldstein JL, Brown MS. Critical review. Most 2002;109(9):1125−31.

[90] Ferré P, Foufelle F. Hepatic steatosis: a role for de novo lipogenesis and the transcription factor SREBP-1c. Diabetes Obes Metab 2010;12(Suppl. 2):83−92.

[91] Dentin R, Benhamed F, Hainault I, Fauveau V, Foufelle F, Dyck JRB, et al. Liver-specific inhibition of ChREBP improves hepatic steatosis and insulin resistance in ob/ob mice. Diabetes 2006;55(8):2159−70.

[92] Houten SM, Wanders RJA. A general introduction to the biochemistry of mitochondrial fatty acid β-oxidation. J Inherit Metab Dis 2010;33(5):469−77.

[93] Bechmann LP, Hannivoort RA, Gerken G, Hotamisligil GS, Trauner M, Canbay A. The interaction of hepatic lipid and glucose metabolism in liver diseases. J Hepatol 2012;56(4):952−64. European Association for the Study of the Liver.

[94] Reddy JK, Rao MS. Lipid metabolism and liver inflammation. II. Fatty liver disease and fatty acid oxidation. Am J Physiol Gastrointest Liver Physiol 2006:G852−8.

[95] Serra D, Mera P, Malandrino MI, Mir JF, Herrero L. Mitochondrial fatty acid oxidation in obesity. Antioxid Redox Signal 2013;19(3):269−84.

[96] Nakamuta M, Kohjima M, Morizono S, Kotoh K, Yoshimoto T, Miyagi I, et al. Evaluation of fatty acid metabolism-related gene expression in nonalcoholic fatty liver disease. Int J Mol Med 2005;16(4):631−5.

[97] Blasiole DA, Davis RA, Attie AD. The physiological and molecular regulation of lipoprotein assembly and secretion. Mol Biosyst 2007;3(9):608.

[98] Barrows BR, Parks EJ. Contributions of different fatty acid sources to very low-density lipoprotein-triacylglycerol in the fasted and fed states. J Clin Endocrinol Metab 2006;91(4):1446−52.

[99] Stillemark-Billton P, Beck C, Borén J, Olofsson S-O. Relation of the size and intracellular sorting of apoB to the formation of VLDL 1 and VLDL 2. J Lipid Res 2005;46(1):104−14.

[100] Choi SH, Ginsberg HN. Increased very low density lipoprotein (VLDL) secretion, hepatic steatosis, and insulin resistance. Trends Endocrinol Metab 2011;22(9):353−63. Elsevier Ltd.

[101] Charlton M, Sreekumar R, Rasmussen D, Lindor K, Nair KS. Apolipoprotein synthesis in nonalcoholic steatohepatitis. Hepatology 2002;35(4):898−904.

[102] Rolo AP, Teodoro JS, Palmeira CM. Role of oxidative stress in the pathogenesis of nonalcoholic steatohepatitis. Free Radic Biol Med 2012;52(1):59−69. Elsevier Inc.

[103] Gardner HW. Oxygen radical chemistry of polyunsaturated fatty acids. Free Radic Biol Med 1989;7(1):65−86.

[104] Esterbauer H, Schaur RJ, Zollner H. Chemistry and biochemistry of 4-hydroxynonenal, malonaldehyde and related aldehydes. Free Radic Biol Med 1991:81−128.

[105] Wei Y, Rector RS, Thyfault JP, Ibdah JA. Nonalcoholic fatty liver disease and mitochondrial dysfunction. World J Gastroenterol 2008;14(2):193−9.

[106] Kawahara H, Fukura M, Tsuchishima M, Takase S. Mutation of mitochondrial DNA in livers from patients with alcoholic hepatitis and nonalcoholic steatohepatitis. Alcohol Clin Exp Res 2007;31(Suppl. 1):54−60.

[107] Ribeiro PS, Cortez-Pinto H, Solá S, Castro RE, Ramalho RM, Baptista A, et al. Hepatocyte apoptosis, expression of death receptors, and activation of NF-κB in the liver of nonalcoholic and alcoholic steatohepatitis patients. Am J Gastroenterol 2004;99(9):1708—17.

[108] Caldwell SH, Swerdlow RH, Khan EM, Iezzoni JC, Hespenheide EE, Parks JK, et al. Mitochondrial abnormalities in non-alcoholic steatohepatitis. J Hepatol 1999;31(3):430—4.

[109] Koliaki C, Szendroedi J, Kaul K, Jelenik T, Nowotny P, Jankowiak F, et al. Adaptation of hepatic mitochondrial function in humans with non-alcoholic fatty liver is lost in steatohepatitis. Cell Metab 2015;21(5):739—46. Elsevier Inc.

[110] Abdelmegeed MA, Banerjee A, Yoo S-H, Jang S, Gonzalez FJ, Song B-J. Critical role of cytochrome P450 2E1 (CYP2E1) in the development of high fat-induced non-alcoholic steatohepatitis. J Hepatol 2012;57(4):860—6.

[111] Schulze-Osthoff K, Bakker AC, Vanhaesebroeck B, Beyaert R, Jacob WA, Fiers W. Cytotoxic activity of tumor necrosis factor is mediated by early damage of mitochondrial functions. Evidence for the involvement of mitochondrial radical generation. J Biol Chem 1992;267(8):5317—23.

[112] Schwarz DS, Blower MD. The endoplasmic reticulum: structure, function and response to cellular signaling. Cell Mol Life Sci 2016;73(1):79—94. Springer Basel.

[113] Pagliassotti MJ, Kim PY, Estrada AL, Stewart CM, Gentile CL. Endoplasmic reticulum stress in obesity and obesity-related disorders: an expanded view. Metabolism 2016;65(9):1238—46. Elsevier Inc.

[114] Zhang X-Q, Xu C-F, Yu C-H, Chen W-X, Li Y-M. Role of endoplasmic reticulum stress in the pathogenesis of nonalcoholic fatty liver disease. World J Gastroenterol 2014;20(7):1768—76.

[115] Malhi H, Kaufman RJ. Endoplasmic reticulum stress in liver disease. J Hepatol 2011;54(4):795—809. European Association for the Study of the Liver.

[116] Colgan SM, Tang D, Werstuck GH, Austin RC. Endoplasmic reticulum stress causes the activation of sterol regulatory element binding protein-2. Int J Biochem Cell Biol 2007;39(10):1843—51.

[117] Arruda AP, Pers BM, Parlakgül G, Güney E, Inouye K, Hotamisligil GS. Chronic enrichment of hepatic endoplasmic reticulum-mitochondria contact leads to mitochondrial dysfunction in obesity. Nat Med 2014;20(12):1427—35.

[118] Ratziu V, Charlotte F, Heurtier A, Gombert S, Giral P, Bruckert E, et al. Sampling variability of liver biopsy in nonalcoholic fatty liver disease. Gastroenterology 2005;128(7):1898—906.

[119] Wieckowska A, McCullough AJ, Feldstein AE. Noninvasive diagnosis and monitoring of nonalcoholic steatohepatitis: present and future. Hepatology 2007;46(2):582—9.

[120] Liu Z, Que S, Xu J, Peng T. Alanine aminotransferase-old biomarker and new concept: a review. J Med Sci 2014;11.

[121] Maximos M, Bril F, Sanchez PP, Lomonaco R, Orsak B, Biernacki D, et al. The role of liver fat and insulin resistance as determinants of plasma aminotransferase elevation in nonalcoholic fatty liver disease. Hepatology 2014:153—60.

[122] Prati D, Taioli E, Zanella A, Della Torre E, Butelli S, Del Vecchio E, et al. Article updated definitions of healthy ranges for serum alanine aminotransferase levels. Ann Intern Med 2017:1—10.

[123] Feldstein AE, Alkhouri N, De Vito R, Alisi A, Lopez R, Nobili V. Serum cytokeratin-18 fragment levels are useful biomarkers for nonalcoholic steatohepatitis in children. Am J Gastroenterol 2013;108(9):1526—31.

[124] Caulín C, Salvesen GS, Oshima RG. Caspase cleavage of keratin 18 and reorganization of intermediate filaments during epithelial cell apoptosis. J Cell Biol 1997;138(6):1379—94.

[125] Weng Y, Cui Y, Fang J. Biological functions of cytokeratin 18 in cancer. Mol Cancer Res 2012:1—10.

[126] Kwok R, Tse Y-K, Wong GL-H, Ha Y, Lee AU, Ngu MC, et al. Systematic review with meta-analysis: non-invasive assessment of non-alcoholic fatty liver disease — the role of transient elastography and plasma cytokeratin-18 fragments. Aliment Pharmacol Ther 2014;39(3):254—69.

[127] Cusi K, Chang Z, Harrison S, Lomonaco R, Bril F, Orsak B, et al. Limited value of plasma cytokeratin-18 as a biomarker for NASH and fibrosis in patients with non-alcoholic fatty liver disease. J Hepatol 2014;60(1):167—74.

[128] Saadeh S, Younossi ZM, Remer EM, Gramlich T, Ong JP, Hurley M, et al. The utility of radiological imaging in nonalcoholic fatty liver disease. Gastroenterology 2002;123(3):745—50.

[129] Hernaez R, Lazo M, Bonekamp S, Kamel I, Brancati FL, Guallar E, et al. Diagnostic accuracy and reliability of ultrasonography for the detection of fatty liver: a meta-analysis. Hepatology 2011;54(3):1082—90.

[130] Fishbein M, Castro F, Cheruku S, Jain S, Webb B, Gleason T, et al. Hepatic MRI for fat quantitation: its relationship to fat morphology, diagnosis, and ultrasound. J Clin Gastroenterol 2005;39(7):619—25.

[131] Ziol M, Handra-Luca A, Kettaneh A, Christidis C, Mal F, Kazemi F, et al. Noninvasive assessment of liver fibrosis by measurement of stiffness in patients with chronic hepatitis C. Hepatology 2005;41(1):48—54.

[132] Beaugrand M. Fibroscan: instructions for use. Gastroenterol Clin Biol 2006;30(4):513—4.

[133] Mikolasevic I, Orlic L, Franjic N, Hauser G, Stimac D, Milic S. Transient elastography (FibroScan®) with controlled attenuation parameter in the assessment of liver steatosis and fibrosis in patients with nonalcoholic fatty liver disease — where do we stand? World J Gastroenterol 2016;22(32):7236—51.

[134] Bedogni G, Bellentani S, Miglioli L, Masutti F, Passalacqua M, Castiglione A, et al. The fatty liver index: a simple and accurate predictor of hepatic steatosis in the general population. BMC Gastroenterol 2006;6(1):33.

[135] Bedogni G, Kahn HS, Bellentani S, Tiribelli C. A simple index of lipid overaccumulation is a good marker of liver steatosis. BMC Gastroenterol December 25, 2010;10(1):98.

[136] Lee J-H, Kim D, Kim HJ, Lee C-H, Yang JI, Kim W, et al. Hepatic steatosis index: a simple screening tool reflecting nonalcoholic fatty liver disease. Dig Liver Dis 2010;42(7):503—8.

[137] Cheung C-L, Lam KS, Wong IC, Cheung BM. Non-invasive score identifies ultrasonography-diagnosed non-alcoholic fatty liver disease and predicts mortality in the USA. BMC Med 2014;12(1):154.

[138] Ratziu V, Giral P, Charlotte F, Bruckert E, Thibault V, Theodorou I, et al. Liver fibrosis in overweight patients. Gastroenterology 2000;118(6):1117—23.

[139] Harrison SA, Oliver D, Arnold HL, Gogia S, Neuschwander-Tetri BA. Development and validation of a simple NAFLD clinical scoring system for identifying patients without advanced disease. Gut 2008;57(10):1441—7.

[140] Ryan MC, Itsiopoulos C, Thodis T, Ward G, Trost N, Hofferberth S, et al. The Mediterranean diet improves hepatic steatosis and insulin sensitivity in individuals with non-alcoholic fatty liver disease. J Hepatol 2013;59(1):138—43.

[141] Trovato FM, Catalano D, Martines GF, Pace P, Trovato GM. Mediterranean diet and non-alcoholic fatty liver disease: the need of extended and comprehensive interventions. Clin Nutr 2015;34(1):86—8.

[142] Parker HM, Johnson NA, Burdon CA, Cohn JS, Connor HTO, George J. Review Omega-3 supplementation and non-alcoholic fatty liver disease: a systematic review and meta-analysis. J Hepatol 2012;56(4):944—51. European Association for the Study of the Liver.

[143] Li S, Tan H-Y, Wang N, Zhang Z-J, Lao L, Wong C-W, et al. The role of oxidative stress and antioxidants in liver diseases. Int J Mol Sci 2015;16(11):26087—124.

[144] Ros E, Martínez-gonzález MA, Estruch R, Salas-salvadó J, Martínez JA, Corella D. Mediterranean diet and cardiovascular health: teachings of the PREDIMED study. Adv Nutr 2014;1—3.

[145] Estruch R. Anti-inflammatory effects of the Mediterranean diet: the experience of the PREDIMED study. Proc Nutr Soc 2010;69(3):333—40.

[146] Cantero I, Abete I, Babio N, Arós F, Corella D, Estruch R, et al. Dietary inflammatory index and liver status in subjects with different adiposity levels within the PREDIMED trial. Clin Nutr 2017:1—8.

[147] Buckley JD, Howe PRC. Long-chain omega-3 polyunsaturated fatty acids may be beneficial for reducing obesity—a review. Nutrients 2010;2(12):1212—30.

[148] Salomone F, Godos J, Zelber-Sagi S. Natural antioxidants for non-alcoholic fatty liver disease: molecular targets and clinical perspectives. Liver Int 2016;36(1):5—20.

[149] Alkhouri N, Feldstein AE. The TONIC trial: a step forward in treating pediatric nonalcoholic fatty liver diseaseGroszmann JR, Iwakiri Y, Taddei TH, editors. Hepatology 2012;55(4):1292—5.

[150] Sanyal AJ, Mofrad PS, Contos MJ, Sargeant C, Luketic VA, Sterling RK, et al. A pilot study of vitamin E versus vitamin E and pioglitazone for the treatment of nonalcoholic steatohepatitis. Clin Gastroenterol Hepatol 2004;2(12):1107—15.

Chapter 7

Kidney Damage in Obese Subjects: Oxidative Stress and Inflammation

Elia Escasany, Adriana Izquierdo-Lahuerta and Gema Medina-Gómez
Universidad Rey Juan Carlos, Madrid, Spain

1. INTRODUCTION

Obesity is a worldwide epidemic affecting more than 600 million adults and up to 17% of children and youth. Moreover, its prevalence has been predicted to grow by 40% in the next decade [1]. The increment in obese patients parallels the increase in the incidence of chronic kidney disease (CKD), independent of the presence of hypertension or diabetes. Both obesity and CKD are associated with higher mortality, mainly due to cardiovascular events. It is not clear how obesity accounts for many of the CKD patients independently of hypertension and diabetes, since all these conditions often coexist. Moreover, studies designed to examine the cause—effect relationship are lacking. To study the real impact of obesity in renal disease, it is necessary to study morbidly obese patients who do not present with diabetes or hypertension.

Nowadays it has been proven that obese patients are at increased risk of developing kidney disease, among other conditions such as hypertension, heart disease, insulin resistance (IR), dyslipidemia, and type 2 diabetes. Under normal circumstances a surplus of calories in the body is stored as triglycerides (TGs) in the adipose tissue. However, once the storage capacity is exceeded, lipids accumulate ectopically in different organs, including the kidney, contributing to their damage through toxic processes named lipotoxicity [2].

The pathological situation in which lipids are deposited in the kidneys has recently started to be known as fatty kidney, reminiscent of fatty liver [3]. Renal lipotoxicity affects the normal functioning of the kidney in several ways. First, the incremental endocrine activity of the adipose tissue leads to an increment in the production and release of several bioactive substances known as adipokines, including leptin and resistin, while diminishing the production of others, such as adiponectin. Some of these adipokines are involved in kidney damage through mediating endothelial dysfunction, inducing oxidative stress and inflammation, and stimulating the renal sympathetic nervous activity [4]. Fat cells also secrete the components of the renin—angiotensin aldosterone system (RAAS), and thus the increased amount of adipose tissue and lipids in obese patients lead to overactivation of the RAAS axis. This translates into hyperfiltration and damage to the glomerular filtration barrier (GFB) [5].

Second, the IR that usually comes with obesity and the altered adipokine secretion also affects the kidney, especially the podocytes, which lose their structure [6]. The loss of podocytes leaves the GFB partially denuded, allowing leakage of several macromolecules and thus leading to proteinuria. Moreover, renal lipid metabolism is affected by the lipid deposition. Renal lipotoxicity usually leads to increased lipid synthesis and decreased oxidation, exacerbating the lipid deposition and leading to energy depletion and thus apoptosis [7].

Third, the adipose tissue secretes chemokines that attract the immune system, leading to a low-level chronic inflammation state [8]. The high concentration of working immune cells leads to a respiratory burst that increases the production of reactive oxygen species (ROS). ROS are known to have detrimental effects on the kidney, leading to endoplasmic reticulum (ER) stress, fibrosis, and even cancer. Having such an important role in the development of renal damage, oxidative stress has been proposed not only as a biomarker for diagnosis and prognosis but also as a plausible target to treat CKD. Many dietary and synthetic antioxidants have been and are currently being investigated, showing promising results. Nevertheless, as obesity the primary cause of the renal damage, weight loss seems like the best therapeutic approach.

Obesity. https://doi.org/10.1016/B978-0-12-812504-5.00007-6

2. PHYSIOLOGICAL STATE OF THE KIDNEY: FROM NORMAL FUNCTION TO CHANGES DURING DISEASE

Kidneys are organs functionally divided into nephrons and collecting tubules. Each kidney contains around 1 million functional nephrons, which are responsible for filtration, excretion, and resorption. Under normal conditions the kidney filters out small molecules from plasma and later selectively reabsorbs most of the water and some of the molecules, with urine as the end product. All these processes allow the regulation of ion balance and water content, thus helping to stabilize blood pressure. Each nephron consists of a renal corpuscle, a proximal collecting tubule, a Henle loop, and a distal collecting tubule. Filtration of the blood plasma takes place in the renal corpuscle, while reabsorption happens into the tubules.

Structurally, kidneys are divided into the medulla, which is the inner part that contains only tubules, and a cortex, which surrounds the medulla and contains the renal corpuscles. Every renal corpuscle contains a glomerulus, which is a compact mass of looped fenestrated capillaries, and a Bowman's capsule, which is the proximal part of the renal tubule that wraps around the glomerulus [9]. Glomeruli receive blood for filtering from the afferent arteriole and drain it through the efferent arteriole. The fenestrations in the capillaries enable the filtration of blood and are wrapped around by very specialized epithelial cells known as podocytes, functioning as a selective barrier. Podocytes are terminally differentiated epithelial cells, which, like neurons, do not divide. Thus podocyte loss is an irreversible event, and it is extremely important to unravel the mechanisms that lead to podocyte damage. Podocytes are one of the three constituents of the GFB, and their role is to allow the selective filtration of water and small solutes while avoiding the flow of large molecules such as albumin. Each podocyte consists of a cell body, primary processes, and foot processes. The feet interdigitate with those from other podocytes to form filtration slits that are only 20–30 nm wide. Several transmembrane proteins, among which podocin and nephrin are the most important, maintain the contacts between foot processes. This way, molecules from the blood need to pass through the fenestrated capillaries, the basement membrane, and the podocyte slits. Only molecules that are under 70 kDa and positively charged can pass through, since a negative charge of heparan sulphate proteoglycan in the glomerular basement membrane (GBM) repels negatively charged proteins, such as albumin.

There are many kidney diseases, each caused by a different etiology ranging from autoimmunity to hypertension; they include diabetic nephropathy (DN), Fabry's disease, minimal change disease (MCD), IgA nephropathy, obesity-related glomeruloscleropathy, lupus nephritis, and polycystic kidney disease. Independently of the etiology, all these diseases if not cured result in CKD, defined as a glomerular filtration rate (GFR) of 60% or less. GFR loss is currently irreversible and can only be slowed down by pharmacological intervention. The end point is kidney failure, known as end-stage renal disease (ESRD), which requires either dialysis or renal transplantation.

3. THE ADIPOSE TISSUE EXPANDABILITY HYPOTHESIS AND RENAL LIPOTOXICITY

In obese patients lipid accumulation in the kidney promotes the so-called renal lipotoxicity, which can be explained by the adipose tissue expandability hypothesis. This hypothesis states that as an individual gains weight, a certain point will be reached when adipose tissue cannot store any more lipids and will thus release them into blood [2]. This leads to ectopic accumulation of lipids in metabolically important organs, like the kidney. This hypothesis explains why some obese patients are insulin-sensitive and have no metabolic complications, since they have not reached their limit of expandability. These patients are labeled as "metabolically healthy obese." This hypothesis is supported by data collected from mouse models, for instance the AdTG-*ob/ob* mice, which overexpress adiponectin in an obese *ob/ob* background and seem to have limitless adipose tissue expandability. These mice, despite having 50% greater body weight than the ob/ob group, remain insulin-sensitive and show no ectopic depositions of lipids [10].

The association between lipids and renal disease was first suggested by Virchow in 1858, studying Bright's disease [11]. Nowadays it is well established that renal lipid accumulation appears in several human diseases such as hypertensive nephrosclerosis, focal segmental glomerulosclerosis (FSGS), Fabry's disease, and MCD, a pathology of unknown etiology that involves the presence of lipid droplets in the urine. In 1982 Moorhead [12] went one step further and proposed a link between dyslipidemia, an alteration in lipids and lipoprotein levels in blood that appears in obese patients, and kidney disease. Moreover, studies in the general population have associated the presence of hyperlipidemia with the development of CKD, characterized by both oxidative stress and ER stress [13]. It is known that the accumulation of nonesterified free fatty acids (NEFAs) leads to systemic inflammation and increased oxidative stress. These two processes are common features in CKD, as well as being risk factors for higher morbidity and mortality. Finally, the uncontrolled production of oxidants in renal cells leads to irreversible cellular damage due to oxidation of proteins and lipids. There are several pathways involved in renal injury by oxidation, mediated by Nicotinamide Adenine Dinucleotide Phosphate (NADPH) oxidase, myeloperoxidase (MPO), nitric oxide (NO) synthase, and superoxide dismutase (SOD) [14].

4. MECHANISMS OF ACTION UNDERLYING THE PATHOLOGICAL RENAL EFFECTS OF OBESITY

The exact mechanisms that link obesity to CKD remain unclear. Since obesity leads to a great variety of complex metabolic changes with wide-ranging effects, some of the deleterious renal effects may be a cause of comorbid conditions such as diabetes mellitus or hypertension. However, some obese patients develop renal disease without presenting any other condition, which suggests that adiposity alone could have a direct impact on kidneys. These deleterious effects of adiposity include increased inflammation, oxidative stress, and insulin levels, IR, and RAAS overactivation, among others. All these are extensively discussed in this chapter.

4.1 The Role of Adipokines and Proinflammatory Factors From Adipose Tissue in Renal Injury

Adipose tissue is now known to be more than a passive organ that stores fat, and is considered as an endocrine organ that has an impact on the whole body. White adipose tissue is in fact probably the largest endocrine organ in humans, since it is distributed extensively in the body. It is responsible for synthesizing many hormones, chemokines, and cytokines, known as "adipokines," that can modulate food intake, IR, inflammatory processes, and many other pathways [15]. Unbalanced production of proinflammatory and antiinflammatory adipokines in obese adipose tissue may contribute to many aspects of metabolic syndrome. Excessive lipid storage in the adipose tissue leads to an overwhelming production of these molecules, which promotes a chronic inflammation state that is characterized by an increased production of proinflammatory cytokines such as interleukins (ILs), mainly IL-1 and IL-6, and tumor necrosis factor-α (TNF-α) by the hypertrophic adipocytes [16] and hyposecretion of beneficial adipocytokines such as adiponectin. The lack of adiponectin leads to inhibited expansibility of the adipose tissue, which as a consequence gives rise to the appearance of bigger adipocytes. Larger adipocytes are known to secrete more proinflammatory cytokines than antiinflammatory ones compared to small adipocytes, which fuels the inflammatory state [5]. Under normal circumstances, adiponectin exerts antiinflammatory effects by suppressing nuclear factor kappa-light-chain-enhancer of activated B cells (NF-κB) activation and avoiding macrophage infiltration through the inhibition of vascular cell adhesion molecule-1 and intercellular adhesion molecule-1. In its absence two inflammatory mediators that are involved in the initiation and progression of atherosclerosis and renal injury, C-reactive protein (CRP) and IL-6, express strongly. Adiponectin knockout mouse models have provided evidence that adiponectin regulates podocyte function and albuminuria [5]. Treatment of these mice with exogenous adiponectin was able to rescue podocyte morphology and decrease albuminuria. Hyperadiponectemia has proven to increase nephrin and decrease the plasminogen activator inhibitor-1 (PAI-1), thus protecting kidney function. On the other hand, the GFB is affected by adipokine levels. A negative correlation has been shown between adiponectin levels and proteinuria in obese patients and animal models [17].

One of the main hormones produced by adipose tissue is leptin. Kidneys express abundant concentrations of the short-form leptin receptor as well as a small amount of the long-form receptors. Thus leptin is likely to affect renal function and structure directly. Obesity-induced leptin resistance leads to increased plasma leptin levels which injure many peripheral tissues, including the kidney. By binding to its receptors, leptin promotes cellular proliferation, hypertrophy, and increased extracellular matrix (ECM) expression, as a response to transcriptional growth factor β1 (TGF-β-1) stimulation that leads to fibrosis in both glomerular endothelial cells and mesangial cells [18]. Thus leptin plays a direct role in the development of glomerulosclerosis. Moreover, it plays an indirect role in kidney injury by exerting proinflammatory effects through its interaction with innate and adaptive immunity and CRP as well as increasing sodium retention, which may cause hypertension—a risk factor for CKD [18].

Resistin is another molecule secreted by white adipocytes in rodents and by infiltrated macrophages in humans that has been shown to be elevated in animal obesity models. Resistin strongly upregulates IL-6 and TNF-α, two of the key inflammatory mediators of renal damage [19]. Studies have demonstrated a positive correlation between IL-6 and body mass index (BMI), and this IL is known to stimulate the synthesis of CRP, an important risk factor of atherosclerosis in CKD patients. IL-6 also stimulates the RAAS axis and enhances TGF-β-1 signaling, thereby promoting hyperfiltration and fibrosis. Moreover, transgenic IL-6 knockout mice show less renal injury as measured by creatinine and histological changes [20]. On the other hand, TNF-α, which can also be produced by the kidney mainly stimulated by angiotensin II, enhances PAI-1 expression, reducing fibrinolysis and leading to renal fibrosis [21]. Of note, TNF-α negatively regulates the expression of klotho, a molecule expressed by renal cells that controls insulin sensitivity and aging. The lack of klotho leads to premature aging and therefore to premature renal injury [22].

Another novel adipokine, visfatin, mainly expressed in visceral adipose tissue, is implicated in obesity-related renal disease. In contrast to adiponectin, the higher the plasma levels of visfatin, the more severe the CKD. High plasma levels of visfatin predict a higher mortality rate in CKD patients. Visfatin induces glomerular endothelial cell dysfunction by a mechanism associated with assembling and activation of NADPH oxidase in ceramide-enriched domains and the formation of lipid raft redox signaling platforms, promoting the rearrangement of the microtubule network [6].

Two other recently discovered adipokines are apelin and chemerin. Apelin was discovered as the ligand of the orphan G-protein-coupled receptor APJ, and is highly expressed on the glomeruli. Apelin levels correlate with inflammation in CKD patients [4]. However, in a type 1 diabetes mouse model, administration of apelin retarded the progression of DN [23], suggesting a possible protective role. Chemerin, on the other hand, is elevated in both type 2 diabetes patients with macroalbuminuria and patients on dialysis [24]. Whether chemerin is only a marker of renal function or plays a role in the renal pathology development needs further research.

Moreover, during obesity there is an increased secretion of proinflammatory factors from adipose tissue that recruit macrophages to other tissues, like macrophage chemoattractant protein-1 (MCP-1), macrophage migration inhibition factor (MIF-1), macrophage inflammatory proteins-1α, chemokine CCL5, and macrophage colony-stimulating factor. Microarray profiling of over 23,500 genes showed differential expression of at least 60 inflammatory genes in diet-induced obese mice. Among those, MCP-1 showed the greatest increase. Expression trended up as soon as 2 days after introducing a high-fat diet (HFD) and reached statistical significance at day 7. After 4 weeks of HFD the levels were sevenfold higher than in the control diet. This increment preceded the expression of CD38, a marker of macrophage infiltration, which suggests that MCP-1 may lead the process [8]. In this same study, inhibition of food intake stimuli through the cannabinoid-1 receptor resulted in a reduction of MCP-1 expression levels, most likely secondary to the loss of weight. This data supports the idea that MCP-1 levels correlate with adiposity. MIF also plays an important role in the pathogenesis of renal disease; indeed, treatment with antiMIF antibodies was shown to reduce proteinuria, prevent loss of renal function, and diminish leukocyte infiltration into the kidney [25]. The recruited macrophages can also produce proinflammatory cytokines, which leads to a vicious cycle of inflammation if the stimulus lasts long enough. Obesity is now viewed as a state of systemic, chronic, low-grade inflammation (Fig. 7.1).

4.2 Lipid Accumulation Promotes Changes in Renal Lipid Metabolism

The kidney is, along with the heart, the organ with the highest energy demand per gram of tissue. Thus it is logical that most renal cells rely on lipids as their source of energy, the main ones being TGs and NEFAs, since lipids hold up to four times more energy than glucose. Kidneys are therefore very susceptible to lipotoxic effects. Under normal circumstances, β-oxidation is the main source of adenosine triphosphate (ATP) for the kidney. When excess fatty acids (FAs) are not oxidized, they are esterified with glycerol and become lipid droplets. It is very common to find these lipid droplets inside podocytes, mesangial cells and tubular cells in obesity-related kidney diseases. In CKD, renal lipid metabolism is altered, mainly leading to increased synthesis and uptake and decreased FA oxidation, which results in lipid accumulation and thus lipotoxicity (Fig. 7.2).

The pathways by which kidneys acquire FAs under normal conditions are not yet well established. Most organs can acquire FAs either through de novo synthesis or by uptaking them from circulation. According to the Human Protein Atlas, under normal conditions in the kidney the expression of the FA synthase (FASN) is very low and thus is most likely that they normally acquire them by uptake [26]. Renal cells are special in this aspect, since they can uptake lipids from both the circulation and the filtrate. Most NEFAs in circulation are bound to the carrier protein albumin and are uptaken by the cluster of differentiation 36 (CD36) transporter and chemokine (C−C motif) ligand 16 (CCL16) transporter, which are the latest specific of the podocytes.

In CKD renal cells are exposed to increased levels of NEFAs due to leakage of albumin into the filtrate. It has been observed that increased FA uptake through CD36 leads to cell apoptosis via activation of the p38 mitogen-activated protein kinase (MAPK) pathway [26]. Moreover, increasing amounts of NEFAs bound to albumin lead to defects in mitochondrial respiration and thus oxidative stress, resulting in induction of apoptotic pathways. In CKD, in addition to increased FA uptake, synthesis plays a role in lipid accumulation. FASN and the sterol regulatory element-binding proteins (SREBP) are markedly increased in diabetic kidney disease (DKD) in animal models [27]. Results showing increased lipogenesis and decreased lipolysis as causes of renal injury are homogeneous in many animal models. Cell cultures studies have proven

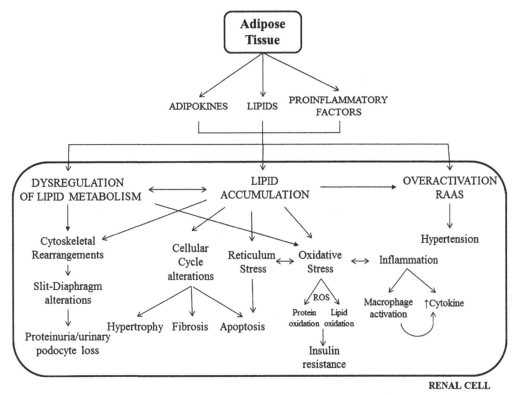

FIGURE 7.1 Renal effects of obesity. In obese people, when the limit of expandability of the adipose tissue is reached, the adipose tissue releases high amounts of adipokines and proinflammatory factors that lead to renal damage through lipid accumulation, renal lipid metabolism dysregulation, and overactivation of the RAAS. *RAAS*, renin—angiotensin aldosterone system; *ROS*, reactive oxygen species.

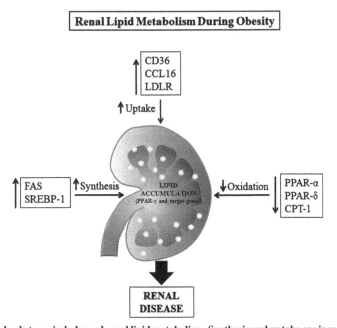

FIGURE 7.2 Lipid accumulation leads to an imbalanced renal lipid metabolism. Synthesis and uptake are increased while oxidation is decreased leading to further lipid accumulation, energy depletion and renal disease.

that high glucose levels lead to increased SREBP1 expression [28]. Controversially, in human samples SREBP1 seems to be downregulated [29].

All three nuclear peroxisome proliferator-activated receptors (PPARs) α, β/δ, and γ, are expressed in the kidney. PPARγ regulates glucose and lipid metabolism and has been shown to play a crucial role in renal disease associated with obesity in both animal models and podocytes [30,31]. The POKO (obtained by crossing the peroxisome proliferator-activated receptor gamma 2 (PPARγ2) knockout (KO) mouse into a genetically obese *ob/ob* background) mouse, a model of metabolic syndrome and deficient in PPARγ2 and leptin, showed accelerated kidney damage, exhibiting renal lipid accumulation, alteration of lipid metabolism, and an incipient IR associated with decreased adiponectin renal expression. Moreover, POKO mice exhibited faster progression of kidney disease compared with ob/ob mice, with increased inflammation, TGF-β, and other profibrotic markers [30].

Regarding FA oxidation, genome-wide transcriptome analysis of patients' samples showed decreased expression of enzymes responsible for oxidation [26]. The rate-limiting step in FA oxidation is its transfer into the mitochondria, which requires the carnitine acetyltranferase 1 (CPT1) transporter. After this, the nuclear receptors PPAR and PPAR gamma coactivator 1 transcriptional regulatory complex play a key role in oxidation. PPARα is involved in the regulation of protein-degradation systems through maintenance of ATP homeostasis, control of FA β-oxidation, and regulation of cytochrome P450. PPARδ is involved in FA oxidation. Several reports indicate that agonists of PPARα, PPARβ/δ, and PPARγ aminorated renal damage [32], highlighting the importance of these nuclear receptors in the maintenance of renal lipid homeostasis.

It is well known that in some organs, such as the heart, glucose oxidation is activated upon lipid oxidation depletion. However, in the kidneys no glucose activation is observed, leading to energy depletion which causes activation of apoptotic and dedifferentiation pathways, fibrosis, and CKD progression [26].

A central component of lipid metabolism is adenine monophosphate kinase (AMPK). When AMPK is activated, it leads to a reduction in FA synthesis and an increase in uptake and oxidation of FAs by mitochondria. When subjected to an HFD, AMPK decreases its activity in many tissues, including the kidney, leading to an imbalance in the lipid metabolism, which translates in renal lipid accumulation. Treatment with the AMPK activator 5-aminoimidazole-4-carboxamide-1-β-D-ribonucleoside prevents glomerulopathy and tubuloinsterstitial fibrosis [33].

Very importantly, decreased expression of FA oxidation enzymes may generate harmful lipid intermediates as well as ROS, leading to lipid peroxidation. The main toxic lipid intermediates are diacylglycerol, ceramides, and fatty acyl-CoA. Altered expression of the carnitine O-acyl transferase, which transports acyl-CoA out of the mitochondria, may cause accumulation of these incompletely oxidized FAs inside the mitochondria, leading to superoxide formation and lipid peroxidation. Lipid peroxidation end products such as 4-hydroxynonenal (4-HNE) and isoprostanes are well-known biomarkers for diabetes, but their role in renal pathophysiology is not well studied. They do correlate with cardiovascular disease, and according to recent studies with kidney disease as well [33a]. Thus lipid peroxidation end products are under investigation, as they may have an important role in the kidney [34,35].

Metabolomic and lipidomic analyses have identified metabolite changes in CKD models. Lipids seem to account for the vast majority of metabolites affected [36], which again suggests that lipid metabolism is significantly disturbed in CKD. Identification of these lipid species could be very useful for diagnostic purposes. It seems that saturated FAs are increased in the plasma of CKD rats while polyunsaturated fatty acids (PUFAs) are decreased. This same pattern has been reported in prehemodialysis patients. It has been hypothesized that the reduction in PUFAs is due to their susceptibility to ROS-mediated peroxidation, which makes them the target of endocytosis by macrophages. This could explain the beneficial effects of supplementation with omega-3, one of the most studied PUFAs [37].

Importantly, dysregulation of renal lipid metabolism and circulating adipokines leads to an imbalance of lipid rafts in podocytes and glomerular endothelial cells, contributing to GFB dysfunction. In podocytes it has been shown that segments rich in cholesterol (lipid rafts) are inserted in the slit diaphragm of podocytes between podocin and nephrin, helping to maintain the link between podocin—nephrin and transient receptor potential nephrin-channel-6 [38]. It has been observed that patients with mutations in the genes that code for enzymes involved in lipid metabolism develop kidney diseases. In this regard, mutations in the acid sphingomyelinase (ASM)-like phosphodiesterase 3b gene, which is involved in conversion of sphingomyelin to ceramide, are associated with FSGS [39]. A similar outcome has been observed for the phospholipase A2 receptor, a transmembrane glycoprotein involved in lipid metabolism that binds to phospholipase A2. Mutations in this protein occur in individuals with primary membranous nephropathy.

Lipid deposition also promotes podocyte loss, albuminuria [40], and cytoskeletal rearrangement, which translates into podocyte foot processes flattening, widening, and retraction. These changes are termed "foot process effacement" and are indicative of podocyte injury and loss. Foot process effacements, unlike podocyte loss, are reversible events. Thus it is very important to understand how lipotoxicity promotes these changes so as to prevent subsequent podocyte loss and CKD appearance. Moreover, nephrin and podocin are not only structural proteins but also play a signaling role. Nephrin acts as signaling scaffold that recruits proteins such as phosphoinositide-3-kinase and Src (SRC proto-oncogene family tyrosine kinases) family proteins, which regulate cytoskeletal changes. On the other hand, nephrin regulates podocyte insulin sensitivity by docking insulin receptors [41]. Actin cytoskeletal changes are also regulated by the Rho family of small Guanosine triphosphate (GTP)ases. Hyperglycemia, ROS, and oxidized low-density lipoprotein (LDL) among others stimulate these GTPases, promoting cytoskeletal changes and foot process effacement [42].

4.3 Inflammation and Oxidative Stress Relationship in Kidney Disease

Obesity has long been associated with an increased production of ROS. Possible mechanisms are the increase in oxygen consumption, FA oxidation, and mitochondrial respiration to deal with the excess of fat. Furthermore, fat itself is able to stimulate NADPH oxidase activity, contributing to ROS generation [5]. ROS in turn promote the expression of NADPH oxidase subunits, such as Nox4, establishing a vicious cycle [43]. Studies performed on cultured tubular cells have shown that when stimulated with the two most frequent NEFAs found in diabetic kidney biopsies, linoleate and palmitate, superoxide production is imbalanced by the activation of the early-response oxidative stress element, the nuclear factor (erythroid-derived 2)-like 2 (Nrf2). Importantly, since kidneys produce most of their ATP through oxidative phosphorylation, they naturally produce higher levels of ROS and are thus exposed to higher levels of oxidative stress than other organs.

Animal studies have shown that, under an HFD, mitochondria from glomerular endothelial cells, podocytes, and proximal tubular endothelial cells suffer drastic structural changes that alter their optimal function, leading to ROS production and lipid accumulation. Under normal conditions renal cells should contain numerous mitochondria with an elongated shape and densely stacked cristae membranes. However, under an HFD mitochondria are small and disorganized, with undefined cristae membranes and often ruptures in the outer membrane. Treatment with SS-31, a tetrapeptide that targets cardiolipin (a phospholipid exclusively found in the inner mitochondrial membrane which protects mitochondrial cristae structure) showed a great variety of nephroprotective properties [44]. In this study, SS-31 completely prevented the upregulation of TGF-β-1 collagen deposition and thus glomerulosclerosis, preserved podocyte number and foot processes, reduced macrophage infiltration by 50%, prevented lipid accumulation in tubular cells, autophagy, apoptosis, mitochondrial damage, and ER stress in podocytes, and restored AMPK activity. Thus targeting mitochondria looks a very promising approach to obesity-related glomerulopathy (ORG).

ROS plays a crucial role in the development of renal injury. The main source of ROS in the kidney is the activity of the NADPH oxidase family, including Nox1, Nox2, and Nox4. One of the many functions that ROS can affect is renal tubule ion transport, thus ROS can alter renal pressure and blood pressure in general while causing oxidative injury to the proximal tubules at the same time. Altogether, these changes lead to proteinuria and IR. Through the NF-κB, ROS induce the expression of profibrotic molecules such as TGF-β-1, and, through the NADPH oxidase pathway, the PAI-1. Thus ROS play a major role in the development of glomerulosclerosis and tubulointerstitial fibrosis.

Inflammation and oxidative stress have a bidirectional and synergistic relationship, which becomes a vicious cycle. During inflammation, large amounts of mast cells and leukocytes are recruited to the site of damage. This concentration of cells increases oxygen uptake in the area, leading to a "respiratory burst." This increment in oxygen consumption results in an increased release and accumulation of ROS at the site of damage. Furthermore, inflammatory cells also produce soluble mediators, such as cytokines and chemokines, which act by further recruiting inflammatory cells to the site of damage and producing more reactive species. On the other hand, inflammation is a redox-sensitive mechanism, as oxidative stress is able to activate transcriptional factors such as NF-κB, activator protein (AP)-1, p53, hypoxia inducible factor (HIF)-1α, PPARγ, β-catenin/Wnt, and Nrf2, which regulate expression of inflammatory mediator genes [45]. Oxidative stress seems to affect some of the activation steps of the NF-κB cascade, such as the phosphorylation and degradation of inhibitor I-κB, as well as antioxidants preventing NF-κB activation [46]. H_2O_2 is able to degrade I-κB and to stimulate Il-4 and IL-6 expression. ROS also increase the PAI-1 and MCP-1 through the NADPH oxidase pathway [43]. Moreover, oxidized products such as oxidized LDL promote TNF-α synthesis in renal cells, fueling the inflammatory status which, in turn, leads to more oxidative stress, creating a vicious cycle [43].

During a respiratory burst, stimulated neutrophils and monocytes generate superoxide and its dismutation product hydrogen peroxide, and simultaneously release the heme enzyme MPO. MPO belongs to the peroxidases enzyme family and has very strong prooxidative and proinflammatory properties. MPO is most abundantly present in azurophilic granules of neutrophils, followed by monocytes and some macrophage subpopulations, and in the presence of hydrogen peroxide is capable of converting chloride to hypochlorous acid (HOCl). HOCl is cytotoxic and is used by neutrophils to kill pathogens. However, over time it also causes oxidative damage in healthy tissue. Reactions of hypohalous acids with proteins contribute to protein unfolding, which causes ER stress and leads to unfolded protein response (UPR). Importantly for the kidney, the sulfhydryl group (−SH) of albumin is very sensitive to the influence of HOCl and chloramine. Biochemical analyses showed that the largest part of serum advanced oxidation protein products (AOPPs) consists of oxidized albumin, and its modification depends on MPO chlorination activity [47]. Modified albumin irreversibly losses its biological properties. In patients undergoing maintenance hemodialysis treatment, the higher basal serum MPO was associated with inflammation, advanced atherosclerosis, and poorer prognosis. Moreover, MPO deficiency was recently demonstrated [47a] to retard the progression of CKD in five out of six nephrectomized mice, thereby confirming the role of MPO in kidney damage.

MPO modulates vascular inflammation by regulating NO bioavailability, which is linked to the development of atherosclerosis. Controversially, some studies show decreased levels of MPO in CKD patients, indicating that this enzyme may not play a role in the etiology of cardiovascular complications in patients with CKD [48].

4.4 Endoplasmic Reticulum Stress Is Also Associated With Renal Lipotoxicity

As seen in the previous section, oxidative stress can contribute to protein unfolding, with the development of ER stress and UPR. At the same time, intracellular lipid accumulation leads to oxidative stress, ER stress, and cytoskeletal changes [31]. Both oxidative stress and ER stress are known to be important agents in the development of lipotoxicity. However, the pathway involved, the cross-talk, the sequence of events, and the exact cellular consequences remain to be clarified. ER stress affects protein assembly and trafficking, leading to an upregulation of UPR genes. The UPR is activated to degrade misfolded proteins and increase synthesis of chaperones, which help in the protein-folding process. If UPR is not enough to overcome the ER stress, the cell enters apoptosis. Oxidative stress can activate UPR as part of a survival process, but long-term exposure leads to excessive protein misfolding and subsequent apoptosis [49]. It is also reported that oxidant paraquat, the commercial name for N,N′-dimethyl-4,4′-bipyridinium dichloride, which is a superoxide producer, can promote chaperone degradation by caspases, specifically the cochaperone p23, and inhibits proteosomal activity, which leads to misfolded protein accumulation and subsequently activates UPR [50].

It is well known that ER stress plays a role in the development and progression of kidney injury. It has been shown that a dietary saturated free fatty acid (FFA) induces ER stress in animal models [51] and culture cells [52]. In podocytes, treatment with palmitic acid promotes ER stress that could be associated with insulin resistant and lead to apoptosis [31]. Although it has been observed that RAAS activation mediates FA-induced ER stress in proximal tubular cells, the intracellular pathways involved in the development of FA-mediated ER stress within the kidney are not fully understood [51].

4.5 Oxidative Stress and Autophagy in the Context of Renal Lipotoxicity

Autophagy is a highly dynamic biological process that removes and recycles damaged and long-lived molecules, serving as a prosurvival mechanism. Autophagy is especially important in long-lived cells, such as podocytes, that need to reuse their intracellular components for a long time. Indeed, podocytes show a high basal level of autophagy [53]. The process involves five major steps: the formation of the isolation membrane or phagophore; elongation of the phagophore and cargo recruitment; closure of the mature autophagosome; fusion between autophagosome and lysosome; and degradation of the autolysosome [53]. The process is initiated upon Unc-51-like kinase-1 (ULK-1) activation. ULK-1 can be phosphorylated by AMPK, a metabolic sensor that gets stimulated upon ATP depletion.

Mitophagy is a selective autophagy that is involved in removal of dysfunctional mitochondria. The canonical pathway involves PTEN-induced putative kinase 1 (PINK1) and Parkin. Activation of this pathway via ROS has been reported, suggesting an interrelation between mitochondrial degradation and oxidative stress [54]. The fact that kidneys are organs rich in mitochondria indicates that they are highly vulnerable to oxidative stress damage.

On the other hand, autophagy seems to play a renoprotective function. Indeed, renal fibrosis is regulated by autophagy, since TGF-β-1 levels are regulated by autophagic degradation [55]. Moreover, autophagy-specific knockout mouse models exhibit FSGS, highlighting the important role of autophagy in podocytes [56]. Supporting this, in one study inhibition of autophagy leads to podocyte apoptosis by activating ER stress [57]. Dysregulation in the autophagic flux in podocytes seems to be detrimental due to their longevity. The inability of the ubiquitin-proteasome system (UPS) to compensate for these protein accumulation results in ER stress and contributes to podocyte death. Controversially, some studies suggest that autophagy contributes to cell death. In human embryonic kidney cells, inhibition of the mitochondrial electronic chain induces cell death, with no activation of caspases [57].

Although oxidative stress and autophagy have long been studied individually, further research is needed to gain a detailed understanding of the molecular links in renal disease.

4.6 Oxidative Stress and Renal Fibrosis

Glomerulosclerosis and tubulointerstitial fibrosis are common final pathological features in the etiology of kidney diseases. Fibrosis, the excessive scarring of tissues, is the result of ECM accumulation due to an increased synthesis of collagen and fibronectin and a decrease in the degradation enzymes, the metalloproteinases (MMPs). The main players in this process are myofibroblasts, which differ from interstitial fibroblasts. However, there is evidence to support the idea that other cells, such as tubular epithelial cells, may go through epithelial-to-mesenchymal transition (EMT) and contribute to the pathogenesis of fibrosis by behaving like myofibroblasts. Moreover, some authors support the idea that macrophages can also transform into myofibroblast, a process named macrophage-to-mesenchymal transition (MMT), and thus contribute to fibrosis [58].

It is generally accepted that TGFβ1 is the protein responsible for fibroblast activation to myofibroblasts, EMT or MMT regulation, and ECM accumulation; also, the regulation of MMPs is known to be through the PAI-1. So when the PAI-1 gets stimulated fibrinolysis decreases, leading to accumulation of ECM and thus to fibrosis. Some authors hypothesize that ROS may exert profibrotic effects through the TGFβ pathway. An in vitro experiment demonstrated that hydrogen peroxide (H_2O_2) increases TGFβ1, collagen III, and collagen IV synthesis and inhibits growth. Treatment with the panselective antiTGFβ1 antibody completely abrogated the H_2O_2-induced increase in ECM proteins [59]. Some studies show that ROS are also capable of stimulating the PAI-1, leading to less fibrinolysis and thus fueling the profibrotic state [43]. Oxidized products, such as oxidized LDL, have also been shown to stimulate secretion of ECM and PAI-1 by mesangial cells, leading to renal fibrosis.

The increment in adipose tissue that is present in obese patients, especially the visceral and perirenal, may lead to obstruction of the renal hilum and thus to some degree of ischemia. This ischemic state brings an accumulation of ROS and increments fibrosis. Moreover, everything that accompanies obesity (discussed above) has an effect on fibrosis. Several adipokines released by the incremented adipose tissue contribute to fibrosis. Leptin and resistin increment TGF-β-1 expression, while TNF-α and adiponectin modulate PAI-1 expression by incrementing and decreasing it, respectively. On a different note, the energy depletion that results from deregulation of the lipid metabolism in the kidney leads to an increase in fibrosis. Indeed, treatment with the AMPK activator 5-aminoimidazole-4-carboxamide-1-β-D-ribonucleoside, which increases lipid oxidation, prevents glomerulopathy and tubulointerstitial fibrosis [33] as well as PPARα agonists do [60]. Likewise, omega-3 administration decreases both TGF-β and PAI-1 expression [61].

4.7 Overactivation of Renin—Angiotensin Aldosterone System in Obesity

Very importantly for the kidney, adipose tissue expresses all components of the RAAS, including angiotensinogen, renin, angiotensin I-converting enzyme, and angiotensin II type 1 receptor [5]. All these components are increased in the plasma of obese patients due to not only synthesis by adipose tissue but also sympathetic stimulation, likely related to hyperleptinemia and hemodynamic alterations as a result of compression of the renal hilum by visceral fat. Angiotensin II is one of the most deleterious components of the RAAS, and can produce ROS via NADPH oxidase [13]. This system regulates vascular tone, aldosterone secretion from the adrenal gland, and sodium and water reabsorption from the kidney, all of which contribute to blood pressure regulation. An RAAS overactivated by obesity leads to excessive tubular reabsorption. The kidney within the macula densa feels a decrease in the sodium excreted in the urine, and activates a response to compensate this by filtering more urine. This is known as hyperfiltration, an early-stage characteristic of renal damage. Hyperfiltration puts the glomerulus under a big physical stress that generally ends up damaging the podocytes and leading to FSGS. Loss of podocytes drives a chain reaction that leads to loss of glomerulus and, therefore, loss of nephrons, which makes the kidney lose filtration capacity, leading to decreased GFR. When GFR reaches a value under 60%, it is considered to be pathologic. If the GFR continues decreasing, patients are at risk of entering ESRD, which requires dialysis and supposes a major risk of cardiovascular events and death. In summary, obesity can trigger and promote renal damage by changing hemodynamic and nonhemodynamic pathways in the kidney regulated by the RAAS (Fig. 7.3).

5. OBESITY AS INDEPENDENT RISK FACTOR FOR RENAL DISEASE: OBESITY-RELATED GLOMERULOPATHY

ORG is the best example that lipids alone can cause a detrimental damage to the kidney, and is an increasing cause of ESRD. Glomerular hypertrophy and FSGS are the two main pathological features of ORG. Glomerular hypertrophy appears in response to an increase in the GFR. Since podocytes cannot proliferate, as glomeruli get bigger the relative density of podocytes decreases. As an adaptive response, podocytes suffer hypertrophy too. This adaptation centers on mammalian

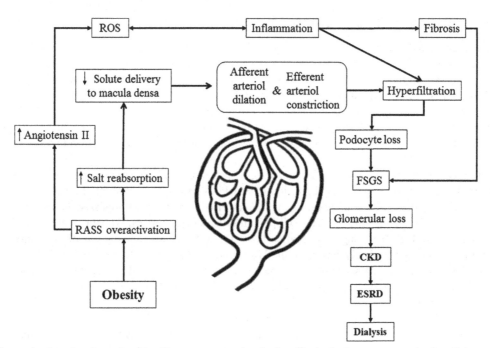

FIGURE 7.3 Overactivation of renin-angiotensin aldosterone system by obesity. Obesity leads to an overactivation of the renin—angiotensin aldosterone (RAAS) system that results in a change in the hemodynamics of the renal filtration, leading to podocyte loss and, if sustained over time, CKD and ESRD. *CKD*, chronic kidney disease; *ESRD*, end-stage renal disease; *FSGS*, focal segmental glomerulosclerosis; *ROS*, reactive oxygen species.

target of rapamycin (mTOR) pathways. However, the hypertrophy capacity of podocytes is limited and lower than that of the glomeruli, thus reaching a breakpoint in which the podocyte stretch tension is too big. Moreover, being the first filtration barrier, hypertrophic podocytes suffer extremely large mechanical stress, which ends up leading to podocyte failure and detachment, leaving the GBM denuded and resulting in FSGS. Podocyte loss is thought to cause further podocyte loss due to the release of proapoptotic signaling. Patients with ORG show up to 45% diminished density of podocytes. The appearance of FSGS means the loss of that functional glomerulus, which sets off a chain reaction. The glomeruli left suffer greater hyperfiltration in compensation, which leads to loss of other glomeruli. Finally, this string of events leads to progressive loss of GFR, which can result in kidney failure and ESRD, requiring dialysis in up to one-third of ORG patients [7]. However, in ORG patients the proteinuria increases very slowly and can actually go undetected for years, which suggests that these events happen at a slow rate.

ORG patients also show an increase in mesangial matrix, interstitial fibrosis, and a thickening of the GBM. By electron microscopy, lipid droplets can be identified inside the podocytes, where they might cause oxidative stress and ER stress. Mesangial cells also accumulate lipids and may transform into a type of foam cell that contributes to loss of glomerular integrity. All these pathological changes occur in ORG patients at the subclinical level, which suggests that many patients with obesity and no clinically evident renal disease do already have established renal alterations [62].

There are two hypotheses to explain obesity-related hyperfiltration. In the first, the primary event is the dilation of the afferent arteriole caused by a transmission of the increased arterial pressure present in hypertensive patients. The second hypothesis is tubelurocentric, and states that the primary event is the increased proximal salt reabsorption resulting in decreased solute delivery to the macula densa, which then leads to the afferent arteriole vasodilation and consequent hyperfiltration [63]. However, it could be that due to hyperfiltration the filtered sodium load is increased, and there is therefore increased salt reabsorption along the nephron to avoid volume depletion. Either way, this exacerbated reabsorption leads to an aggravation of hypertension, a condition highly prevalent in obese patients, resulting in a vicious circle. Moreover, adipokines released by the adipocytes such as leptin, adiponectin, and resistin are known to play a role in cellular hypertrophy and renal fibrosis. Unhealthy obesity may lead to maladaptive changes of renal cells to cope with the mechanical stress of hyperfiltration.

Human biopsies have shown that ORG is present before hypertension, diabetes, or any other clinical feature of renal disease. Thus it is likely that lipids alone can cause renal damage, without any of the concomitant features that are normally present in metabolic syndrome [7]. Nevertheless, the development of ORG does not preclude the development of other kidney diseases and it is generally treated by RAAS blockade. However, the best response is observed after weight loss, which induces a significant decrease in proteinuria and reverses hyperfiltration. Several genes involved in lipid metabolism, such as SREBP and PPARα, show an abnormal expression that causes higher lipid deposition in the kidney [29]. Thus antagonists and agonists respectively for these proteins hold promise for treatment of ORG.

Since no early biomarkers for renal damage currently exist and ORG manifestations seem to appear even earlier that diabetes, albuminuria, hypertension, or hyperglycemia, fatty kidney (ectopic lipid accumulation in the kidney) could be a promising biomarker. With the new noninvasive imaging techniques, such as proton magnetic resonance spectroscopy, measuring the lipid content in the kidney for prevention or diagnosis could indeed be feasible.

6. OBESITY COMPLICATIONS IN KIDNEY DISEASE

Although obesity can be an independent risk factor and cause of renal disease, it usually presents with other comorbidities. Metabolic syndrome is defined as the group of metabolic alterations caused by obesity, low high-density lipoprotein cholesterol, hypertriglycemia, high blood pressure, and hyperglycemia [64]. Metabolic syndrome is usually accompanied by hyperinsulinemia and type 2 diabetes mellitus. All metabolic complications associated with obesity derive from a common molecular pathogenesis that is characterized by two independent stages: IR and lipotoxicity. It is recognized that IR is an integral feature of metabolic syndrome and a major predictor of the development of type 2 diabetes. IR in the kidney, and more specifically in the podocytes, is a key event leading to loss of GFR and thence to renal disease. Furthermore, the most common CKD etiology is DN, which accounts for more than half of all CKD cases.

Obesity and the chronic inflammatory and oxidative status that it promotes in CKD patients lead to other problems, among which the most important are cardiovascular complications and renal cancer. Most CKD patients die as result of cardiovascular events, rather than progressing to ESRD. Thus the study of cardiovascular complications in the context of obese CKD patients is an area of great scientific and medical interest.

6.1 Insulin Resistance in the Development of Renal Disease

It has long been recognized that obesity is associated with type 2 diabetes. The major basis for this link is the ability of obesity to induce IR. IR is a marker of excessive nutrient intake and is known to aggravate lipid deposition ectopically since it leads to a state of hyperinsulinemia to try to overcome the resistance, which promotes TG synthesis [65].

Individuals with metabolic syndrome are at risk of developing CKD. Renal injury in these individuals may be a result of altered lipid metabolism. Studies in the general population have shown that, overall, patients with metabolic syndrome are 3.75 times more likely to suffer from kidney disease. Moreover, ectopic lipid accumulation strongly correlates with IR. Accumulation of NEFAs inside podocytes has been linked to IR and apoptosis, since it seems to play a critical role in podocyte function. At the same time, IR has been linked to renal hyperfiltration and CKD in several studies.

Insulin signaling is vital in the kidney. Under physiological circumstances, podocytes use their insulin receptors to sense postprandial changes and adapt their morphology through actin skeleton conformational changes to the new pressure and filtration rate. When kidneys become insulin resistant, the GFB starts leaking and renal disease develops. Podocytes have been shown to be the only insulin-sensitive cells in the glomerulus. This process is dependent on the nephrin and other proteins, like the lipid phosphatase SHIP2 and septin 7 [66]. When insulin signaling is lost in podocytes, they undergo a reorganization of their actin fibers that leads them to lose their foot processes. This change is dependent on the MAPK and phosphatidylinositol-4,5-bisphosphate 3-kinase cascade through the activation of the small GTPase RhoA. Moreover, insulin may control podocyte depolarization and contractility as well as inducing oxidative stress in podocytes [66]. Since podocytes are key cells in the maintenance of the GFB, loss of their foot processes leads to hyperfiltration and kidney damage in general, recapitulating features of DN [67]. Thus insulin signaling is critical for the normal functioning of the kidney. Adipokines and other inflammatory molecules released in great amounts in obesity inhibit insulin signaling at several levels, including the receptor and receptor substrate levels. The insulin receptor expression and function in the podocytes is really important, since it has been shown that podocyte-specific insulin receptor knockout mice develop a DKD-like phenotype in the absence of hyperglycemia [67].

6.2 Diabesity and Diabetic Nephropathy

Recently it has been proven that obesity and diabetes mellitus type 2 occurring in the context of obesity, known as "diabesity," are the leading causes of CKD.

Maintaining an adequate concentration of glucose in the blood is vital to preserve a constant supply of glucose to all organs, especially the brain, which uses almost only glucose as its source of energy. When glucose levels are not maintained within the healthy band and an individual becomes hyperglycemic, the pancreas tries to compensate for this elevation of glucose concentration by secreting more insulin. This results in a state of hyperinsulinemia. Organs then become insulin resistant, which in the end leads to diabetes.

The liver and the kidney are the only two organs capable of synthesizing glucose de novo. Originally it was thought that the liver was the only organ, since measurements in the kidney showed no differences between arterial and venous glucose concentrations. Later it was discovered that the net equilibrium was due to the renal glucose released by the cortex that was uptaken by the medulla. Now it is known that the kidney is responsible for 20% of all glucose produced via gluconeogenesis in the human body [68]. Conversely, the kidney lacks glucose-6-phosphatase, the enzyme required to break down glycogen. Indeed, kidneys do not store much glycogen.

In patients with type 2 diabetes, which is very common in obese patients, this production of glucose can increase up to 300%, equaling production from the liver. Proximal tubules are the only part of the kidney with the adequate enzymes for gluconeogenesis. Renal gluconeogenesis differs from liver gluconeogenesis in some aspects, such as substrate affinity and regulation. For instance, glucose ingestion stimulates renal gluconeogenesis even further, which contributes to the high postprandial glucose levels typically present in diabetic patients. Also, the kidney contributes to plasma glucose homeostasis by controlling reabsorption from renal tubules upon glomerular filtration. The kidney filters 180 g of free glucose per day; if not recovered through tubular reabsorption, this would be an enormous loss of glucose. This reabsorption is performed through the sodium—glucose cotransporters in the lumen and glucose transporter (GLUT) transporters on the interstitial side. The ability of the tubules to reabsorb is likely regulated according to need by increasing expression of these transporters. The expression of these transporters increases when glucose increases in the filtered load by elevation of either plasma glucose or GFR. However, when a threshold is reached and the glucose in the filtrate keeps increasing, glycosuria develops. Thus in patients with hyperfiltration, glycosuria may appear when blood glucose levels are relatively low, while in CKD patients, when the filtration rate slows down glycosuria may be absent until blood glucose levels are fairly high. Likewise, patients with diabetes can experience hyperglycemia without any glycosuria [69].

DN is the leading cause of CKD, accounting for more than 50% of cases. Obesity or ectopic accumulation of lipids can sometimes be the cause of the diabetes. When the limit of expansibility is reached and lipids begin to accumulate ectopically, they accumulate not only in the kidney but also in other organs such as liver, muscle, heart, and pancreas. When the latter is affected by this deposition, the development of IR and type 2 diabetes mellitus begins. This fact implies that lipotoxicity and glucotoxicity are two linked phenomena, and so using the glucolipotoxicity concept seems reasonable. Furthermore, sustained hyperglycemia caused by the diabetic status promotes both FA synthesis and TG accumulation, which further complicates the already obesogenic background of the majority of these patients. Importantly, very frequently diabetic patients present not only hyperglycemia but also dyslipidemia.

Lipotoxicity seems to play a role in the pathogenesis of DN. In animal models of DN it is well established that lipid accumulation in the kidney occurs and leads to glomerulosclerosis and tubulointerstitial injuries. However, this "fatty kidney" concept is not so clear in humans. In a study carried out by Herman-Edelstein et al., a strong correlation was observed between lipid metabolism dysregulation, lipid accumulation, podocyte dysfunction, fibrosis, inflammation, and loss of GFR [29]. They observed heavy lipid deposition in DN human samples, especially in the podocytes. However, the amount of lipids decreased in very fibrotic samples, perhaps due to a similar process of "burn-out" cirrhotic liver. The accumulation is caused by a dysregulation of TGs and cholesterol metabolism, which promotes increased uptake and decreased oxidation or efflux of both TGs and cholesterol. In the case of TGs this is demonstrated by increased expression of CD36 uptake transporter, and a decrease in lipoprotein lipase (LPL), PPARα, and PPARδ, which are catabolic enzymes, and the mitochondrial transporter CPT-1. For cholesterol, upregulation was observed for most lipoprotein receptors (LDLR, oxLDLR, CD36, and CCL16) specific of podocytes, as well as downregulation of the cholesterol efflux genes ABCA1, ABCG1 and apoE. However, synthesis genes were downregulated in both cases: fatty acid synthase (FAS), acetyl-CoA carboxylase (ACC), and SREBP1 in the case of TGs and SREBP2 for cholesterol.

Even when diabetes has not been established, hyperglycemia can have deleterious effects on kidney functioning. Hyperglycemia induces glomerular hyperfiltration, increases vascular permeability, stimulates the sympathetic nervous system leading to higher sodium reabsorption, alters renal metabolism, and promotes hypertrophy, among many other actions. Hyperglycemia itself can be directly toxic to cells, primarily by incrementing reactive oxygen radicals.

Under high glucose levels podocytes die via apoptosis, and ROS seem to play a key role in the activation of the p38 MAPK cascade leading to this [70]. Dysregulation in the autophagic flux in podocytes seems to be detrimental due to their longevity. The inability of the UPS to compensate for these protein accumulations results in ER stress and contributes to podocyte death. As happens in ORG, podocyte loss leads to podocyte hypertrophy, a process that seems to be regulated via mTOR. This new podocyte disposition translates into more sheer stress caused by the filtration flow, which in the end causes further podocyte loss. Hence while hypertrophy is essential, limiting it may ameliorate the rate of podocyte loss and thus progression of the disease. When podocyte loss reaches 20% the remaining cells start to die, causing glomerulosclerosis even if the causing stimulus is no longer present.

In the early stages of DKD, hyperglycemia produces an inhibition of NO synthesis, which is compensated by an increase in the vascular endothelial growth factor (VEGF) production by podocytes. This induces growth and proliferation of mesangial and endothelial cells to maintain the GBM structure. However, as DKD progresses podocytes are lost and thus less VEGF is produced, resulting in a loss of endothelial fenestration and putting the normal functioning of the GFB at risk. Thus podocyte injury is also decisive for endothelial health. Since podocytes are unable to renew, further research in this area is crucial to develop therapeutics targeting podocyte injury to prevent GFR decline in CKD patients.

6.3 Cardiovascular Risk in Chronic Kidney Disease Patients

Cardiovascular disease is the leading cause of death worldwide, not only in the general population but also in CKD patients. Most patients with CKD stage 3 or 4 die due to cardiovascular events, rather than progressing to ESRD. This is a result of endothelial dysfunction and left ventricular hypertrophy that are very likely triggered by oxidative stress and inflammation. Traditional risk factors are generally used in practice to predict the outcome of CKD patients, including diabetes mellitus, age, hypertension, and hyperlipidemia. However, these factors frequently fail to predict morbidity and mortality. This is where nontraditional risk factors, such as oxidative stress and inflammation, could be of help [71]. In fact, oxidative stress is known to induce endothelial dysfunction and progression to atherosclerosis by reducing NO availability. Oxidative stress reacts very rapidly with NO, reducing its bioavailability. Oxidative stress, endothelial dysfunction, dyslipidemia, and inflammation represent the key factors in the development of atherosclerosis, which is the main cause of cardiovascular disease [72]. Importantly, all these nontraditional risk factors are prevalent in CKD patients, meaning that oxidative stress and inflammatory markers could be of help to predict the morbidity and mortality of these patients.

Moreover, it is known that atherosclerosis development is greatly increased upon LDL oxidation, which happens in the presence of ROS. On the other hand, C-reactive protein (CRP), which is an increased marker of inflammation in renal impairment, also reduces NO production and diminishes endothelin-1, both key events in the development of atherosclerosis [73]. MPO released by immune cells during the respiratory burst caused by obesity modulates vascular inflammation by regulating NO bioavailability. Some studies suggest [73a] that MPO may be a link between CKD and the increased cardiovascular risk. Controversially, other studies show decreased levels of MPO in CKD patients, suggesting that this enzyme may not play a role in the etiology of cardiovascular complications in patients with CKD [48].

6.4 Obesity and Renal Cancer

Among kidney cancers, renal cell carcinoma (RCC) is the most common, accounting for up to 85% of cases. Interestingly, RCC is the third cancer most robustly associated with increased BMI, after endometrial and esophageal tumors. Indeed, up to 40% RCC tumors are associated with excessive body weight. Clear-cell RCC seems to be the subtype most strongly associated. However, the mechanisms underlying the relationship between adipose tissue and RCC are not well understood. Importantly for this chapter, inflammation and oxidative stress could be the missing links. Supporting this hypothesis, the inherited genetic type accounts for as little as 2% of RCC cases, which suggests that exogenous factors play a major role in the development of this type of cancer.

Several cytokines secreted by the adipose tissue are known to have angiogenic properties: Il-6, TNF-α, VEGF, and leptin among many others. It is worth noting that the hypertrophy of the adipose tissue provoked by an obesogenic context leads to a situation of local hypoxia. Thus the master regulator of hypoxia, HIF-1, increases. HIF-1 is a gene deeply implicated in RCC; it also stimulates TNF-α among other inflammatory molecules aggravating the inflammatory status. In addition to obesity, diabetes type 2 and hypertension, both of which are related to metabolic syndrome, are risk factors for RCC. Furthermore, the hyperfiltration state caused by obesity could be a risk factor for RCC since it exposes the kidneys to higher levels of oncogenic nephrotoxins.

Chronic inflammation has been linked to various steps involved in carcinogenesis, including cell transformation, promotion, survival, proliferation, invasion, angiogenesis, and metastasis. CRP, which is elevated in obese patients, has been shown as a potent prognostic factor in RCC patients, although the underlying mechanisms are unknown. In recent years considerable evidence has demonstrated that ROS are involved in this link between chronic inflammation and cancer. Indeed, an important characteristic of tumor promoters is their ability to recruit inflammatory cells and stimulate them to generate ROS. Since cancer has many risk factors that can be the etiology, including CKD, the contribution of oxidative stress alone in neoplastic transformation in renal cells is not so clear. Some studies performed on the established kidney cell line HK-2 have shown that chronic exposure to high levels of oxidative stress is enough to induce malignant transformation, including acquisition of stem-cell-like characteristics and EMT, which suggests invasive and aggressive behavior [74]. Direct effects of ROS include DNA strand breaks, point mutations, aberrant DNA cross-linking, and mutations in proto-oncogenes and tumor-suppressor genes, thus promoting neoplastic transformation. The DNA base modifications observed are characteristic of an attack by hydroxyl radical (OH). Moreover, ROS can specifically activate certain signaling pathways and thereby contribute to tumor development through the regulation of cellular proliferation, angiogenesis, and metastasis. The AP-1, which is involved in cell transformation and proliferation, is one of these ROS-activated pathways. Angiogenesis in tumors is a key event, since it allows the transition from low invasive and poorly vascularized tumors to highly invasive and angiogenic tumors. ROS are important stimuli of angiogenic signaling, stabilizing HIF-1α protein and inducing production of angiogenic factors by tumor cells. Moreover, lymphocyte-induced angiogenesis is triggered by ROS stimulation, and can be blocked by the administration of a free radical scavenger in tumor-bearing mice [75].

In vitro and in vivo experiments have shown that lipid peroxidation, an event very common in obesity due to an increased oxidative status, promotes renal tumorigenesis, while inhibition with antioxidants protects against this malignant transformation. Statins have proven to give protection from RCC due to their effect in reducing lipid peroxidation [76].

Ironically, ROS can induce DNA damage, leading to genetic lesions that initiate tumorigenicity and subsequent tumor progression, but can also induce cellular senescence and cell death and thereby function as antitumorigenic agents. Whether ROS promote tumor cell survival or act as antitumorigenic agents depends on the cell and tissues, the location of ROS production, and the concentration of individual ROS. There is also the "obesity paradox," in which obesity increases the risk of developing RCC but is also associated with a better prognosis.

In the context of diabesity, insulin exerts a proliferative effect on target tissues both directly and indirectly through the increment of insulin growth factor-1 (IGF-1). It has been observed that insulin and IGF-1 receptors are overexpressed in the kidneys of RCC patients. IGF-1 also has tumorigenic properties [77].

The most likely option is that the etiology of RCC in obese patients is multifactorial, and thus both inflammation and oxidative stress, plus other factors present in the obesogenic context, contribute to the onset and progression of RCC.

7. OXIDATIVE STRESS AND INFLAMMATION AS BIOMARKERS FOR RENAL DISEASE DURING OBESITY

It seems that ROS increase in a graded manner as renal function is lost, according to several studies that show an inverse correlation between different markers of oxidative stress and GFR [78]. Thus ROS could be an excellent biomarker of the progression or stage of kidney diseases and cardiovascular events in CKD patients. However, ROS are highly reactive compounds with a half-life of few seconds, which makes evaluating oxidative stress in the clinic very difficult. Measuring more stable markers with longer half-lives, such as molecules that are modified by ROS (lipids, proteins, carbohydrates, or DNA) could be a helpful way to evaluate oxidative stress. Some of the possibilities are reviewed below.

7.1 Lipid Peroxidation

The molecular structure of lipids makes them susceptible to oxidation. Acrolein, malondialdehyde, 4-HNE, and thiobarbituric acid reactive substances (TBARS) are produced during lipid peroxidation. All these molecules are water-soluble, low-molecular-weight products, which make them easy to remove in hemodialysis; hence their value as a marker of oxidative stress during hemodialysis is limited. In contrast, lipid hydroperoxide, which is another product of lipid peroxidation, is lipid-soluble and difficult to remove by hemodialysis; thus it is a more reliable biomarker of oxidative stress in ESRD patients [34]. Arachidonic acid-derived oxidation could also be a good marker. F2-isoprostanes are formed by nonenzymatic oxidation of arachidonic acid, a PUFA present in phospholipids of cell membranes, and could be detected in serum and urine samples. As renal clearance and hemodialysis could alter plasma levels of free isoprostanes, the esterified F2-isoprostanes would be a more reliable marker of oxidative stress in this clinical setting [35].

7.2 Protein Oxidation

AOPPs and advanced glycated end products (AGEs) are markers of protein oxidation. Plasma elevation of MPO, an enzyme that contributes to ROS generation, is indicative of oxidative stress. Moreover, MPO generates chlorinated oxidants, which are important in the formation of AOPPs. AOPPs are oxidative markers but also proinflammatory mediators, since they are able to induce monocyte activation [79]. AOPPs show a positive correlation with malondialdehyde, a lipid peroxidation marker, and a negative correlation with the antioxidant glutathione peroxidase (GPx). Moreover, high levels of AOPPs have been reported in patients with carotid artery plaques and correlate with CRP, indicating a role in the pathogenesis of atherosclerosis. Thus AOPPs could be markers for cardiovascular prognosis in CKD patients. On the other hand, AGEs, which are carbohydrate-derived compounds formed nonenzymatically, are markers of protein glycation. AGEs are able to activate the NF-κB pathway by binding to its receptor, leading to the monocyte-mediated inflammatory syndrome associated with uremia [79].

Protein carbonyls are formed by oxidation of amino acid residues on proteins. During kidney failure, mainly albumin carbonylation is increased and even intensified during hemodialysis. Albumin carbonylation correlates with CRP and fibrinogen, which again links oxidative stress with inflammation and atherosclerosis [80].

7.3 Nucleic Acid Oxidation

The marker of leukocyte DNA damage, 8-hydroxy-2′-deoxyguanosine, is increased as a result of interaction between oxidative compounds with nucleic acids. 8-hydroxy-2′-deoxyguanosine levels gradually increase with progression of kidney failure [81]. The negative correlation between plasma oxidative DNA damage and endothelial function and the positive correlation with carotid artery intima-media thickness show that 8-hydroxy-2′-deoxyguanosine could be a predictor of atherosclerosis and cardiovascular events in CKD patients [82].

7.4 Antioxidants

Total antioxidant status is a good biomarker, since a reduction in the antioxidant defense capacity means an increase in relative oxidative stress. Endogenous enzymatic and nonenzymatic antioxidant mechanisms diminish due to the damaging effects of oxidative products. Vitamin E, β-carotene, and coenzyme Q are fat-soluble antioxidants existing in the cellular membrane. Water-soluble antioxidants include vitamin C, GPx, SOD, and catalase. Ferritin, transferrin, and albumin also exert a nonenzymatic antioxidant effect by sequestering transition of metal ions.

The first line of enzymatic antioxidant defense is SOD, which converts superoxide anion (O_2^-) to hydrogen peroxide (H_2O_2). Then either catalase or GPx reduces H_2O_2 to water and oxygen. The enzymatic activity status of these three enzymes is indicative of the oxidative stress level in CKD patients; however, measures are not very stable.

Paraoxonase/arylesterase, also known as aromatic esterase-1 or serum aryl dialkyl phosphatase-1, is an enzyme that has esterase and more specifically paraoxonase activity. It has a protective effect against lipoprotein oxidation and is a sensitive antioxidant status marker, but there is limited data about it. A reduction in paraoxonase activity was reported in CKD patients, and it was observed that a decrease in antioxidant activity such as paraoxonase and GPx correlated with increased oxidative stress measured by F2-isoprostanes, selenium, and oxidized LDL concentrations [83]. Another enzyme, the gamma glutamyl transferase, which plays a major role in the extracellular catabolism of glutathione, has proven to have a high predictive value for all-cause mortality in ESRD patients [84].

The main nonenzymatic antioxidant is reduced glutathione, which is dependent on GPx activity. Decreased glutathione levels have been reported in CKD patients, consistent with the reduced activity of GPx. This parameter is a more stable indicator than SOD activity. Also lycopene, a carotenoid with effective exogenous antioxidant properties, has been reported to have a negative correlation with malondialdehyde, which suggest that it could be a good biomarker [85]. Vitamins C and E are important and abundant nonenzymatic antioxidants that are normally decreased in CKD patients as a result of dietary restriction, or in ESRD patients due to hemodialysis removal [86]. Both are considered good predictors of adverse cardiovascular outcomes [87].

7.5 Hydrogen Sulfide

Hydrogen sulfide is an endogenous signaling gas with antioxidant, antiinflammatory, and antihypertensive activity. Its deficiency can potentially contribute to CKD progression, since reduced plasma levels of it were reported in CKD patients [88].

7.6 Glutathionyl Hemoglobin

Hemoglobin gets glutathionylated under oxidative stress stimuli, thus it is considered to be an oxidative stress marker. Moreover, increased levels of glutathionyl hemoglobin have been reported in ESRD patients [89].

7.7 Asymmetric Dimethyl Arginine

Asymmetric dimethyl arginine (ADMA) inhibits endothelial NO synthase, leading to decrease NO production in the endothelium and increased superoxide; thus it is an important stress marker in CKD patients, as levels are increased in patients undergoing hemodialysis. Reduced renal excretion and reduced catabolism by dimethyl arginine dimethyl aminohydrolase contribute to increased plasma and tissue levels of ADMA in CKD patients [90].

7.8 Kynurenine Pathway

Kynurenine is produced as a result of tryptophan degradation. There is an association between kynurenine pathway activation and increased oxidative stress, inflammation, and endothelial dysfunction. Moreover, increased levels of this metabolite have been reported in CKD patients. It is a good predictor of the development of atherosclerosis and thus adverse cardiovascular outcomes in these patients [91].

7.9 Inflammation Markers

In addition to markers of oxidative stress there are markers of inflammation, such as high-sensitivity CRP and IL-6, that independently predict the state of renal patients. Recently in this sense, It has been recently described other early inflammation biomarkers of renal injury under HFD conditions that can be detected in urine even before the presence of morphological renal changes [92].

Among all these biomarkers, the most practical and recommended for use in clinical practice are glutathione, the glutathione redox ratio, intracellular enzymatic antioxidants such as SOD or GPx, LDL oxidation, and AOPPs.

8. THERAPIES IN OBESITY-RELATED KIDNEY DISEASE

For several decades targeting the RAAS has been the main therapeutic approach to kidney disease. Angiotensin-converting enzyme inhibitors (ACEIs) and angiotensin II receptor blockers are the two main choices. Their therapeutic benefit relies on their ability to slow down the decline in kidney function and reduce proteinuria. However, these treatments do not reverse the loss of GFR and are associated with some side effects, among which hyperkalaemia is the most limiting. For ESRD patients, dialysis or transplantation are the only options. Thus any new therapies that can augment these existing approaches are of great interest.

Very importantly, weight loss is the most effective intervention in the first stages to reduce proteinuria and hyperfiltration, either by hypocaloric diet, exercise, or bariatric surgery. This clearly shows the importance of lipotoxicity in the development of kidney disease.

8.1 Weight Loss: Dietary Food Restriction and Bariatric Surgery

In obesity-associated renal disease the best therapeutic response is observed after weight loss, which induces a significant decrease in proteinuria and reverses hyperfiltration. Thus weight loss can be considered as a treatment on its own. An animal study performed in obese rats showed that dietary restriction, even in an obesogenic background, was able to prevent the development of the disease or protect from further damage, depending on the life stage when the dietary restriction was imposed [93]. Rats were followed up for 60 weeks. The groups that were restricted in food at an age of 6 or 12 weeks showed more beneficial effects and were indeed very similar to lean animals, whereas rats that were restricted at week 26 did not show that many beneficial effects, although still being in better condition than the obese group fed ad libitum. Interestingly, animals that were restricted in food as old as week 50 still showed an improvement compared to obese ad libitum fed rats, suggesting that caloric restriction has beneficial effects even when imposed late in life. The group restricted at week 6 showed a similar kidney and heart weight and glomerular volume to the lean group, as well as lower insulin and leptin levels, TGs, GFR, and proteinuria. However, cholesterol levels remained higher than in the lean group. Importantly, survival was equal to the lean group. In the rat group restricted at 12 weeks old, weight and glomerular size were similar to the lean group and animals restricted at 6 weeks. However, insulin and leptin levels, TGs, cholesterol, GFR, and proteinuria remained elevated. Nevertheless, the survival was equal to that of rats restricted at week 6 and lean rats. In the group restricted at week 26, all parameters improved compared to the ad libitum fed group with the exception of cholesterol levels. Survival was still better than in the nonrestricted group, although slightly worse than in the 6 and 12 weeks restricted groups and the lean rats. In the case of the rats restricted at 50 weeks old, the progression of the disease was slower and some parameters did indeed improved.

Altogether, this data demonstrates that caloric restriction when initiated early in life has a huge effect on the development of the disease, completely preventing the appearance of proteinuria in some cases. Very importantly, even when initiated later in life caloric restriction results in either reduction or prevention of further progression of the disease. Based on the reduction in proteinuria, it can be hypothesized that even remodeling and repairing of the glomeruli occurs upon restriction [93]. Thus it is of extreme importance to educate CKD patients on the importance of their diet for their outcome and survival. Of course, dietary restriction is not the only lifestyle modification that these patients can adopt; exercise is another efficient approach for weight loss, whether or not accompanied by dietary restriction.

However, it is challenging for patients to achieve sustained weight loss through lifestyle modifications. Bariatric surgery is an alternative method for sustained weight loss that has proven effective and is becoming more common for patients with morbid or severe obesity. Currently the most common bariatric procedures performed worldwide are laparoscopic Roux-en-Y gastric bypass (RYGB) and laparoscopic vertical sleeve gastrectomy (LSG). Laparoscopic adjustable gastric banding (LAGB) is another purely restrictive procedure that involves the insertion of an adjustable ring immediately below the gastroesophageal junction on the proximal stomach. RYGB and LSG, apart from achieving significant weight loss, promote favorable effects for various hormones linked to hunger, satiety, and food preferences, unlike LAGB. This, together with a lower success in achieving weight loss, has make LAGB fall out of favor during the past few years.

Bariatric surgery is able to lower the two main risk factors for CKD: diabetes and hypertension. In a trial of obese patients with uncontrolled type 2 diabetes who were randomized to either bariatric surgery plus intensive medical therapy or intensive medical therapy alone, bariatric surgery resulted in better glycemic control. Impressive effects on blood pressure have also been reported. Interestingly, increased GFR after surgery seems to be significantly associated with decreases in leptin [94]. Some procedures report extraordinary outcomes: two case reports observed complete resolution of proteinuria after bariatric surgery in patients with obesity-related FSGS [95].

However, there are some important risks after bariatric surgery, including infection, respiratory failure, acute kidney injury (AKI), and death. This is why CKD patients have not been considered as candidates for bariatric surgery until recently. Risk factors for AKI after bariatric surgery include higher BMI, lower estimated Glomerular Filtration Rate (eGFR), preoperative use of ACEIs and angiotensin receptor blockers, and intraoperative hypotension [96]. The problem is that obesity is a contraindication for ESRD patients to go on the waiting list for kidney transplantation; thus bariatric surgery may be an important instrument in improving access to kidney transplantation for the increasing number of severely obese ESRD patients. Surprisingly, bariatric surgery appears to be relatively safe in patients with CKD, with an incidence of postoperative complications only slightly higher than in the general bariatric surgery population. However, all studies on this topic are of short duration (1−2 years), and often lack comparison groups, so more research needs to be done.

If it is not possible to lose weight, another way to deal with the obesity is increasing the storage capacity of the adipose tissue, thus avoiding ectopic accumulation and its detrimental effects. This could be achieved either by targeting the adipose tissue fibroinflammatory environment or by increasing the recruitment capability of adipose tissue precursors. A different approach could be targeting the thermogenic capacity of the adipose tissue by increasing the brown adipose tissue mass and/or activity, potentiating the browning capacity of white adipose tissue, or beige adipocyte recruitment to maximize the energy-dissipating potential of thermogenic brown and beige fat [97].

8.2 Peroxisome Proliferator-Activated Receptor Agonists as Therapy

Enhancing FA oxidation and inhibiting inflammation may be a good therapeutic approach. Indeed, PPAR agonists show benefits by reducing albuminuria. Different isoforms of PPARs exist: PPARα, PPARβ/δ, and PPARγ, and different agonists for each isoform, such as fenofibrates or thiazides, could be used as therapy in obesity-associated renal disease.

PPARα is highly expressed in the kidneys and plays a key role in lipid and glucose homeostasis by promoting FA oxidation. Very importantly, PPARα also seems to exert antioxidant and antiinflammatory effects by antagonizing the NF-κB pathway. Rescuing PGC-1 and PPARα with fenofibrates protects against renal fibrosis [26]. In an animal model study, treatment with fenofibrates attenuated albumin excretion, slowed fibrosis by inhibiting myofibroblasts differentiation, and reduced oxidative stress by increasing SOD activity and inflammation [60].

Thiazolidinediones (TZDs), including rosiglitazone or pioglitazone, are synthetic exogenous PPARγ agonists. PPARγ is predominantly expressed in podocytes and may play an important role in the development of albuminuria. PPARγ agonists are thought to act mainly by inhibiting inflammation and oxidative stress, likely by a mitochondrial-protective effect. Unfortunately, use of this group of agonists is greatly restricted due to their severe side effects, which include bone loss, edema, fluid retention, and increased cardiovascular risk. Among TZDs, pioglitazone seems to have less adverse effects. Some groups support the theory that optimizing a lower TZD dose could protect the kidney without the adverse effects [98]. Some preliminary animal approaches have been successful [30,99], but extensive studies and clinical trials are required to validate the data. Other suggested approaches are the use of endogenous PPARγ agonists such as nitro-oleic acid or selective ones that preserve the capability of regulating antidiabetic genes but not adverse-effect-associated genes. Positive results have been observed in both cases; indeed, a selective PPARγ agonist, balaglitazone, is now on clinical trial phase II and holds promise [100]. It is also worth considering the strategy of increasing PPARγ agonists' efficacy by combining them with other effective therapies. Using endogenous PPARγ agonists with RAAS blockers could be the perfect approach. There is already one example with this dual property, telmisartan, but it still needs to be proved in clinical trials. Combining PPARγ agonist with PPARα agonists or COX2 inhibitors has also shown beneficial effects [98].

It is worth noting that is not fully clear whether the beneficial effects of PPAR agonists in obesity-associated renal disease are due to their role in oxidizing lipids, their insulin-sensitizing effects, or the additive effect of both actions.

Renal lipid metabolism definitely plays an important role in its physiology, since lipids are the main source of energy for the kidneys. Further research needs to be done in this line to understand fully the contribution of lipid metabolism abnormalities to CKD development and progression during obesity.

8.3 Antioxidant Therapies

Since different oxidative stress biomarkers have proven to correlate with different aspects of kidney disease associated with obesity, oxidative stress may be an excellent candidate for a new therapeutic target. The most practical way to reduce total oxidative stress is to increase the antioxidant capacity rather than targeting ROS to reduce it. Supplementation of some of these antioxidants is dietary. Components such as vitamin C, vitamin E, β-carotene, copper, iron, selenium, and zinc are present in many foods, which implies that patients could improve by simply following a specific diet. Red grape juice, green tea, and other infusions such as that from the milk thistle have already proved to have beneficial antioxidant effects.

8.3.1 Natural Antioxidants

Being a source of polyphenols, red grape juice increases antioxidant capacity and decreases LDL. It actually had a higher effect on lowering NADPH oxidase activity than vitamin E in hemodialysis patients [101]. Studies on the administration of grape seed proanthocyanidin extract, an efficient phytochemical antioxidant, have shown nephroprotective effects [102]. Resveratrol is another phenolic compound found in various plants, including grapes, berries, and peanuts. Originally resveratrol was used as a cardioprotective, but in recent years it has attracted attention as a renoprotective therapy due to its implication in antioxidant and antiinflammatory processes. Resveratrol reduces inflammation and oxidative stress through SIRT-1 action, mTOR pathway inactivation, and Nrf2 and NF—B factor modulation. Another fruit with proven renal antioxidant properties, such as decreasing lipid oxidation and oxidized LDL, is garcinia, also known as tamarind [103].

Quercetin is a plant polyphenol from the flavonoid group with antioxidant properties that can be found in many foods, such as cranberry, broccoli, and red kidney beans, among many others [104]. Green tea has also proved to be a safe antioxidant that prevents cardiac hypertrophy and ROS production, likely due to the presence of quercetin.

Sylimarin, the main component of the plant *Cardus marianus* or milk thistle, in combination with vitamin E has proved to decrease malondialdehyde and increase GPx activity and hemoglobin levels in ESRD patients [105].

8.3.2 Vitamin C and Vitamin E

Vitamins C and E are probably the most common dietary antioxidants. Vitamin E protects the cell membrane from lipid peroxidation by forming a low-reactivity tocopheroxyl radical thanks to the major components alpha and gamma tocopherol, while vitamin C directly scavenges O_2 and hydroxyl radical. Supplementation with vitamins C and E has proved to have an antioxidant effect in both animal models and humans. In cats with renal insufficiency, a 4-week administration reduced serum 8-hydroxy-2′-deoxyguanosine, the marker of DNA damage [106]. In humans, while short-term administration of vitamin C did not show any effect on oxidative stress biomarkers, a 1-year administration showed a trend toward a decrease of the oxidant status [107]. Moreover, coadministration of vitamins C and E for 6 months in patients undergoing hemodialysis decreased lipid peroxidation [108], and in peritoneal dialysis patients improved all biomarkers [109]. Using vitamin-E-coated cellulose acetate dialysis membranes gives long-term suppression of oxidative biomarkers and inflammation [110]. Also, long-term administration of vitamin E increased LDL resistance to oxidation. Interestingly, administration of γ-tocopherol alone had no significant effect on any oxidative stress biomarker, despite being the major component of vitamin E. However, it did reduce some inflammatory markers.

8.3.3 Omega-3 Fatty Acid

Consumption of omega-3 has proven to mitigate atherosclerosis. In addition to the beneficial effect on controlling hypertriglyceridemia, administration of omega-3 ameliorates oxidative stress, inflammation, and fibrosis. In a rat model with reduced renal mass, it showed lowered COX2, NADPH oxidase, PAI-1, TGF-β, CTGF, α-SMA, fibronectin, MCP-1, ERK1/2, and NFκB [61]. In humans, omega-3 was shown to ameliorate oxidative stress by increasing serum SOD, GPx, and catalase activities in CKD patients with dyslipidemia. In hemodialysis patients, 2-month omega-3 FA supplementation reduced malondialdehyde levels and increased antioxidant status (GPx and SOD) [37].

8.3.4 N-Acetylcysteine

The thiol group on this molecule has scavenging properties, which help to mitigate oxidative stress effects in CKD patients. This beneficial effect has been observed both alone and in combination with vitamin E. Beyond the antioxidant properties, it also deals with inflammation and increases the hematocrit, which helps patients with anemia. In hemodialysis patients a decrease in 8-hydroxy-2'-deoxyguanosine and oxidized LDL was observed [111]. However, this molecule has low clearance for ESRD patients, which limits its use in long-term therapies.

8.3.5 Carnitine

Carnitine supplementation showed beneficial effects in dialysis patients by reducing oxidative stress and chronic inflammation. This compound proved to increase glutathione and GPx activity and decrease malondialdehyde and protein carbonyl [112].

8.3.6 Coenzyme Q10

Administration of coenzyme Q10 showed suppression of oxidative stress indices by lowering AOPPs and malondialdehyde in hemodialysis patients. Unfortunately, it also suppressed the antioxidant capacity, which makes this molecule only partially effective in lowering the general oxidative stress status [113].

8.3.7 Folic Acid

Also known as vitamin B9, folic acid acts against lipoperoxidation in patients on hemodialysis. Moreover, it helps to reduce hyperhomocysteinemia. Homocysteine is a nonprotein α-amino acid that is associated with cardiovascular events since it degrades and inhibits the formation of the three main structural components of arteries: collagen, elastin, and proteoglycans. Thus administration of this molecule could help to reduce cardiovascular risk in CKD patients [114].

8.3.8 Statins

Statins do not exert only hypolipidemic effects. Although the number of studies evaluating the effect of statins in patients with renal failure is limited, post hoc analyses of large trials such as the Anglo—Scandinavian Cardiac Outcomes Trial, the Cholesterol and Recurrent Events Study, and the Pravastatin Pooling Project show a benefit that increases as renal function declines [115]. This beneficial effect seems to involve modulation of endothelial dysfunction, inflammatory processes, and oxidative stress. Indeed, a study showed a 40% reduction in plasma levels of CRP, 38% in IL-1β, and 26% in TNF-α [115]. In this study, changes in CRP and cholesterol showed no correlation, suggesting that the effect of the statins is independent of the lipid-lowering action. This inflammatory reduction was accompanied by an amelioration of the oxidative stress suggested by a reduction in lipid hydroperoxide and oxidized LDL plasma levels, which supports the inflammation—oxidative stress link. This improvement seems to be a consequence of ROS synthesis reduction by preventing NADPH oxidase function rather than by increasing antioxidant defense, since no changes in the total antioxidant capacity were observed. However, statins were also able to improve the total antioxidant status in hemodialysis patients in whom it had earlier been reduced [116]. Altogether, this data suggests that statins can improve the oxidative stress status in CKD patients.

8.3.9 Trace Elements: Selenium and Zinc

Selenium plays an important role in cellular protection as a free radical scavenger. It performs this by incorporating with GPx as selenocysteine [117]. Interestingly, selenium administration failed to increase GPx activity in ESRD patients. This suggests that GPx protein deficiency is a result of a decrease in its synthesis from damaged kidneys, rather than selenium deficiency. However, in CKD patients an improvement of GFR was reported after administration of an oral supplement of sodium selenite [118], and in hemodialysis patients it improved GPx activity and tocopherol and prevented DNA damage [119].

Zinc supplementation in patients on long-term dialysis increased selenium concentration and decreased plasma aluminum and oxidative stress by lowering malondialdehyde and increasing SOD activity [120].

8.3.10 Synthetic Antioxidants

Ebselen, a peroxynitrate scavenger that mimics GPx, ameliorates proteinuria and renal focal and segmental sclerosis [121]. Other synthetic antioxidants that have proven useful in kidney diseases are idebenone and lazaroids, among many others. Idebenone works as an analog of the coenzyme Q10, which is an essential element in mitochondrial functioning. Lazaroids, on the other hand, inhibit ROS-induced lipid peroxidation. By doing so, they have proven to reduce the vasoconstriction and hypoperfusion that ROS sometimes produce in renal circulation [122].

8.4 Antiinflammatory Therapy

Antiinflammatory therapy may be a potential treatment for renal injury associated to obesity. IL-6 and TNF-α are two of the main key inflammatory molecules in obesity-associated renal diseases. The antiIL-6 receptor antibody MR16-1 has shown promising results in reducing proteinuria, renal lipid deposition, and mesangial cell proliferation in a hypercholesterolemia-induced renal model in apolipoprotein E-deficient mice [123]. Inhibition of TNF-α by the antagonist etanercept protected the kidney through the reduction of renal NF-κB, oxidative stress, and blood pressure [124]. Treatment with exogenous adiponectin as well as the introduction of adenovirus-mediated adiponectin has also had promising results in mouse models [17].

Knowing the role of macrophage infiltration in the development of the inflammatory state present during obesity, one could think that targeting its recruitment could be a great therapy. However, studies in mice deficient in the chemokine receptor-2, for which MCP-1 is a ligand, have shown no decrease in macrophage infiltration and, conversely, have produced an elevation in MCP-1 levels as an attempt to compensate for the lack of receptor [8].

Obviously, weight loss must be the best method to reduce all inflammation and its consequences, since obesity is the primary cause.

8.5 Dialysis

Dialysis is the main therapeutic procedure used for patients with ESRD. It is a process by which the waste and extra chemicals and fluid accumulated in the blood are removed. There are two major types of dialysis: hemodialysis and peritoneal dialysis. The main difference between them is that in hemodialysis the cleaning is done externally while peritoneal dialysis is done inside the patient's body. Hemodialysis is the most common type; during the procedure blood passes along a tube that is attached to the patient's arm into an external machine, a hemodialyzer, that filters it before its passed back into the patient's arm along another tube. This is usually carried out 3 days a week, with each session lasting around 4 h. In peritoneal dialysis the peritoneum is used as a filter thanks to its thousand small vessels. To perform this type of dialysis, minor surgery has to be done beforehand to place a catheter in the peritoneal cavity. This cavity is filled with fluid, and after a few hours it has to be drained into a bag. Changing the fluid usually takes about 30—40 min and normally needs to be done around four times a day; it can also be done by a machine overnight while the patient sleeps. The choice of peritoneal dialysis or hemodialysis is usually based on patient motivation, desire, geographic distance from a hemodialysis unit, physician and/or nurse bias, patient education, and economic issues, since peritoneal dialysis costs significantly less than hemodialysis.

Although both techniques are equally effective in cleaning the blood, there are important differences in the oxidative stress and inflammation profiles of each group of patients [13]. Hemodialysis is believed to contribute to chronic inflammation due to exposure of blood to a bioincompatible system causing activation of the immune system. Materials of the hemodialysis membrane may affect both the formation of reactive species by activating mast cells and monocytes and the weakening of the antioxidant capacity of the body due to the loss of hydrophilic antioxidants during dialysis. Higher levels of oxidized LDL cholesterol, TBARS, and protein carbonyl have been reported in hemodialysis patients compared to peritoneal dialysis patiernts, indicative of a higher oxidative profile in hemodialysis patients [125]. Zinc deficiency seems to be greater in hemodialysis patients, too. Moreover, hemodialysis may not increase oxidants but it does reduce the antioxidant reservoir. However, other studies show similar degrees of inflammation and oxidative stress status in hemodialysis and peritoneal dialysis patients as well as equally lowered total antioxidant capacity and SOD. In contrast, with regard to antioxidant therapies hemodialysis patients seem to respond better to vitamin E supplementation than peritoneal dialysis patients [126]. More research needs to be carried out to clarify which type of dialysis could benefit patients most.

There are also different types of hemodialysis membranes and differences in the oxidative stress and inflammatory profiles of different patients [127]. The first membranes used were cellulose, since they were cheap to produce and had thin walls. However, cellulose membranes present cross-reactive immune responses and produce an inflammatory response in patients including activation of complement, neutrophil superoxide production, and cytokine induction. Moreover, the pore size is too small, so they only allow the passage of small molecules, which is a problem in the long term because of the lack of removal of β2-microglobulin, accumulation of which contributes to amyloid formation. Next to appear were modified cellulosic membranes. These are cellulose-based membranes but with different substitutions, such as copper and acetate. They are less inflammatory to the host and can be produced with slightly larger pore sizes, but the biocompatibility problem is not completely solved. Later, synthetic membranes appeared which can be manufactured with different pore sizes, thus most allow good clearance of larger molecules such as β2-microglobulin. The biocompatibility is excellent due to the use of compounds such as polyamide, polymethylmethacrylate, polysulfone, and polyacrylonitrile. Another variation is membranes with the backbone of a common membrane, such as cellulose or polysulfone, but coated with an additional compound for putative benefit. The most common are vitamin E-coated membranes, which have potential benefits in terms of reduced oxidative stress. Vitamin-E-coated polysulfone membranes have been proved to exert antioxidant activity by reducing ADMA accumulation in hemodialysis patients [110].

In recent years another type of membrane has appeared: the superflux membrane. These are synthetic membranes with large pores that allow the passage of larger molecules, especially proteins. They tend to allow the loss of some albumin during dialysis, which may show some benefits. However, more research at the biochemical level needs to be done to find the best membrane for ESRD patients that not only cleans their blood but also preserves their antioxidant reservoir while decreasing their oxidant and inflammatory levels.

9. CONCLUSION

When the limit of expansion and lipid accumulation of the adipose tissue is exceeded (a common feature during obesity), an inflammatory state associated with other processes, such as reticulum stress, oxidative stress, and fibrosis, leads to complications at systemic level and, of note for this chapter, affects the kidney (Fig. 7.4). Traditional approaches are not good enough to detect and treat renal disease. Oxidative stress and inflammation are alternatives to explain several features of renal disease. A joint action that diminishes both the oxidative stress and the lipid excess could improve the inflammatory state and consequently the damage at systemic and kidney levels. However, further investigations in animal models, or specific renal cell lines, as well as in human samples are necessary to understand better the pathways involved in the early signaling events. It is worth remarking that early detection is especially important in kidney disease, since the consequences of most renal injuries are largely irreversible, especially those injuries affecting the podocytes, and lead to loss of renal function. The more that is known about the early steps of renal disease, the earlier we will be able to detect and stop the progression to CKD. Taking into consideration the elevated rates of obesity, which are likely to keep increasing rapidly, preventing CKD or ESRD in patients would not only save lives but also diminish the economic burden imposed on the health system. The cost of treating CKD and its complications are unaffordable for many governments and individuals around the world. According to the International Society of Nephrology, annual costs of dialysis and kidney transplantation are increasing per patient [128]. In low-income and middle-income countries, most people with kidney failure have insufficient access to life-saving dialysis and transplantation. Worldwide it is estimated that only half of ESRD patients can be treated, leaving 2.5−5 million patients untreated.

Moreover, not all patients respond equally to all treatments, so more efforts must be made to ascertain the etiology of CKD in each individual. Ideally, in the proximate future analysis of kidney biopsies should be used to stratify CKD patients into different subgroups to ensure the most appropriate therapy.

GLOSSARY

Chronic kidney disease (CKD) Process of progressive loss of kidney function over a period of months or years. It is diagnosed by measuring the GFR. All patients with a GFR of less than 60% for 3 months are considered to have CKD. There are several stages depending on the GFR status; the last is stage 5, also known as end-stage renal disease, when GFR is less than 15%.

Diabesity Situation in which diabetes develops in the context of obesity. This situation is becoming very common due to the global epidemic of obesity.

Diabetic nephropathy (DN) Kidney-related complication of type 1 and type 2 diabetes. Around 40% of people with diabetes develop this pathology; it is the leading cause of CKD and accounts for more than half of all cases.

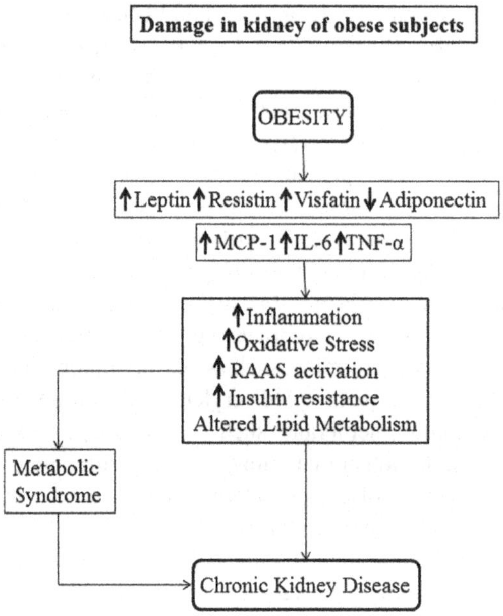

FIGURE 7.4 Damage in kidneys of obese subjects. A surplus of lipids leads to elevated systemic levels of adipokines and proinflammatory factors that promote changes involving inflammation, oxidative stress, RAAS overactivation, insulin resistance, and altered lipid metabolism. These can directly affect the kidney, leading to the development of chronic kidney disease, or indirectly through the development of metabolic syndrome. *IL*, interleukin; *MCP*, macrophage chemoattractant protein; *RAAS*, rennin—angiotensin aldosterone system; *TNF*, tumor necrosis factor.

Dialysis Treatment for acute renal insufficiency in ESRD patients to remove waste products and excess fluid from the blood. There are two major types: hemodialysis and peritoneal dialysis.

End-stage renal disease (ESRD) Last stage of CKD where a complete loss of renal function occurs. At this point, dialysis and kidney transplantation are the only two therapeutic approaches.

Focal segmental glomerulosclerosis (FSGS) Glomerular lesion present in most kidney diseases, by which scarring of the glomerular tuft happens due to extracellular matrix accumulation and leads to loss of function of that glomerulus.

Glomerular filtration barrier (GFB) Highly selective filter located in the renal glomerulus and constituted of three distinctive layers: a fenestrated endothelium with its glycocalyx, glomerular basement membrane, and podocytes.

Glomerular filtration rate (GFR) Parameter that estimates how much blood passes through the glomeruli per minute. It is calculated by measuring creatinine serum levels and adjusting for age, gender, and race. This parameter is used to determine kidney function and stage of renal disease.

Lipotoxicity Pathological situation generated by the ectopic accumulation of lipids in organs that are unable to store fat.

Podocytes Highly specialized perivascular cells in the glomeruli. These cells present multiple interdigitating foot processes and are crucial in the maintenance of the glomerular filtration barrier.

LIST OF ACRONYMS AND ABBREVIATIONS

4-HNE 4-hydroxynonenal
ACEI Angiotensin-converting enzyme inhibitor
AGE Advanced glycation end product
AKI Acute kidney injury
AMPK Adenine monophosphate kinase
AOPP Advanced oxidation protein product
ATP Adenosine triphosphate
CCL16 Chemokine (C—C motif) ligand 16
CD36 Cluster of differentiation 36
CKD Chronic kidney disease
CRP C-reactive protein
DKD Diabetic kidney disease
DN Diabetic nephropathy
ECM Extracellular matrix

EMT Epithelial to mesenchymal transition
ER Endoplasmic reticulum
ESRD End-stage renal disease
FASN Fatty acid synthase
FFA Free fatty acid
FSGS Focal segmental glomerulosclerosis
GBM Glomerular basement membrane
GFB Glomerular filtration barrier
GFR Glomerular filtration rate
GPx Glutathione peroxidase
HFD High-fat diet
HIF-1 Hypoxia inducible factor-1
IGF-1 Insulin growth factor-1
IL Interleukin
IR Insulin resistance
LAGB Laparoscopic adjustable gastric banding
LDL Low-density lipoprotein
LPL Lipoprotein lipase
LSG Laparoscopic vertical sleeve gastrectomy
MAPK Mitogen-activated protein kinase
MCD Minimal change disease
MCP-1 Monocyte chemoattractant protein-1
MIF-1 Macrophage migration inhibitory factor-1
MMP Metalloproteinase
MMT Macrophage to mesenchymal transition
MPO Myeloperoxidase
mTOR Mammalian target of rapamycin
NADPH Nicotinamide adenine dinucleotide phosphate
NEFA Nonesterified fatty acid
NF-κB Nuclear factor kappa-light-chain-enhancer of activated B cells
NO Nitric oxide
ORG Obesity-related glomerulopathy
PAI-1 Plasminogen activator inhibitor-1
PINK1 PTEN-induced putative kinase 1
PPAR Peroxisome proliferator-activated receptor
PUFA Polyunsaturated fatty acid
RAAS Renin−angiotensin aldosterone system
RCC Renal cell carcinoma
ROS Reactive oxygen species
RYGB Roux-en-Y gastric bypass
SOD Superoxide dismutase
SREBP Sterol regulatory element-binding proteins
TBARS Thiobarbituric acid reactive substances
TG Tryglyceride
TGF-β Transforming growth factor-β
TNF-α Tumor necrosis factor-α
TZD Thiazolidinedione
ULK-1 Unc-51-like kinase-1
VEGF Vascular endothelial growth factor

REFERENCES

[1] Kovesdy CP, Furth S, Zoccali C. Obesity and kidney disease: hidden consequences of the epidemic. Indian J Nephrol March−April 2017;27(2):85−92.

[2] Virtue S, Vidal-Puig A. Adipose tissue expandability, lipotoxicity and the metabolic syndrome−an allostatic perspective. Biochim Biophys Acta March 2010;1801(3):338−49.

[3] de Vries AP, Ruggenenti P, Ruan XZ, Praga M, Cruzado JM, Bajema IM, et al. Fatty kidney: emerging role of ectopic lipid in obesity-related renal disease. Lancet Diabetes Endocrinol May 2014;2(5):417−26.

[4] Ruster C, Wolf G. Adipokines promote chronic kidney disease. Nephrol Dial Transplant November 2013;28(Suppl. 4):iv8—14.

[5] Kershaw EE, Flier JS. Adipose tissue as an endocrine organ. J Clin Endocrinol Metab June 2004;89(6):2548—56.

[6] Boini KM, Krishna M, Zhang C, Chun XM, Han WQ, et al. Visfatin-induced lipid raft redox signaling platforms and dysfunction in glomerular endothelial cells. Biochim Biophys Acta December 2010;1801(12):1294—304.

[7] D'Agati VD, Chagnac A, de Vries AP, Levi M, Porrini E, Herman-Edelstein M, et al. Obesity-related glomerulopathy: clinical and pathologic characteristics and pathogenesis. Nat Rev Nephrol August 2016;12(8):453—71.

[8] Chen A, Mumick S, Zhang C, Lamb J, Dai H, Weingarth D, et al. Diet induction of monocyte chemoattractant protein-1 and its impact on obesity. Obes Res August 2005;13(8):1311—20.

[9] Cui D. Atlas of histology with functional and clinical correlations. Wolters Kluwer; 2010.

[10] Kim JY, van de Wall E, Laplante M, Azzara A, Trujillo ME, Hofmann SM, et al. Obesity-associated improvements in metabolic profile through expansion of adipose tissue. J Clin Invest September 2007;117(9):2621—37.

[11] Virchow R. A more precise account of fatty metamorphosis. Cellular pathology, as based upon physiological and pathological histology. 1860. p. 342—6.

[12] Moorhead JF, Chan MK, El-Nahas M, Varghese Z. Lipid nephrotoxicity in chronic progressive glomerular and tubulo-interstitial disease. Lancet December 11, 1982;2(8311):1309—11.

[13] Modaresi A, Nafar M, Sahraei Z. Oxidative stress in chronic kidney disease. Iran J Kidney Dis May 2015;9(3):165—79.

[14] Okamura DM, Pennathur S. The balance of powers: redox regulation of fibrogenic pathways in kidney injury. Redox Biol December 2015;6:495—504.

[15] Coelho M, Oliveira T, Fernandes R. Biochemistry of adipose tissue: an endocrine organ. Arch Med Sci April 20, 2013;9(2):191—200.

[16] Virtue S, Vidal-Puig A. It's not how fat you are, it's what you do with it that counts. PLoS Biol 2008;6(9):237.

[17] Sharma K, Ramachandrarao S, Qiu G, Usui HK, Zhu Y, Dunn SR, et al. Adiponectin regulates albuminuria and podocyte function in mice. J Clin Invest May 2008;118(5):1645—56.

[18] Tang J, Yan H, Zhuang S. Inflammation and oxidative stress in obesity-related glomerulopathy. Int J Nephrol 2012;2012:608397.

[19] Bokarewa M, Nagaev I, Dahlberg L, Smith U, Tarkowski A. Resistin, an adipokine with potent proinflammatory properties. J Immunol May 1, 2005;174(9):5789—95.

[20] Zoccali C, Mallamaci F, Tripepi G. Adipose tissue as a source of inflammatory cytokines in health and disease: focus on end-stage renal disease. Kidney Int Suppl May 2003;(84):S65—8.

[21] Cao YL, Wang YX, Wang DF, Meng X, Zhang J. Correlation between omental TNF-alpha protein and plasma PAI-1 in obesity subjects. Int J Cardiol August 29, 2008;128(3):399—405.

[22] Moreno JA, Izquierdo MC, Sanchez-Niño MD, Suarez-Alvarez B, Lopez-Larrea C, Jakubowski A, et al. The inflammatory cytokines TWEAK and TNFÎalpha reduce renal klotho expression through NFkappaB. J Am Soc Nephrol July 2011;22(7):1315—25.

[23] Day RT, Cavaglieri RC, Feliers D. Apelin retards the progression of diabetic nephropathy. Am J Physiol Renal Physiol March 15, 2013;304(6):F788—800.

[24] Pfau D, Bachmann A, Lössner U, Kratzsch J, Blüher M, Stumvoll M, et al. Serum levels of the adipokine chemerin in relation to renal function. Diabetes Care January 2010;33(1):171—3.

[25] Lan HY, Bacher M, Yang N, Mu W, Nikolic-Paterson DJ, Metz C, et al. The pathogenic role of macrophage migration inhibitory factor in immunologically induced kidney disease in the rat. J Exp Med April 21, 1997;185(8):1455—66.

[26] Stadler K, Goldberg IJ, Susztak K. The evolving understanding of the contribution of lipid metabolism to diabetic kidney disease. Curr Diab Rep July 2015;15(7):40.

[27] Sun L, Halaihel N, Zhang W, Rogers T, Levi M. Role of sterol regulatory element-binding protein 1 in regulation of renal lipid metabolism and glomerulosclerosis in diabetes mellitus. J Biol Chem May 24, 2002;277(21):18919—27.

[28] Jiang T, Liebman SE, Lucia MS, Li J, Levi M. Role of altered renal lipid metabolism and the sterol regulatory element binding proteins in the pathogenesis of age-related renal disease. Kidney Int December 2005;68(6):2608—20.

[29] Herman-Edelstein M, Scherzer P, Tobar A, Levi M, Gafter U. Altered renal lipid metabolism and renal lipid accumulation in human diabetic nephropathy. J Lipid Res March 2014;55(3):561—72.

[30] Martinez-Garcia C, Izquierdo A, Velagapudi V, Vivas Y, Velasco I, Campbell M, et al. Accelerated renal disease is associated with the development of metabolic syndrome in a glucolipotoxic mouse model. Dis Model Mech September 2012;5(5):636—48.

[31] Martinez-Garcia C, Izquierdo-Lahuerta A, Vivas Y, Velasco I, Yeo TK, Chen S, et al. Renal lipotoxicity-associated inflammation and insulin resistance affects actin cytoskeleton organization in podocytes. PLoS One November 6, 2015;10(11):e0142291.

[32] Khurana S, Bruggeman LA, Kao HY. Nuclear hormone receptors in podocytes. Cell Biosci 2012;2:33.

[33] Decleves AE, Mathew AV, Cunard R, Sharma K. AMPK mediates the initiation of kidney disease induced by a high-fat diet. J Am Soc Nephrol October 2011;22(10):1846—55.

[33a] Pedraza-Chaverri J, Sánchez-Lozada LG, Osorio-Alonso H, Tapia E, Scholze A. New Pathogenic Concepts and Therapeutic Approaches to Oxidative Stress in Chronic Kidney Disease. Oxidative Medicine and Cellular Longevity 2016;6043601. https://doi.org/10.1155/2016/6043601.

[34] Lucchi L, Iannone A, Bergamini S, Stipo L, Perrone S, Uggeri S, et al. Comparison between hydroperoxides and malondialdehyde as markers of acute oxidative injury during hemodialysis. Artif Organs October 2005;29(10):832—7.

[35] Handelman GJ, Walter MF, Adhikarla R, Gross J, Dallal GE, Levin NW, et al. Elevated plasma F2-isoprostanes in patients on long-term hemodialysis. Kidney Int May 2001;59(5):1960—6.

[36] Chen DQ, Chen H, Chen L, Vaziri ND, Wang M, Li XR, et al. The link between phenotype and fatty acid metabolism in advanced chronic kidney disease. Nephrol Dial Transplant July 1, 2017;32(7):1154−66.

[37] Tayyebi-Khosroshahi H, Houshyar J, Tabrizi A, Vatankhah AM, Razzagi Zonouz N, Dehghan-Hesari R. Effect of omega-3 fatty acid on oxidative stress in patients on hemodialysis. Iran J Kidney Dis October 2010;4(4):322−6.

[38] Schermer B, Benzing T. Lipid−protein interactions along the slit diaphragm of podocytes. JASN 2009;20(3):473−8.

[39] Fornoni A, Sageshima J, Wei C, Merscher-Gomez S, Aguillon-Prada R, Jauregui AN, et al. Rituximab targets podocytes in recurrent focal segmental glomerulosclerosis. Sci Transl Med June 1, 2011;3(85):85ra46.

[40] Pagtalunan ME, Miller PL, Jumping-Eagle S, Nelson RG, Myers BD, FRennke HG, et al. Podocyte loss and progressive glomerular injury in type II diabetes. J Clin Invest January 15, 1997;99(2):342−8.

[41] Lin JS, Susztak K. Podocytes: the weakest link in diabetic kidney disease? Curr Diab Rep May 2016;16(5):45.

[42] Peng F, Wu D, Gao B, ngram AJ, Zhang B, Chorneyko K, et al. RhoA/Rho-kinase contribute to the pathogenesis of diabetic renal disease. Diabetes June 2008;57(6):1683−92.

[43] Furukawa S, Fujita T, Shimabukuro M, Iwaki M, Yamada Y, Nakajima Y, et al. Increased oxidative stress in obesity and its impact on metabolic syndrome. J Clin Invest December 2004;114(12):1752−61.

[44] Szeto HH, Liu S, Soong Y, Alam N, Prusky GT, Seshan SV. Protection of mitochondria prevents high-fat diet-induced glomerulopathy and proximal tubular injury. Kidney Int November 2016;90(5):997−1011.

[45] Li N, Karin M. Is NF-kappaB the sensor of oxidative stress? FASEB J July 1999;13(10):1137−43.

[46] Schreck R, Rieber P, Baeuerle PA. Reactive oxygen intermediates as apparently widely used messengers in the activation of the NF-kappa B transcription factor and HIV-1. EMBO J August 1991;10(8):2247−58.

[47] Kisic B, Miric D, Dragojevic I, Rasic J, Popovic L. Role of myeloperoxidase in patients with chronic kidney disease. Oxid Med Cell Longev 2016;2016:1069743.

[47a] Lehners A, Lange S, Niemann G, Rosendahl A, Meyer-Schwesinger C, Oh J, StahlR Ehmke H, Benndorf R, Klinke A, Baldus S, Wenzel UO. Myeloperoxidase deficiencyameliorates progression of chronic kidney disease in mice. Am J Physiol RenalPhysiol August 15, 2014;307(4):F407−17. https://doi.org/10.1152/ajprenal.00262.2014.

[48] Madhusudhana Rao A, Anand U, Anand CV. Myeloperoxidase in chronic kidney disease. Indian J Clin Biochem January 2011;26(1):28−31.

[49] Malhotra JD, Kaufman RJ. Endoplasmic reticulum stress and oxidative stress: a vicious cycle or a double-edged sword? Antioxid Redox Signal December 2007;9(12):2277−93.

[50] Chinta SJ, Rane A, Poksay KS, Bredesen DE, Andersen JK, Rao RV. Coupling endoplasmic reticulum stress to the cell death program in dopaminergic cells: effect of paraquat. NeuroMolecular Med 2008;10(4):333−42.

[51] Li C, Lin Y, Luo R, Chen S, Wang F, Zheng P, et al. Intrarenal renin-angiotensin system mediates fatty acid-induced ER stress in the kidney. Am J Physiol Renal Physiol March 1, 2016;310(5):F351−63.

[52] Sieber J, Lindenmeyer MT, Kampe K, Campbell KN, Cohen CD, Hopfer H, et al. Regulation of podocyte survival and endoplasmic reticulum stress by fatty acids. Am J Physiol Renal Physiol October 2010;299(4):F821−9.

[53] Sureshbabu A, Ryter SW, Choi ME. Oxidative stress and autophagy: crucial modulators of kidney injury. Redox Biol April 2015;4:208−14.

[54] Wang Y, Nartiss Y, Steipe B, McQuibban GA, Kim PK. ROS-induced mitochondrial depolarization initiates PARK2/PARKIN-dependent mitochondrial degradation by autophagy. Autophagy October 2012;8(10):1462−76.

[55] Ding Y, Sl K, Lee SY, Koo JK, Wang Z, Choi ME. Autophagy regulates TGF-beta expression and suppresses kidney fibrosis induced by unilateral ureteral obstruction. J Am Soc Nephrol December 2014;25(12):2835−46.

[56] Kawakami T, Gomez IG, Ren S, Hudkins K, Roach A, Alpers CE, et al. Deficient autophagy results in mitochondrial dysfunction and FSGS. J Am Soc Nephrol May 2015;26(5):1040−52.

[57] Chen Y, McMillan-Ward E, Kong J, Israels SJ, Gibson SB. Mitochondrial electron-transport-chain inhibitors of complexes I and II induce autophagic cell death mediated by reactive oxygen species. J Cell Sci December 1, 2007;120(Pt 23):4155−66.

[58] Meng XM, Wang S, Huang XR, Yang C, Xiao J, Zhang Y, et al. Inflammatory macrophages can transdifferentiate into myofibroblasts during renal fibrosis. Cell Death Dis December 2016;7(12):e2495.

[59] Iglesias-De La Cruz MC, Ruiz-Torres P, Alcami J, Diez-Marques L, Ortega-Velazquez R, Chen S, et al. Hydrogen peroxide increases extracellular matrix mRNA through TGF-beta in human mesangial cells. Kidney Int January 2001;59(1):87−95.

[60] Hou X, Shen YH, Li C, Wang F, Zhang C, Bu P, et al. PPARalpha agonist fenofibrate protects the kidney from hypertensive injury in spontaneously hypertensive rats via inhibition of oxidative stress and MAPK activity. Biochem Biophys Res Commun April 9, 2010;394(3):653−9.

[61] An WS, Kim HJ, Cho KH, Vaziri ND. Omega-3 fatty acid supplementation attenuates oxidative stress, inflammation, and tubulointerstitial fibrosis in the remnant kidney. Am J Physiol Renal Physiol October 2009;297(4):F895−903.

[62] D'Agati VD, Markowitz GS. Supersized kidneys: lessons from the preclinical obese kidney. Kidney Int April 2008;73(8):909−10.

[63] Vallon V, Richter K, Blantz RC, Thomson S, Osswald H. Glomerular hyperfiltration in experimental diabetes mellitus: potential role of tubular reabsorption. J Am Soc Nephrol December 1999;10(12):2569−76.

[64] Eckel RH, Grundy SM, Zimmet PZ. The metabolic syndrome. Lancet April 16−22, 2005;365(9468):1415−28.

[65] Chavez JA, Summers SA. Lipid oversupply, selective insulin resistance, and lipotoxicity: molecular mechanisms. Biochim Biophys Acta March 2010;1801(3):252−65.

[66] Coward R, Fornoni A. Insulin signaling: implications for podocyte biology in diabetic kidney disease. Curr Opin Nephrol Hypertens January 2015;24(1):104−10.

[67] Welsh GI, Hale LJ, Eremina V, Jeansson M, Maezawa Y, Lennon R, et al. Insulin signaling to the glomerular podocyte is critical for normal kidney function. Cell Metab October 6, 2010;12(4):329−40.

[68] Meyer C, Stumvoll M, Dostou J, Welle S, Haymond M, Gerich J. Renal substrate exchange and gluconeogenesis in normal postabsorptive humans. Am J Physiol Endocrinol Metab February 2002;282(2):E428−34.

[69] Mogensen CE. Maximum tubular reabsorption capacity for glucose and renal hemodynamcis during rapid hypertonic glucose infusion in normal and diabetic subjects. Scand J Clin Lab Invest September 1971;28(1):101−9.

[70] Susztak K, Raff AC, Schiffer M, Bottinger EP. Glucose-induced reactive oxygen species cause apoptosis of podocytes and podocyte depletion at the onset of diabetic nephropathy. Diabetes January 2006;55(1):225−33.

[71] Himmelfarb J. Linking oxidative stress and inflammation in kidney disease: which is the chicken and which is the egg? Semin Dial 2004 ;17(6):449−54.

[72] Heitzer T, Schlinzig T, Krohn K, Meinertz T, Munzel T. Endothelial dysfunction, oxidative stress, and risk of cardiovascular events in patients with coronary artery disease. Circulation November 27, 2001;104(22):2673−8.

[73] Labarrere CA, Zaloga GP. C-reactive protein: from innocent bystander to pivotal mediator of atherosclerosis. Am J Med October 1, 2004;117(7):499−507.

[73a] Kisic B, Miric D, Dragojevic I, Rasic J, Popovic L. Role of myeloperoxidase in patients with chronic kidney disease. Oxid Med Cell Longev 2016;2016:1069743.

[74] Mahalingaiah PK, Ponnusamy L, Singh KP. Chronic oxidative stress leads to malignant transformation along with acquisition of stem cell characteristics, and epithelial to mesenchymal transition in human renal epithelial cells. J Cell Physiol August 2015;230(8):1916−28.

[75] Reuter S, Gupta SC, Chaturvedi MM, Aggarwal BB. Oxidative stress, inflammation, and cancer: how are they linked? Free Radic Biol Med December 1, 2010;49(11):1603−16.

[76] Gago-Dominguez M, Castelao JE. Lipid peroxidation and renal cell carcinoma: further supportive evidence and new mechanistic insights. Free Radic Biol Med February 15, 2006;40(4):721−33.

[77] Kellerer M, von Eye Corleta H, Mühlhöfer A, Capp E, Mosthaf L, Bock S, et al. Insulin-and insulin-like growth-factor-I receptor tyrosine-kinase activities in human renal carcinoma. Int J Cancer 1995;62(5):501−7.

[78] Dounousi E, Papavasiliou E, Makedou A, Ioannou K, Katopodis KP, Tselepis A, et al. Oxidative stress is progressively enhanced with advancing stages of CKD. Am J Kidney Dis November 2006;48(5):752−60.

[79] Witko-Sarsat V, Descamps-Latscha B. Advanced oxidation protein products: novel uraemic toxins and pro-inflammatory mediators in chronic renal failure? Nephrol Dial Transplant July 1997;12(7):1310−2.

[80] Dalle-Donne I, Rossi R, Giustarini D, Milzani A, Colombo R. Protein carbonyl groups as biomarkers of oxidative stress. Clin Chim Acta March 2003;329(1−2):23−38.

[81] Handelman G. Evaluation of oxidant stress in dialysis patients. Blood Purif 2000;18:343−9.

[82] Ari E, Kaya Y, Demir H, Cebi A, Alp HH, Bakan E, et al. Oxidative DNA damage correlates with carotid artery atherosclerosis in hemodialysis patients. Hemodial Int October 2011;15(4):453−9.

[83] Johnson-Davis KL, Fernelius C, Eliason NB, Wilson A, Beddhu S, Roberts WL. Blood enzymes and oxidative stress in chronic kidney disease: a cross sectional study. Ann Clin Lab Sci 2011;41(4):331−9.

[84] Postorino M, Marino C, Tripepi G, Zoccali C. Gammaglutamyltransferase in ESRD as a predictor of all-cause and cardiovascular mortality: another facet of oxidative stress burden. Kidney Int Suppl December 2008;(111):S64−6.

[85] Roehrs M, Valentini J, Paniz C, Moro A, Charão M, Bulcão R, et al. The relationships between exogenous and endogenous antioxidants with the lipid profile and oxidative damage in hemodialysis patients. BMC Nephrol 2011;12:59.

[86] Wang S, Eide TC, Sogn EM, Berg KJ, Sund RB. Plasma ascorbic acid in patients undergoing chronic haemodialysis. Eur J Clin Pharmacol September 1999;55(7):527−32.

[87] Deicher R, Ziai F, Bieglmayer C, Schillinger M, Horl WH. Low total vitamin C plasma level is a risk factor for cardiovascular morbidity and mortality in hemodialysis patients. J Am Soc Nephrol June 2005;16(6):1811−8.

[88] Aminzadeh MA, Vaziri ND. Downregulation of the renal and hepatic hydrogen sulfide (H2S)-producing enzymes and capacity in chronic kidney disease. Nephrol Dial Transplant February 2012;27(2):498−504.

[89] Takayama F, Tsutsui S, Horie M, Shimokata K, Niwa T. Glutathionyl hemoglobin in uremic patients undergoing hemodialysis and continuous ambulatory peritoneal dialysis. Kidney Int February 2001;59:S155−8.

[90] Baylis C. Arginine, arginine analogs and nitric oxide production in chronic kidney disease. Nat Clin Pract Nephrol April 2006;2(4):209−20.

[91] Pawlak K, Domaniewski T, Mysliwiec M, FPawlak D. The kynurenines are associated with oxidative stress, inflammation and the prevalence of cardiovascular disease in patients with end-stage renal disease. Atherosclerosis May 2009;204(1):309−14.

[92] Bayrasheva VK, Babenko AY, Dobronravov VA, Dmitriev YV, Chefu SG, Pchelin IY, et al. Uninephrectomized high-fat-fed nicotinamide-streptozotocin-induced diabetic rats: a model for the investigation of diabetic nephropathy in type 2 diabetes. J Diabetes Res 2016;2016:8317850.

[93] Maddox DA, Alavi FK, Santella RN, Zawada Jr ET. Prevention of obesity-linked renal disease: age-dependent effects of dietary food restriction. Kidney Int July 2002;62(1):208−19.

[94] Navaneethan SD, Malin SK, Arrigain S, Kashyap SR, Kirwan JP, Schauer PR. Bariatric surgery, kidney function, insulin resistance, and adipokines in patients with decreased GFR: a cohort study. Am J Kidney Dis February 2015;65(2):345−7.

[95] Huan Y, Tomaszewski JE, Cohen DL. Resolution of nephrotic syndrome after successful bariatric surgery in patient with biopsy-proven FSGS. Clin Nephrol January 2009;71(1):69—73.

[96] Chang AR, Grams ME, Navaneethan SD. Bariatric surgery and kidney-related outcomes. Kidney Int Rep March 2017;2(2):261—70.

[97] Carobbio S, Pellegrinelli V, Vidal-Puig A. Adipose tissue function and expandability as determinants of lipotoxicity and the metabolic syndrome. Adv Exp Med Biol 2017;960:161—96.

[98] Arora MK, Reddy K, Balakumar P. The low dose combination of fenofibrate and rosiglitazone halts the progression of diabetes-induced experimental nephropathy. Eur J Pharmacol June 25, 2010;636(1—3):137—44.

[99] Medina-Gomez G, Gray SL, Yetukuri L, Shimomura K, Virtue S, Campbell M, et al. PPAR gamma 2 prevents lipotoxicity by controlling adipose tissue expandability and peripheral lipid metabolism. PLoS Genet April 27, 2007;3(4):e64.

[100] Agrawal R, Jain P, Dikshit SN. Balaglitazone: a second generation peroxisome proliferator-activated receptor (PPAR) gamma (gamma) agonist. Mini Rev Med Chem February 2012;12(2):87—97.

[101] Castilla P, Davalos A, Teruel JL, Cerrato F, Fernandez-Lucas M, Merino JL, et al. Comparative effects of dietary supplementation with red grape juice and vitamin E on production of superoxide by circulating neutrophil NADPH oxidase in hemodialysis patients. Am J Clin Nutr April 2008;87(4):1053—61.

[102] Safa J, Argani H, Bastani B, Nezami N, Rahimi Ardebili B, Ghorbanihaghjo A, et al. Protective effect of grape seed extract on gentamicin-induced acute kidney injury. Iran J Kidney Dis October 2010;4(4):285—91.

[103] Amin KA, Kamel HH, Abd Eltawab MA. Protective effect of garcinia against renal oxidative stress and biomarkers induced by high fat and sucrose diet. Lipids Health Dis January 14, 2011;10:6.

[104] Liu CM, Ma JQ, Sun YZ. Quercetin protects the rat kidney against oxidative stress-mediated DNA damage and apoptosis induced by lead. Environ Toxicol Pharmacol November 2010;30(3):264—71.

[105] Roozbeh J, Shahriyari B, Akmali M, Vessal G, Pakfetrat M, Raees Jalali GA, et al. Comparative effects of silymarin and vitamin E supplementation on oxidative stress markers, and hemoglobin levels among patients on hemodialysis. Ren Fail 2011;33(2):118—23.

[106] Yu S, Paetau-Robinson I. Dietary supplements of vitamins E and C and beta-carotene reduce oxidative stress in cats with renal insufficiency. Vet Res Commun May 2006;30(4):403—13 (0165-7380 (Print); 0165-7380 (Linking)).

[107] Ramos R, Martinez-Castelao A. Lipoperoxidation and hemodialysis. Metabolism October 2008;57(10):1369—74.

[108] Sato M, Matsumoto Y, Morita H, Takemura H, Shimoi K, Amano I. Effects of vitamin supplementation on microcirculatory disturbance in hemodialysis patients without peripheral arterial disease. Clin Nephrol July 2003;60(1):28—34.

[109] Boudouris G, Verginadis II, Simos YV, Zouridakis A, Ragos V, SCh K, et al. Oxidative stress in patients treated with continuous ambulatory peritoneal dialysis (CAPD) and the significant role of vitamin C and E supplementation. Int Urol Nephrol August 2013;45(4):1137—44.

[110] Takouli L, Hadjiyannakos D, Metaxaki P, Sideris V, Filiopoulos V, Anogiati A, et al. Vitamin E-coated cellulose acetate dialysis membrane: long-term effect on inflammation and oxidative stress. Ren Fail January 2010;32(3):287—93.

[111] Hsu SP, Chiang CK, Yang SY, Chien CT. N-acetylcysteine for the management of anemia and oxidative stress in hemodialysis patients. Nephron Clin Pract 2010;116(3):c207—16.

[112] Fatouros IG, Douroudos I, Panagoutsos S, Pasadakis P, Nikolaidis MG, Chatzinikolaou A, et al. Effects of L-carnitine on oxidative stress responses in patients with renal disease. Med Sci Sports Exerc October 2010;42(10):1809—18.

[113] Sakata T, Furuya R, Shimazu T, Odamaki M, Ohkawa S, Kumagai H. Coenzyme Q10 administration suppresses both oxidative and antioxidative markers in hemodialysis patients. Blood Purif 2008;26(4):371—8.

[114] Chiarello PG, Vannucchi MT, Moyses Neto M, Vannucchi H. Hyperhomocysteinemia and oxidative stress in hemodialysis: effects of supplementation with folic acid. Int J Vitam Nutr Res November 2003;73(6):431—8.

[115] Cachofeiro V, Goicochea M, de Vinuesa SG, Oubina P, Lahera V, Luno J. Oxidative stress and inflammation, a link between chronic kidney disease and cardiovascular disease. Kidney Int Suppl December 2008;(111):S4—9.

[116] Mastalerz-Migas A, Reksa D, Pokorski M, Steciwko A, Muszynska A, Bunio A, et al. Comparison of a statin vs. hypolipemic diet on the oxidant status in hemodialyzed patients with chronic renal failure. J Physiol Pharmacol November 2007;58(Suppl. 5(Pt 1):363—70.

[117] Dubois F, Belleville F. Selenium: physiologic role and value in human pathology. Pathol Biol 1988;36:1017—25.

[118] Bellisola G, Perona G, Galassini S, Moschini G, Guidi GC. Plasma selenium and glutathione peroxidase activities in individuals living in the Veneto region of Italy. J Trace Elem Electrolytes Health Dis December 1993;7(4):242—4.

[119] Zachara BA, Gromadzinska J, Palus J, Zbrog Z, Swiech R, Twardowska E, et al. The effect of selenium supplementation in the prevention of DNA damage in white blood cells of hemodialyzed patients: a pilot study. Biol Trace Elem Res September 2011;142(3):274—83.

[120] Guo CH, Chen PC, Hsu GS, Wang CL. Zinc supplementation alters plasma aluminum and selenium status of patients undergoing dialysis: a pilot study. Nutrients April 22, 2013;5(4):1456—70.

[121] Chander PN, Gealekman O, Brodsky SV, Elitok S, Tojo A, Crabtree M, et al. Nephropathy in Zucker diabetic fat rat is associated with oxidative and nitrosative stress: prevention by chronic therapy with a peroxynitrite scavenger ebselen. J Am Soc Nephrol September 2004;15(9):2391—403.

[122] Krysztopik RJ, Bentley FR, Spain DA, Wilson MA, Garrison RN. Free radical scavenging by lazaroids improves renal blood flow during sepsis. Surgery October 1996;120(4):657—62.

[123] Tomiyama-Hanayama M, Rakugi H, Kohara M, Mima T, Adachi Y, Ohishi M, et al. Effect of interleukin-6 receptor blockage on renal injury in apolipoprotein E-deficient mice. Am J Physiol 2009;297(3):679—84.

[124] Venegas-Pont M, Manigrasso MB, Grifoni SC, LaMarca BB, Maric C, Racusen LC, et al. Tumor necrosis factor-alpha antagonist etanercept decreases blood pressure and protects the kidney in a mouse model of systemic lupus erythematosus. Hypertension October 2010;56(4):643−9.

[125] Sozer V, Guntas G, Konukoglu D, Dervisoglu E, Gelisgen R, Tabak O, et al. Effects of peritoneal-and hemodialysis on levels of plasma protein and lipid oxidation markers in diabetic patients. Minerva Med 2013;104(84):75−84.

[126] Islam KN, O'Byrne D, Devaraj S, Palmer B, Grundy SM, Jialal I. Alpha-tocopherol supplementation decreases the oxidative susceptibility of LDL in renal failure patients on dialysis therapy. Atherosclerosis May 2000;150(1):217−24.

[127] Kerr P, Huang L. Review: membranes for haemodialysis. Nephrology 2010;15(4):381−5.

[128] Levin A, Tonelli M, Bonventre J, Coresh J, Donner JA, Fogo AB, et al. Global kidney health 2017 and beyond: a roadmap for closing gaps in care, research, and policy. Lancet October 21, 2017;390(10105):1888−917.

Chapter 8

Inflammatory and Oxidative Stress Markers in Skeletal Muscle of Obese Subjects

Victoria Catalán[1,2,3], Gema Frühbeck[1,2,3] and Javier Gómez-Ambrosi[1,2,3]
[1]Clínica Universidad de Navarra, Pamplona, Spain; [2]Centro de Investigación Biomédica en Red-Fisiopatología de la Obesidad y Nutrición (CIBEROBN), Instituto de Salud Carlos III, Pamplona, Spain; [3]Instituto de Investigación Sanitaria de Navarra (IdiSNA), Pamplona, Spain

1. INTRODUCTION

Obesity has become one of the leading causes of death and disability in recent decades, threatening many of the health achievements of the past century. The World Health Organization estimates that over 1 billion people are overweight worldwide, of whom 300 million are obese. It has also declared obesity to be the major chronic health problem among adults, saying its relevance will outstrip malnutrition globally [1]. Despite the alarm and the progress made in understanding the disease, the pandemic continues to grow unstoppably [2]. Obesity is considered a serious public health problem associated with high morbidity and mortality due to comorbidities such as type 2 diabetes, cardiovascular diseases, stroke, hypertension, hyperlipidemia, steatohepatitis, and several types of cancer, among other illnesses [1].

There has been epidemiological evidence for decades of a relationship between obesity and a proinflammatory status. However, until few years ago no pathophysiological link had been established to demonstrate that excess adipose tissue triggers chronic inflammation [3,4]. The classic concept of inflammation refers to the body's response to infection or injury, characterized by swelling, flushing, pain, and fever, which aims to restore homeostasis [5]. In general the inflammatory response is considered to be beneficial, providing, for example, protection against infection, but if it is not resolved, uncontrolled chronic inflammation may be detrimental, providing no survival advantage to the individual [6]. Obesity is frequently accompanied by inflammation, considered as low-grade chronic inflammation or para-inflammation, which has not to date been found to produce a positive counterpart. This inflammation differs from classical inflammation in that it does not present the described signs, but is similar in that it shares the alterations in typical inflammatory mediators and signaling pathways [5]. Some authors consider that pathologies presenting with low-grade chronic inflammation and not due to infection or tissue damage could be due to environmental changes that were not present at the dawn of human evolution, such as nutrient excess, exposure to certain toxic compounds, and aging [7].

The low-grade chronic inflammation that accompanies obesity becomes apparent at the circulating level in an increase in classical inflammatory markers such as C-reactive protein, tumor necrosis factor-α (TNF-α), and fibrinogen [8,9]. In the proinflammatory state associated with obesity, the expansion of adipose tissue plays a determining role. One of the processes that take place in inflamed adipose tissue is infiltration of cells of the immune system, such as leukocytes and macrophages. The adipocyte hypertrophy that occurs in obesity leads to an increase in the production of chemokines and cytokines by adipocytes and other cells present in the adipose tissue (stromovascular fraction). The increased accumulation of immune cells in adipose tissue plays a key role in increasing mediators of inflammation, which together with the elevated oxidative stress, hypoxia, and altered lipolysis will affect metabolic homeostasis. Thus as adipose tissue increases, the production of adipokines is modified and a series of pathophysiological processes related to inflammation are triggered, leading to an increased risk of cardiovascular disease, type 2 diabetes, and cancer, among other comorbidities [10].

Obesity. https://doi.org/10.1016/B978-0-12-812504-5.00008-8

The trigger for obesity-associated low-grade chronic inflammation in skeletal muscle is not clear but could emanate from the gut, from a nutrient or metabolite, or, more probably, from the expanding and inflamed adipose tissue. Several intrinsic signals trigger inflammation in adipose tissue, including adipocyte death, hypoxia, and mechanotransduction coming from interactions between the cells and the extracellular matrix [11].

On the other hand, obesity involves high levels of circulating glucose and lipids, which can result in an excessive supply of energy substrates to metabolic pathways. This oversupply of nutrients may in turn increase the production of reactive oxygen species (ROS), promoting oxidative stress and subsequent oxidative cellular damage [12]. Several redox species have an impact on oxidative stress. ROS are chemically reactive molecules containing oxygen, including superoxide anion radical ($O_2^{-\cdot}$), hydroxyl radical ($^{\bullet}OH$), and hydrogen peroxide (H_2O_2), among others [13,14]. In addition to ROS, other relevant reactive species may have an impact on oxidative stress, including for example reactive nitrogen species, reactive sulphur species, and reactive carbonyl species [14]. ROS have extremely short half-lives, making direct measurement of ROS and other reactive species costly and laborious. For that reason, simpler determinations that quantify biomarkers or end products are used to estimate oxidative stress [13]. For example, thiobarbituric acid reactive substances (TBARS) or F2-isoprostanes may be used as estimators of lipid peroxidation. Another measure of oxidative stress comes from the study of antioxidant enzymes, which are defense systems against the excessive accumulation of ROS. Superoxide dismutase (SOD), catalase, and glutathione peroxidase (GPx) are the most frequently studied. Finally, nonenzymatic antioxidant defenses against ROS accumulation, such as vitamins E and C, β-carotene, α-lipoic acid, or the total antioxidant status, are also frequently used to study oxidative stress [12−14].

2. INFLAMMATORY MARKERS IN SKELETAL MUSCLE IN OBESITY

Although the obesity-associated proinflammatory condition has been traditionally associated with inflammation of the adipose tissue, a considerable amount of evidence indicates that myocytes in skeletal muscle may also show signs of inflammation. As depicted in Fig. 8.1, skeletal muscle expresses and secretes a large number of cytokines and other molecules, collectively called myokines, that together with infiltrated immune cells regulate the skeletal muscle obesity-associated inflammation [15,16] (Table 8.1).

2.1 Tumor Necrosis Factor-α

TNF-α is a cytokine involved in the metabolic disturbances of chronic inflammation, and has a major role in the development of insulin resistance. Although adipose tissue is a major source of TNF-α, expression of this proinflammatory

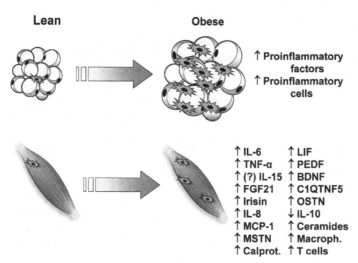

FIGURE 8.1 Obesity-associated changes in markers of inflammation in skeletal muscle. With the expansion of adipose tissue the expression and release of several proteins and lipid molecules in adipose tissue and skeletal muscle are altered. Moreover, some immune cells will be recruited, playing an important role in the regulation of immunometabolism. These molecules have an autocrine or paracrine effect, and many of them are secreted, playing an endocrine role as well. A complex cross-talk between skeletal muscle and adipose tissue, and with other organs such as liver, pancreas, heart, and brain, is established, exerting important influences on insulin sensitivity and other major physiological functions. The changes that take place in adipose tissue have been simplified. *BDNF*, brain-derived neurotrophic factor; *C1QTNF5*, C1q and tumor necrosis factor related protein 5; *Calprot.*, calprotectin; *FGF21*, fibroblast growth factor 21; *FNDC5*, fibronectin type III domain-containing protein 5; *IL*, interleukin; *LIF*, leukemia inhibitory factor; *Macroph.*, macrophages; *MCP-1*, chemotactic protein 1; *MSTN*, myostatin; *OSTN*, osteocrin; *PEDF*, pigment epithelium-derived factor; *TNF-α*, tumor necrosis factor-α.

TABLE 8.1 Major Factors Involved in Inflammation in Skeletal Muscle in Obesity

Factor or Cell Type	Role	References
BDNF	Favors the survival of neurons. Regulates positively skeletal muscle regeneration. Exerts antiinflammatory actions.	[50,51,53]
C1QTNF5	Promotes FFA uptake by adipocytes and hepatocytes. Potential antiinflammatory actions.	[54,55]
Calprotectin	Recruitment of monocytes to the site of inflammation.	[46,47]
Ceramides	Lipid molecules, composed of sphingosine and a fatty acid, involved in the regulation of inflammation. Involved also in the regulation of insulin resistance and increased in the skeletal muscle of obese humans.	[68,69,71]
FGF21	Major regulator of energy homeostasis. Secreted by skeletal muscle, in particular under stress conditions. Exerts antiinflammatory actions, inhibiting NF-κB.	[32,35]
IL-10	Exerts antiinflammatory actions. Protects from TNF-α-induced insulin resistance.	[31]
IL-15	Regulates skeletal muscle and adipose tissue mass. Mediates the positive effects of physical activity. Apparent proinflammatory effect, although its exact role in obesity-associated inflammation is not clear.	[15,26]
IL-6	Increases glucose utilization and fatty acid oxidation. Lipolytic factor in skeletal muscle. Unclear role in the development of insulin resistance and may exert proinflammatory as well as antiinflammatory effects.	[15,16,20,24]
IL-8	Neutrophil chemotactic factor. Potent inducer of angiogenesis. Major mediator of the inflammatory response.	[15,16]
Irisin (FNDC5)	Promotes mitochondrial biogenesis in myocytes. Induces the browning of white adipose tissue. Exhibits antiinflammatory properties.	[36,39]
LIF	Induces skeletal muscle cell proliferation. Inhibitor of inflammation.	[48,49]
Macrophages	Proinflammatory actions. Involved in the recruitment of other proinflammatory cells.	[16,74]
MCP-1	Promotes macrophage and T lymphocyte infiltration. Plays a clear proinflammatory role. Seems to be necessary for skeletal muscle regeneration.	[33]
MSTN	Regulates skeletal muscle and adipose tissue mass. Triggers inflammation in skeletal muscle.	[15,44]
OSTN	Enhances physical endurance. Expression increased by proinflammatory stimulus.	[64,67]
PEDF	Plays a major role in organogenesis and homoeostasis of adult tissues. Antiangiogenic and antifibrotic effect. Induces the proliferation of skeletal muscle cells. Activates several proinflammatory signaling proteins such as JNK and NF-κB in skeletal muscle.	[59–61]
T cells	Proinflammatory effects (T_H1 and $CD8^+$ T cells). Antiinflammatory actions (T_{reg} cells).	[16,72]
TNF-α	Major proinflammatory factor. Involved in the development of obesity-associated insulin resistance.	[17]

BDNF, brain-derived neurotrophic factor; *C1QTNF5*, C1q and tumor necrosis factor related protein 5; *FFA*, free fatty acid; *FGF21*, fibroblast growth factor 21; *FNDC5*, fibronectin type III domain containing protein 5; *IL*, interleukin; *JNK*, c-Jun N-terminal kinase; *LIF*, leukemia inhibitory factor; *MCP-1*, monocyte chemotactic protein 1; *MSTN*, myostatin; *NF-κB*, nuclear factor-κB; *OSTN*, osteocrin; *PEDF*, pigment epithelium-derived factor; *TNF-α*, tumor necrosis factor-α.

molecule is increased in skeletal muscle in obesity [17]. It seems that TNF-α is critical for the macrophage classical M1 proinflammatory polarization in skeletal muscle. Moreover, TNF-α induces inflammation through the activation of the IκB kinase/nuclear factor-κB (NF-κB) and c-Jun N-terminal kinase (JNK) pathways [16].

2.2 Interleukin-6

Interleukin-6 (IL-6) was the first myokine identified and is the best studied. It is released by skeletal muscle and its serum concentrations may increase up to 100-fold in response to physical exercise. IL-6 exerts pleiotropic actions on a variety of tissues, including stimulation of acute-phase protein synthesis and regulation of glucose and lipid metabolism [15,18]. IL-6 activates AMP-activated protein kinase (AMPK) and phosphatidylinositol-3-kinase (PI3K) in an autocrine fashion within the skeletal muscle to increase glucose utilization and fatty acid oxidation, but at the same time may increase hepatic glucose production and induce insulin resistance under chronic overproduction, as is the case in obesity [19]. It is also considered a lipolytic factor, although at physiological concentrations it triggers lipolysis in skeletal muscle without affecting adipose tissue. Although increased levels of IL-6 have been observed in obese patients, it exerts antiobesity effects centrally by increasing energy expenditure. Mice lacking IL-6 exhibit adult-onset obesity, although the exact role of IL-6 in metabolism remains unclear [20]. IL-6 has been considered traditionally as exerting proinflammatory effects. Its expression is increased in the skeletal muscle of obese individuals [21], and is also stimulated in response to palmitic acid in human myotubes promoting inflammation in skeletal muscle [22]. However, in recent years the proinflammatory effect of IL-6 has been questioned by studies showing, for example, that IL-6 signaling suppresses hepatic inflammation [20,23] through promoting alternative M2 activation of macrophages [24].

2.3 Interleukin-15

IL-15 is an anabolic factor for skeletal muscle which belongs to the IL-2 superfamily involved in the skeletal muscle—adipose tissue cross-talk. Besides its role in the regulation of skeletal muscle mass, it has been shown that IL-15 may regulate adipose tissue mass in humans [25]. IL-15 is believed to be secreted after exercise and to participate in the positive effects of physical activity. In this sense, IL-15 may be involved in the physical-activity-induced shift of skeletal muscle toward a more oxidative pattern.

IL-15 is generally considered a proinflammatory cytokine which plays a major role in chronic inflammation by the stimulation of T-lymphocyte recruitment and growth. However, paradoxically, a previous study has shown that the physical-activity-induced production of IL-15 may help to reduce or even suppress the negative effects of TNF-α in diabetic subjects with low-grade chronic systemic inflammation [26]. Moreover, it has been suggested that IL-15 deficiency confers resistance to obesity by reducing inflammation in adipose tissue, although other studies have suggested that IL-15 administration promotes resistance to obesity induced by a high-fat diet and fatty liver, and improves glucose homeostasis [27]. More studies are needed to clarify the role of IL-15 in energy metabolism and the regulation of obesity-associated inflammation.

2.4 Interleukin-8

IL-8 or chemokine (C-X-C motif) ligand 8 (CXCL8) is a member of the CXC chemokine family. It is produced by several cell types, such as macrophages and epithelial and endothelial cells, but also by skeletal muscle and cultured myotubes [15]. Skeletal muscle IL-8 expression is induced after physical activity, but the increase in its expression is even higher in the liver. IL-8 is also known as neutrophil chemotactic factor since it is involved in the chemotaxis of neutrophils to the site of infection or inflammation and is also known to be a potent inducer of angiogenesis [16]. The circulating concentrations of IL-8 are significantly increased in obese subjects [28,29]. This chemokine is one of the major mediators of the inflammatory response. IL-8 expression is induced by ROS, causing the recruitment of proinflammatory cells and promoting a further increase in oxidative stress. The exact role of IL-8 in obesity-associated inflammation still has to be determined.

2.5 Interleukin-10

IL-10 is a class 2 cytokine expressed primarily in monocytes and to a lesser extent in lymphocytes. IL-10 exerts antiinflammatory actions and plays a major role in inflammatory diseases, repressing proinflammatory responses and limiting unnecessary tissue damage caused by inflammation [30]. It downregulates the expression of Th1 cytokines, enhances B cell survival, inhibits NF-κB activity, and protects from TNF-α-induced insulin resistance. Circulating levels of IL-10 protect against the development of type 2 diabetes and hepatic steatosis, and are decreased in obesity. It has been reported that IL-10 is also expressed in skeletal muscle, and blood levels are increased after physical activity [31].

2.6 Fibroblast Growth Factor 21

Fibroblast growth factor 21 (FGF21) is a pleiotropic hormone considered as a major regulator of energy homeostasis. FGF21 is mainly secreted by the liver, but it may also be expressed in skeletal muscle [32]. In this sense, FGF21 protein expression is induced by insulin in C2C12 myocytes, and FGF21 mRNA is upregulated by hyperinsulinemia in skeletal muscle in young healthy men [33]. Moreover, it has been suggested that FGF21 is a signal secreted by the skeletal muscle to communicate with adipose tissue under stress conditions [34]. FGF21 has been shown to be a major regulator of hepatic lipid metabolism, with FGF21 overexpressing mice being resistant to diet-induced obesity. Interestingly, recent studies suggest that FGF21 may exert antiinflammatory actions in the pancreas, heart, and skeletal muscle. A reduction in the JNK and NF-κB signaling pathways has been proposed as the potential mechanism implicated in the FGF21 antiinflammatory effects [35].

2.7 Irisin

Irisin is a myokine released into the bloodstream by cleavage of the fibronectin type III domain-containing protein 5 (FNDC5) triggered by muscle contraction. The expression of FNDC5 is under the control of the peroxisome proliferator-activated receptor γ coactivator 1-α, a master regulator of genes involved in metabolism. In this sense, irisin promotes mitochondrial biogenesis in myocytes, and also induces the browning of white adipose tissue [36,37]. Moreover, irisin increases the metabolic rate of adipocytes and myocytes. Several studies have shown that irisin possesses protective properties against obesity, insulin resistance, and nonalcoholic fatty liver disease, showing in some of these metabolic alterations a correlation with inflammatory markers, which suggests that irisin may regulate the inflammatory response. Interestingly, a direct role as regulator of inflammation in skeletal muscle has not been analyzed, although irisin does not seem to activate NF-κB in myocytes [38]. Irisin exhibits antiinflammatory properties via the downregulation of toll-like receptor 4 (TLR4)/myeloid differentiation primary response 88 in macrophages [39], and reduces the expression of inflammatory genes via inhibiting the p38 mitogen-activated protein kinase (p38 MAPK)/NF-κB in endothelial cells [40]. Furthermore, irisin reduces oxidative stress in macrophages and endothelial cells [40,41].

2.8 Monocyte Chemotactic Protein-1

The monocyte chemotactic protein-1 (MCP-1), also known as C−C motif chemokine ligand 2 (CCL2), is a chemokine involved in immunoregulatory and inflammatory processes. MCP-1 signals through chemokine CC motif receptor 2 (CCR2) that is expressed in macrophages, adipocytes, and skeletal muscle cells. MCP-1 mRNA in skeletal muscle and circulating levels of MCP-1 increase after a bout of exercise [33]. MCP-1 has been reported to promote macrophage and T lymphocyte infiltration after tissue injury, and therefore MCP-1 colocalizes with infiltrated macrophages in skeletal muscle biopsies. The circulating levels of MCP-1 are increased in obese subjects [29]. MCP-1 plays a clear proinflammatory role in skeletal muscle, since specific muscular overexpression of MCP-1 in mice increases the expression of IL-1β and the macrophage markers F4/80 and CD68 in the gastrocnemius muscle [42]. On the other hand, MCP-1 seems to be necessary for skeletal muscle reparative processes and MCP-1-deficient mice show impaired skeletal muscle regeneration [43].

2.9 Myostatin

Myostatin (MSTN) is a secreted member of the transforming growth factor-β (TGF-β) family. Also known as growth differentiation factor 8, MSTN signals through the activin receptors and functions as a negative regulator of skeletal muscle growth [18]. MSTN is produced by skeletal muscle, circulates in the bloodstream, and acts to limit muscle mass. Overexpression of MSTN in mice produces a dramatic loss of skeletal muscle and body fat. Paradoxically, mice lacking MSTN exhibit increased muscle mass but, surprisingly, reduced adipose tissue mass [15]. This observation was explained by increased fatty acid oxidation. Physical activity reduces MSTN production, and inhibition of MSTN has been related to the positive effects of physical activity on metabolism and skeletal muscle mass. Interestingly, skeletal muscle MSTN expression and plasma circulating concentrations are increased in obesity. A link between MSTN and proinflammatory cytokines has been previously suggested [44]. MSTN expression is increased in C2C12 myotubes treated with TNF-α, while myotubes treated with MSTN increase the expression and secretion of IL-6. These relations provide new clues to the mechanisms potentially linking inflammation with the loss of muscle mass [44]. Moreover, systemic levels of TNF-α and IL-6 are not increased after a high-fat diet in MSTN-deficient mice as compared to wild-type animals [45].

2.10 Calprotectin

Calprotectin is a heterodimer comprising the S100A8 (S100 calcium-binding protein A8, calgranulin A, MRP8) and S100A9 (S100 calcium-binding protein A9, calgranulin B, MRP14) subunits, which are members of a subfamily of S100 calcium-binding proteins called calgranulins. The S100A8/A9 complex is constitutively expressed in monocytes, neutrophils, and macrophages at early-differentiation states. In addition, expression of calprotectin may be induced in mature macrophages, fibroblasts, and endothelial cells [46]. It has been reported that plasma calprotectin increased fivefold following physical exercise in humans [47]. Several pathological conditions associated with inflammation in humans are associated with elevated calprotectin concentrations. Circulating concentrations and visceral adipose tissue expression of calprotectin are increased in both normoglycemic and type 2 diabetic obese patients [46]. Moreover, proinflammatory molecules such as IL-1 and TNF-α induce the expression and secretion of calprotectin. Potential mechanisms explaining the role of calprotectin in inflammation are an upregulation of CD11b expression in human monocytes and an increased recruitment of monocytes to the site of inflammation. Furthermore, calprotectin serves as a regulator for nicotinamide adenine dinucleotide phosphate oxidase and may increase the generation of ROS. The exact role of calprotectin in the development of obesity-associated inflammation still has to be elucidated.

2.11 Leukemia Inhibitory Factor

Leukemia inhibitory factor (LIF) is a cytokine which belongs to the IL-6 superfamily. LIF derives its name from its ability to inhibit proliferation of myeloid leukemia cells in culture. LIF signals through the binding to the specific LIF receptor (LIFR-α), which forms a heterodimer with the glycoprotein 130. LIF is involved in a wide variety of biological functions, such as cell growth and differentiation, neural development, bone formation, and acute-phase protein production [15]. Expression of LIF is acutely induced in skeletal muscle after physical activity, and it promotes skeletal muscle satellite cell and myoblast proliferation. LIF-deficient mouse muscles exhibit a reduced regenerative response to muscle injury, while local administration of LIF exerts the opposite effect [48]. LIF has been shown to have antiinflammatory properties. LIF may downregulate TNF-α expression induced by lipopolysaccharide (LPS), while antagonism of the LIFR-α during the inflammatory phase of skeletal muscle regeneration induces an inflammatory response that inhibits myotube formation. In line with this, it has been proposed that the major role of LIF in skeletal muscle regeneration is inhibition of the inflammatory response rather than stimulation of the proliferation of myogenic cells [49].

2.12 Brain-Derived Neurotrophic Factor

Brain-derived neurotrophic factor (BDNF) is a pleiotropic protein member of the neurotrophic factor family with effects on the central nervous system as well as the endocrine and immune systems. BDNF favors the survival of existing neurons, and promotes the growth and differentiation of new ones [50]. Binding of BDNF to its receptor promotes neuronal survival in the adult brain. In addition to neurobiology, BDNF plays a role in metabolism [19]. It has been shown that expression of BDNF increases in skeletal muscle in response to contraction and physical exercise. Moreover, the exercise-induced increase in serum BDNF is positively correlated with an increment in muscle strength. Studies performed in mice lacking BDNF or mice in which BDNF is specifically depleted from skeletal muscle cells suggest that BDNF regulates positively the expression of several molecular markers of regeneration, thus playing a crucial role in regulating satellite cell function, particularly during early stages of skeletal muscle regeneration [51]. BDNF seems to be induced by inflammation; for example, it is expressed in infiltrated immune cells in inflamed skeletal muscle [52]. Moreover, TNF-α and IL-6 increase BDNF secretion by human monocytes. The antiinflammatory nature of the effects of BDNF is evidenced by the fact that BDNF administration produces an increase in IL-6 at the same time as a decrease in TNF-α, counteracts LPS-induced neuron loss, and inhibits C-reactive protein expression in endothelial and hepatic cells [50,53].

2.13 C1QTNF5/Myonectin

C1q and tumor necrosis factor related protein 5 (C1QTNF5), also known as myonectin or CTRP5, is a member of the C1q/TNF superfamily expressed and secreted predominantly by skeletal muscle, although expression has also been detected in adipose tissue, retinal pigment epithelium, and the brain [54]. C1QTNF5 has been proposed as a myokine involved in the cross-talk between skeletal muscle and other metabolic organs, such as adipose tissue and the liver, to coordinate the integration of whole-body energy metabolism [55]. In particular, recombinant C1QTNF5 administration in mice reduced circulating concentrations of free fatty acids (FFAs) without altering adipose tissue lipolysis in relation to the promotion of FFA uptake by adipocytes and hepatocytes, via the regulation of the expression of genes that promote lipid uptake [55]. A long-term exercise program increases the circulating levels of C1QTNF5 in obese women [56]. Although the role of C1QTNF5 in the regulation of inflammation in skeletal muscle has not been analyszed, a closely related member of the same family, C1QTNF3, blocks LPS-, TLR4-, and FFA-induced proinflammatory effects in monocytes and adipocytes [54]. Moreover, C1QTNF5 has been proposed as a potential novel inflammatory biomarker in chronic obstructive pulmonary disease [57].

2.14 Pigment Epithelium-Derived Factor

Pigment epithelium-derived factor (PEDF), also known as SERPIN family F member 1, is a member of the serine proteinase inhibitor (SERPIN) family and is a neurotrophic factor expressed in most organs, including the eye, liver, adipose tissue, skeletal muscle, testis, uterus, heart, and placenta, among others [58]. PEDF plays major roles in organogenesis and homeostasis of adult tissues and is a potent endogenous antiangiogenic and antifibrotic factor. PEDF is secreted from human myotubes and may also be a skeletal muscle trophic factor with autocrine or paracrine effects. In this regard, it has been reported that PEDF induces the proliferation of satellite cells and C2C12 myoblasts in vitro [59]. PEDF has shown to exert proinflammatory actions in several cell types, including skeletal muscle cells, as it directly activates several proinflammatory signaling proteins such as JNK and NF-κB in skeletal muscle [60,61].

2.15 Osteocrin/Musclin

Osteocrin (OSTN), also known as musclin, is a protein expressed in skeletal muscle [62] and bone [63] that acts as a regulator of dendritic growth in the developing brain, as a soluble osteoblast regulator, and as a myokine. In skeletal muscle OSTN is stimulated by exercise, enhancing physical endurance. Disruption of OSTN in mice results in reduced exercise tolerance that can be reversed by treatment with recombinant OSTN [64]. Circulating levels of OSTN are increased in obese subjects [65] and have been related to the development of hypertension [66]. A direct role of OSTN in the regulation of skeletal muscle inflammation has not been studied, but OSTN administration increases endoplasmic reticulum stress in the skeletal muscle [65], and palmitate increases OSTN expression in C2C12 myotubes through the activation of protein kinase R-like endoplasmic reticulum kinase (PERK) signaling pathways [67].

2.16 Ceramides

Ceramides are lipids composed of sphingosine and a fatty acid varying in length from C14 to C26, and represent important signaling molecules involved in the regulation of inflammation, obesity-associated insulin resistance, impaired fatty acid oxidation, and liver steatosis [68]. Circulating concentrations of ceramides are increased in obesity, although blood levels appear to have little impact on tissue ceramide levels [69]. It has been reported that ceramides accumulate in liver and skeletal muscle in mice shortly after beginning a high-fat diet [70]. Ceramide levels are increased in the *vastus lateralis* of obese women [71], and it has been suggested that modulating ceramide metabolism may be an interesting novel tool for the prevention and/or treatment of obesity-associated comorbidities [69].

2.17 Infiltrated Immune Cells

Several studies published in recent years have evidenced that besides adipose tissue, skeletal muscle is also a place of immune cell accumulation during obesity-associated inflammation [16,31,72,73]. Skeletal muscle from mice and humans with obesity exhibits increased amounts of macrophages and T cells. Eosinophils and mast cells are detected in mouse skeletal muscle, but they show normal levels in obesity. Other immune cells such as B cells, neutrophils, natural killer (NK) cells, and invariant NK T cells have not been described in skeletal muscle from mice or humans with obesity [16].

2.17.1 Macrophages

Similarly as in adipose tissue, obesity induced by a high-fat diet increases macrophage accumulation in skeletal muscle. Macrophages in skeletal muscle are located in the intermuscular or perimuscular adipose tissue depots, or between myocytes [16]. However, the amount of macrophages present in skeletal muscle in obesity is far less than the adipose tissue content [74]. Myocytes can express chemokines such as MCP-1 that will allow the recruitment of macrophages, with mice deficient in MCP-1 being protected against obesity-induced macrophage accumulation in skeletal muscle [16]. In addition, molecules such as the leukotriene B4, whose levels are increased in skeletal muscle from obese mice, may also contribute to macrophage infiltration [16]. Subsequently, factors such as increased interferon-γ, TNF-α, JNK, or palmitic acid and decreased IL-10 are responsible for macrophage activation and M1 polarization [16]. The skeletal muscle proinflammatory macrophages are characterized by being positive for F4/80, CD11b, and CD11c and exhibiting a classical M1 activation phenotype [74]. Most macrophages present in skeletal muscle are CD11c$^+$ and overexpress proinflammatory cytokines in comparison with CD11c$^-$ macrophages, which express higher levels of the antiinflammatory cytokine IL-10 [75]. Moreover, CD11c$^+$ macrophages are more sensitive to FFA-induced increases in inflammatory responses. The important role of macrophages in skeletal muscle inflammation is evidenced in mice with ablation of CD11c$^+$ cells. These mice show reduced levels of mRNA and protein of TNF-α, IL-6, and MCP-1 under a high-fat diet despite exhibiting increased intramuscular triglyceride content and a normal insulin sensitivity, which suggests that the presence of proinflammatory macrophages and the release of proinflammatory cytokines released by them play a more crucial role in the development of insulin resistance than the detrimental effect of lipotoxicity [75].

2.17.2 T Cells

Macrophage infiltration in skeletal muscle precedes T-cell infiltration [16]. Chemokines produced by myocytes, adipocytes resident in skeletal muscle, or recruited macrophages are required for infiltration of T cells from the circulation. The β$_2$ integrin lymphocyte function-associated antigen-1 secreted by immune cells appears to play an important role in skeletal muscle T-cell recruitment process, in which interaction with intercellular adhesion molecule-1 also seems to be necessary [16]. Obese subjects exhibit increased expression of T-cell markers CD3, CD4, and CD8 in the *vastus lateralis* [72]. Furthermore, it has been reported that mice fed a high-fat diet exhibit increased amounts of proinflammatory IFN-γ-producing CD4$^+$ T cells (T$_H$1) as well as CD8$^+$ T cells (cytotoxic T cells) in skeletal muscle [72]; the latter have previously been shown to contribute to macrophage recruitment and adipose tissue inflammation in obesity [76]. In contrast, obese mice exhibit reduced amounts of regulatory T cells (T$_{reg}$) [72], which have antiinflammatory effects and are also reduced in adipose tissue from obese mice [77]. The levels of IL-secreting CD4$^+$ T cells (T$_H$2), which exhibit antiinflammatory properties, have not been studied. In addition to the increase in number in obesity, skeletal muscle T cells exhibit a proinflammatory phenotype. The role of infiltrated T cells in skeletal muscle in metabolic disturbances such as obesity has been less studied than the role of macrophages, and the impact of the increased amount of T cells in the skeletal muscle in humans needs to be better addressed.

Finally, although its exact role in skeletal muscle inflammation has not been fully clarified, the proinflammatory actions of the inflammasome have to be taken into consideration. The inflammasome is a multiprotein complex which controls IL-1β maturation [78]. The NLR family pyrin domain containing 3 (NLRP3) inflammasome is the best characterized of the inflammasomes. In addition to the activation of IL-1β, NLRP3 inflammasome has been involved in the maturation of IL-18. IL-18 plays important metabolic roles in skeletal muscle, since mice deficient in IL-18 receptor exhibit obesity accompanied by increased lipid deposition and inflammation in skeletal muscle, which lead to the development of insulin resistance [79]. Furthermore, NLRP3 inflammasome can be activated by ROS, suggesting a link between oxidative stress and inflammation [80].

3. ROLE OF INFLAMMATION-RELATED FACTORS IN THE DEVELOPMENT OF OBESITY-ASSOCIATED SKELETAL MUSCLE INSULIN RESISTANCE

Following the understanding of the connection between obesity-associated low-grade chronic inflammation and the development of insulin resistance and altered glucose homeostasis (metabolic disease), and the critical role played by the adipose tissue in this connection, the term metaflammation was coined to describe the metabolically triggered inflammation [5]. However, it is crucial to emphasize that adipose tissue is not the sole site of metaflammation. Obesity-related influx of immune cells occurs in many other tissues, such as the hypothalamus, liver, pancreas, and skeletal muscle [5,6]. Skeletal muscle represents 40% of total body mass and in normal circumstances is responsible for up to 80% of insulin-stimulated whole-body glucose disposal; it is the largest glycogen reservoir, and a major determinant of energy expenditure. Alterations in skeletal muscle metabolism may strongly influence whole-body glucose homeostasis. In this sense, skeletal muscle inflammation is a key factor underlying insulin resistance in the context of established obesity [16,70].

Studies on the effects of obesity on the expression of myokines have sometimes reported inconsistent data. Myocytes from skeletal muscle of obese patients with type 2 diabetes expressed lower IL-6 levels than those from lean controls [81].

However, other studies found increased IL-6 expression in skeletal muscle of obese subjects with type 2 diabetes compared with healthy controls [16,70], suggesting the involvement of this cytokine in the development of obesity-associated insulin resistance. Another proinflammatory cytokine, TNF-α, has been shown to impair the action of insulin in skeletal muscle in vitro and in vivo; TNF-α-deficient mice exhibit protection against the development of obesity-induced insulin resistance [82]. Circulating concentrations of IL-8, profoundly involved in the inflammatory response, are also increased in obesity and show a positive correlation with the homeostasis model assessment (HOMA), an index of insulin resistance, as well as with C-reactive protein and IL-6, which suggests its involvement in the pathogenesis of insulin resistance and also in obesity-associated cardiovascular risk [29]. In this regard, IL-8 content of skeletal muscle and myotubes is higher in individuals with type 2 diabetes than in subjects with normoglycemia, which has been related to a microenvironment that reduces capillary density, limiting substrate availability, and thus exacerbating impaired muscle glucose uptake [83]. In contrast, IL-15 might exert beneficial effects on insulin resistance, probably through the inhibition of endoplasmic reticulum stress induced by a high-fat diet. IL-15 administration may promote adiponectin secretion from adipocytes [84], which supports an insulin sensitizer mechanism of IL-15 with opposing effects to those of TNF-α. Similarly, acute treatment with IL-10 prevents lipid-induced insulin resistance [85], and mice with muscle-specific overexpression of IL-10 are protected from inflammatory response induced by a high-fat diet [86], showing increased glucose turnover [87]. In contrast, mice with muscle-specific ablation of IL-10 receptor develop insulin resistance with decreased glucose metabolism as compared to wild-type mice [87]. All together, these findings suggest the role of IL-10 as an antiinflammatory cytokine for the treatment of type 2 diabetes.

Circulating levels of FGF21 are increased in obesity, suggesting that obesity is an FGF21-resistant state, and further elevated in obesity-associated type 2 diabetes [88]. However, chronic administration of this gut hormone and myokine decreases serum glucose concentrations in obese and diabetic *ob/ob* and *db/db* mice [89], in part through the increase in glucose disposal, the inhibition of hepatic glucose production by a PI3K-dependent activation of protein kinase C ι/λ, and the diminishment of oxidative stress [90,91]. The expression of another myokine, irisin, has been shown to be generally higher in muscle cells from individuals with type 2 diabetes than in cells from obese or lean normoglycemic individuals [92]. Through actions on skeletal muscle, liver, and adipose tissue, irisin contributes to normoglycemia. However, the exact mechanism by which irisin helps to maintain glucose homeostasis has yet to be clarified [92]. In addition, it has been reported that irisin improves endothelial dysfunction in mice with type 2 diabetes via reducing oxidative stress and NF-κB/inducible nitric oxide synthase, suggesting that irisin may be a promising tool for the treatment of diabetes-related vascular problems [93].

LIF reduces body fat mass in ovariectomized mice [94], potentially contributing to an improvement in glucose homeostasis. A recent study showed that LIF acutely stimulates skeletal muscle glucose uptake through a mechanism involving the PI3K/mammalian target of rapamycin complex 2/AKT serine-threonine kinase (Akt) pathway, and this action is preserved in the skeletal muscle from obese insulin-resistant mice [95]. However, human studies have revealed that although LIF and LIFR-α are increased in skeletal muscle and myoblasts from subjects with type 2 diabetes, LIF signaling is impaired in diabetic myoblasts, suggesting a novel mechanism by which muscle physiology is compromised in type 2 diabetes [96].

PEDF is increased in obesity in the liver, but not in adipose tissue, which has been proposed as the source of increased circulating PEDF linked to obesity-associated insulin resistance [97]. Acute administration of PEDF promotes insulin resistance in skeletal muscle and liver [60]. PEDF in an autocrine, paracrine, or endocrine fashion may inhibit insulin signaling through mechanisms both dependent upon and independent of Akt/protein kinase B (PKB) in human and mouse skeletal muscle cell lines [98]. In contrast, circulating concentrations of another neurotrophic factor expressed by the skeletal muscle, BDNF, are decreased in obesity and further decreased by type 2 diabetes [99], and BDNF administration lowers blood glucose concentrations in obese mice [100].

Calgranulin B (S100A9), one of the components of calprotectin, has been shown to be upregulated in the skeletal muscle of mice with type 2 diabetes as well as in skeletal muscle from subjects with impaired glucose tolerance [101], which has been proposed as a compensatory mechanism to counterbalance the increase in inflammatory factors.

Serum concentrations of C1QTNF5 are significantly increased in obese mice with type 2 diabetes [102] and in obese children [103]. The expression of C1QTNF5 is positively correlated with inflammatory markers, at least in adipose tissue [103]. Moreover, levels of C1QTNF5 behave in parallel to that of HOMA. Together, this data suggests a detrimental effect on insulin sensitivity that may be related to a proinflammatory action [104]. In contrast, other studies indicate that this protein is in some degree homologous in its amino acid sequence to that of adiponectin, suggesting that the two molecules may share functions in metabolism [102]. Similarly, increased in obesity, but with a potential different role, OSTN has been shown to be upregulated in the skeletal muscle of mice with severe obesity and type 2 diabetes [62], as well as those fed a high-fat diet [65]. Mechanistically, OSTN inhibits insulin-stimulated glucose uptake and glycogen synthesis in mouse myocytes [62], apparently through a decrease in activation of the insulin-signaling cascade by protein kinase B (Akt/PKB) inhibition [105] and a downregulation of the glucose transporter type 4 [65]. It has recently been reported that OSTN is increased in patients newly diagnosed with type 2 diabetes strongly related to insulin resistance, representing a major pathological component of this condition [106].

Ceramides have been shown to play a central role in the link between obesity and the development of lipid-induced inflammation, insulin resistance, and steatosis, in a process known as lipotoxicity. The rise in total and ceramide subspecies concentrations in obese subjects with type 2 diabetes is closely correlated with insulin resistance and increased TNF-α concentrations [107]. Moreover, ceramide content is increased in skeletal muscle from obese insulin-resistant subjects [108]. The proposed mechanisms by which ceramides might contribute to the development of insulin resistance are the inhibition of insulin receptor substrate-1 and Akt/PKB [108]. In this regard, it has been reported that inhibition of ceramide de novo synthesis improves insulin resistance in skeletal muscles induced by a high-fat diet, improving glucose homeostasis [109].

Circulating levels of MCP-1 are increased in obese subjects and correlate with HOMA, suggesting its relation with insulin resistance [29]. MCP-1 has been reported to promote macrophage and T-lymphocyte infiltration. In this sense, overexpression of MCP-1 in skeletal muscle induces local inflammation and impairs insulin signaling and glucose metabolism [110]. Moreover, MCP-1 expression is increased in the skeletal muscle of obese individuals, showing positive correlation with CD68, a macrophage-specific antigen, suggesting that MCP1-mediated skeletal muscle macrophage recruitment is involved in the pathogenesis of type 2 diabetes [110]. Macrophage accumulation in skeletal muscle modifies the inflammatory state of muscle cells in the context of obesity, impairing insulin signaling. Obesity and type 2 diabetes have been associated with the presence of M1 polarized macrophages, which exhibit a more inflammatory profile than M2 macrophages in both adipose tissue and skeletal muscle [111]. In this sense, mice with conditional deletion of CD11c-expressing cells, a marker of specific macrophages which are responsive to high-fat diet and have a strong proinflammatory profile, show marked reduction in adipose tissue and skeletal muscle macrophages after a high-fat diet, exhibiting a local and systemic decrease in proinflammatory cytokine levels. This improvement of inflammation is accompanied by a rapid amelioration of insulin resistance [75]. Finally, besides macrophages, different types of T cells are recruited to the skeletal muscle in the obesity milieu, as noted in the previous section, which might contribute to the development of insulin resistance. For example, T cells impair metabolic functions of skeletal muscle cells through paracrine mechanisms. In particular, proinflammatory T_H1 cells may increase inflammation and promote insulin resistance through a janus tyrosine kinase (JAK) signal transducer and activator of transcription (STAT) pathway mechanism [72]. Another study reported that mice deficient in γδ T cells (TCRδ$^{-/-}$) showed reduced mRNA expression of TNF-α and MCP-1 expression under a high-fat diet as compared to wild-type mice, accompanied by significant improvements in systemic insulin resistance [112].

4. OXIDATIVE STRESS MARKERS IN SKELETAL MUSCLE IN OBESITY

There is overwhelming evidence leading to the conclusion that obesity is a state of increased oxidative stress [12,13,113–115]. Similarly, as for inflammation, most studies linking oxidative stress with obesity have been performed in adipose tissue, paying much less attention to oxidative stress in skeletal muscle. Excessive intake of high-calorie, rapidly digestible food produces abnormal excursions in blood FFA and glucose concentrations, which may result in increased generation of ROS [116]. In this sense, it has been proposed that the lack of increased lipid peroxidation in skeletal muscle of mice on a high-fat diet suggests that in obesity, increased oxidative stress in plasma is only due to increased ROS production from accumulated fat [113]. However, as can be seen in Fig. 8.2, there is solid evidence indicating that oxidative stress also increases in skeletal muscle in obesity [114,117–121] (Table 8.2).

4.1 Thiobarbituric Acid Reactive Substances

TBARS are formed as a by-product of lipid peroxidation. Malondialdehyde (MDA) is one of several end products formed through the decomposition of lipid peroxidation products. The TBARS method is nonspecific for MDA; fatty peroxide-derived decomposition products other than MDA are Thiobarbituric Acid (TBA) positive. In general, MDA/TBA reactivity is a reliable estimator of lipid peroxidation [122]. Increased circulating concentrations of TBARS have been observed in leptin-deficient obese mice [123], as well as in men and women with obesity [113] and with metabolic syndrome [124,125]. Besides the reported obesity-associated increase in systemic TBARS, several studies have found increased levels of TBARS in muscle tissues. For example, increased levels of TBARS have been observed in cardiac muscle of obese Zucker Fatty rats and in diet-induced obese Wistar rats, which were returned to normality by treatment with statins [126].

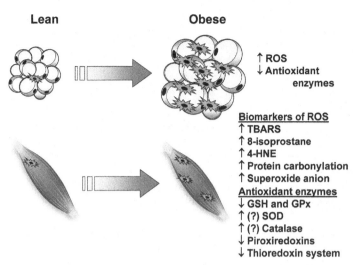

FIGURE 8.2 Obesity-associated changes in markers of oxidative stress in skeletal muscle. With the expansion of adipose tissue, the levels of diverse ROS and antioxidant enzymes in adipose tissue and skeletal muscle are altered. These altered ROS and antioxidant enzymes have an effect on skeletal muscle physiology but also on other peripheral organs. The obesity-related changes in oxidative and antioxidant systems play important roles in the development of insulin resistance and the maintenance of skeletal muscle mass. The changes that take place in adipose tissue have been simplified. *4-HNE*, 4-hydroxynonenal; *GPx*, glutathione peroxidase; *GSH*, glutathione; *ROS*, reactive oxygen species; *SOD*, superoxide dismutase; *TBARS*, thiobarbituric acid reactive substances. Question marks indicate that some discrepancies between mice and humans have been observed.

Levels of TBARS are also increased in the soleus muscle of rats fed ad libitum with a high-fat diet for 12 weeks [127]. Importantly, TBARS levels are elevated in skeletal muscle of *ob/ob* mice, and return to normality after leptin replacement but not after pair feeding, suggesting a direct positive effect of leptin on oxidative stress in the skeletal muscle [128].

4.2 8-Isoprostane

8-isoprostane (8-iso-PGF$_{2\alpha}$) is a prostaglandin isomer derived nonenzymatically through free radical catalyzed metabolism of arachidonic acid; it is considered a reliable biomarker of lipid peroxidation, and is used as a marker of antioxidant deficiency and oxidative stress [129]. Serum circulating concentrations of 8-isoprostane are increased in congenitally obese *ob/ob* mice [123], as well as in rats on a high-fat diet [127,130]. Similar elevated levels of 8-isoprostane have been described in the urine of obese subjects [131,132] and obese Zucker rats [133]. Furthermore, 8-isoprostane levels are significantly increased by a high-fat diet in the *soleus* and cardiac muscles of Sprague—Dawley rats [130] and the hind limb of wild-type mice [134].

4.3 Glutathione and Glutathione Peroxidase Activity

Glutathione (GSH) is the major antioxidant molecule in cells. It is ubiquitous, and helps to protect cells from ROS. GSH and GSH-dependent enzymes, such as GPx whose functions are to reduce lipid hydroperoxides to alcohols and hydrogen peroxide to water, are involved in the development of obesity [135]. However, the role of the glutathionyl system in energy balance is not well understood. Mice deficient in one of the subunits (modifier subunit) of the glutamate—cysteine ligase gene (Gclm$^{-/-}$), which are deficient in GSH, exhibit marked systemic and hepatic oxidative stress but are resistant to fat accretion induced by a high-fat diet, as well as development of type 2 diabetes and hepatic steatosis [136]. Similarly, mice lacking Gpx1 are protected from insulin resistance induced by a high-fat diet [137], while mice overexpressing this protein involved in the reduction of hydrogen peroxide develop obesity and insulin resistance [138]. This data suggests that it is the ROS generation rate which determines the ROS effect on insulin sensitivity. While transient ROS generation may be beneficial, sustained ROS production may induce insulin resistance [137]. Moreover, the ROS generation rate will determine the obesity-associated alterations in the activity of the main antioxidant enzymes. In the initial steps of obesity development there is an elevation in ROS production, which is counteracted by an increase in antioxidant enzymes. Thereafter, when obesity becomes chronic, there is a depletion of antioxidant enzymes [13].

Systemic GPx expression and activity are significantly decreased in obese individuals, and return to normality after weight loss induced by bariatric surgery [139,140]. While the gene expression and enzymatic activity of GPx are markedly

TABLE 8.2 Major Factors Involved in Oxidative Stress in Skeletal Muscle in Obesity

Factor or Enzyme	Role	References
Direct or Indirect Biomarkers of Free Radicals and ROS		
4-HNE	Increased up to three times in the *vastus lateralis* of obese subjects. Involved in the development of insulin resistance.	[117]
8-isoprostane	Considered a reliable biomarker of lipid peroxidation and used as a marker of antioxidant deficiency and oxidative stress. Increased in the urine of obese subjects and in the skeletal muscle of rodents under a high-fat diet.	[123,134]
Protein carbonylation	Most frequent type of protein modification in response to ROS. Elevated in the serum and white adipose tissue in obesity. Increased in skeletal muscle in human obesity.	[117,147,148]
Superoxide anion	Increased in adipose and muscle cell models of insulin resistance as well as in skeletal muscle of obese mice fed on a high-fat diet. Paradoxically decreased in the skeletal muscle of men with central obesity.	[155–157]
TBARS	By-products of lipid peroxidation. Increased in obesity at the systemic level as well as in skeletal muscle.	[113,128]
Antioxidant Enzymes		
Catalase	Involved in the prevention of cellular oxidant damage by metabolizing hydrogen peroxide to water and oxygen. Increased systemically and in visceral adipose tissue of obese individuals. Unaltered in skeletal muscle in obese rodents.	[158,159]
GSH and GPx	GSH is the major antioxidant molecule. GPx reduces lipid hydroperoxides to alcohols and hydrogen peroxide to water. Decreased systemically and altered in skeletal muscle in obesity.	[139,140,142]
Peroxiredoxins	Antioxidant enzymes involved in the scavenging of cytokine-produced hydrogen peroxide. Prx3 and Prx5 play an important role mediating the antioxidant effects of adiponectin in skeletal muscle.	[161]
SOD	Catalyzes the dismutation of $O_2^{-\bullet}$ into hydrogen peroxide and molecular oxygen. Decreased activity at the systemic level and in white adipose tissue. The activity of Cu/ZnSOD is increased in the *vastus lateralis* muscle of obese individuals.	[131,144–146]
Thioredoxin system	TXNs are proteins that function as antioxidants by facilitating the reduction of other proteins. TXNIP is an inhibitor of thioredoxins. TXN1 is decreased in the liver of mice fed on a high-fat diet. TXNIP modulates glucose uptake in human skeletal muscle.	[163,166]

4-HNE, 4-hydroxynonenal; *GPx*, glutathione peroxidase; *GSH*, glutathione; *ROS*, reactive oxygen species; *SOD*, superoxide dismutase; *TBARS*, thiobarbituric acid reactive substances; *TXN*, thioredoxin; *TXNIP*, hioredoxin interacting protein; *TXNRD1*, thioredoxin reductase-1.

decreased in white adipose tissue of mice with severe obesity [113], the effect of obesity on skeletal muscle is quite heterogeneous, showing no change [113], an increase [141], or a decrease [142] in GPx activity. Whether GPx expression levels or activity are modified by obesity in human skeletal muscle needs to be determined.

4.4 Superoxide Dismutase

SOD is the enzyme which catalyzes the dismutation of the superoxide anion radical ($O_2^{-\bullet}$), into hydrogen peroxide (H_2O_2) and molecular oxygen. There are three families of SOD which perform the same reaction and are defined by the metals used for stability and catalysis: Fe or Mn, Cu and Zn, or Ni. The different isoforms exhibit specific cellular localization patterns. The manganese-containing MnSOD (SOD2) localizes to the mitochondrial matrix, while the copper/zinc-containing type Cu/ZnSOD localizes in the cytosol, mitochondrial intermembrane space, and nucleus (SOD1). A fraction of cytoplasmic SOD is secreted into the extracellular space (SOD3). As happens with other ROS-generating or scavenging enzymes, mice genetic models overexpressing or lacking these proteins are contradictory. Mice overexpressing

MnSOD develop obesity and insulin resistance after a high-fat diet, while adipocyte-specific deletion of MnSOD protects mice from diet-induced obesity [143]. Obese patients exhibit lower circulating concentrations of SOD [144,145], suggesting an obesity-associated systemic deficit of cytoprotective antioxidant enzymes. Reduced serum SOD activity is also a hallmark of metabolic syndrome [124]. Analyses of SOD in tissues show that while both expression and activity of Cu/ZnSOD are greatly reduced in white adipose tissue of mice with severe obesity, no changes were found in skeletal muscle [113]. This observation seems to indicate that the obesity-associated defective antioxidant defense system is specific to adipose tissue. Interestingly, contrary to what is observed in obese mice, obese patients exhibit an increase in Cu/ZnSOD protein content in the *vastus lateralis* muscle which is not observed in MnSOD [131,146]. This different regulation of SOD isoforms may be dependent on the source of increased $O_2^{-\cdot}$, since Cu/ZnSOD is located mainly in the cytosol while MnSOD is located within the mitochondria [131].

4.5 4-Hydroxynonenal

4-Hydroxy-2-nonenal, 4-hydroxynonenal, (4-HNE or HNE) is a well-studied aldehyde product of phospholipid peroxidation, exhibiting high reactivity and toxicity. 4-HNE is more stable than ROS and is able to amplify oxidative injury. 4-HNE regulates a number of signaling processes by establishing covalent adducts with functional groups in lipids, proteins, and nucleic acids. Levels of 4-HNE are elevated in the serum and white adipose tissue of mice and humans with obesity, as it is involved in the development of the metabolic syndrome [147,148]. In this sense, disruption of mGsta4, the gene encoding the 4-HNE conjugating enzyme mGSTA4-4, produces raised 4-HNE tissue levels and leads to age-dependent development of obesity which results in the development of insulin resistance, although this effect seems to be dependent on the mouse strain [149]. Obesity also increases the levels of 4-HNE in skeletal muscle as compared with healthy normoponderal subjects [117,131,146]. Levels of 4-HNE are increased up to three times in the *vastus lateralis* of obese subjects [117], which correlates with several anthropometric variables such as body mass index, body fat percentage, and waist circumference, as well as with proinflammatory markers such as C-reactive protein [146].

4.6 Protein Carbonylation

Protein carbonylation, the most frequent type of ROS-induced protein modification, is considered irreversible and aims to induce protein degradation [150]. Two of the most reactive products of lipid peroxidation involved in protein carbonylation are 4-HNE and trans-4-oxo-2-nonenal (4-ONE). These aldehydes can diffuse from the membrane into the cytoplasm and nucleus, and react with a variety of proteins as well as nucleic acids. In the case of proteins, 4-HNE and 4-ONE may be covalently bound to cysteine, histidine, or lysine residues in a process generically termed secondary protein carbonylation, which in most cases leads to the loss of protein function [151]. Studies performed in rodents have shown that serum as well as skeletal muscle protein carbonylation is significantly increased by obesity induced by a high-fat diet [152,153]. In humans, obesity is accompanied by an increase in the carbonylation of several proteins in adipose tissue, representing a potential mechanistic link between elevated oxidative stress and the development of insulin resistance [154]. In addition, protein carbonylation is observed in the *vastus lateralis* muscle of obese men [146]. This finding is readily detectable as early as 3 days after the beginning of overfeeding, suggesting that this nonreversible phenomenon may be an early event during overnutrition in humans [132].

4.7 Superoxide Anion

It has been reported that $O_2^{-\cdot}$ is increased in adipose and muscle cell models of insulin resistance as well as in the skeletal muscle of obese mice with type 2 diabetes fed a high-fat diet, and that pharmacologic or genetic strategies that block mitochondrial $O_2^{-\cdot}$ elevation increase or restore insulin sensitivity [155,156]. This observation has led to suggestions that the development of insulin resistance may be part of the antioxidant defense mechanism to protect cells from further oxidative damage [155]. Paradoxically, it has been shown that the $O_2^{-\cdot}$ production rate in the *vastus lateralis* decreases with increasing waist circumference in healthy sedentary men [157].

4.8 Catalase

Catalase is involved in the prevention of cellular oxidant damage by metabolizing hydrogen peroxide to water and oxygen. Blood catalase activity is reduced in the blood of obese female rats [153] and in the adipose tissue of mice with severe genetic obesity [113], suggestive of an altered antioxidant defense mechanism in response to increased ROS due to the nutrient surplus. Interestingly, no alterations due to obesity were found in skeletal muscle catalase activity of obese mice [113]. However, a significant positive correlation with body weight was observed in catalase activity in the blood of postmenopausal women [158] and catalase activity was increased in the visceral adipose tissue of centrally obese men, but not in the subcutaneous depot [159]. These apparent discrepancies between species could be explained by time-specific differences in the course of obesity or by depot-specific disparities. Further research will help in better understanding the role of catalase activity in the obesity-associated alterations in oxidative stress.

4.9 Peroxiredoxins

Peroxiredoxins are antioxidants enzymes that have been suggested to be involved in the scavenging of cytokine-produced hydroxiperoxide, preventing the formation of lipid aldehydes. The family of peroxiredoxins has at least six members. Prx3, expressed exclusively localized in the mitochondria, has been shown to increase during adipogenesis and decrease in white adipose tissues of obese rodent and human individuals [160]. Moreover, it has been shown that Prx3 and Prx5 play an important role in the antioxidant effects of adiponectin in skeletal muscle in mice [161].

4.10 Thioredoxins

Thioredoxins are proteins that function as antioxidants by facilitating the reduction of other proteins. In humans there are two thioredoxins, thioredoxin 1 and 2, encoded by TXN1 and TXN2, respectively. Thioredoxins are essential for life in mammals, and mutations producing loss of function in these genes are lethal. Thioredoxin reductase-1 (TXNRD1), an enzyme involved in the reduction of thioredoxins, and TXN are positively correlated with body fat percentage in nondiabetic obese subjects, suggesting an activation of oxidative stress defense mechanisms in subcutaneous adipose tissue [162]. Interestingly, TXN1 and TXNRD1 expression and activity are decreased in the liver of mice fed on a high-fat diet, a phenomenon that can be due at least in part to the increase in 4-HNE levels in the liver [163]. Thioredoxin-interacting protein (TXNIP), also known as thioredoxin-binding protein 2, is an α-arrestin inhibitor of thioredoxins that has been involved in the development of insulin resistance through the regulation of cellular oxidative stress and the inhibition of glucose uptake in fat and muscle. Lack of TXNIP promotes adiposity in mice on a high-fat diet, but simultaneously enhances insulin responsiveness in adipose tissue and skeletal muscle [164]. TXNIP mediates β cell death induced by endoplasmic reticulum stress through initiation of the inflammasome in mice and human islets [165]. Moreover, TXNIP modulates both insulin-dependent and insulin-independent glucose uptake in human skeletal muscle, suggesting that this α-arrestin might play a key role in the impairment of glucose homeostasis preceding the appearance of type 2 diabetes [166]. Furthermore, a reduction in the expression of TXNIP in skeletal muscle has been involved in the beneficial effects of caloric restriction [167] and liraglutide [168] in humans.

5. ROLE OF OXIDATIVE STRESS FACTORS IN THE DEVELOPMENT OF OBESITY-ASSOCIATED SKELETAL MUSCLE INSULIN RESISTANCE

ROS have been traditionally considered as toxic by-products of oxygen consumption. Massive accumulations of ROS may cause organ dysfunction. However, at low doses they may be essential for some physiological processes [120]. Although in different cellular models of insulin resistance it has been shown that increased ROS concentrations impair insulin signaling [169], other studies indicate the opposite, showing that H_2O_2 is able to stimulate insulin signaling depending on the concentration of H_2O_2 [137]. Thus ROS are required for insulin to exert its functions, but at high concentrations, as in the case of obesity, may impair insulin action, leading to the development of insulin resistance [120,170]. In line with this, it has been suggested that insulin resistance may be part of an antioxidant defense mechanism aimed to protect cells from excessive oxidative damage, so insulin resistance could be considered as a compensatory response to increased nutrient accumulation [155].

Obesity is associated with an increase in oxidative stress at the systemic level [13], but also in the adipose tissue [113], the liver [171], and the skeletal muscle [119,120,172]. For example, levels of 4-HNE are elevated in the serum and adipose tissue of mice and humans, playing a role in the development of insulin resistance. 4-HNE produces carbonylation-mediated degradation of proteins involved in insulin signaling, thereby reducing the metabolic actions of insulin [173]. Another circulating oxidative stress marker elevated in obesity, 8-isoprostane, is increased in the serum of subjects with type 2 diabetes [129]. Excessive ROS have been reported to affect several signaling pathways involving JNK, forkhead fox, MAPK, JAK/STAT, p53, phospholipase C, and PI3K. Moreover, ROS activate transcription factors such as NF-κB and activator protein-1 involved in the regulation of inflammation increase the expression of proinflammatory factors such as TNF-α, IL-6, MCP-1, and C-reactive protein, which further aggravate the development of insulin resistance [31,119].

Hydrogen peroxide, as noted above, has been shown to induce insulin resistance when its concentration exceeds a certain threshold in different cellular models [169]. Excess of H_2O_2 is scavenged by catalase, GPx, or peroxiredoxins. In this regard, it has been shown that reducing H_2O_2 levels by genetic overexpression of catalase in mitochondria of muscle in mice completely preserves insulin sensitivity despite a high-fat diet [174]. In the same line, mice overexpressing perox-iredoxin 3 show increased resistance to stress-induced cell death and apoptosis, being protected against hyperglycemia and glucose intolerance induced by a high-fat diet [175]. Moreover, reduced plasma GPx3 concentrations are found in patients with type 2 diabetes and in severely obese mice with type 2 diabetes. GPx3 has been reported to be a central mediator of the effect of thiazolidinediones, a class of peroxisome proliferator-activated receptor γ agonists which improve insulin sensitivity, in human skeletal muscle cells. However, the protein content of catalase in the *vastus lateralis* of obese subjects appears to be normal as compared to lean subjects [146]. Finally, hyperglycemia and ROS may induce TXNIP expression and availability for activation of the NLRP3 inflammasome, which finally leads to IL-1β maturation driving to the development of insulin resistance [176].

The observations presented above suggest that antioxidant therapy might be a useful strategy in type 2 diabetes. Although some antioxidant agents have been tested, their clinical utility has been limited so far. The development of more effective antioxidant agents would help to alleviate the health burden of conditions associated with insulin resistance.

6. EFFECT OF AGING ON INFLAMMATION AND OXIDATIVE STRESS IN SKELETAL MUSCLE

Aging influences many physiological functions, producing important changes in body composition. With aging, skeletal muscle and bone decrease, body fat accumulation shifts from subcutaneous to visceral adipose depots, and triglycerides deposit ectopically on liver, skeletal muscle, pancreas, and heart [177]. At the same time aging is associated with decreased muscle performance in obese subjects despite having increased muscle mass, although the mechanisms for this are not fully elucidated. Independent of obesity, skeletal muscle protein synthesis and mitochondrial function decrease with age [178]. Moreover, levels of insulin-like growth factor (IGF-1) are reduced with both obesity and aging. Older adults exhibit higher inflammation with increased expression of TNF-α and IL-6 in skeletal muscle, which together with the low levels of IGF-1 are associated with a significant decrease in protein synthesis and an increase in muscle degradation, which translates in low muscle strength [178,179]. The main aging-dependent changes in muscle proteolysis are a lack of responsiveness of the ubiquitin—proteasome-dependent proteolytic and the caspase-dependent pathways to both anabolic and catabolic stimuli, and modifications in the control of autophagy [180]. Aging further promotes the infiltration of adipose tissue in skeletal muscle that takes place in obesity, aggravating the inflammatory situation [178]. Cumulative evidence suggests that another mechanism, in addition to increased inflammation, that might link aging with obesity-associated insulin resistance is an elevation of oxidative stress in skeletal muscle [114]. Dietary intake and absorption of antioxidants are frequently reduced in the elderly in parallel to the increase in skeletal muscle ROS production. Age-associated proteolysis and muscle wasting may result from the oxidative damage to proteins in skeletal muscle, aimed at the oxidized proteins that are more rapidly eliminated than normal proteins [180]. In summary, aging-associated increased inflammatory stimuli and oxidative stress in skeletal muscle will produce insulin resistance and increased muscle wasting that will translate into elevated frailty and mobility disability, with increased mortality in elders—a phenomenon that is undoubtedly aggravated by obesity.

7. EFFECT OF PROINFLAMMATORY AND OXIDATIVE STRESS FACTORS ON THE DEVELOPMENT OF SARCOPENIC OBESITY

Sarcopenia is defined as an age-related decline in skeletal muscle mass, with lower muscular strength or low physical performance, resulting in elevated risk of adverse outcomes such as falls, reduced mobility, and frailty, producing an increase in morbidity and mortality. Previous studies have evidenced that sarcopenia is frequently associated with obesity, especially in older people, suggesting that the two conditions are pathophysiologically connected [181]. Importantly, the concomitant presence of the two conditions confers a markedly worse outcome for physical functioning, with elevated rate of functional decline [182].

Aging, as noted in the previous section, is one of the major contributors to the development of sarcopenia [183]. Excessive obesity-associated ectopic intramuscular lipid accumulation may lead to pathological conditions, such as an impairment of mitochondria characterized by their reduced biogenesis, finally leading to muscle fiber insufficiency and dysfunction [183]. Moreover, obesity exacerbates the fall in anabolic hormone secretion and testosterone concentrations, which are lower in sarcopenic adults with obesity compared to their older obese counterparts [178]. Systemic chronic low-grade inflammation is reportedly increased in sarcopenic obesity, as evidenced, for example, by the significantly increased circulating concentrations of MCP-1 [182]. Serum concentrations of both IL-6 and C-reactive protein also become elevated [184]. This systemic chronic low-grade inflammation and inflammation in adipose tissue and skeletal muscle clearly contribute to explaining the skeletal muscle dysfunction and increased morbidity associated with sarcopenic obesity [183]. Importantly, excess caloric intake that leads to obesity might also contribute to the development of sarcopenia by producing high levels of oxidative stress. Sustained consumption of a high-calorie diet may not only exacerbate obesity but also induce oxidative cellular damage in skeletal muscle [116]. In this regard, increased surrogate markers of systemic oxidative stress, such as urine 8-isoprostane, are associated with reduced skeletal muscle mass in elderly subjects with obesity. This increase in oxidative stress has been proposed as a mechanism underlying atherosclerosis development in subjects with sarcopenic obesity [185]. Observational studies indicate that aging-related TNF-α elevations show a consistent association with declines in muscle mass and strength [184]. Imbalance of the intracellular ROS and antioxidant systems appears to be a primary causal factor for sarcopenic obesity-related skeletal muscle inflammation. It has been suggested that the activation of NF-κB by ROS promotes the expression of IL-6 and TNF-α [184]. In summary, sarcopenic obesity, characterized by the presence of excess adiposity and decreased muscle mass, may contribute to the increased risk of cardiometabolic diseases through the complex interrelationship between elevated proinflammatory factors, insulin resistance, and increased oxidative stress [116].

8. THERAPEUTIC EFFECT OF DIET ON INFLAMMATION AND OXIDATIVE STRESS IN SKELETAL MUSCLE IN OBESITY

The type and amount of macronutrients of the diet exert a profound influence on the degree of systemic and local inflammation and oxidative stress [186,187]. It must be emphasized that caloric restriction and the resulting weight loss have a beneficial effect on obesity-associated inflammation and oxidative stress; but while this effect is clear at the systemic level, its impact on skeletal muscle is not so clear. In this regard, a 15-week hypocaloric diet in severely obese subjects improved insulin sensitivity and reduced low-grade chronic inflammation. Inflammatory markers, such as circulating levels of C-reactive protein, IL-6, IL-8, and MCP-1, were decreased and the expression of IL-6, IL-8, and MCP-1 in adipose tissue was downregulated. However, the impact on skeletal muscle was minor, with significant effects only on IL-6. Several nutritional strategies aimed at decreasing inflammation and oxidative stress have been proposed, in particular in the context of the prevention or treatment of obesity and metabolic syndrome [186].

8.1 Reduce Saturated Fats and Transfats From Diet

The consumption of transfatty acids from partially hydrogenated oils presents considerable potential for harm and increases cardiometabolic risk. Higher intake of transfat has been associated with increased levels of TNF-α, IL-6, and C-reactive protein in overweight women, suggesting that the inflammatory properties of transfats may account in part for their effects on cardiovascular health [188]. Moreover, high intake of saturated fats has been related to increased expression of inflammatory genes in skeletal muscle [78,189], as well as with a marked reduction in the expression of genes regulating skeletal muscle glucose transport and oxidation [190]. Several studies have shown that replacement of saturated fats and transfats by unsaturated fat improves insulin resistance and oxidative stress in subjects with abdominal obesity [100]. Furthermore, dietary fatty acids may regulate inflammatory factors. For example, C-reactive protein and E-selectin concentrations are higher after consumption of a diet rich in transfats, while IL-6 levels are lower after consumption of a diet rich in oleic acid than after eating a diet rich in transfats and saturated fats [186].

8.2 Omega-3 Fatty Acids

Several animal and clinical studies have shown that omega-3 (n-3) fatty acids exert important antiinflammatory effects, improving disease outcome in diverse inflammatory pathologies [191]. Dietary intake of eicosapentaenoic acid (EPA), docosahexaenoic acid (DHA), and alpha-linolenic acid is inversely related to circulating concentrations of markers of inflammation such as TNF-α, C-reactive protein, and IL-6 [186]. Moreover, emulsions containing EPA and DHA inhibited inflammation and fever in response to the endotoxin challenge [192]. Importantly, DHA does not reduce macrophage number in obesity-induced inflamed adipose tissue, but significantly changes macrophage polarization from an M1 proinflammatory phenotype to an M2 antiinflammatory one [193]. In healthy individuals, omega-3 fatty acid supplementation increased fat oxidation in the skeletal muscle at the expense of glucose utilization [194]. Moreover, diets rich in fish oil result in a lower degree of systemic inflammation and insulin resistance, accompanied by decreased lipotoxicity, inflammation, and insulin resistance in skeletal muscle [195]. Diets rich in omega-3 fatty acids reduce both endoplasmic reticulum stress and oxidative stress in skeletal muscle [196]. Surprisingly, although the antiinflammatory effects of omega-3 fatty acids seem to be proved, daily treatment with omega-3 fatty acids does not decrease cardiovascular mortality and morbidity in patients with multiple cardiovascular risk factors [197].

8.3 Increase the Amount of Fruits and Vegetables in Diet

Numerous studies have shown an inverse correlation between fruit and vegetable consumption and circulating concentrations of inflammatory markers, resulting in a reduction of cardiometabolic disease risk [186]. The addition of vegetables to the diet has been reported to reverse the increase in circulating proinflammatory molecules such as TNF-α and IL-6, as well as the endothelial dysfunction induced by the consumption of a diet rich in saturated fat [198]. Moreover, diets rich in fruits and vegetables reportedly increase the serum antioxidant capacity and inhibit in vivo lipid peroxidation [199]. These positive effects of fruits and vegetables on inflammation and oxidative stress are produced by vitamins, flavonoids, and fiber, among other nutrients [186]. The specific effects of a global diet rich in fruits and vegetables on skeletal muscle inflammatory and oxidative stress markers need to be better characterized.

8.4 Increase Foods Rich in Antioxidants

Extensive studies have analyzed the effect of antioxidant-rich supplements or foods rich in natural antioxidants on inflammatory and oxidative stress markers, in particular in the context of obesity [114]. Diets rich in vitamins E and C, β-carotene, lycopene, resveratrol, folic acid, or polyphenols, among others, or these nutrients individually or combined in dietary supplements, have been shown to reduce systemic levels of inflammatory and oxidative stress factors even in the absence of weight loss [114,115]. For example, vitamins C and E supplementation improves levels of oxidative stress associated with repetitive loading exercise and aging in the skeletal muscle of rats through an elevation of the levels of endogenous antioxidant enzymes [200]. Even vitamin D has been shown to exert some protective effects against oxidative-stress-induced proteolysis in skeletal muscle [201]. Resveratrol has been suggested as a promising therapy or preventive tool for inflammation in skeletal muscle, since it inhibits palmitate-induced inflammation in myotubes by reducing oxidative stress and JNK/NF-κB pathways through mechanisms independent of sirtuin 1 [202]. Finally, grape polyphenol supplementation might be beneficial for reducing muscle atrophy, as indicated in a mouse model of chronic inflammation [203].

9. ROLE OF EXERCISE IN THE REGULATION OF INFLAMMATION AND OXIDATIVE STRESS IN SKELETAL MUSCLE IN OBESITY

While acute exercise may induce a transitory state of increased oxidative stress and inflammation, chronic physical activity promotes favorable oxidative adaptations and antiinflammatory responses. Exercise or regular physical activity improves systemic markers of inflammation and oxidative stress as well as the antioxidant capacity [204]. An optimal level of oxidative stress production may actually serve as the primary stimulus for antioxidant defenses, thus protecting against future detrimental action of ROS and the development of oxidative-stress-related diseases [205]. In a similar way, IL-6 increases extraordinarily after acute exercise, up to 100-fold (but still is not clear whether this has proinflammatory effects), which is necessary to trigger the release of cytokine inhibitors such as IL-1 receptor antagonist and soluble tumor necrosis factor receptor, as well as the antiinflammatory cytokine IL-10 [206].

Contracting muscle can induce the secretion of many myokines that allow cross-talk with other organs such as adipose tissue, liver, and pancreas to exert beneficial effects of physical activity on the whole-body level [207]. Exercise upregulates gene expression and secretion of IL-6, IL-8, and IL-15. Exercise-induced changes in these molecules promote metabolic changes in skeletal muscle, increasing glucose uptake and fatty acid oxidation. Exercise-induced downregulation of MSTN expression, a negative regulator of skeletal muscle mass, might mediate hypertrophic adaptive responses in the muscle [208]. Interestingly, it has been shown that the impact of exercise on circulating concentrations and skeletal muscle expression of inflammatory factors is different than the impact of weight loss. Diet-induced weight loss reduces circulating levels of C-reactive protein, but has no effect on the expression of inflammatory markers in skeletal muscle. Conversely, 12 weeks of exercise (aerobic and resistance) reduces the expression of TLR-4, IL-6, and TNF-α, but produces no changes in circulating concentrations of C-reactive protein, IL-6, or TNF-α [209]. Moreover, inactivity leads to increased oxidative stress both in skeletal muscle and at the systemic level, and exercise reverts this harmful condition. For example, 3 months of moderate-intensity endurance exercise reduces oxidative stress on both skeletal muscle and at the systemic level in previously sedentary obese men, showing reduced urine concentrations of 8-isoprostane and 4-HNE [146]. Moreover, exercise produces an elevation in the activities of both SOD and GPx, along with increased cellular concentrations of GSH in skeletal muscle [210]. In addition, the inhibitor of thioredoxins TXNIP, which is involved in the development of insulin resistance, is acutely upregulated after a single exercise session while it is downregulated in the skeletal muscle by exercise training in both mice and humans [211]. Interestingly, ceramides and other sphingolipids which are increased in skeletal muscle in obesity are significantly reduced after recovery from an exercise bout, representing a potential mechanism improving insulin sensitivity [212].

In summary, chronic exercise reduces inflammation and oxidative stress in skeletal muscle by diverse mechanisms. These positive effects of exercise lead to an improvement in insulin sensitivity both in the skeletal muscle and at the systemic level [120].

10. CONCLUSIONS

The incidence and prevalence of obesity worldwide continue to grow at alarming levels without symptoms of abatement. This implies serious health consequences and the obliteration of health achievements made in recent decades. Obesity is associated with an increased risk of developing cardiovascular disease, type 2 diabetes, and cancer. Two central processes involved in the etiopathogenesis of obesity are the elevations in inflammation and oxidative stress (Fig. 8.3). Obesity-associated inflammation and increased oxidative stress can be found systemically but also at the tissue level, in particular in white adipose tissue and skeletal muscle. The trigger for this increased inflammation and oxidative stress is uncertain, but there is little doubt about the tight relation between obesity and both processes. Several animal and clinical studies have shown that the degree of inflammation and oxidative stress in skeletal muscle correlates well with the severity

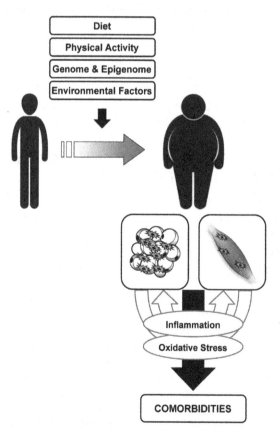

FIGURE 8.3 The etiopathogenesis of obesity is of multifactorial origin. Diet, amount of physical activity, genetic and epigenetic modifications, and environmental factors determine the development of obesity. Obesity produces profound alterations in adipose tissue and skeletal muscle inflammation and oxidative stress, establishing a cross-talk between both organs. This dysregulation in inflammation and oxidative stress increases the risk of obesity-associated comorbidities such as type 2 diabetes, cardiometabolic diseases, nonalcoholic fatty liver disease, and several types of cancer, among others.

of insulin resistance and type 2 diabetes. Several strategies have been proposed to curtail the increased inflammation and unbalanced redox in the obesity milieu, encompassing diverse nutritional measures as well as an increase in physical activity. Better understanding of the pathophysiological mechanisms involved in the obesity-associated inflammatory response as well as in the pathways that lead to the elevation of oxidative stress might lead to the development of new approaches for preventing and treating these devastating obesity-associated comorbidities.

LIST OF ACRONYMS AND ABBREVIATIONS

4-HNE 4-hydroxynonenal
4-ONE Trans-4-oxo-2-nonenal
Akt AKT serine-threonine kinase
AMPK AMP-activated protein kinase
AP-1 Activator protein 1
BDNF Brain-derived neurotrophic factor
BMI Body mass index
C1QTNF5 C1q and tumor necrosis factor related protein 5
CCL2 C−C motif chemokine ligand 2
CCR2 Chemokine CC motif receptor 2
CNS Central nervous system
CXCL8 Chemokine (C-X-C motif) ligand 8
DHA Docosahexaenoic acid
EPA Eicosapentaenoic acid
FFA Free fatty acid
FGF21 Fibroblast growth factor 21
FNDC5 Fibronectin type III domain-containing protein 5
FOXO Forkhead fox
GDF8 Growth differentiation factor 8
GLUT4 Glucose transporter type 4
GP130 Glycoprotein 130
GPx Glutathione peroxidase
GSH Glutathione
HOMA Homeostasis model assessment
ICAM-1 Intercellular adhesion molecule-1
IGF-1 Insulin-like growth factor
IKK IκB kinase
IL-6 Interleukin-6
INF-γ Interferon-γ
iNKT Invariant NK T
iNOS Inducible nitric oxide synthase
IRS-1 Insulin receptor substrate-1
JAK Janus tyrosine kinase
JNK c-Jun N-terminal kinase
LIF Leukemia inhibitory factor
LIFR-α LIF receptor
LPS Lipopolysaccharide
LTB4 Leukotriene B4
MAPK Mitogen-activated protein kinase
MCP-1 Monocyte chemotactic protein 1
MDA Malondialdehyde
MSTN Myostatin
mTORC2 Mammalian target of rapamycin complex 2
MyD88 Myeloid differentiation primary response 88
NADPH Nicotinamide adenine dinucleotide phosphate
NAFLD Non-alcoholic fatty liver disease
NF-κB Nuclear factor-κB
NK Natural killer
NLRP3 NLR family pyrin domain containing 3
OSTN Osteocrin

p38 MAPK p38 mitogen-activated protein kinase
PEDF Pigment epithelium-derived factor
PERK Protein kinase R-like endoplasmic reticulum kinase
PGC-1α Peroxisome proliferator-activated receptor γ coactivator 1-α
PI3K Phosphatidylinositol-3-kinase
PKB Protein kinase B
PKCι/λ Protein kinase C ι/λ
RCS Reactive carbonyl species
RNS Reactive nitrogen species
ROS Reactive oxygen species
RSS Reactive sulfur species
S100A8 S100 calcium binding protein A8
S100A9 S100 calcium binding protein A9
SERPIN Serine proteinase inhibitor
SERPINF1 Serpin family F member 1
SOD Superoxide dismutase
STAT Signal transducer and activator of transcription
sTNFR Tumor necrosis factor receptor
TAS Total antioxidant status
TBARS Thiobarbituric acid reactive substances
TGF-β Transforming growth factor-β
TLR4 Toll-like receptor 4
TNF-α Tumor necrosis factor-α
TXN Thioredoxin
TXNIP Hioredoxin interacting protein
TXNRD1 Thioredoxin reductase-1

ACKNOWLEDGMENTS

Supported by project grants FIS PI16/01217, PI17/02183 and PI17/02188 integrated in the Plan Estatal I+D+I 2013-16 from the Spanish Instituto de Salud Carlos III—Subdirección General de Evaluación y Fomento de la investigación—FEDER, and Centro de Investigación Biomédica en Red Fisiopatología de la Obesidad y Nutrición, CIBEROBN, ISCIII, Spain. All authors have contributed to the writing and revision of the text and have approved the final manuscript. There are no conflicts of interest to declare.

REFERENCES

[1] Bray GA, Frühbeck G, Ryan DH, Wilding JP. Management of obesity. Lancet 2016;387(10031):1947−56.
[2] The GBD 2015 Obesity Collaborators. Health effects of overweight and obesity in 195 countries over 25 years. N Engl J Med 2017;377(1):13−27.
[3] Hotamisligil GS, Shargill NS, Spiegelman BM. Adipose expression of tumor necrosis factor-α: direct role in obesity-linked insulin resistance. Science 1993;259(5091):87−91.
[4] Wellen KE, Hotamisligil GS. Obesity-induced inflammatory changes in adipose tissue. J Clin Invest 2003;112(12):1785−8.
[5] Hotamisligil GS. Inflammation and metabolic disorders. Nature 2006;444(7121):860−7.
[6] Hotamisligil GS. Inflammation, metaflammation and immunometabolic disorders. Nature 2017;542(7640):177−85.
[7] Medzhitov R. Origin and physiological roles of inflammation. Nature 2008;454(7203):428−35.
[8] Gómez-Ambrosi J, Salvador J, Silva C, Pastor C, Rotellar F, Gil MJ, et al. Increased cardiovascular risk markers in obesity are associated with body adiposity: role of leptin. Thromb Haemost 2006;95(6):991−6.
[9] Catalán V, Gómez-Ambrosi J, Ramírez B, Rotellar F, Pastor C, Silva C, et al. Proinflammatory cytokines in obesity: impact of type 2 diabetes mellitus and gastric bypass. Obes Surg 2007;17(11):1464−74.
[10] Schwartz MW, Seeley RJ, Zeltser LM, Drewnowski A, Ravussin E, Redman LM, et al. Obesity pathogenesis: an endocrine society scientific statement. Endocr Rev 2017;38(4):267−96.
[11] Reilly SM, Saltiel AR. Adapting to obesity with adipose tissue inflammation. Nat Rev Endocrinol 2017;13(11):633−43.
[12] McMurray F, Patten DA, Harper ME. Reactive oxygen species and oxidative stress in obesity-recent findings and empirical approaches. Obesity (Silver Spring) 2016;24(11):2301−10.
[13] Vincent HK, Taylor AG. Biomarkers and potential mechanisms of obesity-induced oxidant stress in humans. Int J Obes 2006;30(3):400−18.
[14] Sies H, Berndt C, Jones DP. Oxidative stress. Annu Rev Biochem 2017;86:715−48.
[15] Pedersen BK, Febbraio MA. Muscles, exercise and obesity: skeletal muscle as a secretory organ. Nat Rev Endocrinol 2012;8(8):457−65.
[16] Wu H, Ballantyne CM. Skeletal muscle inflammation and insulin resistance in obesity. J Clin Invest 2017;127(1):43−54.

[17] Saghizadeh M, Ong JM, Garvey WT, Henry RR, Kern PA. The expression of TNFα by human muscle. Relationship to insulin resistance. J Clin Invest 1996;97(4):1111–6.

[18] Lancha A, Frühbeck G, Gómez-Ambrosi J. Peripheral signalling involved in energy homeostasis control. Nutr Res Rev 2012;25(2):223–48.

[19] Pedersen BK. The diseasome of physical inactivity - and the role of myokines in muscle - fat cross talk. J Physiol 2009;587(Pt 23):5559–68.

[20] Pedersen BK, Febbraio MA. Muscle as an endocrine organ: focus on muscle-derived interleukin-6. Physiol Rev 2008;88(4):1379–406.

[21] Reyna SM, Ghosh S, Tantiwong P, Meka CS, Eagan P, Jenkinson CP, et al. Elevated toll-like receptor 4 expression and signaling in muscle from insulin-resistant subjects. Diabetes 2008;57(10):2595–602.

[22] Wen H, Gris D, Lei Y, Jha S, Zhang L, Huang MT, et al. Fatty acid-induced NLRP3-ASC inflammasome activation interferes with insulin signaling. Nat Immunol 2011;12(5):408–15.

[23] Wunderlich FT, Strohle P, Konner AC, Gruber S, Tovar S, Bronneke HS, et al. Interleukin-6 signaling in liver-parenchymal cells suppresses hepatic inflammation and improves systemic insulin action. Cell Metab 2010;12(3):237–49.

[24] Mauer J, Chaurasia B, Goldau J, Vogt MC, Ruud J, Nguyen KD, et al. Signaling by IL-6 promotes alternative activation of macrophages to limit endotoxemia and obesity-associated resistance to insulin. Nat Immunol 2014;15(5):423–30.

[25] Nielsen AR, Hojman P, Erikstrup C, Fischer CP, Plomgaard P, Mounier R, et al. Association between interleukin-15 and obesity: interleukin-15 as a potential regulator of fat mass. J Clin Endocrinol Metab 2008;93(11):4486–93.

[26] Duan Y, Li F, Wang W, Guo Q, Wen C, Li Y, et al. Interleukin-15 in obesity and metabolic dysfunction: current understanding and future perspectives. Obes Rev 2017;18(10):1147–58.

[27] Sun H, Liu D. Hydrodynamic delivery of interleukin 15 gene promotes resistance to high fat diet-induced obesity, fatty liver and improves glucose homeostasis. Gene Ther 2015;22(4):341–7.

[28] Straczkowski M, Dzienis-Straczkowska S, Stepien A, Kowalska I, Szelachowska M, Kinalska I. Plasma interleukin-8 concentrations are increased in obese subjects and related to fat mass and tumor necrosis factor-alpha system. J Clin Endocrinol Metab 2002;87(10):4602–6.

[29] Kim CS, Park HS, Kawada T, Kim JH, Lim D, Hubbard NE, et al. Circulating levels of MCP-1 and IL-8 are elevated in human obese subjects and associated with obesity-related parameters. Int J Obes (Lond) 2006;30(9):1347–55.

[30] Ouyang W, Rutz S, Crellin NK, Valdez PA, Hymowitz SG. Regulation and functions of the IL-10 family of cytokines in inflammation and disease. Annu Rev Immunol 2011;29:71–109.

[31] Wei Y, Chen K, Whaley-Connell AT, Stump CS, Ibdah JA, Sowers JR. Skeletal muscle insulin resistance: role of inflammatory cytokines and reactive oxygen species. Am J Physiol Regul Integr Comp Physiol 2008;294(3):R673–80.

[32] Itoh N. FGF21 as a hepatokine, adipokine, and myokine in metabolism and diseases. Front Endocrinol 2014;5:107.

[33] Raschke S, Eckel J. Adipo-myokines: two sides of the same coin - mediators of inflammation and mediators of exercise. Mediat Inflamm 2013;2013:320724.

[34] Luo Y, McKeehan WL. Stressed liver and muscle call on adipocytes with FGF21. Front Endocrinol (Lausanne) 2013;4:194.

[35] Lee MS, Choi SE, Ha ES, An SY, Kim TH, Han SJ, et al. Fibroblast growth factor-21 protects human skeletal muscle myotubes from palmitate-induced insulin resistance by inhibiting stress kinase and NF-κB. Metabolism 2012;61(8):1142–51.

[36] Rodríguez A, Becerril S, Méndez-Giménez L, Ramírez B, Saínz N, Catalán V, et al. Leptin administration activates irisin-induced myogenesis via nitric oxide-dependent mechanisms, but reduces its effect on subcutaneous fat browning in mice. Int J Obes (Lond) 2015;39(3):397–407.

[37] Rodríguez A, Becerril S, Ezquerro S, Méndez-Giménez L, Frühbeck G. Crosstalk between adipokines and myokines in fat browning. Acta Physiol (Oxf) 2017;219(2):362–81.

[38] Vaughan RA, Gannon NP, Mermier CM, Conn CA. Irisin, a unique non-inflammatory myokine in stimulating skeletal muscle metabolism. J Physiol Biochem 2015;71(4):679–89.

[39] Mazur-Bialy AI, Pochec E, Zarawski M. Anti-inflammatory properties of irisin, mediator of physical activity, are connected with TLR4/MyD88 signaling pathway activation. Int J Mol Sci 2017;18(4).

[40] Zhang Y, Mu Q, Zhou Z, Song H, Zhang Y, Wu F, et al. Protective effect of irisin on atherosclerosis via suppressing oxidized low density lipoprotein induced vascular inflammation and endothelial dysfunction. PLoS One 2016;11(6):e0158038.

[41] Mazur-Bialy AI. Irisin acts as a regulator of macrophages host defense. Life Sci 2017;176:21–5.

[42] Evers-van Gogh IJ, Oteng AB, Alex S, Hamers N, Catoire M, Stienstra R, et al. Muscle-specific inflammation induced by MCP-1 overexpression does not affect whole-body insulin sensitivity in mice. Diabetologia 2016;59(3):624–33.

[43] Shireman PK, Contreras-Shannon V, Ochoa O, Karia BP, Michalek JE, McManus LM. MCP-1 deficiency causes altered inflammation with impaired skeletal muscle regeneration. J Leukoc Biol 2007;81(3):775–85.

[44] Zhang L, Rajan V, Lin E, Hu Z, Han HQ, Zhou X, et al. Pharmacological inhibition of myostatin suppresses systemic inflammation and muscle atrophy in mice with chronic kidney disease. FASEB J 2011;25(5):1653–63.

[45] Wilkes JJ, Lloyd DJ, Gekakis N. Loss-of-function mutation in myostatin reduces tumor necrosis factor alpha production and protects liver against obesity-induced insulin resistance. Diabetes 2009;58(5):1133–43.

[46] Catalán V, Gómez-Ambrosi J, Rodríguez A, Ramírez B, Rotellar F, Valentí V, et al. Increased levels of calprotectin in obesity are related to macrophage content: impact on inflammation and effect of weight loss. Mol Med 2011;17(11–12):1157–67.

[47] Mortensen OH, Andersen K, Fischer C, Nielsen AR, Nielsen S, Akerstrom T, et al. Calprotectin is released from human skeletal muscle tissue during exercise. J Physiol 2008;586(14):3551–62.

[48] Hunt LC, White J. The role of leukemia inhibitory factor receptor signaling in skeletal muscle growth, injury and disease. Adv Exp Med Biol 2016;900:45–59.

[49] Hunt LC, Upadhyay A, Jazayeri JA, Tudor EM, White JD. An anti-inflammatory role for leukemia inhibitory factor receptor signaling in regenerating skeletal muscle. Histochem Cell Biol 2013;139(1):13−34.

[50] Papathanassoglou ED, Miltiadous P, Karanikola MN. May BDNF be implicated in the exercise-mediated regulation of inflammation? Critical review and synthesis of evidence. Biol Res Nurs 2015;17(5):521−39.

[51] Clow C, Jasmin BJ. Brain-derived neurotrophic factor regulates satellite cell differentiation and skeltal muscle regeneration. Mol Biol Cell 2010;21(13):2182−90.

[52] Colombo E, Bedogni F, Lorenzetti I, Landsberger N, Previtali SC, Farina C. Autocrine and immune cell-derived BDNF in human skeletal muscle: implications for myogenesis and tissue regeneration. J Pathol 2013;231(2):190−8.

[53] Noren Hooten N, Ejiogu N, Zonderman AB, Evans MK. Protective effects of BDNF against C-reactive protein-induced inflammation in women. Mediat Inflamm 2015;2015:516783.

[54] Schäffler A, Buechler C. CTRP family: linking immunity to metabolism. Trends Endocrinol Metab 2012;23(4):194−204.

[55] Seldin MM, Peterson JM, Byerly MS, Wei Z, Wong GW. Myonectin (CTRP15), a novel myokine that links skeletal muscle to systemic lipid homeostasis. J Biol Chem 2012;287(15):11968−80.

[56] Choi HY, Park JW, Lee N, Hwang SY, Cho GJ, Hong HC, et al. Effects of a combined aerobic and resistance exercise program on C1q/TNF-related protein-3 (CTRP-3) and CTRP-5 levels. Diabetes Care 2013;36(10):3321−7.

[57] Li D, Wu Y, Tian P, Zhang X, Wang H, Wang T, et al. Adipokine CTRP-5 as a potential novel inflammatory biomarker in chronic obstructive pulmonary disease. Medicine (Baltimore) 2015;94(36):e1503.

[58] He X, Cheng R, Benyajati S, Ma JX. PEDF and its roles in physiological and pathological conditions: implication in diabetic and hypoxia-induced angiogenic diseases. Clin Sci (Lond) 2015;128(11):805−23.

[59] Ho TC, Chiang YP, Chuang CK, Chen SL, Hsieh JW, Lan YW, et al. PEDF-derived peptide promotes skeletal muscle regeneration through its mitogenic effect on muscle progenitor cells. Am J Physiol Cell Physiol 2015;309(3):C159−68.

[60] Crowe S, Wu LE, Economou C, Turpin SM, Matzaris M, Hoehn KL, et al. Pigment epithelium-derived factor contributes to insulin resistance in obesity. Cell Metab 2009;10(1):40−7.

[61] Famulla S, Lamers D, Hartwig S, Passlack W, Horrighs A, Cramer A, et al. Pigment epithelium-derived factor (PEDF) is one of the most abundant proteins secreted by human adipocytes and induces insulin resistance and inflammatory signaling in muscle and fat cells. Int J Obes (Lond) 2011;35(6):762−72.

[62] Nishizawa H, Matsuda M, Yamada Y, Kawai K, Suzuki E, Makishima M, et al. Musclin, a novel skeletal muscle-derived secretory factor. J Biol Chem 2004;279(19):19391−5.

[63] Thomas G, Moffatt P, Salois P, Gaumond MH, Gingras R, Godin E, et al. Osteocrin, a novel bone-specific secreted protein that modulates the osteoblast phenotype. J Biol Chem 2003;278(50):50563−71.

[64] Subbotina E, Sierra A, Zhu Z, Gao Z, Koganti SR, Reyes S, et al. Musclin is an activity-stimulated myokine that enhances physical endurance. Proc Natl Acad Sci USA 2015;112(52):16042−7.

[65] Chen WJ, Liu Y, Sui YB, Yang HT, Chang JR, Tang CS, et al. Positive association between musclin and insulin resistance in obesity: evidence of a human study and an animal experiment. Nutr Metab (Lond) 2017;14:46.

[66] Li YX, Cheng KC, Asakawa A, Kato I, Sato Y, Amitani H, et al. Role of musclin in the pathogenesis of hypertension in rat. PLoS One 2013;8(8):e72004.

[67] Gu N, Guo Q, Mao K, Hu H, Jin S, Zhou Y, et al. Palmitate increases musclin gene expression through activation of PERK signaling pathway in C2C12 myotubes. Biochem Biophys Res Commun 2015;467(3):521−6.

[68] Fucho R, Casals N, Serra D, Herrero L. Ceramides and mitochondrial fatty acid oxidation in obesity. FASEB J 2017;31(4):1263−72.

[69] Aburasayn H, Al Batran R, Ussher JR. Targeting ceramide metabolism in obesity. Am J Physiol Endocrinol Metab 2016;311(2):E423−35.

[70] Lee YS, Li P, Huh JY, Hwang IJ, Lu M, Kim JI, et al. Inflammation is necessary for long-term but not short-term high-fat diet-induced insulin resistance. Diabetes 2011;60(10):2474−83.

[71] Coen PM, Hames KC, Leachman EM, DeLany JP, Ritov VB, Menshikova EV, et al. Reduced skeletal muscle oxidative capacity and elevated ceramide but not diacylglycerol content in severe obesity. Obesity (Silver Spring) 2013;21(11):2362−71.

[72] Khan IM, Perrard XY, Brunner G, Lui H, Sparks LM, Smith SR, et al. Intermuscular and perimuscular fat expansion in obesity correlates with skeletal muscle T cell and macrophage infiltration and insulin resistance. Int J Obes (Lond) 2015;39(11):1607−18.

[73] Lackey DE, Olefsky JM. Regulation of metabolism by the innate immune system. Nat Rev Endocrinol 2016;12(1):15−28.

[74] Olefsky JM, Glass CK. Macrophages, inflammation, and insulin resistance. Annu Rev Physiol 2010;72:219−46.

[75] Patsouris D, Li PP, Thapar D, Chapman J, Olefsky JM, Neels JG. Ablation of CD11c-positive cells normalizes insulin sensitivity in obese insulin resistant animals. Cell Metab 2008;8(4):301−9.

[76] Nishimura S, Manabe I, Nagasaki M, Eto K, Yamashita H, Ohsugi M, et al. CD8+ effector T cells contribute to macrophage recruitment and adipose tissue inflammation in obesity. Nat Med 2009;15(8):914−20.

[77] Feuerer M, Herrero L, Cipolletta D, Naaz A, Wong J, Nayer A, et al. Lean, but not obese, fat is enriched for a unique population of regulatory T cells that affect metabolic parameters. Nat Med 2009;15(8):930−9.

[78] Ralston JC, Lyons CL, Kennedy EB, Kirwan AM, Roche HM. Fatty acids and NLRP3 inflammasome-mediated inflammation in metabolic tissues. Annu Rev Nutr 2017;37:77−102.

[79] Netea MG, Joosten LA, Lewis E, Jensen DR, Voshol PJ, Kullberg BJ, et al. Deficiency of interleukin-18 in mice leads to hyperphagia, obesity and insulin resistance. Nat Med 2006;12(6):650−6.

[80] Abais JM, Xia M, Zhang Y, Boini KM, Li PL. Redox regulation of NLRP3 inflammasomes: ROS as trigger or effector? Antioxid Redox Signal 2015;22(13):1111–29.

[81] Green CJ, Pedersen M, Pedersen BK, Scheele C. Elevated NF-κB activation is conserved in human myocytes cultured from obese type 2 diabetic patients and attenuated by AMP-activated protein kinase. Diabetes 2011;60(11):2810–9.

[82] Uysal KT, Wiesbrock SM, Marino MW, Hotamisligil GS. Protection from obesity-induced insulin resistance in mice lacking TNF-α function. Nature 1997;389:610–4.

[83] Amir Levy Y, Ciaraldi TP, Mudaliar SR, Phillips SA, Henry RR. Excessive secretion of IL-8 by skeletal muscle in type 2 diabetes impairs tube growth: potential role of PI3K and the Tie2 receptor. Am J Physiol Endocrinol Metab 2015;309(1):E22–34.

[84] Quinn LS, Strait-Bodey L, Anderson BG, Argilés JM, Havel PJ. Interleukin-15 stimulates adiponectin secretion by 3T3-L1 adipocytes: evidence for a skeletal muscle-to-fat signaling pathway. Cell Biol Int 2005;29(6):449–57.

[85] Kim HJ, Higashimori T, Park SY, Choi H, Dong J, Kim YJ, et al. Differential effects of interleukin-6 and -10 on skeletal muscle and liver insulin action in vivo. Diabetes 2004;53(4):1060–7.

[86] Hong EG, Ko HJ, Cho YR, Kim HJ, Ma Z, Yu TY, et al. Interleukin-10 prevents diet-induced insulin resistance by attenuating macrophage and cytokine response in skeletal muscle. Diabetes 2009;58(11):2525–35.

[87] Dagdeviren S, Jung DY, Lee E, Friedline RH, Noh HL, Kim JH, et al. Altered interleukin-10 signaling in skeletal muscle regulates obesity-mediated inflammation and insulin resistance. Mol Cell Biol 2016;36(23):2956–66.

[88] Gómez-Ambrosi J, Gallego-Escuredo JM, Catalán V, Rodríguez A, Domingo P, Moncada R, et al. FGF19 and FGF21 serum concentrations in human obesity and type 2 diabetes behave differently after diet- or surgically-induced weight loss. Clin Nutr 2017;36(3):861–8.

[89] Kharitonenkov A, Shiyanova TL, Koester A, Ford AM, Micanovic R, Galbreath EJ, et al. FGF-21 as a novel metabolic regulator. J Clin Invest 2005;115(6):1627–35.

[90] Kong LJ, Feng W, Wright M, Chen Y, Dallas-yang Q, Zhou YP, et al. FGF21 suppresses hepatic glucose production through the activation of atypical protein kinase ι/λ. Eur J Pharmacol 2013;702(1–3):302–8.

[91] Gómez-Sámano MA, Grajales-Gómez M, Zuarth-Vázquez JM, Navarro-Flores MF, Martínez-Saavedra M, Juárez-León OA, et al. Fibroblast growth factor 21 and its novel association with oxidative stress. Redox Biol 2017;11:335–41.

[92] Perakakis N, Triantafyllou GA, Fernández-Real JM, Huh JY, Park KH, Seufert J, et al. Physiology and role of irisin in glucose homeostasis. Nat Rev Endocrinol 2017;13(6):324–37.

[93] Zhu D, Wang H, Zhang J, Zhang X, Xin C, Zhang F, et al. Irisin improves endothelial function in type 2 diabetes through reducing oxidative/nitrative stresses. J Mol Cell Cardiol 2015;87:138–47.

[94] Jansson JO, Movérare-Skrtic S, Berndtsson A, Wernstedt I, Carlsten H, Ohlsson C. Leukemia inhibitory factor reduces body fat mass in ovariectomized mice. Eur J Endocrinol 2006;154(2):349–54.

[95] Brandt N, O'Neill HM, Kleinert M, Schjerling P, Vernet E, Steinberg GR, et al. Leukemia inhibitory factor increases glucose uptake in mouse skeletal muscle. Am J Physiol Endocrinol Metab 2015;309(2):E142–53.

[96] Broholm C, Brandt C, Schultz NS, Nielsen AR, Pedersen BK, Scheele C. Deficient leukemia inhibitory factor signaling in muscle precursor cells from patients with type 2 diabetes. Am J Physiol Endocrinol Metab 2012;303(2):E283–92.

[97] Moreno-Navarrete JM, Touskova V, Sabater M, Mraz M, Drapalova J, Ortega F, et al. Liver, but not adipose tissue PEDF gene expression is associated with insulin resistance. Int J Obes (Lond) 2013;37(9):1230–7.

[98] Carnagarin R, Dharmarajan AM, Dass CR. PEDF attenuates insulin-dependent molecular pathways of glucose homeostasis in skeletal myocytes. Mol Cell Endocrinol 2016;422:115–24.

[99] Krabbe KS, Nielsen AR, Krogh-Madsen R, Plomgaard P, Rasmussen P, Erikstrup C, et al. Brain-derived neurotrophic factor (BDNF) and type 2 diabetes. Diabetologia 2007;50(2):431–8.

[100] Das UN. Is there a role for bioactive lipids in the pathobiology of diabetes mellitus? Front Endocrinol (Lausanne) 2017;8:182.

[101] Ortega FJ, Mercader JM, Moreno-Navarrete JM, Sabater M, Pueyo N, Valdés S, et al. Targeting the association of calgranulin B (S100A9) with insulin resistance and type 2 diabetes. J Mol Med (Berl) 2013;91(4):523–34.

[102] Park SY, Choi JH, Ryu HS, Pak YK, Park KS, Lee HK, et al. C1q tumor necrosis factor alpha-related protein isoform 5 is increased in mitochondrial DNA-depleted myocytes and activates AMP-activated protein kinase. J Biol Chem 2009;284(41):27780–9.

[103] Schwartze JT, Landgraf K, Spielau U, Rockstroh D, Loffler D, Kratzsch J, et al. Adipocyte C1QTNF5 expression is BMI-dependently related to early adipose tissue dysfunction and systemic CTRP5 serum levels in obese children. Int J Obes (Lond) 2017;41(6):955–63.

[104] Lim S, Choi SH, Koo BK, Kang SM, Yoon JW, Jang HC, et al. Effects of aerobic exercise training on C1q tumor necrosis factor alpha-related protein isoform 5 (myonectin): association with insulin resistance and mitochondrial DNA density in women. J Clin Endocrinol Metab 2012;97(1):E88–93.

[105] Liu Y, Huo X, Pang XF, Zong ZH, Meng X, Liu GL. Musclin inhibits insulin activation of Akt/protein kinase B in rat skeletal muscle. J Int Med Res 2008;36(3):496–504.

[106] Chen WJ, Liu Y, Sui YB, Zhang B, Zhang XH, Yin XH. Increased circulating levels of musclin in newly diagnosed type 2 diabetic patients. Diabetes Vasc Dis Res 2017;14(2):116–21.

[107] Haus JM, Kashyap SR, Kasumov T, Zhang R, Kelly KR, Defronzo RA, et al. Plasma ceramides are elevated in obese subjects with type 2 diabetes and correlate with the severity of insulin resistance. Diabetes 2009;58(2):337–43.

[108] Adams 2nd JM, Pratipanawatr T, Berria R, Wang E, DeFronzo RA, Sullards MC, et al. Ceramide content is increased in skeletal muscle from obese insulin-resistant humans. Diabetes 2004;53(1):25–31.

[109] Kurek K, Miklosz A, Lukaszuk B, Chabowski A, Gorski J, Zendzian-Piotrowska M. Inhibition of ceramide de novo synthesis ameliorates diet induced skeletal muscles insulin resistance. J Diabetes Res 2015;2015:154762.

[110] Patsouris D, Cao JJ, Vial G, Bravard A, Lefai E, Durand A, et al. Insulin resistance is associated with MCP1-mediated macrophage accumulation in skeletal muscle in mice and humans. PLoS One 2014;9(10):e110653.

[111] Kraakman MJ, Murphy AJ, Jandeleit-Dahm K, Kammoun HL. Macrophage polarization in obesity and type 2 diabetes: weighing down our understanding of macrophage function? Front Immunol 2014;5:470.

[112] Mehta P, Nuotio-Antar AM, Smith CW. γδ T cells promote inflammation and insulin resistance during high fat diet-induced obesity in mice. J Leukoc Biol 2015;97(1):121−34.

[113] Furukawa S, Fujita T, Shimabukuro M, Iwaki M, Yamada Y, Nakajima Y, et al. Increased oxidative stress in obesity and its impact on metabolic syndrome. J Clin Invest 2004;114(12):1752−61.

[114] Vincent HK, Innes KE, Vincent KR. Oxidative stress and potential interventions to reduce oxidative stress in overweight and obesity. Diabetes Obes Metab 2007;9(6):813−39.

[115] Huang CJ, McAllister MJ, Slusher AL, Webb HE, Mock JT, Acevedo EO. Obesity-related oxidative stress: the impact of physical activity and diet manipulation. Sports Med Open 2015;1(1):32.

[116] Kim TN, Choi KM. The implications of sarcopenia and sarcopenic obesity on cardiometabolic disease. J Cell Biochem 2015;116(7):1171−8.

[117] Russell AP, Gastaldi G, Bobbioni-Harsch E, Arboit P, Gobelet C, Deriaz O, et al. Lipid peroxidation in skeletal muscle of obese as compared to endurance-trained humans: a case of good vs. bad lipids? FEBS Lett 2003;551(1−3):104−6.

[118] Vincent HK, Powers SK, Stewart DJ, Shanely RA, Demirel H, Naito H. Obesity is associated with increased myocardial oxidative stress. Int J Obes Relat Metab Disord 1999;23(1):67−74.

[119] Samocha-Bonet D, Heilbronn LK, Lichtenberg D, Campbell LV. Does skeletal muscle oxidative stress initiate insulin resistance in genetically predisposed individuals? Trends Endocrinol Metab 2010;21(2):83−8.

[120] Di Meo S, Iossa S, Venditti P. Improvement of obesity-linked skeletal muscle insulin resistance by strength and endurance training. J Endocrinol 2017;234(3):R159−81.

[121] Di Meo S, Iossa S, Venditti P. Skeletal muscle insulin resistance: role of mitochondria and other ROS sources. J Endocrinol 2017;233(1):R15−42.

[122] Janero DR. Malondialdehyde and thiobarbituric acid-reactivity as diagnostic indices of lipid peroxidation and peroxidative tissue injury. Free Radic Biol Med 1990;9(6):515−40.

[123] Frühbeck G, Catalán V, Rodríguez A, Ramírez B, Becerril S, Portincasa P, et al. Normalization of adiponectin concentrations by leptin replacement in *ob/ob* mice is accompanied by reductions in systemic oxidative stress and inflammation. Sci Rep 2017;7(1):2752.

[124] Yokota T, Kinugawa S, Yamato M, Hirabayashi K, Suga T, Takada S, et al. Systemic oxidative stress is associated with lower aerobic capacity and impaired skeletal muscle energy metabolism in patients with metabolic syndrome. Diabetes Care 2013;36(5):1341−6.

[125] Frühbeck G, Catalán V, Rodríguez A, Ramírez B, Becerril S, Salvador J, et al. Involvement of the leptin-adiponectin axis in inflammation and oxidative stress in the metabolic syndrome. Sci Rep 2017;7(1):6619.

[126] Ansari JA, Bhandari U, Haque SE, Pillai KK. Enhancement of antioxidant defense mechanism by pitavastatin and rosuvastatin on obesity-induced oxidative stress in Wistar rats. Toxicol Mech Methods 2012;22(1):67−73.

[127] Tian YF, Hsia TL, Hsieh CH, Huang DW, Chen CH, Hsieh PS. The importance of cyclooxygenase 2-mediated oxidative stress in obesity-induced muscular insulin resistance in high-fat-fed rats. Life Sci 2011;89(3−4):107−14.

[128] Sáinz N, Rodríguez A, Catalán V, Becerril S, Ramírez B, Gómez-Ambrosi J, et al. Leptin administration downregulates the increased expression levels of genes related to oxidative stress and inflammation in the skeletal muscle of *ob/ob* mice. Mediat Inflamm 2010;2010:784343.

[129] Kaviarasan S, Muniandy S, Qvist R, Ismail IS. F$_2$-isoprostanes as novel biomarkers for type 2 diabetes: a review. J Clin Biochem Nutr 2009;45(1):1−8.

[130] Li G, Liu JY, Zhang HX, Li Q, Zhang SW. Exercise training attenuates sympathetic activation and oxidative stress in diet-induced obesity. Physiol Res 2015;64(3):355−67.

[131] Devries MC, Hamadeh MJ, Glover AW, Raha S, Samjoo IA, Tarnopolsky MA. Endurance training without weight loss lowers systemic, but not muscle, oxidative stress with no effect on inflammation in lean and obese women. Free Radic Biol Med 2008;45(4):503−11.

[132] Samocha-Bonet D, Campbell LV, Mori TA, Croft KD, Greenfield JR, Turner N, et al. Overfeeding reduces insulin sensitivity and increases oxidative stress, without altering markers of mitochondrial content and function in humans. PLoS One 2012;7(5):e36320.

[133] Ndisang JF, Lane N, Jadhav A. The heme oxygenase system abates hyperglycemia in Zucker diabetic fatty rats by potentiating insulin-sensitizing pathways. Endocrinology 2009;150(5):2098−108.

[134] Liu Y, Qi W, Richardson A, Van Remmen H, Ikeno Y, Salmon AB. Oxidative damage associated with obesity is prevented by overexpression of CuZn- or Mn-superoxide dismutase. Biochem Biophys Res Commun 2013;438(1):78−83.

[135] Picklo MJ, Long EK, Vomhof-DeKrey EE. Glutathionyl systems and metabolic dysfunction in obesity. Nutr Rev 2015;73(12):858−68.

[136] Kendig EL, Chen Y, Krishan M, Johansson E, Schneider SN, Genter MB, et al. Lipid metabolism and body composition in *Gclm*(−/−) mice. Toxicol Appl Pharmacol 2011;257(3):338−48.

[137] Loh K, Deng H, Fukushima A, Cai X, Boivin B, Galic S, et al. Reactive oxygen species enhance insulin sensitivity. Cell Metab 2009;10(4):260−72.

[138] McClung JP, Roneker CA, Mu W, Lisk DJ, Langlais P, Liu F, et al. Development of insulin resistance and obesity in mice overexpressing cellular glutathione peroxidase. Proc Natl Acad Sci USA 2004;101(24):8852−7.

[139] Lee YS, Kim AY, Choi JW, Kim M, Yasue S, Son HJ, et al. Dysregulation of adipose GPx3 in obesity contributes to local and systemic oxidative stress. Mol Endocrinol 2008;22(9):2176–89.

[140] Monzo-Beltran L, Vazquez-Tarragón A, Cerdà C, Garcia-Perez P, Iradi A, Sánchez C, et al. One-year follow-up of clinical, metabolic and oxidative stress profile of morbid obese patients after laparoscopic sleeve gastrectomy. 8-oxo-dG as a clinical marker. Redox Biol 2017;12:389–402.

[141] Barazzoni R, Zanetti M, Semolic A, Cattin MR, Pirulli A, Cattin L, et al. High-fat diet with acyl-ghrelin treatment leads to weight gain with low inflammation, high oxidative capacity and normal triglycerides in rat muscle. PLoS One 2011;6(10):e26224.

[142] Madani Z, Sener A, Malaisse WJ, Dalila AY. Sardine protein diet increases plasma glucagon-like peptide-1 levels and prevents tissue oxidative stress in rats fed a high-fructose diet. Mol Med Rep 2015;12(5):7017–26.

[143] Han YH, Buffolo M, Pires KM, Pei S, Scherer PE, Boudina S. Adipocyte-specific deletion of manganese superoxide dismutase protects from diet-induced obesity through increased mitochondrial uncoupling and biogenesis. Diabetes 2016;65(9):2639–51.

[144] Olusi SO. Obesity is an independent risk factor for plasma lipid peroxidation and depletion of erythrocyte cytoprotectic enzymes in humans. Int J Obes Relat Metab Disord 2002;26(9):1159–64.

[145] Torkanlou K, Bibak B, Abbaspour A, Abdi H, Saleh Moghaddam M, Tayefi M, et al. Reduced serum levels of zinc and superoxide dismutase in obese individuals. Ann Nutr Metab 2016;69(3–4):232–6.

[146] Samjoo IA, Safdar A, Hamadeh MJ, Raha S, Tarnopolsky MA. The effect of endurance exercise on both skeletal muscle and systemic oxidative stress in previously sedentary obese men. Nutr Diabetes 2013;3:e88.

[147] Farooqui AA, Farooqui T, Panza F, Frisardi V. Metabolic syndrome as a risk factor for neurological disorders. Cell Mol Life Sci 2012;69(5):741–62.

[148] Dasuri K, Ebenezer P, Fernandez-Kim SO, Zhang L, Gao Z, Bruce-Keller AJ, et al. Role of physiological levels of 4-hydroxynonenal on adipocyte biology: implications for obesity and metabolic syndrome. Free Radic Res 2013;47(1):8–19.

[149] Singh SP, Niemczyk M, Saini D, Awasthi YC, Zimniak L, Zimniak P. Role of the electrophilic lipid peroxidation product 4-hydroxynonenal in the development and maintenance of obesity in mice. Biochemistry (Moscow) 2008;47(12):3900–11.

[150] Cattaruzza M, Hecker M. Protein carbonylation and decarboylation: a new twist to the complex response of vascular cells to oxidative stress. Circ Res 2008;102(3):273–4.

[151] Ruskovska T, Bernlohr DA. Oxidative stress and protein carbonylation in adipose tissue – implications for insulin resistance and diabetes mellitus. J Proteomics 2013;92:323–34.

[152] Gómez-Pérez Y, Amengual-Cladera E, Català-Niell A, Thomàs-Moyà E, Gianotti M, Proenza AM, et al. Gender dimorphism in high-fat-diet-induced insulin resistance in skeletal muscle of aged rats. Cell Physiol Biochem 2008;22(5–6):539–48.

[153] Bouanane S, Benkalfat NB, Baba Ahmed FZ, Merzouk H, Mokhtari NS, Merzouk SA, et al. Time course of changes in serum oxidant/antioxidant status in overfed obese rats and their offspring. Clin Sci (Lond) 2009;116(8):669–80.

[154] Grimsrud PA, Picklo Sr MJ, Griffin TJ, Bernlohr DA. Carbonylation of adipose proteins in obesity and insulin resistance: identification of adipocyte fatty acid-binding protein as a cellular target of 4-hydroxynonenal. Mol Cell Proteomics 2007;6(4):624–37.

[155] Hoehn KL, Salmon AB, Hohnen-Behrens C, Turner N, Hoy AJ, Maghzal GJ, et al. Insulin resistance is a cellular antioxidant defense mechanism. Proc Natl Acad Sci USA 2009;106(42):17787–92.

[156] Yokota T, Kinugawa S, Hirabayashi K, Matsushima S, Inoue N, Ohta Y, et al. Oxidative stress in skeletal muscle impairs mitochondrial respiration and limits exercise capacity in type 2 diabetic mice. Am J Physiol Heart Circ Physiol 2009;297(3):H1069–77.

[157] Chanseaume E, Barquissau V, Salles J, Aucouturier J, Patrac V, Giraudet C, et al. Muscle mitochondrial oxidative phosphorylation activity, but not content, is altered with abdominal obesity in sedentary men: synergism with changes in insulin sensitivity. J Clin Endocrinol Metab 2010;95(6):2948–56.

[158] Mittal PC, Kant R. Correlation of increased oxidative stress to body weight in disease-free post menopausal women. Clin Biochem 2009;42(10–11):1007–11.

[159] Akl MG, Fawzy E, Deif M, Farouk A, Elshorbagy AK. Perturbed adipose tissue hydrogen peroxide metabolism in centrally obese men: association with insulin resistance. PLoS One 2017;12(5):e0177268.

[160] Huh JY, Kim Y, Jeong J, Park J, Kim I, Huh KH, et al. Peroxiredoxin 3 is a key molecule regulating adipocyte oxidative stress, mitochondrial biogenesis, and adipokine expression. Antioxid Redox Signal 2012;16(3):229–43.

[161] Jortay J, Senou M, Abou-Samra M, Noel L, Robert A, Many MC, et al. Adiponectin and skeletal muscle: pathophysiological implications in metabolic stress. Am J Pathol 2012;181(1):245–56.

[162] Das SK, Sharma NK, Hasstedt SJ, Mondal AK, Ma L, Langberg KA, et al. An integrative genomics approach identifies activation of thioredoxin/thioredoxin reductase-1-mediated oxidative stress defense pathway and inhibition of angiogenesis in obese nondiabetic human subjects. J Clin Endocrinol Metab 2011;96(8):E1308–13.

[163] Qin H, Zhang X, Ye F, Zhong L. High-fat diet-induced changes in liver thioredoxin and thioredoxin reductase as a novel feature of insulin resistance. FEBS Open Bio 2014;4:928–35.

[164] Chutkow WA, Birkenfeld AL, Brown JD, Lee HY, Frederick DW, Yoshioka J, et al. Deletion of the α-arrestin protein Txnip in mice promotes adiposity and adipogenesis while preserving insulin sensitivity. Diabetes 2010;59(6):1424–34.

[165] Oslowski CM, Hara T, O'Sullivan-Murphy B, Kanekura K, Lu S, Hara M, et al. Thioredoxin-interacting protein mediates ER stress-induced β cell death through initiation of the inflammasome. Cell Metab 2012;16(2):265–73.

[166] Parikh H, Carlsson E, Chutkow WA, Johansson LE, Storgaard H, Poulsen P, et al. TXNIP regulates peripheral glucose metabolism in humans. PLoS Med 2007;4(5):e158.

[167] Johnson ML, Distelmaier K, Lanza IR, Irving BA, Robinson MM, Konopka AR, et al. Mechanism by which caloric restriction improves insulin sensitivity in sedentary obese adults. Diabetes 2016;65(1):74–84.

[168] Koska J, Lopez L, D'Souza K, Osredkar T, Deer J, Kurtz J, et al. Effect of liraglutide on dietary lipid-induced insulin resistance in humans. Diabetes Obes Metab 2018;20(1):69–76. https://doi.org/10.1111/dom.13037.

[169] Houstis N, Rosen ED, Lander ES. Reactive oxygen species have a causal role in multiple forms of insulin resistance. Nature 2006;440(7086):944–8.

[170] Bashan N, Kovsan J, Kachko I, Ovadia H, Rudich A. Positive and negative regulation of insulin signaling by reactive oxygen and nitrogen species. Physiol Rev 2009;89(1):27–71.

[171] Valle A, Catalán V, Rodríguez A, Rotellar F, Valentí V, Silva C, et al. Identification of liver proteins altered by type 2 diabetes mellitus in obese subjects. Liver Int 2012;32(6):951–61.

[172] Newsholme P, Cruzat VF, Keane KN, Carlessi R, de Bittencourt Jr PI. Molecular mechanisms of ROS production and oxidative stress in diabetes. Biochem J 2016;473(24):4527–50.

[173] Boden G, Homko C, Barrero CA, Stein TP, Chen X, Cheung P, et al. Excessive caloric intake acutely causes oxidative stress, GLUT4 carbonylation, and insulin resistance in healthy men. Sci Transl Med 2015;7(304):304re7.

[174] Anderson EJ, Lustig ME, Boyle KE, Woodlief TL, Kane DA, Lin CT, et al. Mitochondrial H_2O_2 emission and cellular redox state link excess fat intake to insulin resistance in both rodents and humans. J Clin Invest 2009;119(3):573–81.

[175] Chen L, Na R, Gu M, Salmon AB, Liu Y, Liang H, et al. Reduction of mitochondrial H_2O_2 by overexpressing peroxiredoxin 3 improves glucose tolerance in mice. Aging Cell 2008;7(6):866–78.

[176] Schroder K, Zhou R, Tschopp J. The NLRP3 inflammasome: a sensor for metabolic danger? Science 2010;327(5963):296–300.

[177] JafariNasabian P, Inglis JE, Reilly W, Kelly OJ, Ilich JZ. Aging human body: changes in bone, muscle and body fat with consequent changes in nutrient intake. J Endocrinol 2017;234(1):R37–51.

[178] Vincent HK, Raiser SN, Vincent KR. The aging musculoskeletal system and obesity-related considerations with exercise. Ageing Res Rev 2012;11(3):361–73.

[179] Jo E, Lee SR, Park BS, Kim JS. Potential mechanisms underlying the role of chronic inflammation in age-related muscle wasting. Aging Clin Exp Res 2012;24(5):412–22.

[180] Combaret L, Dardevet D, Bechet D, Taillandier D, Mosoni L, Attaix D. Skeletal muscle proteolysis in aging. Curr Opin Clin Nutr Metab Care 2009;12(1):37–41.

[181] Stenholm S, Harris TB, Rantanen T, Visser M, Kritchevsky SB, Ferrucci L. Sarcopenic obesity: definition, cause and consequences. Curr Opin Clin Nutr Metab Care 2008;11(6):693–700.

[182] Lim JP, Leung BP, Ding YY, Tay L, Ismail NH, Yeo A, et al. Monocyte chemoattractant protein-1: a proinflammatory cytokine elevated in sarcopenic obesity. Clin Interv Aging 2015;10:605–9.

[183] Kalinkovich A, Livshits G. Sarcopenic obesity or obese sarcopenia: a cross talk between age-associated adipose tissue and skeletal muscle inflammation as a main mechanism of the pathogenesis. Ageing Res Rev 2017;35:200–21.

[184] Sakuma K, Yamaguchi A. Sarcopenic obesity and endocrinal adaptation with age. Int J Endocrinol 2013;2013:204164.

[185] Nakano R, Takebe N, Ono M, Hangai M, Nakagawa R, Yashiro S, et al. Involvement of oxidative stress in atherosclerosis development in subjects with sarcopenic obesity. Obes Sci Pract 2017;3(2):212–8.

[186] Giugliano D, Ceriello A, Esposito K. The effects of diet on inflammation: emphasis on the metabolic syndrome. J Am Coll Cardiol 2006;48(4):677–85.

[187] Halliwell B. Oxidative stress, nutrition and health. Experimental strategies for optimization of nutritional antioxidant intake in humans. Free Radic Res 1996;25(1):57–74.

[188] Mozaffarian D, Katan MB, Ascherio A, Stampfer MJ, Willett WC. Trans fatty acids and cardiovascular disease. N Engl J Med 2006;354(15):1601–13.

[189] Tishinsky JM, De Boer AA, Dyck DJ, Robinson LE. Modulation of visceral fat adipokine secretion by dietary fatty acids and ensuing changes in skeletal muscle inflammation. Appl Physiol Nutr Metab 2014;39(1):28–37.

[190] Turco AA, Guescini M, Valtucci V, Colosimo C, De Feo P, Mantuano M, et al. Dietary fat differentially modulate the mRNA expression levels of oxidative mitochondrial genes in skeletal muscle of healthy subjects. Nutr Metab Cardiovasc Dis 2014;24(2):198–204.

[191] Flock MR, Rogers CJ, Prabhu KS, Kris-Etherton PM. Immunometabolic role of long-chain omega-3 fatty acids in obesity-induced inflammation. Diabetes Metab Res Rev. 2013;29(6):431–45.

[192] Skulas-Ray AC. Omega-3 fatty acids and inflammation: a perspective on the challenges of evaluating efficacy in clinical research. Prostaglandins Other Lipid Mediat 2015;116–117:104–11.

[193] Titos E, Claria J. Omega-3-derived mediators counteract obesity-induced adipose tissue inflammation. Prostaglandins Other Lipid Mediat 2013;107:77–84.

[194] Jeromson S, Gallagher IJ, Galloway SD, Hamilton DL. Omega-3 fatty acids and skeletal muscle health. Mar Drugs 2015;13(11):6977–7004.

[195] Putti R, Migliaccio V, Sica R, Lionetti L. Skeletal muscle mitochondrial bioenergetics and morphology in high fat diet induced obesity and insulin resistance: focus on dietary fat source. Front Physiol 2016;6:426.

[196] Cavaliere G, Trinchese G, Bergamo P, De Filippo C, Mattace Raso G, Gifuni G, et al. Polyunsaturated fatty acids attenuate diet induced obesity and insulin resistance, modulating mitochondrial respiratory uncoupling in rat skeletal muscle. PLoS One 2016;11(2):e0149033.

[197] Risk, Prevention Study Collaborative G, Roncaglioni MC, Tombesi M, Avanzini F, Barlera S, et al. n-3 fatty acids in patients with multiple cardiovascular risk factors. N Engl J Med 2013;368(19):1800—8.

[198] Esposito K, Nappo F, Giugliano F, Giugliano G, Marfella R, Giugliano D. Effect of dietary antioxidants on postprandial endothelial dysfunction induced by a high-fat meal in healthy subjects. Am J Clin Nutr 2003;77(1):139—43.

[199] Miller 3rd ER, Appel LJ, Risby TH. Effect of dietary patterns on measures of lipid peroxidation: results from a randomized clinical trial. Circulation 1998;98(22):2390—5.

[200] Ryan MJ, Dudash HJ, Docherty M, Geronilla KB, Baker BA, Haff GG, et al. Vitamin E and C supplementation reduces oxidative stress, improves antioxidant enzymes and positive muscle work in chronically loaded muscles of aged rats. Exp Gerontol 2010;45(11):882—95.

[201] Bhat M, Ismail A. Vitamin D treatment protects against and reverses oxidative stress induced muscle proteolysis. J Steroid Biochem Mol Biol 2015;152:171—9.

[202] Sadeghi A, Seyyed Ebrahimi SS, Golestani A, Meshkani R. Resveratrol ameliorates palmitate-induced inflammation in skeletal muscle cells by attenuating oxidative stress and JNK/NF-κB pathway in a SIRT1-independent mechanism. J Cell Biochem 2017;118(9):2654—63.

[203] Lambert K, Coisy-Quivy M, Bisbal C, Sirvent P, Hugon G, Mercier J, et al. Grape polyphenols supplementation reduces muscle atrophy in a mouse model of chronic inflammation. Nutrition 2015;31(10):1275—83.

[204] Pesta D, Roden M. The Janus head of oxidative stress in metabolic diseases and during physical exercise. Curr Diabetes Rep 2017;17(6):41.

[205] Fisher-Wellman K, Bloomer RJ. Acute exercise and oxidative stress: a 30 year history. Dyn Med 2009;8:1.

[206] Pedersen BK, Bruunsgaard H. Possible beneficial role of exercise in modulating low-grade inflammation in the elderly. Scand J Med Sci Sports 2003;13(1):56—62.

[207] Huh JY. The role of exercise-induced myokines in regulating metabolism. Arch Pharm Res 2018;41(1):14—29. https://doi.org/10.1007/s12272-017-0994-y.

[208] Lightfoot AP, Cooper RG. The role of myokines in muscle health and disease. Curr Opin Rheumatol 2016;28(6):661—6.

[209] Lambert CP, Wright NR, Finck BN, Villareal DT. Exercise but not diet-induced weight loss decreases skeletal muscle inflammatory gene expression in frail obese elderly persons. J Appl Physiol (1985) 2008;105(2):473—8.

[210] Biolo G, Cederholm T, Muscaritoli M. Muscle contractile and metabolic dysfunction is a common feature of sarcopenia of aging and chronic diseases: from sarcopenic obesity to cachexia. Clin Nutr 2014;33(5):737—48.

[211] Görgens SW, Benninghoff T, Eckardt K, Springer C, Chadt A, Melior A, et al. Hypoxia in combination with muscle contraction improves insulin action and glucose metabolism in human skeletal muscle via the HIF-1α pathway. Diabetes 2017;66(11):2800—7.

[212] Bergman BC, Brozinick JT, Strauss A, Bacon S, Kerege A, Bui HH, et al. Muscle sphingolipids during rest and exercise: a C18:0 signature for insulin resistance in humans. Diabetologia 2016;59(4):785—98.

Chapter 9

Evaluation of Oxidative Stress in Humans: A Critical Point of View

Josep A. Tur, Antoni Sureda and Antoni Pons

University of the Balearic Islands & CIBEROBN, Palma de Mallorca, Spain

An important causative factor in human aging and the development of chronic diseases is the instauration of oxidative stress through the genesis and effects of oxidative-damaged macromolecules or their degradation products. Overproduction of reactive oxygen species (ROS) is usually associated with the pathophysiology of many diseases, including excessive activation of polymorphonuclear neutrophils and macrophages which leads to ROS generation [1]. Antioxidants showed beneficial effects on biological systems, mainly preventing damage associated with oxidative stress. Thus accurate evaluation of oxidative stress status in the body is highly recommended. Blood cells are useful tools to determine functional oxidative status.

1. BLOOD CELLS GIVE INFORMATION ON ANTIOXIDANT ENDOGENOUS STATUS

Neutrophils constitute the most abundant leukocytes in human organisms, playing a central role in antibacterial defense. Neutrophils rapidly migrate to a site of infection and destroy pathogens through generation of ROS by NADPH oxidase complex of the cell membrane nicotinamide adenine dinucleotide phosphate oxidase complex and the release and degranulation of cytosolic granules containing proteolytic enzymes [2]. These cells also initiate the inflammatory response, and produce and release a wide variety of cytokines. To prevent the auto-oxidative process, neutrophils possess antioxidant enzymes, such as superoxide dismutases (SOD-Mn, SOD-Cu/Zn), catalase and glutathione peroxidases, and others in order to decompose ROS and repair oxidized proteins or recycle antioxidant molecules (gluthatione, ascorbate). So, neutrophils have an antioxidant defense mechanism against self-generated ROS and oxidative damage, limiting the destruction of neighboring tissues [3]. The immune cell levels of these enzymes are important and contribute to deactivating ROS [4]. Accordingly, antioxidant defenses are also part of the acute-phase immune response mechanism. Peripheral blood mononuclear cells (PBMCs) comprise the monocytes and lymphocytes, which represent cells of the innate and adaptive immune systems, respectively. In terms of quantity, lymphocytes are the largest cell population within the PBMCs. Lymphocytes, as cells of the adaptive immune system, recognize specific pathogens, contribute to their recognition and destruction, and act to protect against future infections. After immune stimulation these cells significantly increase the oxygen consumption, and consequently lead to an antioxidant adaptation to prevent any cellular oxidative damage.

Reduced glutathione (GSH) is the major intracellular nonprotein thiol redox buffer; GSH and GSH-related enzymes are essential for the maintenance of the cellular redox state [5]. Under oxidizing conditions, two GSH molecules become linked by a disulfide bridge forming glutathione disulfide (GSSG). GSSG can be transformed back to its GSH form by the action of glutathione reductase. In this regard, GSH, GSSG, and the GSH:GSSG ratio are considered as biomarkers of cellular redox metabolism. An oxidative stress situation can overwhelm the capacity of the cell to reduce GSSG to GSH, leading to GSSG accumulation. For instance, it has been reported that blood GSSG levels were significantly increased after performing strenuous physical exercise such as a mountain biking or intense swimming [6]. Decreases in GSH could reflect its consumption by skeletal muscle, causing a lower release from the muscle itself to the plasma [7]. Exercise increases glutathione reductase activity, which is interpreted as a response to exercise-induced oxidative stress, since glutathione reductase regenerates GSH at the expense of GSSG [8]. After running a marathon, the activity of glutathione peroxidase and SOD decreases [9]. Moderate exercises increase glutathione peroxidase activity and a half-marathon increases SOD activity [10] and decreases catalase activity [11].

Despite having the lowest antioxidant enzymatic defense ability compared to the peripheral blood immune cells, erythrocytes also play a role in oxidative stress contributing to ROS elimination. Erythrocytes have enzymes such as SOD, catalase, several peroxidases, glutathione and the mechanisms necessary for their regeneration. Catalase and glutathione peroxidase are the enzymes that in most cases eliminate hydrogen peroxide from erythrocytes [12]. Erythrocyte antioxidant enzymes act like free radical scavengers and other low-molecular-weight antioxidants to maintain cell integrity and functional capacity. Obviously, any alteration in the erythrocyte membrane will be compensated by a new production of erythrocytes, although there is a long recovery period since erythrocytes are not able to synthesize proteins. However, acute regulation of the erythrocytes' antioxidant enzymatic activity is achieved by the action of certain environmental factors; thus micromolar concentrations of H_2O_2 stimulate erythrocyte SOD activity. Similarly, the superoxide anion enzymatically produced by xanthine oxidase activates catalase. There is evidence of acute adaptive changes in antioxidant erythrocyte enzyme activities during exhaustive exercise and after short-term recovery [13]. A biathlon competition and/or its short-term recovery produced a slight hemolysis and increase the activity of catalase and peroxidases but not SOD enzymes. This change in catalase activity is mimicked in vitro by the superoxide-anion-generating system. The changes are required to minimize the oxidative stress induced by exercise. However, strenuous exercises, both long-term and fast, exceed erythrocyte's ability to eliminate ROS, producing oxidative stress and decreasing the intraerythrocyte reserves of catalase and glutathione peroxidase, especially during the recovery period after exercise [11].

The characteristics of aerobic or anaerobic exercise, the previous physical preparation, the duration of the training program, the frequency of the sessions, and the nutritional status of the athlete will modify the activity of the antioxidant enzymes. The training induces an increase in the activities of the antioxidant enzymes contained in the erythrocytes. Variations in enzymatic activity will depend on each enzyme and the type of physical activity performed [14]. These variations are interpreted as a mechanism aimed at maintaining a balance between the increase in oxidative stress induced by physical exercise and the defenses to it.

The determination of enzymatic activities requires fresh blood samples or samples that have undergone only a short period of freezing, since prolonged storage is associated with a progressive loss of activity. In longitudinal studies or investigations in which the collection of samples is prolonged over time, it is preferable to determine the enzyme activities in fresh blood samples throughout the trial or to determine the protein or mRNA levels instead, since they present greater stability.

2. BLOOD CELLS GIVE INFORMATION ON EICOSANOID LEVELS

Prostaglandins (PGs) transient molecules with a half-life of only seconds to minutes are usually mediators; PGs arise from the ciclooxygenase-1 (COX-1) and COX-2 cascade from arachidonic acid or its precursors, and induce central to vascular responses, permitting neutrophils and monocytes to leave post capillary venules. PGs also play a role in the regulation of muscle protein metabolism [15], vasodilation, human skeletal muscle microcirculation, febrile and inflammatory responses [16], and initiation and timely resolution of inflammation [17]. Prostaglandin E1 (PGE1) and prostaglandin E2 (PGE2) are potent vasodilators which account for the increased blood flow in inflamed areas, but PGE1 also regulates neutrophil function by reducing neutrophil activation [18]. Because of these vasodilator and immune properties, PGs are used as treatment for diseases derived from ischemia reperfusion, such as arterial occlusive disease and venous ulcers [18–20].

The response of PGs to exercise has not yet been clearly established. Skeletal muscle produces PGs in response to muscular work, and this production is blocked by the intake of COX inhibitors [20,21]. Plasma PGE2 concentration increases in response to exercise or muscle damage [22]. In other words, exercise increases PGE2 production as part of the inflammatory response, triggered by microtraumas occurring in skeletal muscles [22]. In addition, PGE2 synthesis by infiltrating macrophages in the inflamed muscle increases 24–48 h after an exercise session [23]. It is also noticeable that downhill running for 45 min at 75% VO2 max increases circulating monocyte production of PGE2 [24]. The effects of PGE2 can be described as proinflammatory or antiinflammatory, depending on location, since PGE2 enhances leukotriene B4-mediated neutrophil extravasation and tissue injury, but it can also inhibit the nuclear factor-κB signaling pathway in macrophages [25]. This inhibition plays a critical function in the initiation of resolution via lipid mediator class switching [17].

A new family of lipid mediators produced from the oxidation of ω-3 polyunsaturated fatty acid, including resolvins (Rvs), maresins, and protectins, has been described as proresolving mediators of inflammation [26,27]. The synthesis of these products involves COX and Lipoxygenase (LOX) pathways from docosahexaenoic acid and eicosapentaenoic acid

[27]. Rvs have been reported to reduce inflammation in chronic inflammatory diseases. Specifically, RvE1 and RvD1 inhibit transendothelial migration of neutrophils, preventing the infiltration of neutrophils into sites of inflammation, and RvD1 also inhibits Interleukin-1beta (IL1β) production [28]. Plasma RvE1 and RvD1 have also been demonstrated to increase after acute exercise [20], but the participation of these lipid mediators in the antiinflammatory effects of exercise has not been widely studied.

3. BLOOD CELLS ARE USEFUL TO DEFINE ANTIOXIDANT EXOGENOUS (VITAMIN) STATUS

High plasma levels of exogenous antioxidants are usually associated with low risk of cardiovascular disease and cancer [29,30]. It would thus be useful to find biomarkers showing the status of antioxidant vitamin depots and availability. Balanced diets provide appropriate amounts of all nutrients. Within them, vitamins C and E are key antioxidants in humans, and are exclusively obtained from the diet. Vitamin C is hydrophilic and protects water-soluble components of the body, while vitamin E is a lipid-soluble antioxidant that protects cell membranes from peroxidative damage. It has been demonstrated that these key antioxidants show an in vivo interaction: vitamin C is able to recycle vitamin E. Antioxidant vitamin status depends not only on vitamin intake but may also be influenced by exercise, smoking habits, and levels of other dietary nutrients, modifying the absorption and metabolism of antioxidant vitamins [31–33]. Thus dietary intake cannot accurately reflect plasma vitamin levels. However, the plasma levels of antioxidant vitamins could reflect the acute assimilation of these vitamins [34]. The quantity of antioxidant vitamins required to avoid suboptimal supply and deficiency [35–37], or oxidative damage in persons engaged in physical activity [38], is still controversial. Conflicting results for vitamin E have been explained by increased bioavailability of vitamin E due to fat-rich meals [39], changes in vitamin E absorption according to an individual's ability to absorb fat, supplemental vitamin E malabsorption, and maximal absorption after vitamin E has been given at meals [40].

Plasma vitamin C concentration is controlled by mediated tissue transport, absorption, and excretion. Plasma vitamin C concentration of 60–70 μmol/L has been used as indicative of good dietary intake. Immune blood cells (lymphocytes and neutrophils) contain 1–4 mM of vitamin C and saturate at vitamin C doses of 100–200 mg daily. Lymphocytes are reported to be saturated at plasma concentrations of >50 μmol/L. Thus cells are saturated before plasma. When plasma vitamin C contents approach maximal concentration, additional vitamin C is lost in urine. Higher vitamin C doses than 200 mg daily are unnecessary to avoid oxidative damage in nonrisk population groups [30]. Thus the lymphocyte or neutrophil vitamin C concentration is a good marker of vitamin C status.

Plasma vitamin E is a biomarker to assess vitamin E status. A daily dietary intake of about 15–30 mg α-tocopherol is required to maintain optimal plasma levels. This amount of vitamin E could be obtained from dietary sources if a concerted effort was made to eat foods high in this vitamin. In contrast, the amounts of supplemental vitamin E suggested as protective in epidemiological studies are many times higher than those that could be obtained from the diet. The correlation between α-tocopherol and blood lipids, especially cholesterol, is high. So it is recommended that plasma α-tocopherol concentrations should be lipid corrected. Plasma vitamin E is quickly redistributed between tissues, mainly in the adipose tissue, and hence plasma does not reflect the vitamin E status. However, the adipose tissue vitamin E is a useful measure of vitamin E status [41].

Increased mitochondrial respiration occurs in exercise, allowing for high ROS production through the incomplete reduction of oxygen to water. In response to exercise-induced muscle damage, neutrophils and macrophages migrate to the site, infiltrate the muscle tissue, activate cytokines, and produce additional ROS. Excess generation of ROS may overwhelm natural cellular antioxidant defenses, leading to lipid peroxidation and further contributing to muscle damage [34]. Thus there is a paradox between the benefits of moderate exercise and damaging strenuous exercise. Increased oxidative stress risk and increased antioxidant vitamin demand are usually present in sportspeople who practice exhaustive exercise. Vitamin E depots in tissues are used to counteract ROS production induced by exercise. So exercise is a good model to establish the importance of plasma vitamin E to reflect the tissue status for this vitamin. We have demonstrated elsewhere that the recommended daily intake of vitamin E is not enough to avoid the oxidative stress induced by intense exercise in professional cyclists during a mountain stage, since vitamin E plasma levels fall to values lower than basal levels [42,43].

The dose of antioxidants administered seems to be important to decrease the deleterious effects of exercise. It has been shown that administering 330 mg/day of vitamin E decreases the oxidative stress markers after intensive aerobic training in cyclists [44]; administering low doses of vitamin E (20 mg/day α-tocopheryl succinate) and ascorbic acid (120 mg/day) for 4 weeks decreases muscle damage in triathletes [45].

We have previously evaluated the effects of vitamin C supplementation on this vitamin's plasma and lymphocyte levels after repetitive episodes of hypoxia reoxygenation induced by diving apnea [46]. Seven voluntary male professional apnea divers participated in a double-blind cross-study. The sportsmen were divided randomly into two groups: one was supplemented with vitamin C capsules (1 g/day) for 7 days, while the second group took a placebo. Ten days after the first diving apnea session (wash-out period), the procedure was repeated, but now changing the supplementation, i.e. the group firstly supplemented with vitamin C, was now supplemented with placebo, and vice versa. The subjects dived in apnea for 4 hours and remained under hypoxic conditions. After the supplementation, both groups showed similar plasma and lymphocyte basal values of vitamin C. Plasma and lymphocyte vitamin C concentration increased after diving apnea, but this increase was significant only in the supplemented group.

The combined effects on exercise-induced oxidative stress of 1 month supplementation of antioxidant vitamins C and E were also studied [47], using 14 volunteer male amateur runners who trained for 7.5 ± 1.3 h/week. The subjects did not take antioxidant dietary supplements or routine medication for 1 month before the study. Antioxidant vitamin intake in the supplemented group was 60 ± 1 mg/day for vitamin E and 277 ± 30 mg/day for vitamin C, while in the placebo group vitamin E intake was 14.8 ± 1.2 mg/day and vitamin C was 162 ± 29 mg/day. These antioxidant doses can be provided by a diverse and well-balanced diet. One month later subjects participated in a half-marathon race (21 km), and took 91 ± 10 min to finish the race. Basal plasma and lymphocyte levels of vitamin C and E after supplementation remained unchanged. However, plasma vitamin C concentration increased (+30%) after exercise only in the supplemented group and returned to basal values after 3 h recovery, whereas vitamin E maintained the basal values. Lymphocytes of the supplemented group increased (+40%) their vitamin C content after the exercise and remained high after 3 h of recovery, while lymphocyte vitamin C contents maintained basal levels in the placebo group. After the half-marathon, vitamin E levels in lymphocytes and neutrophils of supplemented subjects were practically twice the levels before exercise, and these levels remained high after recovery. The increase was higher in the supplemented group (about 130%) than in the placebo (about 100%). Neutrophil vitamin E contents in the placebo group were close to those in plasma. However, the contribution of neutrophils and lymphocytes to vitamin E blood contents is low, because most vitamin E blood contents come from plasma.

High antioxidant vitamin availability allows lymphocytes to increase their antioxidant defenses to avoid the deleterious ROS effects induced by intense exercise. Immune blood cells accumulate vitamin E to prevent autooxidative processes and maintain their functionality. These results show that antioxidant vitamins exert a protective effect against oxidative stress on human cells, but also that intense exercise promotes mechanisms to accumulate antioxidant vitamins into cells sensitive to the effects of ROS.

Thus antioxidant vitamin contents in lymphocytes and neutrophils after exercise are a useful tool to assess the functional status of antioxidant vitamins in both individuals and populations, especially among sportspeople.

4. CONCLUSIONS

An accurate evaluation of oxidative stress in the body is highly recommended. Blood cells can provide information on the functional antioxidant status, both endogenous and exogenous, as well as eicosanoid levels.

REFERENCES

[1] Ji LL. Antioxidants and oxidative stress in exercise. PSEBM 1999;222:283−92.

[2] Kovalenko EI, Boyko AA, Semenkov VF, Lutsenko GV, Grechikhina MV, Kanevskiy LM, Azhikina TL, Telford WG, Sapozhnikov AM. ROS production, intracellular HSP70 levels and their relationship in human neutrophils: effects of age. Oncotarget 2014;5:11800−12.

[3] Clarkson PM, Thompson HS. Antioxidants: what role do they play in physical activity and health. Am J Clin Nutr 2000;72:637S−46S.

[4] Pietarinen-Runtti P, Lakari E, Raivio KO, Kinnula VL. Expression of antioxidant enzymes in human inflammatory cells. Am J Physiol 2000;278:C118−25.

[5] Robaczewska J, Kedziora-Kornatowska K, Kozakiewicz M, Zary-Sikorska E, Pawluk H, Pawliszak W, Kedziora J. Role of glutathione metabolism and glutathione-related antioxidant defense systems in hypertension. J Physiol Pharmacol 2016;67:331−7.

[6] Inal M, Akyuz F, Turgut A, Getsfried W. Effect of aerobic and anaerobic metabolism on free radical generation in swimmers. Med Sci Sports Exerc 1999;33:564−7.

[7] Kretzschmar M, Muller D. Aging, training and exercise. A review of effects on plasma glutathione and lipid peroxides. Sports Med 1993;15:196−209.

[8] Boccatonda A, Tripaldi R, Davì G, Santilli F. Oxidative stress modulation through habitual physical activity. Curr Pharm Des 2016;22:3648−80.

[9] Hessel E, Haberland A, Müller M, Lerche D, Schimke I. Oxygen radical generation of neutrophils: a reason for oxidative stress during marathon running. Clin Chim Acta 2000;298:145−56.

[10] Atalay M, Laaksonen DE, Niskanen L, Uusitupa M, Hänninen O, Sen CK. Altered antioxidant enzyme defences in insulin-dependent diabetic men with increased resting and exercise-induced oxidative stress. Acta Physiol Scand 1997;161:195—201.

[11] Marzatico F, Pansarasa O, Bertorelli L, Della Valle G. Blood free radical antioxidant enzymes and lipid peroxides following long distance and lactacidemic performances in highly trained aerobic and sprint athletes. J Sports Med Phys Fit 1997;37:235—9.

[12] Müller S, Riedel HD, Stremmel W. Direct evidence for catalase as the predominant H_2O_2-removing enzyme in human erythrocytes. Blood 1997;90:4973—6.

[13] Tauler P, Gimeno I, Aguiló A, Guix MP, Pons A. Regulation of erythrocyte antioxidant enzyme activities in athletes during competition and short-term recovery. Pflügers Arch — Eur J Physiol 1999;438:782—7.

[14] Miyazaki H, Oh-ishi S, Ookawara T, Kizaki T, Toshinai K, Ha S, Haga S, Ji LL, Ohno H. Strenuous endurance training in humans reduces oxidative stress following exhausting exercise. Eur J Appl Physiol 2001;84:1—6.

[15] Burd NA, Dickinson JM, Lemoine JK, Carroll CC, Sullivan BE, Haus JM, Jemiolo B, Trappe SW, Hughes GM, Sanders Jr CE, Trappe TA. Effect of a cyclooxygenase-2 inhibitor on postexercise muscle protein synthesis in humans. Am J Physiol Endocrinol Metab 2010;298:E354—61.

[16] Uchida MC, Nosaka K, Ugrinowitsch C, Yamashita A, Martins Jr E, Moriscot AS, Aoki MS. Effect of bench press exercise intensity on muscle soreness and inflammatory mediators. J Sports Sci 2009;27:499—507.

[17] Serhan CN. Pro-resolving lipid mediators are leads for resolution physiology. Nature 2014;510:92—101.

[18] Weiss T, Eckstein H, Weiss C, Diehm C. Neutrophil function in peripheral arterial occlusive disease: the effects of prostaglandin E1. Vasc Med (Lond, Engl) 1998;3:171—5.

[19] Frassdorf J, Luther B, Mullenheim J, Otto F, Preckel B, Schlack W, Thamer V. Influence of groin incision, duration of ischemia, and prostaglandin E1 on ischemia-reperfusion injury of the lower limb. J Cardiothorac Vasc Anesth 2006;20:187—95.

[20] Markworth JF, Vella L, Lingard BS, Tull DL, Rupasinghe TW, Sinclair AJ, Maddipati KR, Cameron-Smith D. Human inflammatory and resolving lipid mediator responses to resistance exercise and ibuprofen treatment. Am J Physiol Regul Integr Comp Physiol 2013;305:R1281—96.

[21] Trappe TA, Liu SZ. Effects of prostaglandins and COX-inhibiting drugs on skeletal muscle adaptations to exercise. J Appl Physiol (1985) 2013;115:909—19.

[22] Bassit RA, Curi R, Costa Rosa LF. Creatine supplementation reduces plasma levels of pro-inflammatory cytokines and PGE2 after a half-ironman competition. Amino Acids 2008;35:425—31.

[23] Volek JS, Rawson ES. Scientific basis and practical aspects of creatine supplementation for athletes. Nutrition (Burbank, Los Angeles County, Calif) 2004;20:609—14.

[24] Cannon JG. Inflammatory cytokines in nonpathological states. News Physiol Sci 2000;215:298—303.

[25] Liu Y, Chen LY, Sokolowska M, Eberlein M, Alsaaty S, Martinez-Anton A, Logun C, Qi HY, Shelhamer JH. The fish oil ingredient, docosahexaenoic acid, activates cytosolic phospholipase A2 via GPR120 receptor to produce prostaglandin E2 and plays an anti-inflammatory role in macrophages. Immunology 2014;143:81—95.

[26] Capó X, Martorell M, Sureda A, Tur JA, Pons A. Effects of dietary docosahexanoic, training and acute exercise on lipid mediators. J Int Soc Sports Nutr 2016;13:16—27.

[27] Serhan CN, Clish CB, Brannon J, Colgan SP, Gronert K, Chiang N. Antimicroinflammatory lipid signals generated from dietary N-3 fatty acids via cyclooxygenase-2 and transcellular processing: a novel mechanism for NSAID and N-3 PUFA therapeutic actions. J Physiol Pharmacol 2000;51:643—54.

[28] Serhan CN, Hong S, Gronert K, Colgan SP, Devchand PR, Mirick G, Moussignac RL. Resolvins: a family of bioactive products of omega-3 fatty acid transformation circuits initiated by aspirin treatment that counter proinflammation signals. J Exp Med 2002;196:1025—37.

[29] Morrisey PA, Sheehy PJA. Optimal nutrition: vitamin E. Proc Nutr Soc 1999;58:459—68.

[30] Padayatty SJ, Katz A, Wang Y, Eck P, Kwon O, Lee J, Chen S, Corpe C, Dutta A, Dutta SK, Levine M. Vitamin C as an antioxidant: evaluation of its role in disease prevention. Am J Coll Nutr 2003;22:18—35.

[31] Aguiló A, Tauler P, Guix P, Villa G, Córdova A, Tur JA, Pons A. Effect of exercise intensity and training on antioxidants and cholesterol profile in cyclists. J Nutr Biochem 2003;14:319—25.

[32] Hamilton IM, Gilmore WS, Benzie IF, Mulholland CW, Strain JJ. Interactions between vitamins C and E in human subjects. Br J Nutr 2000;84:261—7.

[33] Traber MG, Winklhofer-Roob BM, Roob JM, Khoschsorur G, Aigner R, Cross C. Vitamin E kinetics in smokers and nonsmokers. Free Radic Biol Med 2001b;31:1368—74.

[34] Tur JA, Sureda A, Pons A. Blood cells as functional markers of antioxidant status. Br J Nutr 2006;96(Suppl. 1):S38—41.

[35] Food and Nutrition Board, Institute of Medicine. Dietary reference intakes for vitamin C, vitamin E, selenium, and carotenoids. Washington (DC): National Academy Press; 2000.

[36] Horwitt MK. Critique of the requirement for vitamin E. Am J Clin Nutr 2001;73:1003—5.

[37] Traber MG. Vitamin E: too much or not enough. Am J Clin Nutr 2001a;73:997—8.

[38] Packer L, Obermüller-Jevic UC. Vitamin E in disease prevention and therapy: future perspectives. In: Packer L, Traber MG, Kraemer, Frei B, editors. The antioxidant vitamins C and E. Illinois: AOCS Press; 2002. p. 255—88.

[39] Leonard SW, Good CK, Gugger ET, Traber MG. Vitamin E bioavailability from fortified breakfast cereal is greater than that from encapsulated supplements. Am J Clin Nutr 2004;79:86—92.

[40] Iuliano L, Micheletta F, Maranghi M, Frati G, Diczfalusy U, Violi F. Bioavailability of vitamin E as a function of food intake in healthy subjects: effects on plasma peroxide-scavenging activity and cholesterol-oxidation products. Arterioscler Thromb Vasc Biol 2001;21:E34—7.

[41] Kayden HJ, Hatam LJ, Traber MG. The measurement of nanograms of tocopherol from needle aspiration biopsies of adipose tissue: normal and abetalipoproteinemic subjects. J Lipid Res 1983;24:652−6.

[42] Aguiló A, Tauler P, Fuentespina E, Tur JA, Córdova A, Pons A. Antioxidant response to oxidative stress induced by exhaustive exercise. Physiol Behav 2005;84:1−7.

[43] Cases N, Sureda A, Tauler P, Aguiló A, Villa G, Córdova A, Pons A, Tur JA. Vitamin E recommended daily intake is not enough to avoid the oxidative stress induced by intense exercise. In: Proceedings of the meeting "oxidants and antioxidants in biology", a joint meeting of the Oxygen Club of California. El Puerto de Santa María, Cádiz: The University of Cádiz (Spain), and The Free Radicals Spanish Group; 2003.

[44] Rokitzki L, Logemann E, Huber G, Keck E, Keul J. Alpha-tocopherol supplementation in racing cyclist during extreme endurance training. Int J Sport Nutr 1994;4:253−64.

[45] Palazzetti S, Rousseau AS, Richard MJ, Favier A, Margaritis I. Antioxidant supplementation preserves antioxidant response in physical training and low antioxidant intake. Br J Nutr 2004;91:91−100.

[46] Sureda A, Batle JM, Tauler P, Aguiló A, Cases N, Tur JA, Pons A. Hypoxia/reoxygenation and vitamin C intake influence NO synthesis and antioxidant defenses of neutrophils. Free Radic Biol Med 2004;37:1744−55.

[47] Cases N, Aguiló A, Tauler P, Sureda A, Llompart I, Pons A, Tur JA. Differential response of plasma and immune cell's vitamin E levels to physical activity and antioxidant vitamin supplementation. Eur J Clin Nutr 2005;59:781−8.

Chapter 10

Benefits of Selenium, Magnesium, and Zinc in Obesity and Metabolic Syndrome

Paulina López-López[1], Loreto Rojas-Sobarzo[2] and Miguel Arredondo-Olguín[1]

[1]*Universidad de Chile, Santiago, Chile;* [2]*Pontificia Universidad Católica de Chile, Santiago, Chile*

1. INTRODUCTION

Globally, the percentage of individuals with a body mass index (BMI) higher than 25 kg/m^2 increased between 1980 and 2013 from 28.8% to 36.9% in men, and from 29.8% to 38% in women [1]. Likewise, the prevalence of obesity in children and adolescents has increased substantially in both developed and developing countries. For this reason the World Health Organization (WHO) has established obesity as one of the priorities in public health [2].

Metabolic syndrome (MS) is a grouping of factors that increase the risk for the development and progression of type 2 diabetes mellitus (T2DM) and cardiovascular disease (CVD). The criteria for identifying MS include three of five markers (ATP III) [3]: abdominal obesity, impaired carbohydrate metabolism, high blood pressure, elevated levels of triglycerides, and decreased levels of high-density lipoprotein (HDL). In developed countries, MS occurs in approximately 25% of the middle-aged population. Environmental exposure to heavy metals, including arsenic [4], lead, and cadmium [5], increases the occurrence of diabetes and CVDs. More commonly, the relationship between MS and the macroelements and microelements vital to life is with magnesium, iron, zinc, copper, selenium, manganese, and chromium [6].

Obesity is classified into three classes for white, Hispanic, and African American adults: obesity class I—BMI of $30-34.9 \text{ kg/m}^2$; obesity class II—BMI of $35-39.9 \text{ kg/m}^2$; and obesity class III (severe obesity)—BMI higher than 40 kg/m^2 (or $>35 \text{ kg/m}^2$ in the presence of comorbidities). Asian and South Asian people classify obesity as a BMI higher than 25 kg/m^2 [7].

Weight gain occurs when energy intake exceeds energy expenditure, resulting in a positive energy balance, which if sustained in time leads to obesity. The availability of cheap calorically dense food and the intake of sugar-sweetened beverages have contributed significantly to the increase in obesity. Furthermore, physical activity makes the largest contribution to significant energy expenditure, but current lifestyles have reduced the time that we dedicate to physical activity [8].

Adipose tissue is the main organ in charge of storing energy as triglycerides in mammals. It has unlimited capacity for expansion and can recycle stored calories when they are required. This tissue expands by increasing the number of cells (hyperplasia) in childhood and adolescence, while in adulthood the tissue is expanded by an increase in the size of individual cells (hypertrophy) [9].

Obesity is characterized by an excess of white adipose tissue (WAT) attained by the production of hyperplasia and hypertrophy adipocytes. WAT has an active endocrine organ function that secretes a variety of adipokines, such as leptin, adiponectin, tumor necrosis factor alpha (TNF-α), and plasminogen activator inhibitor-1 (PAI-1), among others [10]. The production of adipokines is not only mediated by adipocytes but also by adipose tissue stroma cells, which are largely composed of leukocytes: macrophages, T cells, and natural killer (NK) cells. In humans it is showed that stroma-vascular fraction (SVF) cells are the primary source of most inflammatory cytokines, with macrophages being the main source of these [11].

In obese subjects WAT is characterized by a mild chronic inflammation state that presents macrophage infiltration and high production of proinflammatory adipokines [12], evidenced by an increase in the circulating levels of inflammatory

Obesity. https://doi.org/10.1016/B978-0-12-812504-5.00010-6

markers such as high-sensitivity C-reactive protein (hsCRP), interleukin-6 (IL-6), monocyte chemoattractant protein-1, PAI-1, intercellular adhesion molecule (ICAM), and TNF-α [13]. The inflammatory state of WAT plays a key role in the linkage of obesity with T2DM and CVD [14], high blood pressure [15], and some cancers [16]. In addition, epidemiological studies have shown that excess visceral adipose tissue, as compared to subcutaneous adipose tissue, is associated with an increased risk of obesity comorbidities [17].

2. SELENIUM

Selenium (Se) is an essential trace element with biological functions of importance for human health. The four natural oxidation states of Se are elemental selenium [0], selenide [−2], selenite [+4], and selenate [+6]. The +4 and +6 oxidation states are more bioavailable than 0 and −2, being more soluble in water [18].

2.1 Requirements and Absorption

The main route for Se intake is through the diet: the main sources are cereals, meat, fish, eggs, cereals, black tea, mushrooms, soyabeans, lima beans, bamboo shoots, Brazil nuts, broccoli, and milk/dairy products [19]. The distribution of Se species in food varies considerably depending on the plant/animal species, the environment, and the growth conditions. The main Se species in vegetables are selenomethionine (SeMet), selenite, selenocysteine (SeCys), Se-methyl-seleno-cysteine, and γ-glutamyl-Se-methyl-selenocysteine, with the last three found in lower proportions. In animal products the main Se species are selenite, SeMet, and SeCys, in widely variable proportions depending on the animal's diet [19].

The assessment of nutritional Se status in the short term can be evaluated by serum Se concentration, while Se in erythrocytes is a better marker of the long-term status. Other tissues can also be used to measure long-term Se status, including hair and toenails. These determinations are not representative of the real functional activity of Se; hence measurement of the activity of individual Se proteins is a better method to evaluate Se status. The activity of the plasma Se protein glutathione peroxidase 3 (GPx3) is the most frequently used parameter. Plasma selenoprotein P (SelP) has also been proposed as a biomarker, but it reflects mostly the short-term status because it has a half-life in plasma of a few hours (3−4 h in rat plasma). However, an increase in Se concentration does not lead to an increase in GPX3 or SelP concentration, so such Se biomarkers have limited validity [20].

An intake of 20 μg/day for adults is generally accepted as the minimum needed to prevent onset of Keshan's disease [21], an endemic disorder found in Se-deficient areas. The WHO corrected this basal requirement to an average of 19 μg/day (corresponding to 21 μg/day for men and 16 μg/day for women). Other criteria, based on GPx3 activity maximization, recommend a daily intake of 55 μg for adult, 60 μg during pregnancy, and 70 μg during lactation, with an upper limit of 400 μg without adverse effects. The US National Institutes for Health recommended a daily intake of Se according to life stage (see Table 10.1) [22].

For improving Se status, SeMet is one of the most effective organic seleno compounds, as it is nonspecifically incorporated into proteins. However, this compound is a less-efficient metabolic source than inorganic forms since it needs to be reduced, thru the SeCys pathway, to hydrogen selenide (H2Se), which is considered a key precursor in the metabolic interconversions of both organic and inorganic [23].

TABLE 10.1 Daily Intake of Selenium According to Life Stage

Life Stage	Recommended Intake (μg)
Infants up to 6 months of age	15
Infants 7 months to 3 years old	20
Children 4−8 years old	30
Children 9−13 years old	40
Adults from 14 years old	55
Women and adolescents when pregnant	60
Women and adolescents when breastfeeding	70

The four Se states are absorbed in the lower part of the small intestine, but have different mechanisms of absorption. Selenate is absorbed paracellularly via a passive diffusional process. The Se amino acids, SeMet and SeCys, are absorbed through transcellular pathways mediated by transporters. Under normal physiological and intake conditions, the percentage of absorption is close to 70%–90%. Selenite is an exception because its direct absorption does not exceed 60%; this increases in the presence of reduced glutathione (GSH), being converted to hydrogen selenide [24].

2.2 Selenoproteins

Many biological functions of selenium are carried out by selenoproteins. This element is incorporated into proteins by a cotranslational mechanism as part of the amino acid selenocysteine, and is used for selenoproteins synthesis [25]. The utilization of selenium in de novo synthesis of SeCys requires the generation of Se-donor selenophosphate, which is synthesized by selenophosphate synthetases 2. Selenophosphate is enzymatically attached to O-phosphoseryl-tRNA$^{[Ser]Sec}$, which is converted to selenocysteyl-tRNA$^{[Ser]Sec}$ and incorporated in the translation process [26].

These proteins are encoded by 25 human genes, of which 24 contain 1 SeCys residue solely and 1, SelP, contains 10 residues. The position of SeCys in the polypeptide chain defines its biochemical activity. When the amino acid residue is located in the C-terminal region, they are selenoprotein K, S, R, O, I, and thioredoxin reductases. On other hand, if the residue is located in the N-terminal region, they are iodothyronine deiodinases (DIOs), GPxs, selenoprotein M, 15, W, H, T, V, P, and N [27].

The thioredoxin reductases catalyze the reduction of oxidized thioredoxins in a manner dependent on nicotinamide adenine dinucleotide phosphate/H+. Thioredoxins are redox proteins containing a dithiol–disulfide active site that reduces the disulfide bonds present in thioredoxin peroxidase, ribonucleotide reductase, and some transcription factors (gene expression). In mammals threes isoforms of thioredoxin reductases have been identified. Thioredoxin reductase 1 is located in cytosol and has a main role in embryogenesis. Thioredoxin reductase 2 is located in mitochondria and, like isoform 1, participates in embryogenesis to defend the cell from mitochondrial-mediated oxidative stress. Thioredoxin reductase 3 is expressed in male sperm cells and participates in sperm maturation.

Thioredoxin reductase participates in signaling, cell–cell communication, and DNA metabolism and repair. The reduction of proteins is carried out by cysteine thiol–disulfide exchange. Other substrates include the cytotoxic peptide NK-lysine, protein disulfide-isomerase, dehydroascorbic acid, calcium-binding proteins 1 and 2, glutaredoxin 2, the tumor-suppressor protein p53, selenocystine, selenodiglutathione, methylselenate, selenite, ebselen, lipoic acid, and lipid hydroperoxides (LOOHs) [28].

GPx enzymes catalyze the reduction of hydrogen peroxide and LOOHs, using GSH as a reducing cofactor. GPx can neutralize the reactive oxygen species (ROS) and reactive nitrogen species. Five of the eight of the GPx enzyme isoforms of have SeCys residues (Table 10.2). The SeCys residue present in GPxs is oxidized by H_2O_2 or LOOHs, forming

TABLE 10.2 Glutathione Peroxidase (GPx) Family with Selenium Residue

Isoform	Ubication	Action
Glutathione peroxidase 1	Localized in the cytosol and mitochondria. It is expressed in all tissues, but at higher levels in lungs, kidney, erythrocytes, and liver.	Participates in cytokine signaling and apoptosis.
Glutathione peroxidase 2	Localized in the cytoplasm. Expressed in liver and epithelium of the gastrointestinal tract, mainly in the crypt grounds and decreasing toward the luminal surface.	Protect intestinal epithelium from oxidative stress.
Glutathione peroxidase 3	Present in plasma. Secreted by cells of the proximal tubular epithelium and in the parietal cells of Bowman's capsule of the kidney.	Reduce H_2O_2 and the organic hydroperoxides, but 10-fold lower that glutathione peroxidase 1.
Glutathione peroxidase 4	Localized nuclear, mitochondrial, and cytoplasm. Present in various tissues, but mainly expressed in endocrine organs and in the mitochondria in the midpiece of spermatozoa.	Antioxidant in cellular differentiation in embryonic development and spermatogenesis.
Glutathione peroxidase 6	Expressed in embryos and olfactory epithelium.	Function remains unknown.

TABLE 10.3 Human Selenoproteins

Protein	Ubication	Action
Selenoprotein O	Localized in various tissues.	Participates in kinase signaling and redox detection/signaling.
Selenoprotein I (ethanolaminephospho-transferase 1)	Localized in the endoplasmic reticulum (ER). Ubiquitously expressed, but particularly in the cerebellum.	Participates in biosynthesis of phosphatidylethanolamine.
Selenoprotein N	Localized in ER membrane. Ubiquitous, expressed in fetal tissues, skeletal muscle, brain, and lung.	Modulates the activity of ryanodine receptor and protects it against oxidative stress. Potential function in the development of muscle fibers in embryos.
Selenoprotein R	Localized in cytoplasm and nucleus. Expressed in liver, heart, kidney, and skeletal muscle.	Reconversion of methionine residues from their oxidized form.
Selenophosphate synthetase 2 (SPS2)	Localized in cytoplasm. Expressed in liver.	Participates in Se proteins biosynthesis.
Selenoprotein P (SEPP1)	Localized in plasma. Expressed mainly in liver, and to a lesser extent in brain and heart.	Se transport and homeostasis. Antioxidant defense function related to protection of membrane of endothelial cells
Selenoprotein V	Expressed in testes.	Forms mixed disulfides with substrate proteins and bind DNA in a redox-sensitive manner.
Selenoprotein T	Localized in Golgi, endoplasmic reticulum and plasma membrane. Ubiquitous, expressed high level in testes.	Participates in tissue maturation/regeneration, ontogenesis, cellular metabolism and redox action, calcium mobilization and glucose metabolism.
Selenoprotein H	Localized in nucleus. Expressed in various tissues, but an elevated expression reported in brain's embryo, thyroid, lung, stomach, and human liver tumors.	Regulates antioxidant capacity in response to the redox state. Functions in regulating expression levels of genes involved in de novo glutathione synthesis.
Selenoprotein W	Localized in cytoplasm. Expressed in various tissues, but mainly in skeletal muscle.	Antioxidant in muscle tissue and brain. It is highly expressed in first stage of embryogenesis.
Selenoprotein M	Localized in Golgi and in endoplasmic reticulum, and perinuclear. Ubiquitously expressed, mainly in brain.	Functions as thiol−disulfide oxidoreductase.
Selenoprotein 15	Localized in endoplasmic reticulum. Expressed in prostate, liver, kidney, testes, and brain.	Functions as thiol−disulfide oxidoreductase.
Selenoprotein S	Plasma and various tissues.	Transmembrane protein of endoplasmic reticulum. Regulates stress in this organelle.
Selenoprotein K	Several tissues, but mainly in spleen, immune cells, brain, and heart.	Transmembrane protein of endoplasmic reticulum. Regulates stress in this organelle.

selenenic acid, which is then reduced back. The selenolic group is stabilized and activated by hydrogen bonding into a catalytic triad of selenocysteine−glutamine−tryptophan residues [29].

The DIOs are oxide reductases that are involved in thyroid hormone metabolism. Three isoforms have been described: DIO1 is expressed in the pituitary gland, thyroid, liver, and kidney; DIO2 is in the central nervous system, heart, pituitary gland, thyroid, and skeletal muscle; and DIO3 is expressed in the embryonic and neonatal state. DIO1 and DIO2 control circulating triiodothyronine (T3) levels through of the conversion of thyroxine (T4) into T3, which is the active form of the thyroid hormone and plays a key role in normal lipid metabolism; while DIO3 are involved in deiodination processes, inactivating T4 and T3 irreversibly. The amount of Se available for selenoprotein synthesis may be affected by active thyroid hormones, and thus DIOs may play an indirect role in inflammation and immunity. Table 10.3 gives a brief description of the other human selenoproteins, with their locations and functions [30].

2.3 Role of Selenium in Metabolic Syndrome and Obesity

CVD is a major cause of mortality worldwide. ROS and oxidative stress play a key role in the progression of CVDs, including atherosclerosis, hypertension, and congestive heart failure [31]. Se proteins may play a significant role in cellular defense against ROS. It has been suggested that Se has a protective effect against CVDs. Lower blood concentrations of Se in patients with heart failure compared to healthy persons have been reported [31].

Keshan's disease had been linked to the coxsackie B virus and associated with Se deficiency [32]. This pathology is characterized by congestive cardiomyopathy and cardiac dysfunction, and is reversed after Se supplementation. Using a murine model fed with Se-replete or Se-deficient diet and challenged with coxsackie B virus, demonstrated a decreased in the enzymatic activity of GPx1 and an increased in the sensitivity to this viral infection in the animals [33].

There is an inverse correlation between serum selenium, hsCRP, and soluble ICAM-1, which indicates that low Se levels are associated with oxidative stress and decreased protection for the blood vessels against oxidative damage. Plasma level of SelP is correlated with prevention of lipid and low-density lipoprotein peroxidation, which is the major cause of the development of atherosclerotic plaques. However, observational metaanalysis studies found a moderate inverse correlation between blood, serum/plasma or toenail Se concentration, and coronary heart disease [34].

Studies in murine models with cardiac failure, either genetic or induced by drugs, demonstrate the cardio protection effects of Se supplementation. Administration of Se increased Se-containing antioxidant enzyme activity and decreased cardiac oxidative injury, increased cardiac concentrations of GSH and plasma HDL cholesterol, and reduced lipid peroxidation, protein carbonyls, and LDL cholesterol. But an Se deficiency in rats led to increased myocardial damage and altered recovery of the cardiac function after myocardial ischemia/reperfusion (I/R), which is related to decreased GPx activity measured in the blood and cardiomyocytes [35].

In two mice models with induced hypertrophy in cardiomyocytes, it was observed that increasing GPx3, GPx4, thioredoxin reductase 1, and selenoprotein R, reduced the intracellular oxidative damage and did not induced significant increases in phospholipid peroxidation or DNA damage, suggesting that antioxidant systems protect these cells [36]. Se supplementation in a model of myocardial I/R injury results in higher GPxs and thioredoxin reductase (TrxRs) activity and reduced oxidative damage [37]. Studies of $GPx1^{-/-}$ and $GPx3^{-/-}$ carried out in a transgenic mouse model show increased susceptibility of animals to oxidative damage caused by I/R injury [38]. There is evidence that the Trx-1/TrxR1 system regulates the response to ventricular remodeling after myocardial infarction [39].

Alterations in the homeostasis of thyroid hormones may result in cardiovascular perturbations such as hypertrophy and increased heart rate and contractility, along with changes in circulating lipoproteins, increasing the risk of developing atheroma plaques. DIO2 has been described as important for cardiac function, and overexpression of this enzyme enhanced heart function in a murine model. Adequate activity of DIO1 during hypercholesterolemia is relevant to preserve the homeostasis of lipid metabolism through the efficient supply of T3 [40].

Selenoprotein S (SEPS) was found to be associated with CVD, having a protective effect on astrocytes during ischemia, but its mechanism of action is unknown [41]. Polymorphisms in the SEPS1 locus are associated with the development of subclinical CVD risk during type 2 diabetes [42]. Also, selenoprotein R has been related to the regulation of cardiac stress, minimizing the damage produced in stressed cardiomyocytes. This protein is involved in the dynamic actin reorganization during cardiac stress [43]. In murine models of cardiac hypertrophy and I/R an increase of selenoprotein R was observed [44]. Finally, selenoprotein K protects cardiomyocytes from oxidative stress and participates in foam cell formation [45].

In contrast, high serum Se concentrations were associated with higher prevalence of hypertension in a representative sample of adults in the United States, a region with high Se intake [46]. Another study performed on men in Western Europe, an Se-deficient area, concluded that high Se levels might be an underestimated risk factor for the development of high blood pressure or hypertension [47]. Studies have shown that increasing Se levels above the recommended daily intake is not beneficial and can actually cause hypertension, diabetes, and hyperlipidemia [48]. Randomized trials with Se as part of multivitamin supplementation in Se-depleted areas did not reduce the risk of hypertension and CVD. There is no conclusive evidence supporting an association between Se and hypertension [49].

Oxidative stress plays a major role in the pathogenesis and development of complications of T2DM. Hyperglycemia induces free radicals, and impairs the endogenous antioxidant defense system in patients with diabetes. Endogenous antioxidant defense mechanisms include selenoproteins such as GPx. The overexpression of GPx in islets may protect pancreatic β cells from oxidative stress and improve islet function [50]. However, high Se concentrations in the human body may interfere with insulin signaling [51].

The relationship between selenium and T2DM is controversial. Some report that blood Se is negatively associated with T2DM, while others report a positive correlation or no significant association. For example, it has been reported that an increase in erythrocyte GPx1 activity was associated with mild insulin resistance in pregnant women [52]. Other studies have shown that plasma, serum, or blood total Se concentrations, GPx3 level, or GPx3 activity were lower in patients with T2DM than in controls [53].

However, randomized trials shown that Se supplementation could either increase the risk of type 2 diabetes or be ineffective [54]. Wang et al. [55] indicate that the relationship between Se and T2DM has a U-shape, with possible harm occurring both below and above the physiological range for optimal activity of some or all selenoproteins. Se status and intake vary widely in different parts of the world, which might cause the inconsistencies observed in study outcomes.

SelP acts to inhibit the insulin-signaling pathway by inactivating the adenosine monophosphate-activated protein kinase, a positive regulator of insulin synthesis in pancreatic insulin-producing β cells. In vitro studies demonstrated that expression of this protein in human subcutaneous adipocytes is upregulated by insulin [56].

In vitro studies have shown in isolated rat adipocytes that selenate stimulated glucose transport (GLUT) activity in a dose-dependent manner by translocation of GLUT-1 and GLUT-2 to the membrane surface [57]. Cells incubated with selenate induced a concentrated and time-dependent increase in tyrosine phosphorylation of the insulin receptor's β subunit and the insulin receptor substrate-1 (IRS-1). Selenate stimulated cyclic AMP (cAMP) phosphodiesterase activity in rat adipocytes. This enzyme catalyzes decomposition of cAMP into AMP [58].

In vivo studies have demonstrated that Se acts as an insulin mimetic [59]. Oral administration of selenate in a diabetic murine model improved plasma glucose levels, and the glucose tolerance test decreased significantly. Along with these changes, selenate reversed abnormal liver expression of both glycogenic and gluconeogenic enzymes. Fatty acid synthase and glucose 6-phosphate dehydrogenase activity was normalized in the liver of diabetic animals, demonstrating that Se was capable of stimulating lipogenesis in the liver. Diabetic rats treated with selenate improved heart function, plasma lipid levels, triglycerides, cholesterol, and free fatty acids. Transgenic mice overexpressing GPx1 exhibit insulin resistance, whereas knockout of GPx1 improves insulin sensitivity.

Selenocysteine lyase catalyzes the decomposition of SeCys to mobilize Se for utilization in selenoprotein synthesis [60]. Whole-body selenocysteine lyase knockout mice developed metabolic disturbances, such as hepatic steatosis, glucose intolerance, hyperinsulinemia, and hyperleptinemia with an adequate Se intake. When exposed to a low dietary Se intake, the mice developed obesity and MS, with increased hepatic lipogenesis and attenuation of insulin signaling. Selenium metabolism has a significant role in the pathogenesis of obesity [61].

Based on the above, there is wide evidence of the effects of Se on glucose metabolism, obesity, cardiovascular function, and lipid metabolism; however, other studies demonstrate a deleterious association of this element in MS, or simply show no association at all. For this reason, vitamin supplements that incorporate Se must be taken with caution, especially in regions where there is an adequate contribution of this element.

3. MAGNESIUM

Magnesium (Mg) is the second most abundant mineral at intracellular level and acts as cofactor of hundreds of enzymes [62]. Its functions are linked to the role of these enzymes, among which are phosphotransferases and hydrolases, which participate in vital intracellular reactions such as energy metabolism. Mg is also required for nucleic acid synthesis, cytoskeletal and mitochondrial integrity, and substances binding to the plasma membrane. In addition, Mg is a calcium antagonist, influencing and regulating cellular processes in neurological and muscular functioning [63].

3.1 Requirements and Absorption

Mg is absorbed as an ion in the ileum and jejunum, and its absorption is proportional to the amount consumed. Its main mechanism of absorption is passive, through a paracellular pathway. The human body contains about 20–28 g of Mg, which is housed mainly in bones (60%–65%), muscle (27%), and other tissues. Extracellular Mg accounts for <1% of total body magnesium [62].

Mg requirements are in the range of 400–420 mg/day for men and 310–320 mg/day in women. The main food sources are leafy green vegetables, whole grains, legumes, and nuts [64]. Mg bioavailability is approximately 50% [65]. Despite its wide distribution in food, changes in dietary habits in recent years have shifted consumption away from foods rich in Mg toward refined and processed foods high in critical nutrients (sugars, saturated fats, and sodium) [66]. This could be the reason why the population is possibly not meeting the recommended intake of Mg [67], which can produce marginal deficiencies of the mineral and lead to a series of metabolic consequences. In this context, evidence has emerged that relates dietary Mg intake to the development of chronic noncommunicable diseases of nutritional origin [68]. Low Mg intake can lead to metabolic changes related to obesity and MS.

3.2 Role of Magnesium in Metabolic Syndrome and Obesity

Cross-sectional studies have shown the existence of a significant inverse relationship between Mg intake and prevalence or incidence of MS. This relationship has been found in both young and older adults (>60 years). Subjects who consumed less Mg (<221 mg/day) had a higher probability of having MS compared to those who consumed a greater amount of the mineral (>332 mg/day) [69].

He et al. [70] studied in young adults (men and women between 18 and 30 years) the incidence of MS according to dietary Mg intake. The incidence of MS was inversely associated with Mg intake. The risk reduction was 31%, adjusted for confounding variables (age, gender, BMI, physical activity, calorie intake, and dietary fiber intake, among others), for those subjects who had a higher intake of Mg (190.5 mg/1000 kcal daily).

Additionally, the same significant relationship had been found with some of the components of MS: glycemia, triglycerides, and HDL cholesterol [71]. Glucose levels were found to be negatively associated with Mg intake [69] in both apparently healthy subjects and those with diabetes mellitus [72]. This relationship can be explained by the role of Mg as a cofactor of enzymes involved in glucose metabolism [62]. Mg could modify both the secretion of insulin and its intracellular signal. Intracellular Mg would decrease insulin secretion as a result of reduced intracellular calcium concentration in beta cells of the pancreas. In addition, it would favor phosphorylation of the beta subunit of the insulin receptor and other kinases, allowing the translocation of the GLUT-4 transporter to the apical membrane to increase the uptake of intracellular glucose [73]. Mg deficiency could thus decrease insulin sensitivity.

On the other hand, Mg is a cofactor of lipoprotein lipase (LPL), which participates in chylomicron metabolism. Studies in Mg-deficient rats showed a decrease in the clearance of circulating levels of triglycerides and in the activity of LPL, indicating a lower chylomicron clearance [74]. In addition, there was lower activity of the enzyme cholesterol acyltransferase [75], also explaining the role of Mg deficiency in the development of dyslipidemias.

3.3 Magnesium and Inflammation

Low levels of Mg favor a proinflammatory environment, a condition present in MS and obesity. It was postulated that there is an inverse relationship between Mg consumption and levels of C-reactive protein (CRP) [76], a marker indicating the presence of mild and chronic inflammation. Song et al. [77] showed in women older than 45 years a relationship between Mg intake, CRP levels, and prevalence of MS. The authors found two relevant findings. First, there was a significant inverse relationship between CRP levels and dietary Mg intake, especially in women with a BMI >25 kg/m^2 and in those who had ever smoked. Second, there was an inverse association between Mg intake and the prevalence of MS.

Other studies showed that subjects with MS with low plasma levels of Mg would have increased circulating levels of CRP and higher levels of TNF-α [78,79].

Experimental studies in animal models have shown that Mg-deficient rats are characterized by developing a response very like an allergic condition, with increased circulating levels of cytokines, indicating a state of general inflammation [80,81]. The possible contribution of hypomagnesemia to the inflammatory state is shown in Fig. 10.1.

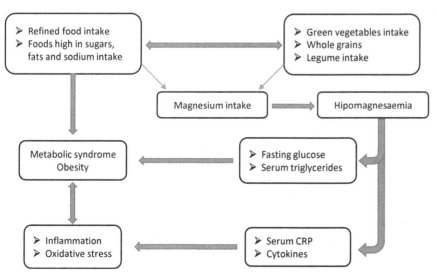

FIGURE 10.1 The figure shows the possible contribution of hypomagnesemia to the inflammatory state, as well as the presence of metabolic syndrome. Increased consumption of refined foods high in sugars and saturated fats displaces consumption of vegetables, whole grains, and legumes. This leads to a low intake of magnesium, which in turn leads to hypomagnesemia. The latter can cause increased levels of fasting blood glucose as well as triglycerides in plasma. In parallel, it may contribute to the inflammatory state and oxidative stress by increasing levels of CRP and circulating cytokines. *CRP*, C-reactive protein.

3.4 Magnesium Consumption: Clinical and Prospective Trials

It is difficult to isolate the individual effect of Mg intake on MS and its constituents since, as mentioned above, the dietary sources of this mineral (whole grains and leafy green vegetables) are also composed of other nutrients or food factors which have beneficial effects. Of particular importance is dietary fiber, which has a positive association with Mg consumption [71,82]; for this reason, the studies must correct the effect of Mg over fiber intake. When the intake of Mg is corrected according to fiber consumption, the association between Mg consumption and MS is attenuated. This inconsistency depends on the type of diet eaten by the population under study, especially if the majority of dietary fiber comes from whole grains. In the study, the authors correct their results according to fiber intake among other variables associated with a healthy lifestyle, which can impact both the prevalence and the development of MS and obesity. However, since foods rich in Mg have other beneficial components, the benefits associated with the consumption of Mg may be due to the type of food (diet) consumed rather than the consumption of the mineral itself. In fact, it has been seen that the adoption of a healthy diet leads to increased intake of some minerals, including Mg [83].

3.5 Magnesium Supplementation

Apparently, there could be beneficial effects from taking Mg supplements. The most used form for mineral supplementation is Mg citrate, since it has better bioavailability than other forms. Simental-Mendía et al. [84], studied in apparently healthy subjects with prediabetes and hypomagnesaemia the oral supplementation of 320 mg of magnesium per day for 3 months. They showed a significant reduction in CRP and blood glucose levels compared to the control group. This effect can be observed in people with hypomagnesemia. However, this result is not found when the same amount of Mg is administered over the same period to diabetic subjects with normal levels of blood Mg [85]. This suggests that subjects with hypomagnesemia would benefit from better metabolic control of glucose [86].

With respect to the effect of Mg supplementation on the lipid profile, the evidence is more controversial and apparently depends on the status of Mg, characteristics of subjects, and the levels of circulating levels of blood lipids. In this context, those with hypertriglyceridemia or hypercholesterolemia and low levels of Mg and without problems in renal function would benefit [87].

On the other hand, Joris et al. [88] show the possible benefits of Mg supplementation for vascular rigidity, an indicator that is independent of risk of cardiovascular events. Supplementation of 350 mg daily of Mg (as citrate) for 24 weeks in overweight and obese men and postmenopausal women produced a significant reduction in vascular rigidity.

Regarding the antioxidative effects of Mg supplementation, there is evidence in animal models [89] but limited data for humans. Decreased urinary 8-isoprotan excretion was shown in subjects with prehypertension or stage I hypertension supplemented with 250 mg daily of Mg for 4 weeks [90].

4. ZINC

Zinc (Zn) belongs to the series of transition elements which also includes chromium, iron, copper, cobalt, manganese, and nickel. It is an essential trace element for the growth and development of most organisms and humans. The essentiality of Zn lies in its irreplaceable functions, which can be classified as catalytic, structural, and regulatory. It is indispensable for the activity of more than 300 enzymes (which participate in the metabolism of nucleic acids, proteins, lipids, carbohydrates, and some vitamins and minerals) [90,91], and regulates the expression of multiple genes (mainly by its key role in the structure of so-called "zinc fingers," which allow protein–DNA interactions). An important number of transcription factors contain these zinc fingers, thus involving this element in gene expression [92]. It also participates in maintaining the structural integrity of proteins and is found in all tissues and bodily fluids. The study of zinc finger functions related to adipogenesis regulations can serve as a theoretical basis for developing novel and efficient antiobesity drugs. Recent studies have looked at the role of zinc fingers in adipose development, especially zinc finger regulators in white adipogenesis (determination/differentiation). The interaction of zinc fingers regulatory networks with other adipogenic factors (such as peroxisome proliferator-activated receptor gamma (PPARγ) and CCAAT/enhancer-binding proteins (C/EBPs)) highlights zinc fingers as potential targets in obesity and associated disease treatment strategies [93]. Zn is also involved in insulin synthesis and secretion [94] and blood pressure regulation [95], and has antioxidant and antiinflammatory properties [96,97].

The regulatory functions refer to the role of the Zn ion (Zn^{2+}) in intracellular signaling cascades; the activity of enzymes such as some phosphatases, phosphodiesterase, and caspases is regulated by the greater or lesser presence of Zn^{2+} in the medium [98]. Consequently, the Zn participates in cell division and multiplication and metabolic–hormonal metabolic and growth regulation systems.

4.1 Requirements and Absorption

The total content of Zn in an adult (70 kg) is about $2-3$ g approximately. The highest proportion of body Zn is found in muscles ($50\%-60\%$) and bones ($25\%-30\%$; this may reach 40% in newborns). Liver and kidney have similar concentrations ($50-60$ µg/g). The highest concentrations of Zn are found in choroids ($250-280$ µg/g) and prostatic secretions ($300-400$ µg/mL). The plasma Zn content is about 0.1% of the total content.

Zn is removed from the body through the kidneys, skin, and intestines. Endogenous intestinal losses vary, depending on Zn intake, from 0.5 mg/day to more than 3 mg/day. Urinary and cutaneous losses are each in the order of $0.5-0.7$ mg/day and depend less on the normal variation of Zn intake.

There is no marker that is sensitive and specific to define groups of humans with Zn deficiency in clinical or population conditions, and thus there is some variability in the suggestions for requirements. The recommendations (lower limits of Zn consumption) are adjusted for diets with low bioavailability (phytate content: >15 mg/day), medium bioavailability (phytate content: $10-15$ mg/day), and high bioavailability (phytate: <15 mg/day) of Zn. Thus the minimum Zn consumption recommendations proposed for low-bioavailability infant diets are 7.9 mg/day between 1 and 3 years, 9.2 mg/day between 3 and 6 years, and 10.7 mg/day between 6 and 10 years.

The main causes of Zn deficiencies are reduced deposits at birth (prematurity, low birth weight), inadequate inputs (deficiency and/or low availability of these microminerals in the diet), increased requirements (growth, pregnancy), and increased losses. Modifications and/or diversification of diet, food fortification, and supplementation are the main strategies used to prevent micronutrient deficiencies.

Zn homeostasis is complex and requires Zn compartmentalization into cellular organelles. Twenty-four proteins (transporters) have been identified, but knowledge of their roles is incomplete. There are 14 members that encode for Zn transporters ZIP $1-14$, which are mainly importers of Zn into the cytoplasm, and 10 members that encode for Zn transporters ZnT1-10, which are mainly exporters of Zn from the cytoplasm to organelles and the extracellular space [99].

4.2 Role of Zinc in Metabolic Syndrome and Obesity

Studies evaluating Zn status in patients with MS have been controversial and have had inconclusive results. Some studies demonstrated an association of Zn with MS, such as fasting blood glucose concentration, blood pressure, and abdominal obesity. However, some authors have shown that greater numbers of MS components are associated with lower plasma Zn concentrations [100].

Zn participates in a number of processes related to insulin function (secretion and activity) in peripheral tissues. Zn is necessary for the correct formation of insulin hexamers, storage, and secretion of insulin by β-cells. Zn^{2+} is present in secretory granules of β-cells, where insulin undergoes a maturation process, aggregating to form 2-Zn$-$hexameric complexes [101]. This dimerization reduces the solubility of the hexamer, inducing crystallization within the granule and the formation of a dense crystalline core. The process increases insulin storage capacity before secretion and reduces susceptibility to enzymatic degradation of insulin. Reconversion to insulin monomer is necessary for its biological action. This process occurs after the exposure of the granule interior to the extracellular milieu, in the presence of Zn^{2+} [102]. Also, Zn is cosecreted along with insulin and is involved in the paracrine regulation of glucagon secretion by α-cells [103,104]. In this association, the ZnT8, which is expressed almost uniquely in the pancreas, is responsible for the transport of Zn into insulin granules from β-cells cytosol. Cytosolic free Zn^{2+} concentrations in pancreatic β-cells range close to 1 nM, but in the secretory granule are much higher (120 nM). The total contents of Zn^{2+} are in the mM and tens of mM range, respectively [102]. In addition, Zn is involved in the phosphorylation of insulin receptors and regulation of signaling by tyrosine-phosphatase [105].

Velázquez-López L et al. [106] showed at the end of an intervention using a Mediterranean diet (MD, which included dietary fiber, proteins, omega-9 fatty acids, Zn, Se, vitamin E, and flavonoids) that the MD group had a significantly reduced proportion of patients exhibiting MS in regard to the basal metabolic rate. These results support the usefulness of providing children exhibiting obesity and MS with an MD aimed at increasing consumption of these elements. However, a limitation of this study was the short intervention and its need for a larger number of participants to adjust the effect by variables such as age, socioeconomic status, physical activity, and sedentary status.

Seo et al. [107] showed, in a Korean population, associations between serum Zn levels and certain MS components. Among them, serum Zn levels in men were negatively associated with elevated fasting glucose and positively associated with elevated triglycerides; in both men and women, as serum Zn levels increased, HDL cholesterol levels showed a decreasing trend; and in women, serum Zn levels decreased as the number of MS components increased, and low serum Zn levels (Q1$-$Q3) showed a greater prevalence than the highest serum Zn levels (Q4) among almost every MS phenotype.

Al-Daghri et al. [108] demonstrate an inverse relationship between insufficient dietary micronutrient intake (including vitamins A, C, E, and K, calcium, Zn, and Mg) and MS risk in females. However, this finding cannot be generalized, due to the small sample size studied. Also, because the cross-sectional design of this study, the micronutrient levels could not be related to the causality of MS.

Azab et al. [109] studied 80 children with obesity and found a significantly lower serum Zn level in the obese children compared to the nonobese controls. They also observed a significant negative correlation between serum leptin and Zn levels in the obese children. It has been observed that Zn concentration is directly associated with serum leptin concentration, an adipokine associated with satiety. Mracek et al. [110] demonstrate that in human subjects zinc-α2-glycoprotein (ZAG) mRNA levels in visceral and subcutaneous fat are negatively associated with increased adiposity and the parameters of insulin resistance and positively correlate with adiponectin, but are negatively associated with leptin mRNA levels in adipose tissue in humans. They conclude that ZAG is a major adipokine that may have a protective role in susceptibility to obesity and its related insulin resistance.

Neprilysin (NEP, a neutral Zn metallo-endopeptidase) is widely expressed on the surface of a variety of cells, including endothelial, epithelial, and smooth muscle cells, cardiac myocytes, and fibroblasts. NEP expression has been associated with regulation of insulin resistance, blood pressure, lipid metabolism, and adipocyte differentiation in obese subjects. The association of NEP with dyslipidemia and elevated blood pressure independent of insulin resistance supports pleiotropic effects of NEP in relation to cardiovascular risk, which may be partly mediated by the development of endothelial dysfunction [111].

Dourado et al. [112] showed that there are alterations in biochemical parameters of Zn in obese women. The levels of Zn in erythrocytes are influenced by components anthropometrics of MS. The BMI and waist circumference showed a negative relation with this mineral. Moreover, there was no relationship between nutritional Zn status and the biochemical markers of MS.

De Oliveira et al. [113] showed that intake of heme iron and Zn from red meat, but not from other sources, was associated with greater risk of CVD and MS. However, they suggest that their findings might reflect an association with other constituents of red meat or that such components might interact with heme iron and Zn, altering their bioavailability and producing the observed associations with disease.

In subjects undergoing bariatric surgery the preexisting malnutrition in calcium, vitamin D, and iron is exacerbated due to reduced bioavailability and malabsorption, poor dietary intake, and compliance with micronutrient supplementation following surgery. However, copper and Zn deficiencies are difficult to diagnose, because laboratory assessment may be confounded by inflammation and signs and symptoms are shared with deficiencies in other nutrients [114].

4.3 The Role of Zinc as an Antioxidant

Zn is known for its antioxidative properties [115], and has been studied as a possible treatment option in the context of diabetes in animal models [116] and human patients [117]. However, the results have been inconclusive, possibly because changes in Zn intake are often too small to alter intracellular levels of Zn^{2+} to an extent that allows a measurable effect on oxidative stress.

Zinc is a cofactor for several antioxidant enzymes, such as Cu−Zn superoxide dismutase (SOD). Zinc supplements have been tested for effects on oxidative stress and T2DM. Jayawardena et al. [118] showed in a systematic review that Zn supplementation in patients with diabetes has beneficial effects on glycemic control and promotes healthy lipid parameters. They conclude that individual studies showed considerable heterogeneity, and thus it is important to conduct well-designed randomized control trials in those with prediabetes to evaluate the potential beneficial effects of Zn supplementation in prevention of diabetes.

Individuals with higher serum SOD and β-carotene levels, and less dietary intake of energy and fat, may have reduced risk of MS. A negative association has been reported between serum antioxidant status and dietary fat, energy, protein, and Zn intake in MS patients. These findings suggest that high antioxidant and low fat and energy intake could beneficially affect serum oxidative status, followed by attenuating MS [119].

5. CONCLUDING REMARKS

- Se, Mg, and Zn are essential metals for living.
- Se proteins may play a significant role in cellular defense against ROS.
- Se may have a protective effect against CVDs.
- Lower blood Se levels have been shown in patients with heart failure compared to healthy persons.

- There are inverse correlations between serum Se, hsCRP, and soluble ICAM-1, which indicates that Se levels are associated with oxidative stress and decreased protection of the blood vessels against oxidative damage.
- High serum Se concentrations were associated with higher prevalence of hypertension.
- The relationship between Se and T2DM is controversial.
- Se may act as an insulin mimetic.
- Mg acts as cofactor of hundreds of enzymes.
- There is an inverse relationship between Mg intake and prevalence or incidence of MS.
- Mg could modify both the secretion of insulin and its intracellular signal.
- Mg deficiency could decrease insulin sensitivity.
- Low levels of Mg favor a proinflammatory environment, a condition present in MS and obesity.
- Subjects with hypomagnesemia would benefit from better metabolic control of glucose.
- Zn is indispensable for the activity of more than 300 enzymes.
- Zn has catalytic, structural, and regulatory functions.
- Zn regulates the expression of multiple genes through the zinc fingers.
- There are 14 members that encode for Zn transporters ZIP 1−14, which are mainly importers of Zn into the cytoplasm.
- There are 10 members that encode for Zn transporters ZnT1-10, which are mainly exporters of Zn from the cytoplasm to organelles and the extracellular space.
- Zn participates in processes related to insulin function.
- Zn is necessary for the correct formation of insulin hexamers, storage, and secretion of insulin by β-cells.
- Patients with MS have high prevalence of inadequate Zn intake and alterations in Zn metabolism.
- Alterations in cardiometabolic components lead to higher zincuria in patients with MS.
- Studying the phenotype of each individual as it relates to Zn biomarkers will provide more reliable answers regarding the role of Zn in the mechanisms involved in MS.
- Adequate dietary ingestion and/or Zn supplementation are essential in the control of T2DM.

LIST OF ABBREVIATIONS

BMI Body mass index
cAMP Cyclic AMP
CRP C-reactive protein
CVD Cardiovascular disease
DIO Iodothyronine deiodinases
GLUT Glucose transport
GPx Glutathione peroxidase
GSH Reduced glutathione
H_2O_2 Hydrogen peroxide
HDL High-density lipoprotein
hsCRP High-sensitivity C-reactive protein
ICAM Intercellular adhesion molecule
IL-6 Interleukin 6
IRS-1 Insulin receptor substrate-1
LDL Low-density lipoprotein
LOOHs Lipid hydroperoxides
LPL Lipoprotein lipase
MD Mediterranean diet
Mg Magnesium
MS Metabolic syndrome
NEP Neprilysin
NK T cells natural killer
PAI-1 Plasminogen activator inhibitor-1
ROS Reactive oxygen species
Se Selenium
SeCys Selenocysteine
SelP Selenoprotein P
SeMet Selenomethionine
SOD Cu−Zn superoxide dismutase

T2DM Type 2 diabetes mellitus
T3 Triiodothyronine
T4 Thyroxine
TNF-α Tumor necrosis factor alpha
WAT White adipose tissue
WHO World Health Organization
ZAG Zinc-α2-glycoprotein
Zn Zinc

REFERENCES

[1] Ng M, et al. Global, regional, and national prevalence of overweight and obesity in children and adults during 1980–2013: a systematic analysis for the Global Burden of Disease Study 2013. Lancet 2014;384(9945):766–81.

[2] Smith KB, Smith MS. Obesity statistics. Prim Care 2016;43(1):121–35.

[3] Beilby J. Definition of metabolic syndrome: report of the National Heart, Lung, and Blood Institute/American Heart Association conference on scientific issues related to definition. Circulation 2004;109:433–8.

[4] Navas-Acien A, et al. Arsenic exposure and prevalence of type 2 diabetes in US adults. J Am Med Assoc 2008;300:814–22.

[5] Lee BK, Kim Y. Blood cadmium, mercury, and lead and metabolic syndrome in South Korea: 2005–2010 Korean National Health and Nutrition Examination Survey. Am J Ind Med 2013;56:682–92.

[6] Rotter I, et al. Relationship between the concentrations of heavy metals and bioelements in aging men with metabolic syndrome. Int J Environ Res Public Health 2015;12:3944–61.

[7] Consultation WHOE. Appropriate body-mass index for Asian populations and its implications for policy and intervention strategies. Lancet 2004;363(9403):157–63.

[8] Peters JC, et al. From instinct to intellect: the challenge of maintaining healthy weight in the modern world. Obes Rev 2002;3(2):69–74.

[9] Becker C, et al. Iron metabolism in obesity: how interaction between homoeostatic mechanisms can interfere with their original purpose. Part I: underlying homoeostatic mechanisms of energy storage and iron metabolisms and their interaction. J Trace Elem Med Biol 2015;30:195–201.

[10] Rosen ED, Spiegelman BM. Adipocytes as regulators of energy balance and glucose homeostasis. Nature 2006;444(7121):847–53.

[11] Capel F, et al. Macrophages and adipocytes in human obesity: adipose tissue gene expression and insulin sensitivity during calorie restriction and weight stabilization. Diabetes 2009;58(7):1558–67.

[12] Zhang X, et al. Adipose tissue-specific inhibition of hypoxia-inducible factor 1{alpha} induces obesity and glucose intolerance by impeding energy expenditure in mice. J Biol Chem 2010;285(43):32869–77.

[13] Hotamisligil GS. Inflammation and metabolic disorders. Nature 2006;444(7121):860–7.

[14] Haffner SM. Abdominal adiposity and cardiometabolic risk: do we have all the answers? Am J Med 2007;120(9 Suppl. 1):S10–6.

[15] Hall JE. The kidney, hypertension, and obesity. Hypertension 2003;41(3 Pt 2):625–33.

[16] Semenza GL, et al. Hypoxia, HIF-1, and the pathophysiology of common human diseases. Adv Exp Med Biol 2000;475:123–30.

[17] Carey VJ, et al. Body fat distribution and risk of non-insulin-dependent diabetes mellitus in women. The Nurses' Health Study. Am J Epidemiol 1997;145(7):614–9.

[18] Barceloux DG. Selenium. J Toxicol Clin Toxicol 1999;37(2):145–72.

[19] Rayman MP, et al. Food-chain selenium and human health: spotlight on speciation. Br J Nutr 2008;100(2):238–53.

[20] Hurst R, et al. Establishing optimal selenium status: results of a randomized, double-blind, placebo-controlled trial. Am J Clin Nutr 2010;91(4):923–31.

[21] Levander OA, Whanger PD. Deliberations and evaluations of the approaches, endpoints and paradigms for selenium and iodine dietary recommendations. J Nutr 1996;126(9 Suppl.):2427S–34S.

[22] Trumbo P, et al. Dietary reference intakes: vitamin A, vitamin K, arsenic, boron, chromium, copper, iodine, iron, manganese, molybdenum, nickel, silicon, vanadium, and zinc. J Am Diet Assoc 2001;101(3):294–301.

[23] Schrauzer GN. Selenomethionine: a review of its nutritional significance, metabolism and toxicity. J Nutr 2000;130(7):1653–6.

[24] Gammelgaard B, et al. Estimating intestinal absorption of inorganic and organic selenium compounds by in vitro flux and biotransformation studies in Caco-2 cells and ICP-MS detection. Biol Trace Elem Res 2012;145(2):248–56.

[25] Low SC, Berry MJ. Knowing when not to stop: selenocysteine incorporation in eukaryotes. Trends Biochem Sci 1996;21(6):203–8.

[26] Wang KT, et al. Crystal structures of catalytic intermediates of human seleno-phosphate synthetase 1. J Mol Biol 2009;390(4):747–59.

[27] Lobanov AV, et al. Eukaryotic selenoproteins and selenoproteomes. Biochim Biophys Acta 2009;1790(11):1424–8.

[28] Arner ES. Focus on mammalian thioredoxin reductases—important selenoproteins with versatile functions. Biochim Biophys Acta 2009;1790(6):495–526.

[29] Gromer S, et al. Human selenoproteins at a glance. Cell Mol Life Sci 2005;62(21):2414–37.

[30] St Germain DL, et al. Minireview: defining the roles of the iodothyronine deiodinases: current concepts and challenges. Endocrinology 2009;150(3):1097–107.

[31] Schnabel R, Blankenberg S. Oxidative stress in cardiovascular disease: successful translation from bench to bedside? Circulation 2007;116(12):1338–40.

[32] MacFarquhar JK, et al. Acute selenium toxicity associated with a dietary supplement. Arch Intern Med 2010;170(3):256−61.

[33] Jun EJ, et al. Selenium deficiency contributes to the chronic myocarditis in coxsackievirus-infected mice. Acta Virol 2011;55(1):23−9.

[34] Zhang X, et al. Selenium status and cardiovascular diseases: meta-analysis of prospective observational studies and randomized controlled trials. Eur J Clin Nutr 2016;70(2):162−9.

[35] Gunes S, et al. Cardioprotective effect of selenium against cyclophosphamide-induced cardiotoxicity in rats. Biol Trace Elem Res 2017;177(1):107−14.

[36] Hoffmann FW, et al. Specific antioxidant selenoproteins are induced in the heart during hypertrophy. Arch Biochem Biophys 2011;512(1):38−44.

[37] Tanguy S, et al. Dietary selenium intake influences Cx43 dephosphorylation, TNF-alpha expression and cardiac remodeling after reperfused infarction. Mol Nutr Food Res 2011;55(4):522−9.

[38] Lim CC, et al. Glutathione peroxidase deficiency exacerbates ischemia-reperfusion injury in male but not female myocardium: insights into antioxidant compensatory mechanisms. Am J Physiol Heart Circ Physiol 2009;297(6):H2144−53.

[39] Ago T, Sadoshima J. Thioredoxin and ventricular remodeling. J Mol Cell Cardiol 2006;41(5):762−73.

[40] Dhingra S, Bansal MP. Hypercholesterolemia and tissue-specific differential mRNA expression of type-1 5′-iodothyronine deiodinase under different selenium status in rats. Biol Res 2006;39(2):307−19.

[41] Fradejas N, et al. SEPS1 gene is activated during astrocyte ischemia and shows prominent antiapoptotic effects. J Mol Neurosci 2008;35(3):259−65.

[42] Auro K, et al. Combined effects of thrombosis pathway gene variants predict cardiovascular events. PLoS Genet 2007;3(7):e120.

[43] Lee BC, et al. MsrB1 and MICALs regulate actin assembly and macrophage function via reversible stereoselective methionine oxidation. Mol Cell 2013;51(3):397−404.

[44] Picot CR, et al. Alterations in mitochondrial and cytosolic methionine sulfoxide reductase activity during cardiac ischemia and reperfusion. Exp Gerontol 2006;41(7):663−7.

[45] Lu C, et al. Identification and characterization of selenoprotein K: an antioxidant in cardiomyocytes. FEBS Lett 2006;580(22):5189−97.

[46] Laclaustra M, et al. Serum selenium concentrations and hypertension in the US population. Circ Cardiovasc Qual Outcomes 2009;2(4):369−76.

[47] Nawrot TS, et al. Blood pressure and blood selenium: a cross-sectional and longitudinal population study. Eur Heart J 2007;28(5):628−33.

[48] Stranges S, et al. Selenium status and cardiometabolic health: state of the evidence. Nutr Metab Cardiovasc Dis 2010;20(10):754−60.

[49] Kuruppu D, et al. Selenium levels and hypertension: a systematic review of the literature. Public Health Nutr 2014;17(6):1342−52.

[50] Robertson RP, Harmon JS. Pancreatic islet beta-cell and oxidative stress: the importance of glutathione peroxidase. FEBS Lett 2007;581(19):3743−8.

[51] Steinbrenner H, et al. High selenium intake and increased diabetes risk: experimental evidence for interplay between selenium and carbohydrate metabolism. J Clin Biochem Nutr 2011;48(1):40−5.

[52] Chen X, et al. Association of glutathione peroxidase activity with insulin resistance and dietary fat intake during normal pregnancy. J Clin Endocrinol Metab 2003;88(12):5963−8.

[53] Roman M, et al. Plasma selenoproteins concentrations in type 2 diabetes mellitus−a pilot study. Transl Res 2010;156(4):242−50.

[54] Stranges S, et al. Effects of long-term selenium supplementation on the incidence of type 2 diabetes: a randomized trial. Ann Intern Med 2007;147(4):217−23.

[55] Wang XL, et al. Association between serum selenium level and type 2 diabetes mellitus: a non-linear dose-response meta-analysis of observational studies. Nutr J 2016;15(1):48.

[56] Zhou J, et al. Selenium and diabetes−evidence from animal studies. Free Radic Biol Med 2013;65:1548−56.

[57] Ezaki O. The insulin-like effects of selenate in rat adipocytes. J Biol Chem 1990;265(2):1124−8.

[58] Stapleton SR, et al. Selenium: potent stimulator of tyrosyl phosphorylation and activator of MAP kinase. Biochim Biophys Acta 1997;1355(3):259−69.

[59] Berg EA, et al. Insulin-like effects of vanadate and selenate on the expression of glucose-6-phosphate dehydrogenase and fatty acid synthase in diabetic rats. Biochimie 1995;77(12):919−24.

[60] Collins R, et al. Biochemical discrimination between selenium and sulfur 1: a single residue provides selenium specificity to human selenocysteine lyase. PLoS One 2012;7(1):e30581.

[61] Seale LA, et al. Disruption of the selenocysteine lyase-mediated selenium recycling pathway leads to metabolic syndrome in mice. Mol Cell Biol 2012;32(20):4141−54.

[62] Vormann J. Magnesium: nutrition and metabolism. Mol Aspect Med 2003;24:27−37.

[63] Nils-Erik S, et al. Magnesium
An update on physiological, clinical and analytical aspects. Clin Chim Acta 2000;294:1−26.

[64] McNeill DA, et al. Mineral analyses of vegetarian, health, and conventional foods: magnesium, zinc, copper, and manganese content. J Am Diet Assoc 1985;85:569−72.

[65] Institute of Medicine (US) Standing Committee on the Scientific Evaluation of Dietary Reference Intakes. Dietary reference intakes for calcium, phosphorus, magnesium, vitamin D, and fluoride. Washington (DC): National Academies Press (US); 1997. Magnesium. Available from: https://www.ncbi.nlm.nih.gov/books/NBK109816/.

[66] Popkin BM, et al. Now and then: the global nutrition transition: the pandemic of obesity in developing countries. Nutr Rev 2012;70(1):3−21.

[67] Ford ES, Mokdad AH. Dietary magnesium intake in a national sample of us adults. J Nutr 2003;133:2879−82.

[68] Wang J, et al. Dietary magnesium intake improves insulin resistance among non-diabetic individuals with metabolic syndrome participating in a dietary trial. Nutrients 2013;5:3910–9.

[69] McKeown NM, et al. Dietary magnesium intake is related to metabolic syndrome in older Americans. Eur J Nutr 2008;47(4):210–6.

[70] He K, et al. Magnesium intake and incidence of metabolic syndrome among young adults. Circulation 2006;113(13):1675–82.

[71] Mirmiran P, et al. Magnesium intake and prevalence of metabolic syndrome in adults: Tehran Lipid and Glucose Study. Public Health Nutr 2012;15(4):693–701.

[72] Yokota K, et al. Clinical efficacy of magnesium supplementation in patients with type 2 diabetes. J Am Coll Nutr 2004;23(5):506S–9S.

[73] Gunther T. The biochemical function of Mg (2)+ in insulin secretion, insulin signal transduction and insulin resistance. Magnes Res 2010;23:5–18.

[74] Rayssiguier Y. Magnesium, lipids and vascular diseases. Experimental evidence in animal models. Magnesium 1986;5:182–90.

[75] Sales CH, et al. Magnesium- deficient high-fat diet: effects on adiposity, lipid profile and insulin sensitivity in growing rats. Clin Nutr 2014;33:879–88.

[76] Dibaba DT, et al. Dietary magnesium intake is inversely associated with serum C-reactive protein levels: meta-analysis and systematic review. Eur J Clin Nutr 2014;68(4):510–6.

[77] Song Y, et al. Magnesium intake, C-reactive protein, and the prevalence of metabolic syndrome in middle-aged and older U.S. women. Diabetes Care 2005;28:1438–44.

[78] Guerrero-Romero F, et al. Severe hypomagnesemia and low-grade inflammation in metabolic syndrome. Magnes Res 2011;24(2):45–53.

[79] Guerrero-Romero F, Rodríguez-Mora M. Hypomagnesemia, oxidative stress, inflammation, and metabolic syndrome. Diabetes Metab Res 2006;22(6):471–6.

[80] Mazur A, et al. Magnesium and the inflammatory response: potential physiopathological implications. Arch Biochem Biophys 2007;458(1):48–56.

[81] Weglicki WB, et al. Role of free radicals and substance P in magnesium deficiency. Cardiovasc Res 1996;31:677–82.

[82] Bo S, et al. Dietary magnesium and fiber intakes and inflammatory and metabolic indicators in middle-aged subjects from a population-based cohort. Am J Clin Nutr 2006;84:1062–9.

[83] Bo S, et al. Magnesium and trace element intake after a lifestyle intervention. Nutrition 2011;27:108–10.

[84] Simental-Mendía LE, et al. Oral magnesium supplementation decreases C-reactive protein levels in subjects with prediabetes and hypomagnesemia: a clinical randomized double-blind placebo-controlled trial. Arch Med Res 2014;45(4):325–30.

[85] Navarrete-Cortes A, et al. No effect of magnesium supplementation on metabolic control and insulin sensitivity in type 2 diabetes patients with normomagnesemia. Magnes Res 2014;27(2):48–56.

[86] Morais JBS, et al. Effect of magnesium supplementation on insulin resistance in humans: a systematic review. Nutrition 2017;38:54–60.

[87] Simental-Mendía LE, et al. Effect of magnesium supplementation on lipid profile: a systematic review and meta-analysis of randomized controlled trials. Eur J Clin Pharmacol 2017;73(5):525–36.

[88] Joris PJ, et al. Long-term magnesium supplementation improves arterial stiffness in overweight and obese adults: results of a randomized, double-blind, placebo-controlled intervention trial. Am J Clin Nutr 2016;103(5):1260–6.

[89] Hans CP, et al. Effect of magnesium supplementation on oxidative stress in alloxanic diabetic rats. Magnes Res 2003;16(1):13–9.

[90] Vongpatanasin W, et al. Effects of potassium magnesium citrate supplementation on 24-hour ambulatory blood pressure and oxidative stress marker in pre-hypertensive and hypertensive subjects. Am J Cardiol 2016;118(6):849–53.

[91] Maret W. Zinc biochemistry: from a single zinc enzyme to a key element of life. Adv Nutr 2013;4(1):82–91.

[92] Ruz M. Zinc: properties and determination. In: Trugo L, Finglas PM, Caballero B, editors. Encyclopedia of food sciences and nutrition. 2nd ed. London: Academic Press; 2003. p. 6267–72.

[93] Wei S, et al. Emerging roles of zinc finger proteins in regulating adipogenesis. Cell Mol Life Sci 2013;70(23):4569–84.

[94] Miao X, et al. Zinc homeostasis in the metabolic syndrome and diabetes. Front Med China 2013;7:31–52.

[95] Tubek S. Role of zinc in regulation of arterial blood pressure and in the etiopathogenesis of arterial hypertension. Biol Trace Elem Res 2007;117:39–51.

[96] Kloubert V, Rink L. Zinc as a micronutrient and its preventive role of oxidative damage in cells. Food Funct 2015;6:3195–204.

[97] Bonaventura P, et al. Zinc and its role in immunity and inflammation. Autoimmun Rev 2015;14:277–85.

[98] Haase H, Rink L. Functional significance of zinc-related signaling pathways in immune cells. Annu Rev Nutr 2009;29:133–52.

[99] Ruz M, et al. Does zinc really metal with diabetes? The epidemiologic evidence. Curr Diabetes Rep 2016;16:111. https://doi.org/10.1007/s11892-016-0803-x.

[100] Freitas E, et al. Zinc status biomarkers and cardiometabolic risk factors in metabolic syndrome: a case control study. Nutrients 2017;9:175. https://doi.org/10.3390/nu9020175).

[101] Steiner DF. Adventures with insulin in the islets of Langerhans. J Biol Chem 2011;286:17399–421.

[102] Gerber PA, Rutter GA. The role of oxidative stress and hypoxia in pancreatic beta-cell dysfunction in diabetes mellitus. Antioxid Redox Signal 2017;26(10). https://doi.org/10.1089/ars.2016.6755).

[103] Emdin SO, et al. Role of zinc in insulin biosynthesis. Some possible zinc-insulin interactions in the pancreatic B-cell. Diabetologia 1980;19(3):174–82.

[104] Zhou H, et al. Zinc, not insulin, regulates the rat alpha-cell response to hypoglycemia in vivo. Diabetes 2007;56(4):1107–12.

[105] Shan Z, et al. Interactions between zinc transporter-8 gene (SLC30A8) and plasma zinc concentrations for impaired glucose regulation and type 2 diabetes. Diabetes 2014;63:1796–803.

[106] Velázquez-López L, et al. Mediterranean-style diet reduces metabolic syndrome components in obese children and adolescents with obesity. BMC Pediatr 2014;14:175.

[107] Seo J-A, et al. The associations between serum zinc levels and metabolic syndrome in the Korean population: findings from the 2010 Korean National Health and Nutrition Examination Survey. PLoS One 2014;9(8):e105990.

[108] Al-Daghri N, et al. Selected dietary nutrients and the prevalence of metabolic syndrome in adult males and females in Saudi Arabia: a pilot study. Nutrients 2013;5:4587—604.

[109] Azab S, et al. Serum trace elements in obese Egyptian children: a case—control study. Ital J Pediatr 2014;40:20.

[110] Mracek T, et al. This association could be explained by the effect of zinc-α2-glycoprotein (ZAG) on leptin concentrations. The adipokine zinc-a2-glycoprotein (ZAG) is downregulated with fat mass expansion in obesity. Clin Endocrinol 2010;72:334—41.

[111] Standeven K, et al. Neprilysin, obesity and the metabolic syndrome. Int J Obes (Lond) 2011;35(8):1031—40.

[112] Dourado F, et al. Biomarkers of metabolic syndrome and its relationship with the zinc nutritional status in obese women. Nutr Hosp 2011;26(3):650—4.

[113] de Oliveira M, et al. Dietary intakes of zinc and heme iron from red meat, but not from other sources, are associated with greater risk of metabolic syndrome and cardiovascular disease. J Nutr January 18, 2012. https://doi.org/10.3945/jn.111.149781).

[114] Gletsu-Miller N, Wright B. Mineral malnutrition following bariatric surgery. Adv Nutr 2013;4:506—17.

[115] Prasad AS. Zinc in human health: effect of zinc on immune cells. Mol Med 2008;14:353—7.

[116] Zhang C, et al. Diabetes-induced hepatic pathogenic damage, inflammation, oxidative stress, and insulin resistance was exacerbated in zinc deficient mouse model. PLoS One 2012;7:e49257.

[117] Foster M, et al. Zinc transporter gene expression and glycemic control in postmenopausal women with type 2 diabetes mellitus. J Trace Elem Med Biol 2014;28:448—52.

[118] Jayawardena R, et al. Effects of zinc supplementation on diabetes mellitus: a systematic review and meta-analysis. Diabetol Metab Syndr 2012;4:13.

[119] Li Y, et al. Serum and dietary antioxidant status is associated with lower prevalence of the metabolic syndrome in a study in Shanghai, China. Asia Pac J Clin Nutr 2013;22(1):60—8.

Chapter 11

Polyphenols in Obesity and Metabolic Syndrome

Belén Pastor-Villaescusa[1], Estefania Sanchez Rodriguez[1] and Oscar D. Rangel-Huerta[2, a]

[1]University of Granada, Granada, Spain; [2]University of Oslo, Oslo, Norway

1. OBESITY AND METABOLIC SYNDROME

Overweight and obesity are considered a world pandemic of the 21st century. Worldwide obesity has nearly doubled since 1980. In 2016, more than 1.9 billion adults, 18 years and older, were overweight. Of these over 650 million were obese [1].

Obesity is a complex multifactorial disease influenced by lifestyle, behavioural, environmental, and genetic factors. Obesity consists of an abnormal or excessive fat accumulation, for which the main cause is a chronic imbalance between energy intake and energy expenditure. Metabolic syndrome (MetS) is a cluster of associated metabolic disturbances which tend to coexist, commonly represented by the combination of obesity (especially abdominal obesity), hyperglycemia, dyslipidemia, and hypertension [2]. MetS is associated with an increased risk of cardiovascular diseases (CVDs), which are the leading cause of disability and death in industrialized countries and are associated with a chronic inflammatory response, characterized by abnormal cytokine production that leads to endothelial dysfunction [3].

2. OXIDATIVE STRESS AND ANTIOXIDANT DEFENSE

Living organisms are constantly producing reactive oxygen species (ROS) in their normal cellular metabolism. ROS can be divided into two groups: free radicals and nonradicals. Molecules containing one or more unpaired electrons and thus giving reactivity to the molecule are called free radicals. When two free radicals share their unpaired electrons, nonradical forms are created. The three major ROS, according to physiological significance, are superoxide anion (O_2^-), hydroxyl radical ($-OH$), and hydrogen peroxide (H_2O_2).

At low to moderate concentrations ROS function in physiological cell processes, but at high concentrations they produce adverse modifications in cell components such as lipids, proteins, and DNA, thus altering their functions. The shift in the balance between oxidant/antioxidant in favor of oxidants is termed *oxidative stress*. Oxidative stress is associated with CVD and its related risk factors, such as obesity and type 2 diabetes (T2D), and also with other chronic degenerative processes such as cancer and other aging-related diseases.

The human body is equipped with a variety of antioxidants that serve to counterbalance the effect of oxidants and protect against the harmful effects of ROS. For all practical purposes these can be divided into two categories: enzymatic and nonenzymatic. The enzymatic defense system comprises molecules of superoxide dismutase (SOD), catalase, glutathione peroxidase (GPx), thioredoxin, peroxiredoxin, and glutathione transferase (GR). The nonenzymatic antioxidants include low-molecular-weight compounds, such as vitamins (C and E), β-carotene, uric acid, and glutathione (GSH).

---

[a] Senior and corresponding author

Obesity. https://doi.org/10.1016/B978-0-12-812504-5.00011-8

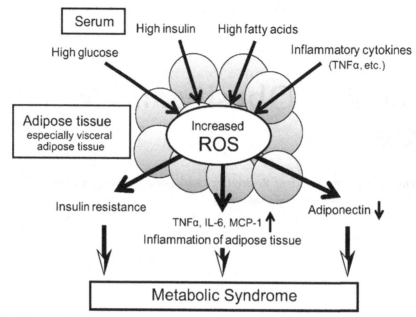

FIGURE 11.1 Factors contributing to increased ROS in adipocytes and linked to IR, inflammation of adipose tissue, and decreased adiponectin. *IL*, interleukin; *IR*, insulin resistance; *MCP*, monocyte chemoattractant protein; *ROS*, reactive oxygen species; *TNF*, tumor necrosis factor.

2.1 Oxidative Stress and Metabolic Syndrome

In pathological conditions the antioxidant systems can be overwhelmed. When ROS generation is out of control or antioxidant defense is damaged, oxidative stress occurs, with extensive molecular and cellular consequences [4]. Concretely, the physiopathology of obesity is characterized by a state of chronic oxidative stress [5], and it is well known that adipose tissue in obese individuals undergoes many pathological changes (Fig. 11.1) due to the accumulation of fat, such as inflammation, hypoxia, and increased oxidative stress [6]. The white adipose tissue (WAT) exerts a pivotal role to warrant the redox homeostasis in the organism. The production of ROS in such adipose tissue can also produce a dysregulation of adipocytokines and the migration of oxidative stress to remote tissues [7]. Hence this phenomenon is a significant cause of insulin resistance (IR), T2D, hypertension, and cardiovascular damage [8].

3. EXOGENOUS ANTIOXIDANTS

Epidemiological evidence indicates that polyphenol-rich diets, such as the Mediterranean diet, are associated with antioxidant, antiinflammatory, and antiobesity effects and a reduction of risk factors for MetS and CVDs. These effects might be related to the high intake of polyphenol-rich foods contained in this type of diet, like fruits and vegetables, which are capable of modulating the nonenzymatic antioxidant defense system. Antioxidants can act as chain breakers or radical scavengers according to their chemical structure. Furthermore, antioxidant-rich foods such as red wine, cocoa, green tea, and berries are shown to aid in the improvement of cardiovascular health. This effect may be attributed to the ability of polyphenols to interact with adipose tissue.

In this chapter we first explain the nature of polyphenols and their classification, and secondly elucidate their potential mechanism of action and the current evidence regarding obesity and MetS.

4. POLYPHENOLS

Polyphenols can be found in nature, mainly in plants, vegetables (Table 11.1), and their derivative products, and are of considerable interest due to their contribution to the taste, color, and nutritional properties of such products. These compounds are abundant in our diet; Scalbert et al. [9] reported that the intake of polyphenols is around 1 g/day, higher than that of other known antioxidants. Products such as grapes, wine, onions, coffee, tea, and chocolate are shown to be rich in polyphenols.

TABLE 11.1 Main Food Sources of Polyphenols

Polyphenol	Class	Main Food Sources
Phenolic Acids	Benzoic acid	American cranberry, chestnut, cloves, pomegranate juice, red raspberry, star anise
	Cinnamic acid	Coffee, common verbena, dried peppermint, dried rosemary, maize oil, potatoes
Stilbenes	Resveratrol	Grapes, nuts, red wine
Lignans		Black sesame oil, bread from whole-grain rye flour, flaxseed, sesame seed oil, whole-grain rye flour, virgin olive oil
Flavonoids	Flavones	Black olives, celery seed, dried common verbena, dried peppermint, oranges, refined-grain wheat-flour bread, whole grain wheat-flour, whole grain wheat-flour bread, virgin olive oil
	Flavonols	Beans, capers, dried oregano, onions, saffron, shallots, spinach
	Flavan-3-ols	Apples, cocoa powder, dark chocolate, nuts, peaches, red wine
	Flavanones	Dried oregano, dried peppermint, fresh rosemary, grapefruit/pomelo juice, oranges
	Isoflavones	Beans and soy products
	Anthocyanins	Almonds, black chokeberry, black elderberry, blueberries, cherries, hazelnuts, olives, red wine

Probably the best known beneficial effect of polyphenols is their antioxidant capacity, which is capable of reducing ROS and various organic substrates and minerals; they are also shown to have antiinflammatory activity and might modulate gene expression of neurodegenerative and anticarcinogenic processes. Dietary polyphenols represent a large family of bioactive compounds with a potentially beneficial effect on noncommunicable diseases, for instance obesity and MetS [10]. Their specific mechanisms of action remain unclear, but it is hypothesized that polyphenols might trigger changes in the signaling pathways and consequently in gene expression.

One must take into consideration that the potential beneficial effects of polyphenols are related to their bioavailability, and this depends on several factors. Environmental, genetic, processing, and technological factors might affect the polyphenol content in food, and polyphenol properties might be greatly affected by interactions with other components of the food matrix. Furthermore, these interactions are likely to influence bioavailability and should be taken into account when designing intervention studies. For instance, the interactions among polyphenols, proteins, and digestive enzymes reduce the protein digestibility and decrease polyphenol bioavailability. Daily cooking processes are shown to reduce the phenolic content, thus reducing antioxidant activity.

5. CLASSIFICATION OF POLYPHENOLS

Polyphenols are known as compounds containing phenolic structural features, but the complexity of these compounds is high and diverse, and it is possible to divide them into several subgroups. There are several categorizations, based on their source of origin, biological function, or chemical structure.

In this chapter, for better comprehension we discuss polyphenols according to their chemical structure (Fig. 11.2), including the nonflavonoids, which are the phenolic acids (C6—C1 and C6—C3), stilbenes (C6—C2—C6), lignans (C6—C3—C3—C6), and curcuminoids ($C_{21}H_{20}O_6$), and the flavonoids (C6—C3—C6) [11]. The chemical structure of flavonoids classifies them into six basic subclasses: flavones, anthocyanins (ACNs), flavanones, flavonols, isoflavones, and flavanols. Flavanols include the flavanol oligomers, the proanthocyanidins (PAs), which are further subdivided into 16 species including the procyanidins, oligomers of the flavan-3-ols catechin and epicatechin, and the prodelphinidins, which are oligomers of the gallocatechins. We also include the open-ring chalcones.

5.1 Nonflavonoids

Nonflavonoids comprise a major group of polyphenols with a broad variety of chemical structures that are responsible for their different properties, including phenolic acids, stilbenes, lignans, and curcuminoids.

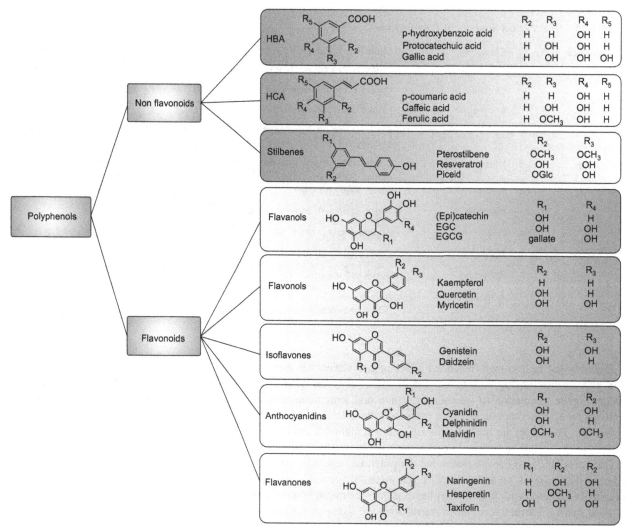

FIGURE 11.2 Classification and chemical structure of some polyphenols. *EGCG*, epigallocatechin 3-gallate.

5.1.1 Phenolic Acids

Phenolic acids are aromatic secondary metabolites that are widespread in the plant kingdom. These compounds contain both hydroxyl and carboxyl groups. The content of phenolic acids in plants, as for other phenolic compounds, depends on many factors, such as climatic conditions, cultivation, fertilization, and time of harvest [12]. Additionally, storage conditions of the plant materials and methods of preparation should be taken into account. Overall phenolic acids can be found in large amounts in fruits and vegetables. The average intake in humans is reported to be 200 mg/day depending on dietary habits and preferences [13]. The main sources of phenolic acids are herbal infusions such as black and green tea, and coffee [14]. Mushrooms have received particular attention, being described as rich sources of phenolic acids, which are among the major contributors to their medicinal properties [15]. Phenolic acids may influence the color, flavor, fragrance, and oxidation stability of food. In this regard, their concentration depends on, among other factors, the type of technological process applied to a given plant material [16].

Extensive knowledge of phenolic acid bioavailability is essential to understand the conjugations and biological properties in the organism. When phenolic acids are absorbed in the free form, their absorption and conjugation (methylation, hydroxylation, sulfation, and especially glucuronidation) follow the same pathways as those of flavonoids and other polyphenols [17]. Within the phenolic acids group, cinnamic and *p*-coumaric acid aromatic rings are hydroxylated and methylated to form their derivatives, ferulic and caffeic acids [18]. Benzoic acid formation can result from degradation of the side chain of cinnamic acid. The same hydroxylation and methylation reactions can occur in the aromatic ring of benzoic acid, giving the correspondent derivatives, gallic, vanillic, and *p*-hydroxybenzoic acids [19]. It is

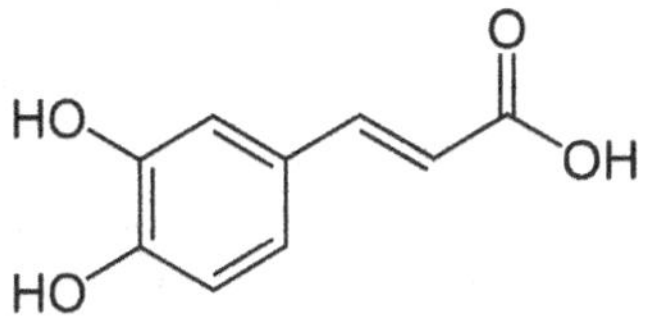

FIGURE 11.3   Chemical structure of caffeic acid.

known that phenolic acids and their derivatives have a high antioxidant activity, which depends on the number of hydroxyl groups found in the molecule [20]. Overall, the hydroxylated cinnamic acids are more effective than their benzoic acids counterparts. Thus methylated polyphenols have a decreased ability to protect low-density lipoprotein (LDL) from in vitro oxidation compared to the respective parental compound [18]. For this reason, much attention has been focused on hydroxylated cinnamic acids and their properties. Caffeic acid (3,4-dihydroxycinnamic acid) (Fig. 11.3) is found in the form of esters: chlorogenic acid is the most frequently encountered in the normal diet [13], and along with ferulic and p-coumaric acids makes coffee the main source of bound phenolic acids. Caffeic acid is also present in many fruits (blueberries, apples, pears, etc.), vegetables (lettuce, potatoes, eggplants, etc.), and beverages, wine, and tea [21]. Recently, two in vitro studies have reported promising results: on the one hand, caffeic acid decreases the expression and secretion of C-reactive protein (CRP), vascular cell adhesion molecules-1 (VCAM-1), and monocyte chemoattractant protein-1 (MCP-1) in human endothelial cells incubated with glycated LDL [22]; on the other hand, caffeic acid decreases inflammation in the same type of cells incubated with high glucose by attenuating nuclear factor-kappa B (NF-κB) signaling [23]. Moreover, coffee consumption is associated with lower CRP levels in plasma of diabetic or obese women [24,25].

p-Coumaric acid is another compound from the hydroxycinnamic acid family which plays a central role in secondary metabolism because it can be subsequently transformed to phenolic acids (e.g., caffeic acid, ferulic acid, chlorogenic acid, and sinapic acid), as well as into flavonoids, lignin precursors, and other secondary metabolites [21]. The content of free p-coumaric acid is very high in some mushroom species, such as *Ganoderma lucidum*, *Termitomyces heimii*, *G. lucidum*, and *Cantharellus cibarius* [26]. It should be highlighted that p-coumaric acid has higher bioavailability than chlorogenic acid, caffeic acid, and ferulic acid, although overall it presents lower antioxidant power [26]. That capacity increases significantly upon conjugation with quinic acid, monosaccharides, and amine. Regarding its effect on health, p-coumaric acid might mitigate diabetes by reducing the intestinal absorption of dietary carbohydrate (by inhibiting glucosidase), modulating the enzymes involved in glucose metabolism, improving β-cell function and insulin action, stimulating insulin secretion, and strengthening antioxidant and antiinflammatory properties [27]. Yoon et al. [28] found that p-coumaric acid in differentiated L6 skeletal muscle cells increases the phosphorylation of AMP-activated protein kinase (AMPK), promotes the β-oxidation of fatty acids by increasing the messenger RNA (mRNA) expression of carnitine palmitoyltransferase-1 and its transcription factor peroxisome proliferator-activated receptor-γ (PPAR-γ), and suppresses oleic acid-induced triacylglyceride (TG) accumulation. Nevertheless, solid evidence in humans on the effect of p-coumaric acid is absent so far.

Gallic acid (3, 4, 5-trihydroxybenzoic acid) (Fig. 11.4) is found both free and as part of tannin compounds, which can be classified into two groups, hydrolyzable tannins and condensed tannins, that differ in their chemical structures (see Section 5.2.7) [13]. Hydrolysable tannins can be further divided into gallotannins, which provide sugar and gallic acid on hydrolysis, and ellagitannins, which on hydrolysis yield sugar, gallic acid, and also ellagic acid [29]. They are one of the main secondary metabolites found in cacao beans, tea, wine (mainly red), fruits, juices, nuts, chocolate, legumes, and cereal grains, and are responsible for the astringent taste of many of them [29].

Focusing on gallic acid properties, it has shown a beneficial effect on MetS [30], and in vivo studies in particular have demonstrated its antiobesity and hypolipidemic effects [31,32]. For instance, in obese and diabetic rats the administration

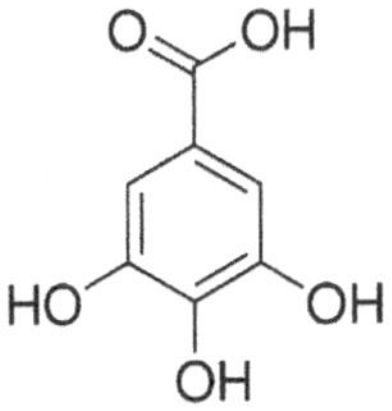

FIGURE 11.4   Chemical structure of gallic acid.

of 20 mg/kg of gallic acid decreased weight gain and blood glucose and insulin levels. Gallic acid also increased levels of PPAR-γ expression in the adipose tissue of these rats [30]. Gallic acid intake significantly improves insulin and glucose homeostasis and ameliorates the risk of metabolic diseases by the decrease of serum TGs, phospholipids, total cholesterol, LDL cholesterol, hepatic TGs, and cholesterol induced by consumption of a high-fat diet (HFD) [31]. Such effects might be associated with one principal mechanism of action, the phosphorylation of AMPK, which shows a dose-dependent response to gallic acid in studies using the cell line HepG2 [33].

Despite the antioxidant activity of phenolic compounds and their possible benefits to human health, until the beginning of the last decade (2005) most studies on these substances looked at their deleterious effects. Indeed, a recent study assessed the phytotoxicity of olive mill solid wastes and the possible influence of phenolic acids [34].

5.1.2 Stilbenes

Stilbenes are among the most relevant polyphenols. This group of polyphenols is characterized by its estrogenic activity and its capability to modulate the signaling pathway of the estrogenic receptors. Plants produce these compounds as a protective response to adverse conditions, against pathogens, damage, or stress [35].

Resveratrol (3,5,4′-trihydroxiestilbene) is considered to be the major stilbene; its name appears to be due to its chemical structure and the plant source used for isolation (a resorcinol derivative or polyphenol in the resin, occurring in *Veratrum* species which contains hydroxyl (−OH) groups (-*ol*)) [35]. The main enzyme responsible for resveratrol biosynthesis is stilbene synthase, which condenses one *p*-coumaroyl-CoA (4-coumaroyl-CoA) and three molecules of malonyl-CoA [36].

The principal sources are red grapes and derived products (red wine, grape juice) containing concentrations up to 14 mg/L; other sources of resveratrol are peanuts (0.02−1.8 mg/g) and several berries [33]. Evidence from animal models and human studies reveals that resveratrol is rapidly and efficiently absorbed following oral administration, although its bioavailability is low due to its metabolism to sulfated and glucuronidated derivates during first-pass metabolism by the liver [37]. Such compounds are produced mainly by the gut microbiota.

Resveratrol has shown antioxidant and antiinflammatory activities, and cardioprotective, antiobesity, and antidiabetic capacities [38]. Although it exists in both *cis* and *trans* form, the *trans* isomer is a more efficient antioxidant [39]. The antioxidant effects of resveratrol are reported to regulate the activity of main antioxidant enzymes such as SOD and catalase, and oxidative stress markers [35,40]. Moreover, it is reported that the antiinflammatory effects of resveratrol are mediated by inhibiting NF-κB signaling [40a]. This polyphenol reduces the expression of proinflammatory cytokines such as interleukin 6 (IL-6), interleukin 8 (IL-8), tumor necrosis factor-α (TNF-α), and MCP-1, and inhibits the cyclooxygenase (COX) protein expression and matrix metalloproteinase-9 protein release in cultured endothelial cells [41]. Additionally, cardioprotective effects have been attributed to resveratrol; it is suggested that it improves endothelial function by its vasodilatory effect, which appears to be mediated via improved bioavailability of nitric oxide (NO) through increasing endothelial nitric oxide synthase (eNOS) expression and activity [42]. eNOS is of particular importance in cardiovascular physiology as it regulates vascular tone via the release of NO in the vascular endothelium [43]. Although not fully delineated, some of the beneficial cardiovascular effects of resveratrol are mediated through activation of silent information regulator 1, AMPK, and endogenous antioxidant enzymes [44]. Besides, resveratrol exerts endothelial protection by stimulation of a nuclear factor erythroid-2 related factor-2 (NRF2) [45] and decreasing the expression of adhesion proteins such as intercellular adhesion molecules-1 [46] and VCAM-1 through NF-κB inhibition [46]. Regarding glucose metabolism, resveratrol enhances glucose transporter 4 (GLUT-4) translocation to the plasma membrane of muscle cells [47] and increases GLUT-4 expression in skeletal muscle of animals with diet-induced IR [48] and in *db/db* mice as well [49].

Regarding the evidence on resveratrol demonstrated in vivo studies, little research has been done so far, but several findings are remarkable. Firstly, high doses of resveratrol (≥150 mg/day) have been reported to reduce systolic blood pressure (SBP) significantly [44]. This effect is more pronounced if resveratrol is administered to hypertensive individuals. Several studies in humans have shown that resveratrol can also inhibit significant steps in the process of thrombogenesis [50]. Interestingly, resveratrol inhibits epinephrine- and collagen-induced aggregation of platelets from aspirin-resistant patients [51], suggesting that it may be a second-line antiplatelet in these patients. This fact is of particular importance from a clinical perspective, since aspirin remains the most clinically used antiplatelet medication and up to 20% of serious vascular events in high-risk vascular patients can be attributed to aspirin resistance [52].

Additionally, some animal studies have shown that resveratrol can lower plasma levels of total and LDL cholesterol, as well as TGs, and increase the level of high-density lipoprotein (HDL) cholesterol [44]. In hypercholesteremic rats a resveratrol administration (20 mg/kg/day) for 20 days inhibited the expression of several markers of platelet activation [53]. However, the effect of resveratrol on plasma lipid profile in humans is not clear. According to a metaanalysis of seven clinical trials, resveratrol has no significant effect on plasma lipid concentrations; but the small size, the heterogeneity of the study populations and study designs, resveratrol dose, and duration of resveratrol supplementation must be considered as potential confounders in those studies [54]. Nevertheless, resveratrol may augment the antiatherosclerotic effect of traditional lipid-lowering medications, which work mainly by lowering the cholesterol and/or TG levels [55]. Regarding the impact on glucose and insulin metabolism impairment, this polyphenol provides significant improvements in the status of multiple clinically relevant biomarkers in diabetic conditions. Concretely, some studies have shown that prolonged administration of this compound reduces blood glucose and improves insulin action in experimental IR and diabetic animal models and diabetic humans [56,57]. A concomitant decrease in a homeostasis model of assessment for β-cell function was observed in T2D patients [58]. According to the evidence reported so far, doses of resveratrol lower than 0.5 g per day may be sufficient to improve insulin action and decrease blood glucose levels. Studies on the toxicity of resveratrol in humans show that this polyphenol is well tolerated, and doses up to 0.5 g/day for extended periods of time may induce only moderate and reversible side effects [59]. Interestingly, it has been found that resveratrol may have a role in preventing obesity, as it has been related to energy metabolism improvement and the compound appears to mimic calorie restriction [56,60]. Qiao et al. observed that supplementation with resveratrol (200 mg/kg/day) for 12 weeks significantly decreased both body and visceral adipose weights, and reduced blood glucose and lipid levels in mice eating an HFD [61].

Nevertheless, due to the lack of clinical data more investigations in humans are required. A recent clinical trial providing 150−1000 mg/day of resveratrol to middle-aged men with MetS for 16 weeks showed no effect on inflammatory status, glucose homeostasis, blood pressure (BP), or hepatic lipid content [62]; the impact on body weight is not clear yet [35]. The resveratrol effects on obesity-related morbidities are inconsistent, perhaps due to differences in design and experimental settings (type of patients, doses, time of intervention, the molecular structure of resveratrol) [62]. Moreover, most studies have been performed in animal models, and more homogenized clinical trials are needed to corroborate these findings in humans. Novel metabolomic analyses performed on blood and urine samples, adipose tissue, and skeletal muscle tissue from middle-aged men with MetS randomized to either resveratrol or placebo treatment (1000 mg/day) for 4 months reveal that certain metabolic pathways, particularly in steroid metabolism and the gut microbiome, could exert a major role in resveratrol's mechanism of action, which might be the focus of future clinical trials of it effects [63]. Qiao et al. [61] also found that resveratrol improves the gut microbiota dysbiosis induced by the HFD (e.g., increasing the *Bacteroidetes*-to-*Firmicutes* ratio).

5.1.3 Lignans

Lignans are diphenolic compounds found in many plants that play a role in plant defense, and belong to the group of phytoestrogens that are structurally similar to 17-estradiol [64]. They are formed by the union of two cinnamic acid residues or their biogenetic equivalents, and are known to be associated with estrogenic activity. After ingestion, lignans are metabolized to enterolignans, enterodiol, and enterolactone by colonic bacteria before they are absorbed [65]. Secoisolariciresinol and matairesinol are the main precursors of enterolignans (Fig. 11.5), although lariciresinol, pinoresinol, and sesamin have been recently proposed as their precursors. Enterolignans have been used as biomarkers in biological fluids (urine, plasma, saliva, semen, and prostatic fluid) of humans and animals to quantify lignan intake [33].

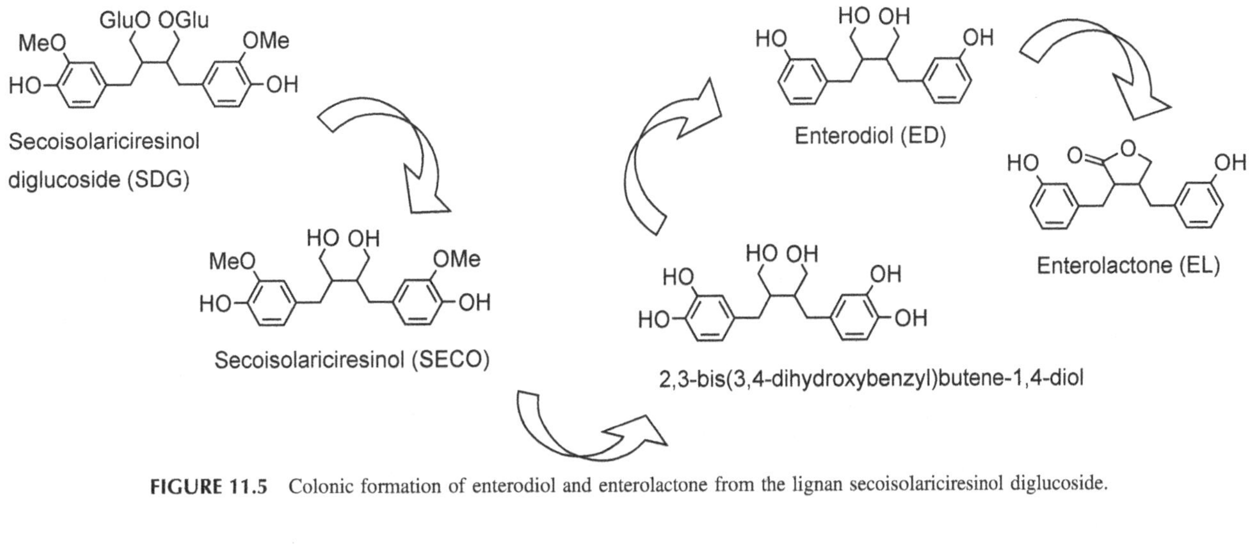

FIGURE 11.5 Colonic formation of enterodiol and enterolactone from the lignan secoisolariciresinol diglucoside.

The primary food group sources of lignans are beverages (coffee, tea, beer, and wine), cruciferous vegetables, nuts, cereals (corn, oats, wheat, rye), fruits (apricots, oranges, kiwi, strawberries) [64], and even some seeds (flaxseed and sesame contain very high concentrations of lignans); although the intake of such foods depends on the country, the population, and its food habits. Technological treatment can affect availability, since lignans are often lost when dehulling seeds and berries, so bioavailability is probably low in processed foods considering that they are typically consumed without crushing the seeds.

Lignans show a diverse spectrum of health-promoting effects, such protective effects against cancer, osteoporosis, and coronary heart disease through their antitumor, antioxidant, and antiestrogenic properties [66] and antidiabetic and antiobesity effects [67]. Lignans appear to act through various mechanisms that modulate pancreatic insulin secretion or through antioxidative actions. They may also act via estrogen-receptor-mediated mechanisms as isoflavones [67,68]. They may bind to estrogen receptors α and β [69], which are expressed in various tissues, as well as inhibit certain enzymes (e.g., aromatase and 5 α-reductase) and stimulate the production of sex-hormone-binding globulin. Plant lignans are considered important supplements for cardiovascular benefits due to their estrogenic activity [70]. Particularly, it was found that sesamin binds to PPAR-α, downregulating the expression of lipogenic enzymes [71], and has been associated with decreased expression of sterol regulatory element-binding protein-1 (SREBP-1), acetyl-CoA carboxylase, and fatty acid synthase [72].

Two major pathways related to estrogen signaling are the Erk1/2 and phosphatidylinositol-3-kinase (PI3K)/Akt pathways. They are almost equally stimulated by each of the enterolignans/precursors examined, although they show differences in cell functions. Signals induced with enterolignans/precursors show similarity at early stages but are differentially and directionally modulated later in the pathways, related to cell proliferation, cell cycle progression, and chemokine secretion. These differences could be explained by the nature of each of the enterolignans/precursors [73]. Some authors note the importance of considering what kind of lignan or precursor is analyzed, as they may show very different biological effects [74].

Sesame lignans are obtained from *Sesamum indicum*, a highly prized oilseed crop cultivated widely in many countries in the East. This plant is the largest source of clinically relevant antioxidant lignans: there are 16 types, including sesamin, a major lignan component of sesame, as well as sesamolin, sesaminol, and sesamol [75]. Another major source of lignans is flaxseed (linseed, *Linum usitatissimum*), an edible oilseed/grain which is emerging as an attractive functional food with a concentration of lignans around 0.2−13.3 mg/g flaxseed [76].

Promising overall evidence has been found in humans. A randomized controlled trial (RCT) evaluated the effects of sesamin supplementation (200 mg/day) for 8 weeks on glycemic status, serum levels of inflammatory markers, and adiponectin in patients with T2D. The authors concluded that the sesamin supplementation led to a significant reduction in fasting glucose, glycated hemoglobin (HbA1c), and TNF-α levels in T2D patients compared with the placebo [77]. According to a recent metaanalysis, the evidence reported so far shows a beneficial effect of sesame consumption on BP. However, the authors declared that the metaanalysis was limited to studies with high methodological quality [78]. Other rigorous metaanalyses, including flaxseed interventions, provided evidence of no general benefit of supplementation with flaxseed or its derivatives on decreasing CRP levels, but the supplementation significantly decreased CRP levels in studies where participants' body mass index (BMI) was over 30 kg/m^2 [79]. Furthermore, Milder et al. [68] suggested that individual matairesinol intake may exert different effects on human health (coronary heart disease, CVDs, cancer, and all-cause mortality) according to the results from a prospective cohort in which 570 men aged 64−84 years were followed for 15 years. Similar results were found in a population-based study, showing an association of a high serum enterolactone level with reduced coronary heart disease [80].

5.1.4 Curcuminoids

Curcuminoids (especially curcumin) are the active ingredients of the dietary Indian spice turmeric and are extracted from the rhizomes of *Curcuma longa*, a plant in the ginger family which has been used for medicinal purposes for years, mostly in Asian countries. The different beneficial properties of curcumin are well known and include antioxidant, antiinflammatory, hypoglycemic, antiinflammatory, and anticancer activities [81], and antithrombotic and hepatoprotective actions [82]. These features can possibly be attributed to the methoxy, hydroxyl, α-, β-unsaturated carbonyl moiety, and diketone groups present in curcumin [83].

The curcumin 1,7-bis-(4-hydroxy-3methoxyphenyl)-hepta-1,6-diene-3,5-dione (known as diferuloylmethane), whose chemical formula is $C_{21}H_{20}O_6$, is the molecule most studied and the most abundant polyphenol in the curcuma [33]. The use of curcumin is mainly limited because of its poor pharmacokinetic and pharmacodynamic profile: poor absorption, short half-life, and rapid metabolism in the gastrointestinal tract [84]. According to the Joint FAO/WHO Expert Committee on Food Additives and the European Food Safety Authority, the appropriate daily intake values of curcumin are 0–3 mg/kg [85]. Previous phase I clinical trials have indicated that curcumin is safe even at a dose of 12 g/day in humans, but exhibits relatively poor bioavailability [86]. Several strategies have been used to improve the bioavailability of curcumin by technological treatments [81]. Among them, a significant increase in its bioaccessibility was obtained by an excipient food emulsions technique [87] and nanotizing curcumin or combining it with piperine [88]. Moreover, several synthetic derivatives of curcumin can be obtained with various chemical modifications, including phenolic hydroxyl groups, acylation, alkylation, glycosylation, and amino acylation, to improve its bioavailability [85].

Regarding the impact on health, experimental studies support the activity of curcumin in promoting weight loss and reducing the incidence of obesity-related diseases [89,90]. Little is known about its exact underlying molecular mechanisms in the treatment of obesity and metabolic diseases. However, evidence agrees with the hypothesis that curcumin directly interacts with WAT to suppress chronic inflammation. This antiinflammatory activity is related to the suppression of protein signaling pathways such as the signal transducer and activator of transcription-3 [33], NF-κB, Wnt/bcatenin, and PPAR-γ and Nrf-2 activation [33,91]. Curcumin has been shown to reduce the expression of potent proinflammatory adipokines, such as IL-6, TNFα, MCP-1 [90,92], and plasminogen activator inhibitor type-1 (PAI-1), and to induce the expression of adiponectin and delay preadipocyte differentiation [90]. All these phenomena might offset the symptoms associated with obesity and metabolic diseases [92,93].

Recently, besides these effects, *C. longa* extract has been shown to improve insulin-mediated lipid accumulation (lipotoxicity) in adipocytes exposed to oxidative stress and increase the secretion of insulin-sensitising adipokines in 3T3-L1 adipose cells [92]. Similarly, Priyanka et al. [94] found that during hypoxia in 3T3-L1 adipose cells, the administration of curcumin reduced the production of inflammatory mediators (e.g., leptin, resistin, TNFα, NF-κB, c-Jun N-terminal kinase, and serine phosphorylation of IRS-1 receptors), restored the antiinflammatory adipokines (e.g., adiponectin) to the normal level, and also improved insulin sensitivity. Na et al. [95] demonstrated that curcuminoid supplementation of 300 mg/day administrated for 3 months led to a significant decrease of the serum adipocyte-fatty acid binding protein, CRP, TNF-α, and IL-6 levels in overweight/obese T2D patients, improving metabolic parameters in these subjects. Moreover, dietary supplementation with curcuminoids is reported to increase the hepatic acyl-CoA and prevent the lipid accumulation induced by an HFD in liver and adipose tissue of rats, as well as improving IR [33]; In HFD-induced obesity and insulin-resistant mice, its oral administration proved to be effective in reducing glucose intolerance [96]. Likewise, Na et al. [95] observed that curcuminoids decrease the blood glucose concentrations in overweight/obese T2D patients. A curcuminoid supplementation of 1 g/day combined with piperine (95%) for 30 days leads to a significant reduction in serum TG concentrations as well but do not on other lipids, neither on BMI or body fat in obese patients [97]. It has been reported that intake of curcumin could reduce atherogenic risks and amend the metabolic profiles of high-risk populations [98]. Another study using 20 mg/day of curcumin for 15 days in human subjects with atherosclerosis significantly lowered the levels of plasma fibrinogen in both men and women [99].

The impact on oxidative stress has been reported, with interesting findings. An important mechanism of curcumin reported in in vitro studies is the activation of Nrf-2, a transcription factor and master regulator of antioxidant responses, affecting the expression of hundreds of cytoprotective genes controlling antioxidant enzymes and immune responses [90]. Septembre-Malaterre et al. [92] observed a reduction in the intracellular levels of ROS and modulation of the expression of genes encoding SOD and catalase antioxidant enzymes by *C. longa* extract. Similarly, Na et al. [95] detected a significantly increased SOD activity after curcuminoid administration in overweight/obese T2D subjects during 3 months.

Despite the promising findings, further evidence is needed to evaluate the impact of curcuminoids on animal models, especially in obese subjects. A study protocol has been recently published regarding the evaluation of the nanocurcumin effects (80 mg/day for 3 months) in obese patients with nonalcoholic fatty liver disease, assessing the impacts on glycemia, lipid profile, inflammatory biomarkers, IR, and liver function [100]. Absorption and bioavailability studies in in vivo condition are required to clarify the beneficial effect of these bioactive compounds in human health.

5.2 Flavonoids

Flavonoids are secondary metabolites that can be found in different parts of fruits, vegetables, and their derived products. These compounds are characterized by a 15-carbon flavan structure in their skeleton containing both aromatic (ring A and B), and heterocyclic (ring C) rings (Fig. 11.6) [101].

There are several classes of flavonoids, classified according to their carbon structure and level of oxidation, including flavanones, flavanols, flavones, flavan-3-ols, ACNs, and isoflavones, as shown in Fig. 11.7. Interestingly, the substitution pattern of the A or B rings is responsible for the radical scavenging and antioxidant activity [102]. Furthermore, the antioxidant capacity is related to the presence and number of free hydroxyl groups contained in their skeleton.

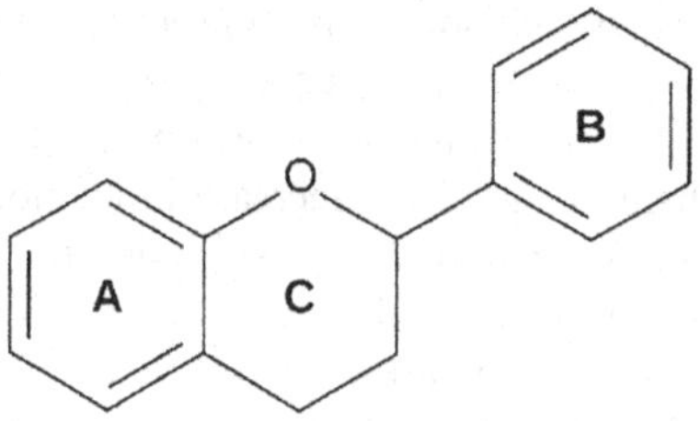

FIGURE 11.6   The basic molecular structure of flavonoids.

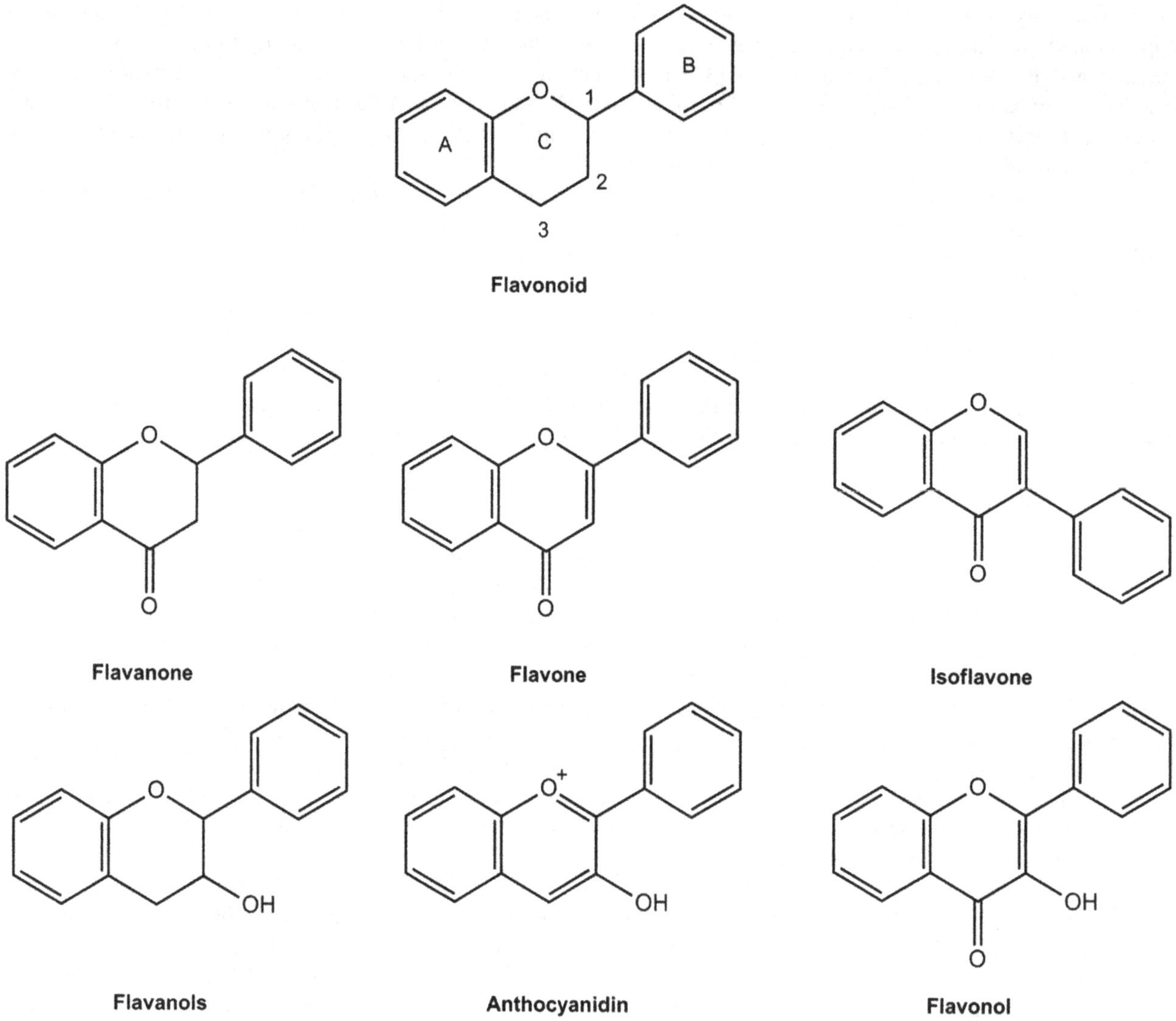

Flavonoid

Flavanone

Flavone

Isoflavone

Flavanols

Anthocyanidin

Flavonol

FIGURE 11.7   Molecular structures of the different types of flavonoids.

These compounds are powerful in vitro antioxidants with antithrombotic and antiinflammatory pharmacological properties [103]. Their consumption has been shown to be inversely associated with morbidity and mortality from coronary heart diseases and the prevention of diverse human diseases such as cancer and T2D [104,105].

Flavonoids might play a role in obesity through the modulation of food intake/absorption, promoting energy expenditure or preventing energy storage. One of the popular approaches to weight loss is appetite control. Food urge and satiety are controlled by serotonin, histamine, dopamine, and their receptors [106]. However, there are other mechanisms to deal with lipid oxidation, for instance the stimulation of energy expenditure to reduce body weight through nonshivering thermogenesis. Thermogenesis activates a cascade of uncoupling proteins, thermogenins, found in the mitochondria of brown adipose tissue. Thermogenins are capable of enhancing lipid oxidation with a low rate of adenosine triphosphate (ATP) production. Furthermore, there are certain protagonist mechanisms during lipid peroxidation: on the one hand, peroxisome PPAR-γ is a transcriptional factor expressed in the adipose tissue which stimulates adipose differentiation, so PPAR-γ agonists are capable of decreasing dyslipidemia and improving adiposity and IR; on the other hand, AMPK, which is an enzyme that regulates the target proteins controlling metabolism and its activation, regulates glucose transport and fatty acid oxidation [107]. In this landscape, the polyphenols might act to mimic caloric restriction and activate AMPK, thereby suppressing processes such as hepatic gluconeogenesis, inducing hepatic fatty acid oxidation, and stimulating glucose transporters in muscle and adipose tissue. So it is possible to observe a reduction in the glucose level in the blood and the lipid content of the liver, and an enhancement of insulin sensitivity. From all the proposed mechanisms, one of the most promising approaches for weight management is the decrease in fat absorption. Due to the capability of flavonoids to interact with digestive enzymes, it is possible to interfere in fat catabolism through the modulation of lipases [107−110].

In the next subsection we present the most representative flavonoid subclass and its role in the treatment of obesity and the alleviation of MetS.

5.2.1 Flavonols

Flavonols are the 3-hydroxy derivatives of flavanones, and probably the most common subclass of flavonoids in the human diet. Flavonols are found in different types of vegetables such as onions, spinach, broccoli, and asparagus, as well as in several types of berries, tea, and cocoa. Among flavonols, quercetin, kempferol, and myricetin are the most common. Quercetin and kempferol have at least 279 and 347 different glycosidic combinations, respectively [101].

Quercetin is commonly found in is glycoside forms, with rutin the principal structure found in nature. Several beneficial effects had been attributed to this compound in the improvement of MetS and its clinical features. The antioxidant properties of quercetin have been associated with an inhibition of lipid peroxidation and augmentation of enzymes such as SOD, CAT, and GPx [111]. The high antioxidant activity is associated with an inhibitory function of the angiotensin II receptor and endothelin. Furthermore, the antiinflammatory effect of this compound is mediated via the attenuation of TNF-α, NF-κB, and mitogen-activated protein kinases (MAPKs), as well as depletion of IL-6, interleukin-1 (IL-1), IL-8, and MCP-1. Likewise, studies in macrophages, which contribute to the chronic inflammation in obese subjects, see quercetin as a potential antiinflammatory compound. The effect is related to a modulation of certain inflammatory genes, such as TNF-α, IL-6, IL-8, interleukin-1β (IL-1β), interferon-γ-inducible protein-10, and cyclooxygenase-2 (COX-2) [112]. A study in primary human adipocytes [113] shows that quercetin is quite effective. In brief, the compound is capable of reducing several events following TNF-α release: phosphorylation of extracellular signal-related kinase and c-Jun-NH$_2$ terminal kinase, NF-κB transcriptional activity, expression of PPAR-γ, serine phosphorylation of insulin receptor substrate-1, and protein tyrosine phosphatase-1B gene expression [113].

Quercetin is shown to inhibit adipogenesis mainly through the activation of AMPK and decreasing the expression of CCAAT enhancer-binding protein, PPAR-γ, and SREBP-1. Additionally, quercetin may ameliorate hyperglycemia by inhibiting glucose transporter 2 (GLUT-2) and insulin-dependent PI3K and blocking tyrosine kinase [111].

Quercetin has been utilized in several animal and human studies of hypertension and endothelial function, obesity, and T2D [114,115]. For instance, 500 mg/day of quercetin can decrease SBP when compared with placebo. Egert et al. [116] found that the supplementation of 150 mg/day for 5 weeks also decreased SBP. However, a study in prehypertensive subjects concluded that there was no effect on BP after quercetin consumption; nevertheless, the authors found that a subgroup analysis revealed a significant decrease in both SBP and diastolic BP in subjects with level 1 hypertension.

Investigations of oxidative stress and inflammation have shown that quercetin ameliorates certain markers, such as NRF2, heme oxygenase-1, and NF-κB, suggesting that the antiinflammatory effects on the adipose tissue can be associated with the reduction of body weight [117]. However, contrary to the initial hypothesis, another study in rats supplemented with 30 mg/kg body weight/day of quercetin saw no impact on body weight or adipose tissue. Furthermore, the authors did not observe any change in the activity of lipogenic enzymes, lipoprotein lipase, or the muscle triacylglycerol content. Nevertheless, it was possible to reduce the basal glucose and insulin, which points to an antidiabetic role [118]. De la Iglesia et al. [111] reviewed in depth the possible mechanisms and suggested that quercetin may increase eNOS, thus contributing to the inhibition of platelet aggregation and the improvement of the endothelial function, but other studies state the opposite [111a].

Kempferol can be found in foods such as broccoli, apples, strawberries, and peas. In the past it had been proposed as a phytoestrogen, and nowadays it is used for the treatment of several human diseases. Nevertheless, the evidence for its effectiveness in reducing hypertension is weak: only a study in rats using 10 mg/kg body weight produced a beneficial effect [119]. The effect could be associated with a vasodilator property of the compound.

Myricetin can be considered one of the major flavonols; the compound is found in grape products, vegetables, herbs, and walnuts. Its high power as an antioxidant and its cytoprotective activity suggest it as a promising bioactive compound in the treatment of MetS. It has been shown to provide consistent protection against hypertension, obesity, and T2D regardless of the dose and length of treatment [120,121].

The consumption of cocoa flavonols, probably the most studied in the clinical field, has been associated with a marked improvement in endothelial function and key markers of MetS such as BP and insulin sensitivity [122]. Furthermore, cocoa flavonols have been reported to enhance thermogenesis and lipolysis, consequently reducing the white adipose tissue weight gain in rats fed a high-fat diet [123]. However, it is necessary to stress that frequently foods containing sufficient flavonols tend to be high in calories, thus consumption must be carefully controlled; in this regard, it seems that the food matrix has an impact on the effect. For instance, Davison et al. found that consuming dark chocolate is eight times more effective than intake of a cocoa powder drink (with an equivalent dose) to reduce BP [124].

5.2.2 Flavones

The principal characteristic of flavones is its double bond between C2 and C3 in the flavonoid skeleton, there is no substitution at the C3 position, being oxidized at the C4 position [125]. The presence of flavanones in dried tealeaves and herbs is common, with chamomile and parsley having the highest content. The most common flavone aglycones are apigenin, acacetin, luteolin, diosmetin, and chysoeriol and their derivatives.

Flavones exhibited antioxidant, antiproliferative, antitumor, antimicrobial, estrogenic, and antiinflammatory activities in several in vivo and in vitro studies [126]. Studies in macrophages and animal models revealed a reduction in the phosphorylation of the NFκB p65 subunit required for its transcriptional activity. Thus reducing the expression of inflammatory cytokines leads to a reduction of the cell damage that occurs during acute inflammation [127,128]. Moreover, the flavones acacetin and wogonin, found in saffron and *Scutellaria* respectively, inhibit COX-2 through NF-κB nuclear localization. Luteolin seems to reduce the Ras homologous (Rho) GTPases activity, thus decreasing the leucocyte migration that serves as a protection against inflammation [129]. Likewise, apigenin inhibits leukocyte migration, modulating the Janus kinase 3 [130]. Also, a novel mechanism related to the antiinflammatory activity of apigenin has been proposed: the regulation of noncoding RNAs, such as the reduction of microRNA155, a main inflammatory regulator [131]. The reduction of microRNA155 suggests that apigenin might decrease inflammation through an alternative mechanism other than antioxidant activity.

Nielsen et al. revealed that apigenin increases the concentration of blood antioxidant enzyme activities, including SOD, GSH, GPx, GR, and catalase [132]. Nonetheless, the consumption of a dried parsley supplement for 7 days seemed to be ineffective in humans, contrary to previous results in vitro [133]. With regard to cholesterol, two studies using different foods rich in the flavones apigenin and vitexin, respectively, saw a lowering of total cholesterol but without a significant modification of HDL or TGs [134,135].

Some authors propose that the lack of effect might be related to the flavone form, because flavones circulate through the bloodstream as glucuronides or sulfate conjugates, while the common form utilized in experiments is aglycones or glucoside conjugates [136]. Several studies have shown that it is possible for flavones to extend greater activity in the lumen than in circulation [137,138]. Therefore the analysis of flavones must be focused on the flavone form, not only the dose, to identify the potential benefits of the compounds. More studies are required due to the lack of evidence in human trials.

5.2.3 Flavanones

In the past, flavanones were considered minor flavonoids, but the discovery during the last decade (2010 and beyond) of up to 350 flavanone aglycones and 100 flavanone glycosides in plants gave them the main role in polyphenol research. Flavanones are extensively distributed in about 42 higher plant families, particularly Compositae, Leguminosae, and Rutaceae [139]. Flavanones are characterized by the absence of a double bond between carbons 2 and 3 of the flavone structure and a chiral centre at carbon 2. These compounds are highly reactive, and thus prone to many O- and/or C-substitutions at the A- or B-ring [139].

The main flavanone aglycones are hesperitin (40-methoxy-5,7,30-trihydroxyflavanone) and naringenin (5,7,40-trihydroxyflavanone); its glycosides, hesperidin (hesperetin 7-rutinoside) and naringin (naringenin-7-neohesperidoside), among others, have also been shown to be effective. Flavanone glycosides are hydrolyzed/deglycosylated in the small intestine and colon by intestinal microbiota, thus producing their respective active aglycones. During absorption, flavanones undergo several modifications, and the released aglycones are converted into their respective glucuronides, sulfates, and sulfoglucuronides on their way through the small intestine and liver. The generated compounds are released to plasma, distributed to different tissues, and excreted in urine [140].

Several studies have shown that naringin could reduce the inflammatory biomarkers CRP, TNF-α, and IL-6 [141−143]. Glycosides such as hesperidin and naringin present potential beneficial effects related to antiinflammatory, hypolipidemic, and vasoprotective properties that might help in the control of BP and LDL cholesterol [9,144,145]. For instance, numerous investigators have demonstrated that doses above 400 mg of hesperidin might improve the blood lipid profile [146−149]. The consumption of flavanones helps to reduce inflammatory biomarkers like CRP, IL-6, and TNF-α [145,150,151]. Furthermore, according to Knekt et al. [120] the joint consumption of hesperetin and naringenin reduces the risk of cerebrovascular disease.

Research using beverages enriched in flavanones has shown several potential benefits, such as a decrease in incidence in coronary heart disease, blood cell DNA oxidative damage, and apolipoprotein B (Apo B) concentration (the principal component of LDL cholesterol), a reduction of LDL oxidability, and the improvement of plasma concentration of inflammation and vascular function biomarkers [150−155]. More recently, Rangel-Huerta et al. [156] used a metabolomics approach, and determined that the consumption of orange juice with a high content of flavanones enhances several oxidative stress and inflammatory biomarkers. All these attributes were associated with the flavanone and its glycosides.

5.2.4 Chalcones

Chalcone, or 1,3-diphenyl-2-propene-1-one, is an open-chain intermediate in flavone synthesis that exists in many conjugated forms in nature (Fig. 11.8). Chalcones are described as minor flavonoids, biochemically related compounds of restricted occurrence in foods. They are the precursors of flavonoids and isoflavonoids containing the benzylidene acetophenone scaffold, where the two aromatic nuclei are joined by a three-carbon α−β unsaturated carbonyl bridge [157].

Chalcones are found in fruits and vegetables, such as in the form of naringenin chalcone, present in tomato skin in only trace amounts (∼5−10 mg/kg fresh weight) [158]. Flavanone−chalcone mixtures have also been reported in *Prunus* spp. [159], and mixtures of prenyl−chalcones in hops and beer [160].

Chalcones might protect from life-threatening diseases. Natural as well as synthetic chalcones act on molecular targets related to beneficial cardiovascular effects, and have shown promising activity as antiplatelet [161], antidiabetic [162], antiinflammatory [163], antioxidant [164], antiobesity [165], and hypolipidemic [166] compounds.

Chalcones isolated from plants have insulin-like activities and improve the glucose uptake in adipocytes [167]. It has been reported that sulfonamide chalcones act as a potent new class of α-glucosidase inhibitors, so chalcones are effective antihyperglycemic or hypoglycemic agents in both in vitro and in vivo experimental models.

Recently, a few chalcone-based products have come on the market for treating hyperlipidemia, hypercholesterolemia, and heart disease [168]. Therapeutic targets such as diacylglycerol acyltransferase (DGAT), lipoprotein lipase, pancreatic lipase, cholesteryl ester transfer protein, and PPAR-α have been associated with lipid synthesis, transfer, and metabolism [169]. Casaschi et al. [170] examined the role of xanthohumol (XN), a plant chalcone, on Apo B and TG synthesis and secretion, using HepG2 cells as the model system. It was observed that XN decreased Apo B secretion in a dose-dependent manner under both basal and lipid-rich conditions (up to 43%). This decrease was associated with increased cellular Apo B degradation and inhibition of TG synthesis in the microsomal membrane, and the transfer of this newly synthesized TG to the microsomal lumen (decrease in 26% and 64%, respectively, under lipid-rich conditions). The inhibition of TG synthesis was caused by a reduction in DGAT activity, which corresponded to a decrease in DGAT-1 mRNA expression [171].

However, evidence on the effect of chalcones in human studies is scarce, thus it is necessary to develop more RCTs to confirm their potential beneficial effects.

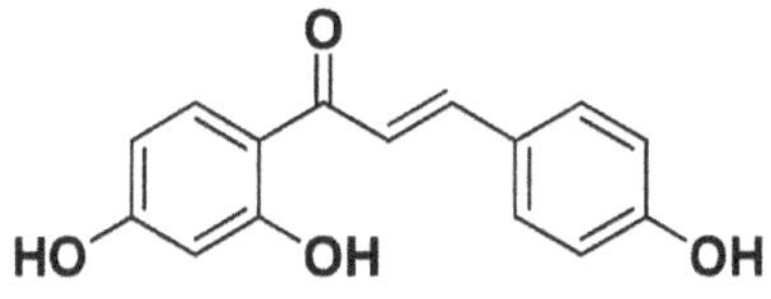

FIGURE 11.8 Molecular scaffold of chalcones.

5.2.5 Anthocyanins

ACNs are water-soluble polyphenols with a high antioxidant capacity, inhibiting or decreasing free radicals by donating or transferring electrons from hydrogen atoms. ACNs include aglycones—anthocyanidins and their glycosides. They differ in the position and number of hydroxyl groups, degree of methylation, number of sugar molecules (monoglycosides, diglycosides, or triglycosides), type of sugars (the most common sugars include glucose, galactose, and arabinose), and type and number of aliphatic or aromatic acids (i.e., p-coumaric, caffeic, and ferulic acids).

ACNs are the most abundant polyphenols in fruits and vegetables, with more than 700 already identified in nature. They are found in berries, teas, honey, nuts, olive oil, cocoa, and cereals, mainly in the external layer of the pericarp. Among berries, blackcurrants, black elderberries, blackberries, and blueberries are particularly rich in ACNs (400–500 mg/100 g), which contain pelargonidin, cyanidin, delphinidin, petunidin, peonidin, and malvidin as the most predominant ACN compounds [172].

ACNs have been shown to exert antioxidant and antiinflammatory activities, depending on their chemical structure [173]. They prevent CVD development by improving the endothelial function via brachial-artery-flow-mediated dilation and HDL cholesterol concentration increase, as well as a decrease in the serum VCAM-1 and LDL cholesterol concentrations [174,175]. ACNs may also prevent T2D development by improving insulin sensitivity. The exact mechanisms by which ACNs exert their antidiabetic effects are not clear, but it has been suggested that an enhancement of the glucose uptake by muscle and adipocyte cells in an insulin-independent manner may be responsible [176].

ACNs are recommended for obesity prevention because they may contribute to weight maintenance in adulthood [177] and avoid body fat accumulation [178]. Basu et al. [179] found that ingestion of 742 mg of blueberry ACNs for 8 weeks significantly improved BP and oxidized LDL cholesterol levels, whereas blood glucose levels, body weight, and waist circumference were not improved in obese individuals.

These polyphenolic compounds may also exert antiinflammatory effects through a reduction of proinflammatory molecules such as IL-8, IL-1, and CRP that seem to attenuate the lipopolysaccharide-induced NF-κB translocation to the nucleus cellular and mediate inflammatory responses [180].

ACNs have been identified as modulators of gut microbiota that contribute to obesity control with a prebiotic action [181]. ACNs might promote intestinal colonization by specific groups of bacteria, particularly Bifidobacterium spp., Lactobacillus spp., and Akkermansia muciniphila [181]. These bacteria contribute to the activation and absorption of provitamins and phenolic compounds. The growth of Bifidobacterium spp. stimulates mucus secretion and thickens the mucus layer through the increase of intestinal production of the fasting-induced adipocyte factor and the degradation of short-chain fatty acids. Hence gut permeability is decreased and the metabolic endotoxemia is lowered, thus modulating low-grade inflammation and obesity-related comorbidities. Together, these contribute to the prebiotic properties of ACNs (Fig. 11.9) [182].

5.2.6 Flavanols/Flavan-3-ols or Catechins

Flavanols or flavan-3-ols are often commonly called catechins. The main structural difference from other flavonoids is the absence of a double bond between C2 and C3 in flavanols, and no C4 carbonyl in ring C. In addition, the hydroxylation at C3 permits flavanols to have two chiral centres on the molecules (located on C2 and C3), thus four possible diastereoisomers. Catechin is the isomer with trans configuration and epicatechin is the isomer with cis configuration. Each of these two configurations has two stereoisomers: (+)-catechin, (−)-catechin, (+)-epicatechin and (−)-epicatechin; of these (+)-catechin and (−)-epicatechin are the two isomers often found in food plants [101].

Catechins are widely available in plant-based products such as chocolate, wine, and tea. Epigallocatechin 3-gallate (EGCG), present in tealeaves from Camellia sinensis, is probably the catechin class most studied. Several benefits had been associated with EGCG, such as reducing body weight, alleviating MetS risk factors like inflammation and oxidative stress, and preventing diabetes and CVD in in vitro animal and human studies [183–186]. The collected evidence on polyphenols and obesity, including several metaanalyses, shows an antiobesity potential of green tea catechins, particularly EGCG, in cell culture, animal, and human studies [183,187]. In brief, it was found that EGCG or green tea extract (GTE) might affect obesity-related parameters such as body weight, adipose mass, total lipids, cholesterol, TGs in liver and plasma, and glucose homeostasis. Earlier animal studies had shown that catechins might lower BP through suppression of the activity of nicotinamide adenine dinucleotide phosphate oxidase, thus reducing ROS production [188]. In this regard, a metaanalysis including 20 RCTs showed a slight decrease in SBP as well as a moderate reduction of LDL cholesterol [189].

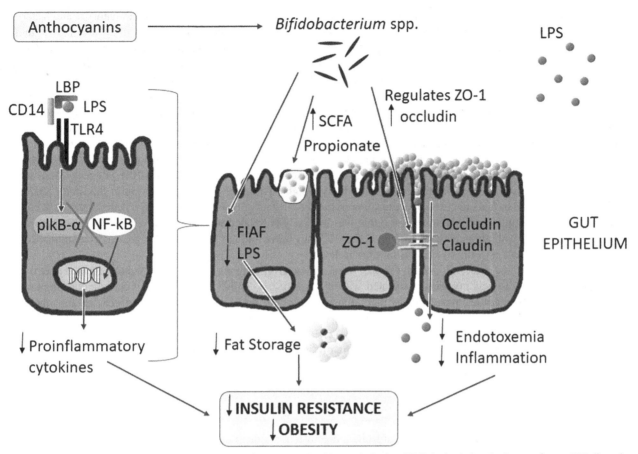

FIGURE 11.9 The potential prebiotic effect of anthocyanins on gut microbiota and obesity. *FIAF*, fasting-induced adipocyte factor; *LBP*, lipopoly-saccharide binding protein; *LPS*, lipopolysaccharide; *NF-κB*, nuclear factor-kappa B; *SCFAs,* short-chain fatty acids.

Yang et al. proposed two major mechanisms for these benefits: catechins act by decreasing absorption of lipids and proteins by tea constituents in the intestine, thus reducing calorie intake; and by activating AMPK by tea polyphenols that are bioavailable in the liver, skeletal muscle, and adipose tissues. The activated AMPK would decrease gluconeogenesis and de novo lipogenesis and increase catabolism, leading to body weight reduction and MetS alleviation [190].

Another hypothesis points out that energy expenditure is enhanced by catechol-O-methyltransferase and phosphodiesterase inhibition, which stimulates the sympathetic nervous system to cause activation of the brown adipose tissue. Fat oxidation is mediated by upregulation of acyl-CoA dehydrogenase and peroxisomal β-oxidation enzymes [111].

Several factors must be taken into account to understand the differences across the studies, including study design, length of study, age, sex, and ethnicity of subjects, and the formulations of the catechin supplement (EGCG, Green tea catechins (GTC), and GTE). In addition, the presence or absence of a weight control factor such as caffeine, exercise, and diet must be monitored. Nevertheless, the evidence from in vitro and animal studies shows that supplementation with EGCG or GTE might be a potential help in the prevention of obesity. However, further better-designed and controlled studies are needed to reinforce the contradictory evidence in humans.

5.2.7 Proanthocyanidins

PAs, also known as condensed tannins, are a group of flavonoids derived from flavan-3-ols, which are very abundant in the human diet. After lignins, they are considered the second most abundant group of natural phenolics. PAs may occur as monomers, dimers, trimers, and oligomers of 20 or more units, although higher-molecular-weight polymers are regularly found [191].

PAs have been identified in cereals (barley, rice, sorghum, and wheat), legumes (pinto beans), seeds (grape seeds and cocoa seeds), fruits (apples, pears, blueberries, and cranberries), vegetables, and beverages such as red wine and tea [192]. Their biological metabolism and pharmacokinetics have been extensively reviewed [193].

PAs present antioxidant [194], vasodilatory, anticarcinogenic, antiallergic, antiinflammatory, antibacterial, cardioprotective, immune-stimulating, antiviral, and estrogenic activities [195]. Furthermore, they are shown to be inhibitors of the enzymes phospholipase A2 [196], COX, and lipoxygenase [197]. The antiinflammatory activity of PAs is widely studied [198]; the mechanisms for this action include modulation of the arachidonic acid and NF-κB pathways, and inhibition of eicosanoid-generating enzymes, inflammatory mediator secretion, and the MAPK pathway [199].

A few studies have reported the relevance and potential of PAs in the treatment of obesity in humans. Salvadó et al. [200] discussed the available literature, focusing on the relationship between obesity and PA-rich extracts. For instance, in a human study subjects received 300 mg of grape-seed extract supplement with more than 90% of PAs, but no differences were found in 24 h energy intake compared with the placebo. Nevertheless, those subjects whose energy requirements were lower than the median showed an effect, reflected in a decrease of 4% in their 24 h energy intake compared to the placebo [201]. In another study, overweight and obese subjects who consumed an isocaloric diet, with 10% of energy from white wine or grape juice, showed a significant reduction of body weight. There was no placebo group in this study [202].

PA-rich foods have shown effects on appetite suppression. For instance, 12 females were given chocolate (85% cocoa) to eat and smell, resulting in a satiation response that was inversely correlated with ghrelin levels [203]. Higher levels of ghrelin are associated with an increase of food intake [204], thus these findings suggest that regular cocoa and chocolate consumption may reduce appetite by decreasing ghrelin levels.

The antihyperglycemic effect of dietary PA has been reviewed in humans [205]. Some studies have reported that consumption of flavan-3-ols is inversely associated with the risk of developing T2D [206] and chronic consumption of pycnogenol (a French maritime pine bark extract), muscadine grape products, chocolate, or green tea PA improves glycemic control in T2D subjects [207–209]. However, other studies showed no significant effect on glucose and/or insulin levels after dietary supplementation with a flavanol-rich cacao drink or a polyphenol-rich chocolate in T2D subjects [210,211]. The discrepancies could have been due to the different PA doses administered in each study.

More studies in humans are necessary to demonstrate the role of PA-rich foods in the decrease of energy intake and body weight; and probably higher amounts of PA are needed to improve glycemia in humans.

5.2.8 Isoflavones

Isoflavones are a subclass within flavonoids. Daidzein and genistein are the most common isoflavones; their characteristic chemical structure (the B ring is linked to the C3 position of the C ring instead of the C2 position) resembles the structure of estrogens, in particular 17-β estradiol [212] (Fig. 11.10). Isoflavones are mainly found in soyabeans, soy foods, and legumes [213].

The physiological effects of flavonoids depend on their bioavailability. Isoflavones are the most absorbable and bioavailable flavonoids, and the bioavailability of genistein is greater than that of daidzein [214]. After ingestion, isoflavone glucosides are hydrolyzed to aglycones by glucosidases in the small intestine, where the metabolites are partially absorbed completely and partially further metabolized into other metabolites, such as equol and O-desmethylangolensin, by intestinal microbiota in the large intestine [215]. Next the metabolites enter the portal vein and undergo further metabolism in the liver [216]. Isoflavones persist in plasma for about 24 h, and the average half-life is 6–8 h [217].

Isoflavones are well known for their phytoestrogenic activity: they can act as a pseudohormonal by binding to estrogen receptors in mammals [218,219]. These compounds also present antioxidant, anticancer, antimicrobial, and antiinflammatory activities, just like other flavonoids.

Yu et al. [220] reviewed the antiinflammatory effects of isoflavones in various animal models and humans. This activity is modulated through increased antioxidative activities, NF-κB regulation, and reduced proinflammatory enzyme activities and cytokine levels, and the authors encourage the application of isoflavones in a range of inflammatory diseases. In this regard, a validated food frequency questionnaire suggests that soy food consumption is related to lower circulating levels of IL-6, TNFα, and soluble TNF receptors 1 and 2 in Chinese women [221]. Moreover, a short-term study revealed that following a soyabean diet (340 mg isoflavones/100 g soyabean) reduced some markers of inflammation (e.g., IL-18 and CRP) and increased plasma NO levels in postmenopausal women with MetS [222]. In postmenopausal women with hypertension, dietary soy nuts (25 g soy protein and 101 mg aglycone isoflavones) reduce VCAM-1 and suggest an improvement in endothelial function that may reflect the underlying inflammatory process [223]. However, another study indicates that soy protein and isoflavone (either alone or together) have no impact on serum lipids or inflammatory markers, and the reason might be that healthy late-postmenopausal women lack the ability to produce equol, which is a metabolite of isoflavones and has more effective biological and pharmacological effects than its prototype [224]. Similar results indicate that cardiovascular risk reduction with soy nuts is not uniform and may be dependent on the ability to produce equol [225].

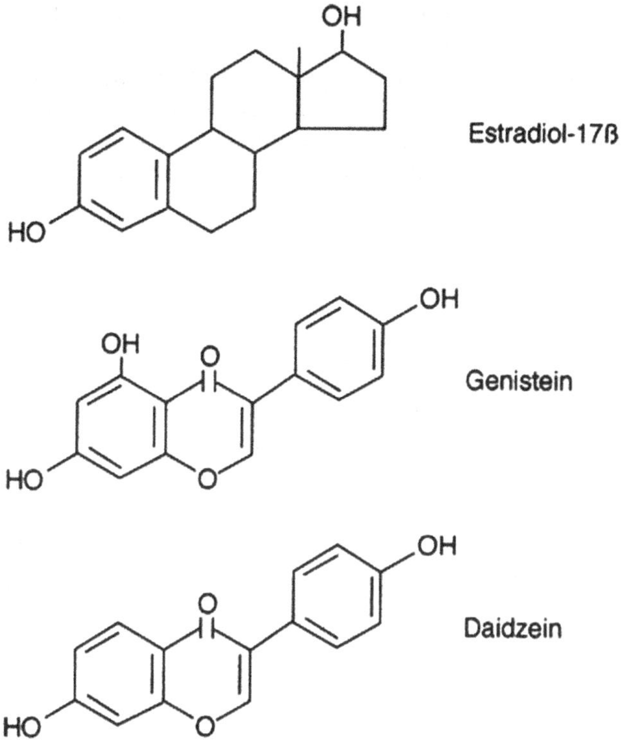

FIGURE 11.10 Structure of estradiol-17β, genistein, and daidzein.

The use of isoflavones for weight loss management and body composition was assessed by Allison et al. [226]. In their intervention, they included subjects with MetS who were followed up at 4-week intervals and checked at 4, 8, and 12 weeks. The participants in the treatment group had a significantly greater loss of body weight at week 12 and body fat at weeks 8 and 12 when compared with the controls. The administration of soy flavones may thus help to decrease body weight and fat accumulation.

Phytoestrogen-rich supplementation in mice (198 ppm daidzein and 286 ppm genistein equivalents in a high-phytoestrogen diet) from conception to adulthood was found to activate AMPK in the liver, WAT, and muscle. This intake would alter mitochondrial metabolism and cause the improvement of fatty acid β-oxidation [227]. Thus dietary soy could prove useful to prevent obesity and associated disorders. Activation of the AMPK pathway by dietary soy is likely involved, and may mediate the beneficial effects of dietary soy in peripheral tissues.

By contrary, there is a lack of evidence related to the effect of isoflavones on BP, but the combination of cocoa polyphenols with soy isoflavones and myoinositol seems to be effective for TG levels [228].

Regarding carbohydrate metabolism, supplementation with 0.2 g/kg of the isoflavones genistein and daidzein reduced blood glucose levels and liver TG concentrations in several mice models [229,230]. The isoflavones reduced glucose-6-phosphatase and phosphoenolpyruvate carboxykinase liver activities and increased glucokinase activities, suggesting that genistein and daidzein suppress liver glucose output.

6. CONCLUSION

The main sources of polyphenols are fruits, vegetables, and their derived products. A diet rich in plant-based products, such as legumes, tea, and coffee in addition to fruits and vegetables might have a beneficial effect for health. The potential effect of polyphenols is related to their antioxidant activity: their ability to scavenge oxygen radicals and other ROS. Their bioavailability is a major concern to guarantee their potential beneficial effect.

The study of polyphenols reveals that these bioactive compounds may contribute in the prevention of obesity and MetS. Although some compounds, such as stilbenes, lignans, flavanols, flavanones, or ACNs, are shown to have a beneficial effect on some features of MetS, like BP, the evidence derived from human studies regarding other compounds is still scarce or confused due to the difficulty in isolating the effect of a compound or its derivatives.

It is thus necessary to develop more and better-quality RCTs (cross-over design, double-blinded, long term, and placebo/controlled) to evaluate the possible preventive effects of a higher consumption of polyphenols. The design of such RCTs must take into account factors like the chemical structure of the polyphenols, the dose, the ideal food matrix, and the mode of supplementation. Moreover, the population included must be clearly identified, given that certain compounds respond better according to type of subjects—for instance, resveratrol has been shown to be effective in hypertensive patients rather than in healthy subjects. Finally, further research is needed to evaluate the effect of these compounds by a combination of their diverse dietary sources (green tea, dark chocolate, berries, citrus fruit, etc.) as well as the isolated compounds.

GLOSSARY

Antioxidant A molecule that inhibits the oxidation of other molecules.
Microbiota The vast number of microbes colonizing a specific entourage.
Oxidative stress The shift in the balance between oxidant/antioxidant in favor of oxidants.
Polyphenol Structural class of mainly natural, but also synthetic or semisynthetic, organic chemicals characterized by the presence of large multiples of phenol structural units.
Reactive oxygen species Chemical reactive chemical species containing oxygen.

LIST OF ACRONYMS AND ABBREVIATIONS

ACN Anthocyanin
AMPK AMP-activated protein kinase
BMI Body mass index
BP Blood pressure
CoA Coenzyme A
COX Cyclooxygenase
CRP C-reactive protein
CVD Cardiovascular disease
DGAT Diacylglycerol acyltransferase
EGCG Epigallocatechin 3-gallate
eNOS Endothelial nitric oxide synthase
ER Estrogen receptor
GLUT-2 Glucose transporter 2
GLUT-4 Glucose transporter 4
GSH Glutathione
GTE Green tea extract
HDL High-density lipoprotein
HFD High-fat diet
IF-γ Interferon-γ
IL-1 Interleukin-1
IL-6 Interleukin-6
IL-8 Interleukin-8
IR Insulin resistance
LDL Low-density lipoprotein
MAPK Mitogen-activated protein kinase
MCP-1 Monocyte chemoattractant protein 1
MetS Metabolic syndrome
NF-κB Nuclear factor-Kappa B
NO Nitric oxide
NRF2 Nuclear factor erythroid-2 related factor-2 or nuclear factor-related factor-2
PA Proanthocyanidin
PAI-1 Plasminogen activator inhibitor type-1
PEPCK Phosphoenolpyruvate carboxykinase
PPAR-α Peroxisome proliferator-activated receptor-α
PPAR-γ Peroxisome proliferator-activated receptor-γ
RCT Randomized controlled trials
RDA Recommended dietary allowance

ROS Reactive oxygen species
SBP Systolic blood pressure
SREBP-1 Sterol regulatory element-binding protein-1
T2D Type 2 diabetes
TG Triacylglycerides
TNFα Tumor necrosis factor-α
VCAM-1 Vascular cell adhesion molecules-1
WAT White adipose tissue

REFERENCES

[1] WHO. Obesity and overweight. World Health Organization, 2017.

[2] Alberti KGMM, Zimmet P, Shaw J. The metabolic syndrome — a new worldwide definition. Lancet 2005;366(9491):1059–62.

[3] Freitas Lima LC, Braga V, do Socorro de França Silva M, Cruz J, Sousa Santos SH, de Oliveira Monteiro MM, et al. Adipokines, diabetes and atherosclerosis: an inflammatory association. Front Physiol 2015;6:304.

[4] Wang X, Hai C. Redox modulation of adipocyte differentiation: hypothesis of "redox chain" and novel insights into intervention of adipogenesis and obesity. Free Radic Biol Med 2015:99–125. Elsevier. Available from: https://doi.org/10.1016/j.freeradbiomed.2015.07.012.

[5] Furukawa S, Fujita T, Shimabukuro M, Iwaki M, Yamada Y, Nakajima Y, et al. Increased oxidative stress in obesity and its impact on metabolic syndrome. J Clin Invest December 2004;114(12):1752–61. American Society for Clinical Investigation.

[6] Trayhurn P. Hypoxia and adipose tissue function and dysfunction in obesity. Physiol Rev 2013;93(1):1–21. Available from: http://www.ncbi.nlm.nih.gov/pubmed/23303904.

[7] Ouchi N, Parker JL, Lugus JJ, Walsh K. Adipokines in inflammation and metabolic disease. Nat Rev Immunol 2011;11(2):85–97. Nature Publishing Group. Available from: http://www.ncbi.nlm.nih.gov/entrez/query.fcgi?cmd=Retrieve&db=PubMed&dopt=Citation&list_uids=21252989.

[8] Bjørklund G, Chirumbolo S. Role of oxidative stress and antioxidants in daily nutrition and human health. Nutrition 2017:311–21. Elsevier Inc.

[9] Scalbert A, Manach C, Morand C, Rémésy C, Jiménez L. Dietary polyphenols and the prevention of diseases. Crit Rev Food Sci Nutr January 2005;45(4):287–306.

[10] Rangel-Huerta OD, Pastor-Villaescusa B, Aguilera CM, Gil A. A systematic review of the efficacy of bioactive compounds in cardiovascular disease: phenolic compounds. Nutrients 2015:5177–216.

[11] Manach C, Scalbert A, Morand C, Rémésy C, Jiménez L. Polyphenols: food sources and bioavailability. Am J Clin Nutr 2004;79(5):727–47.

[12] Robbins RJ. Phenolic acids in foods: an overview of analytical methodology. J Agric Food Chem 2003:2866–87.

[13] Clifford MN, Scalbert A. Review ellagitannins — nature, occurrence and dietary burden. J Sci Food Agric 2000;80(November 1999):1118–25.

[14] Atoui AK, Mansouri A, Boskou G, Kefalas P. Tea and herbal infusions: their antioxidant activity and phenolic profile. Food Chem 2005;89(1):27–36.

[15] Ferreira ICFR, Barros L, Abreu RMV. Antioxidants in wild mushrooms. Curr Med Chem 2009;16(12):1543–60.

[16] Naczk M, Shahidi F. Phenolics in cereals, fruits and vegetables: occurrence, extraction and analysis. J Pharmaceut Biomed Anal 2006:1523–42.

[17] Cremin P, Kasim-karakas S, Waterhouse AL. LC/ES — MS detection of hydroxycinnamates in human plasma and urine. J Agric Food Chem 2001;49:1747–50.

[18] Heleno SA, Martins A, Queiroz MJRP, Ferreira ICFR. Bioactivity of phenolic acids: metabolites versus parent compounds: a review. Food Chem 2015:501–13. Elsevier Ltd. Available from: https://doi.org/10.1016/j.foodchem.2014.10.057.

[19] Gross G. Biosynthesis and metabolism of phenolic acids and monolignols. Biosynthesis and biodegradation of wood components. 1st ed. 1985. p. 229–71 Available from: https://doi.org/10.1016/B978-0-12-347880-1.50011-8.

[20] Piazzon A, Vrhovsek U, Masuero D, Mattivi F, Mandoj F, Nardini M. Antioxidant activity of phenolic acids and their metabolites: synthesis and antioxidant properties of the sulfate derivatives of ferulic and caffeic acids and of the acyl glucuronide of ferulic acid. J Agric Food Chem 2012;60(50):12312–23.

[21] El-Seedi HR, El-Said AMA, Khalifa SAM, Göransson U, Bohlin L, Borg-Karlson AK, et al. Biosynthesis, natural sources, dietary intake, pharmacokinetic properties, and biological activities of hydroxycinnamic acids. J Agric Food Chem 2012:10877–95.

[22] Toma L, Sanda GM, Niculescu LS, Deleanu M, Stancu CS, Sima AV. Caffeic acid attenuates the inflammatory stress induced by glycated LDL in human endothelial cells by mechanisms involving inhibition of AGE-receptor, oxidative, and endoplasmic reticulum stress. BioFactors 2017:1–13. Available from: http://doi.wiley.com/10.1002/biof.1373.

[23] Fratantonio D, Speciale A, Canali R, Natarelli L, Ferrari D, Saija A, et al. Low nanomolar caffeic acid attenuates high glucose-induced endothelial dysfunction in primary human umbilical-vein endothelial cells by affecting NF-κB and Nrf2 pathways. BioFactors 2017;43(1):54–62.

[24] Lopez-Garcia E, Van Dam RM, Qi L, Hu FB. Coffee consumption and markers of inflammation and endothelial dysfunction in healthy and diabetic women. Am J Clin Nutr 2006;84(4):888–93.

[25] Arsenault BJ, Earnest CP, Després J-P, Blair SN, Church TS. Obesity, coffee consumption and CRP levels in postmenopausal overweight/obese women: importance of hormone replacement therapy use. Eur J Clin Nutr 2009;63(12):1419–24. Available from: http://www.pubmedcentral.nih.gov/articlerender.fcgi?artid=2787671&tool=pmcentrez&rendertype=abstract.

[26] Pei K, Ou J, Huang J, Ou S. p-Coumaric acid and its conjugates: dietary sources, pharmacokinetic properties and biological activities. J Sci Food Agric 2016;96(9):2952—62.

[27] Bahadoran Z, Mirmiran P, Azizi F. Dietary polyphenols as potential nutraceuticals in management of diabetes: a review. J Diabetes Metab Disord 2013;12(1):43. Available from: http://www.pubmedcentral.nih.gov/articlerender.fcgi?artid=3751738&tool=pmcentrez&rendertype=abstract.

[28] Yoon SA, Kang SI, Shin HS, Kang SW, Kim JH, Ko HC, et al. P-Coumaric acid modulates glucose and lipid metabolism via AMP-activated protein kinase in L6 skeletal muscle cells. Biochem Biophys Res Commun 2013;432(4):553—7. Available from: https://doi.org/10.1016/j.bbrc.2013.02.067.

[29] Lamy E, Pinherio C, Rodriguez L, Capela e Silva F, Silva Lopez O, Tavares S, et al. Determinants of tannin-rich food and beverage consumption: oral perception vs. psychosocial aspects. Tannins: biochemistry, food sources and nutritional properties. 2016. p. 29—58. Available from: https://www.novapublishers.com/catalog/product_info.php?products_id=56550.

[30] Doan KV, Ko CM, Kinyua AW, Yang DJ, Choi YH, Oh IY, et al. Gallic acid regulates body weight and glucose homeostasis through AMPK activation. Endocrinology 2015;156(1):157—68.

[31] Hsu C-L, Yen G-C. Effect of gallic acid on high fat diet-induced dyslipidaemia, hepatosteatosis and oxidative stress in rats. Br J Nutr 2007;98(4):727—35.

[32] Oi Y, Hou IC, Fujita H, Yazawa K. Antiobesity effects of Chinese black tea (Pu-erh tea) extract and gallic acid. Phytother Res 2012;26(4):475—81.

[33] Gómez Llorente C, Olza Meneses J, Pastor Villaescusa MB. Compuestos bioactivos de los alimentos de origen vegetal. Tratado de Nutrición: Bases fisiológicas y bioquímicas de la nutrición. 2017.

[34] Pinho IA, Lopes DV, Martins RC, Quina MJ. Phytotoxicity assessment of olive mill solid wastes and the influence of phenolic compounds. Chemosphere 2017;185:258—67. Available from: http://www.sciencedirect.com/science/article/pii/S0045653517310457.

[35] Park EJ, Pezzuto JM. The pharmacology of resveratrol in animals and humans. Biochim Biophys Acta — Mol Basis Dis 2015;1852(6):1071—113. Elsevier B.V. Available from: https://doi.org/10.1016/j.bbadis.2015.01.014.

[36] Giovinazzo G, Ingrosso I, Paradiso A, de Gara L, Santino A. Resveratrol biosynthesis: plant metabolic engineering for nutritional improvement of food. Plant Foods Hum Nutr 2012;67(3):191—9.

[37] Boocock DJ, Patel KR, Faust GES, Normolle DP, Marczylo TH, Crowell JA, et al. Quantitation of trans-resveratrol and detection of its metabolites in human plasma and urine by high performance liquid chromatography. J Chromatogr B Anal Technol Biomed Life Sci 2007;848(2):182—7.

[38] Nøhr MK, Dudele A, Poulsen MM, Ebbesen LH, Radko Y, Christensen LP, et al. LPS-enhanced glucose-stimulated insulin secretion is normalized by resveratrol. PLoS One 2016;11(1):1—15.

[39] Mikulski D, Górniak R, Molski M. A theoretical study of the structure-radical scavenging activity of trans-resveratrol analogues and cis-resveratrol in gas phase and water environment. Eur J Med Chem 2010;45(3):1015—27.

[40] Sengottuvelan M, Viswanathan P, Nalini N. Chemopreventive effect of trans-resveratrol — a phytoalexin against colonic aberrant crypt foci and cell proliferation in 1,2-dimethylhydrazine induced colon carcinogenesis. Carcinogenesis 2006;27(5):1038—46.

[40a] Ma C, Wang Y, Dong L, Li M, Cai W. Anti-inflammatory effect of resveratrol through the suppression of NF- B and JAK/STAT signaling pathways. Acta Biochim Biophys Sin (Shanghai). 2015;47(3):207—13.

[41] Scoditti E, Calabriso N, Massaro M, Pellegrino M, Storelli C, Martines G, et al. Mediterranean diet polyphenols reduce inflammatory angiogenesis through MMP-9 and COX-2 inhibition in human vascular endothelial cells: a potentially protective mechanism in atherosclerotic vascular disease and cancer. Arch Biochem Biophys 2012:81—9. Elsevier Inc. Available from: https://doi.org/10.1016/j.abb.2012.05.003.

[42] Wallerath T, Deckert G, Ternes T, Anderson H, Li H, Witte K, et al. Resveratrol, a polyphenolic phytoalexin present in red wine, enhances expression and activity of endothelial nitric oxide synthase. Circulation 2002;106(13):1652—8.

[43] Calvert JW, Lefer DJ. Myocardial protection by nitrite. Cardiovasc Res 2009:195—203.

[44] Zordoky BNM, Robertson IM, Dyck JRB. Preclinical and clinical evidence for the role of resveratrol in the treatment of cardiovascular diseases. Biochim Biophys Acta 2015;1852(6):115—1177. Elsevier B.V. Available from: https://doi.org/10.1016/j.bbadis.2014.10.016.

[45] Carrizzo A, Puca A, Damato A, Marino M, Franco E, Pompeo F, et al. Resveratrol improves vascular function in patients with hypertension and dyslipidemia by modulating NO metabolism. Hypertension 2013;62(2):359—66.

[46] Deng YH, Alex D, Huang HQ, Wang N, Yu N, Wang YT, et al. Inhibition of TNF-α-mediated endothelial cell-monocyte cell adhesion and adhesion molecules expression by the resveratrol derivative, trans-3,5,4'-trimethoxystilbene. Phytother Res 2011;25(3):451—7.

[47] Tan Z, Zhou LJ, Mu PW, Liu SP, Chen SJ, Fu XD, et al. Caveolin-3 is involved in the protection of resveratrol against high-fat-diet-induced insulin resistance by promoting GLUT4 translocation to the plasma membrane in skeletal muscle of ovariectomized rats. J Nutr Biochem 2012;23(12):1716—24. Elsevier Inc. Available from: https://doi.org/10.1016/j.jnutbio.2011.12.003.

[48] Burgess TA, Robich MP, Chu LM, Bianchi C, Sellke FW. Improving glucose metabolism with resveratrol in a swine model of metabolic syndrome through alteration of signaling pathways in the liver and skeletal muscle. Arch Surg 2011;146(5):556—64. Available from: http://archsurg.jamanetwork.com/article.aspx?doi=10.1001/archsurg.2011.100.

[49] Do GM, Jung UJ, Park HJ, Kwon EY, Jeon SM, Mcgregor RA, et al. Resveratrol ameliorates diabetes-related metabolic changes via activation of AMP-activated protein kinase and its downstream targets in db/db mice. Mol Nutr Food Res 2012;56(8):1282—91.

[50] Chu LM, Lassaletta AD, Robich MP, Sellke FW. Resveratrol in the prevention and treatment of coronary artery disease. Curr Atheroscler Rep 2011;13(6):439—46.

[51] Stef G, Csiszar A, Lerea K, Ungvari Z, Veress G. Resveratrol inhibits aggregation of platelets from high-risk cardiac patients with aspirin resistance. J Cardiovasc Pharmacol 2006;48(2):1−5. Available from: http://www.ncbi.nlm.nih.gov/pubmed/16954814.

[52] Gum PA, Kottke-Marchant K, Poggio ED, Gurm H, Welsh PA, Brooks L, et al. Profile and prevalence of aspirin resistance in patients with cardiovascular disease. Am J Cardiol 2001;88(1):230−5.

[53] Göçmen AY, Burgucu D, Gümüşlü S. Effect of resveratrol on platelet activation in hypercholesterolemic rats: CD40-CD40L system as a potential target. Appl Physiol Nutr Metab 2011;36(3):323−30.

[54] Sahebkar A. Effects of resveratrol supplementation on plasma lipids: a systematic review and meta-analysis of randomized controlled trials. Nutr Rev 2013;71(12):822−35.

[55] Tonkin A, Byrnes A. Treatment of dyslipidemia. F1000Prime Rep 2014;6(February):17. Available from: http://www.ncbi.nlm.nih.gov/pubmed/24669298.

[56] Dolinsky VW, Dyck JRB. Calorie restriction and resveratrol in cardiovascular health and disease. Biochim Biophys Acta − Mol Basis Dis 2011;1812(11):1477−89. Elsevier B.V. Available from: https://doi.org/10.1016/j.bbadis.2011.06.010.

[57] Szkudelski T, Szkudelska K. Resveratrol and diabetes: from animal to human studies. Biochim Biophys Acta − Mol Basis Dis 2015:1145−54. Elsevier B.V. Available from: https://doi.org/10.1016/j.bbadis.2014.10.013.

[58] Movahed A, Nabipour I, Lieben Louis X, Thandapilly SJ, Yu L, Kalantarhormozi M, et al. Antihyperglycemic effects of short term resveratrol supplementation in type 2 diabetic patients. Evid Based Complement Altern Med 2013;2013.

[59] Cottart CH, Nivet-Antoine V, Beaudeux JL. Review of recent data on the metabolism, biological effects, and toxicity of resveratrol in humans. Mol Nutr Food Res 2014:7−21.

[60] Milton-Laskibar I, Aguirre L, Macarulla MT, Etxeberria U, Milagro FI, Martínez JA, et al. Comparative effects of energy restriction and resveratrol intake on glycemic control improvement. BioFactors 2017;43(3):371−8.

[61] Qiao Y, Sun J, Xia S, Tang X, Shi Y, Le G. Effects of resveratrol on gut microbiota and fat storage in a mouse model with high-fat-induced obesity. Food Funct 2014;5(6):1241−9. Available from: http://pubs.rsc.org/en/content/articlehtml/2014/fo/c3fo60630a.

[62] Kjær TN, Ornstrup MJ, Poulsen MM, Stødkilde-Jørgensen H, Jessen N, Jørgensen JOL, et al. No beneficial effects of resveratrol on the metabolic syndrome: a randomized placebo-controlled clinical trial. J Clin Endocrinol Metab 2017;102(May):1642−51. Available from: http://www.ncbi.nlm.nih.gov/pubmed/28182820.

[63] Korsholm A, Kjær T, Ornstrup M, Pedersen S. Comprehensive metabolomic analysis in blood, urine, fat, and muscle in men with metabolic syndrome: a randomized, placebo-controlled clinical trial on the effects of resveratrol after four months' treatment. Int J Mol Sci 2017;18(3):554. Available from: http://www.mdpi.com/1422-0067/18/3/554.

[64] Tetens I, Turrini A, Tapanainen H, Christensen T, Lampe JW, Fagt S, et al. Dietary intake and main sources of plant lignans in five European countries. Food Nutr Res 2013;57(July 2017):19805. Available from: http://www.pubmedcentral.nih.gov/articlerender.fcgi?artid=3681209&tool=pmcentrez&rendertype=abstract.

[65] Borriello SP, Setchell KDR, Axelson M, Lawson AM. Production and metabolism of lignans by the human faecal flora. J Appl Bacteriol 1985;58(1):37−43.

[66] Adlercreutz H. Lignans and human health. Crit Rev Clin Lab Sci 2007;44(5−6):483−525.

[67] Bhathena SJ, Velasquez MT. Beneficial role of dietary phytoestrogens in obesity and diabetes. Am J Clin Nutr 2002;76(1):191−1201.

[68] Milder IEJ, Feskens EJM, Arts ICW, Bueno-de-Mesquita HB, Hollman PCH, Kromhout D. Intakes of 4 dietary lignans and cause-specific and all-cause mortality in the Zutphen Elderly Study. Am J Clin Nutr 2006;84(2):400−5.

[69] Martin PM, Horwitz KB, Ryan DS, McGuire WL. Phytoestrogen interaction with estrogen receptors in human breast cancer cells. Endocrinology 1978;103(5):1860−7.

[70] van der Schouw YT, de Kleijn MJ, Peeters PH, Grobbee DE. Phyto-oestrogens and cardiovascular disease risk. Nutr Metab Cardiovasc Dis 2000;10(3):154−67. Available from: http://www.ncbi.nlm.nih.gov/pubmed/11006924.

[71] Peñalvo JL, Hopia A, Adlercreutz H. Effect of sesamin on serum cholesterol and triglycerides levels in LDL receptor-deficient mice. Eur J Nutr 2006;45(8):439−44.

[72] Ide T, Kushiro M, Takahashi Y, Shinohara K, Fukuda N, Sirato-Yasumoto S. Sesamin, a sesame lignan, as a potent serum lipid-lowering food component. Japan Agric Res Q 2003:151−8.

[73] Zhu Y, Kawaguchi K, Kiyama R. Differential and directional estrogenic signaling pathways induced by enterolignans and their precursors. PLoS One 2017;12(2):1−14.

[74] Smeds AI, Eklund PC, Willför SM. Content, composition, and stereochemical characterisation of lignans in berries and seeds. Food Chem 2012;134(4):1991−8. Elsevier Ltd. Available from: https://doi.org/10.1016/j.foodchem.2012.03.133.

[75] Dar AA, Arumugam N. Lignans of sesame: purification methods, biological activities and biosynthesis − a review. Bioorg Chem 2013:1−10. Elsevier Inc. Available from: https://doi.org/10.1016/j.bioorg.2013.06.009.

[76] Bloedon LT, Balikai S, Chittams J, Cunnane SC, Berlin JA, Rader DJ, et al. Flaxseed and cardiovascular risk factors: results from a double blind, randomized, controlled clinical trial. J Am Coll Nutr 2008;27(1):65−74. Available from: http://www.embase.com/search/results?subaction=viewrecord&from=export&id=L351600524.

[77] Mohammad Shahi M, Zakerzadeh M, Zakerkish M, Zarei M, Saki A. Effect of sesamin supplementation on glycemic status, inflammatory markers, and adiponectin levels in patients with type 2 diabetes mellitus. J Diet Suppl 2016;211(September):1−12. Available from: http://www.ncbi.nlm.nih.gov/pubmed/27450646.

[78] Khosravi-Boroujeni H, Nikbakht E, Natanelov E, Khalesi S. Can sesame consumption improve blood pressure? A systematic review and meta-analysis of controlled trials. J Sci Food Agric 2017:3087−94.

[79] Ren G-Y, Chen C-Y, Chen G-C, Chen W-G, Pan A, Pan C-W, et al. Effect of flaxseed intervention on inflammatory marker C-reactive protein: a systematic review and meta-analysis of randomized controlled trials. Nutrients 2016;8(3):136. Available from: http://www.ncbi.nlm.nih.gov/pubmed/26959052%5Cnhttp://www.pubmedcentral.nih.gov/articlerender.fcgi?artid=PMC4808865.

[80] Vanharanta M, Voutilainen S, Rissanen TH, Adlercreutz H, Salonen JT. Risk of cardiovascular disease-related and all-cause death according to serum concentrations of enterolactone: Kuopio Ischaemic Heart Disease Risk Factor Study. Arch Intern Med 2003;163(9):1099−104. Available from: http://archinte.jamanetwork.com/article.aspx?articleid=215486.

[81] Ghosh S, Banerjee S, Sil PC. The beneficial role of curcumin on inflammation, diabetes and neurodegenerative disease : a recent update. Food Chem Toxicol 2015;83(June):1−14. Available from: http://www.sciencedirect.com/science/article/pii/S0278691515001878.

[82] Naik RS, Mujumdar AM, Ghaskadbi S. Protection of liver cells from ethanol cytotoxicity by curcumin in liver slice culture in vitro. J Ethnopharmacol 2004;95(1):31−7.

[83] Aggarwal BB, Deb L, Prasad S. Curcumin differs from tetrahydrocurcumin for molecular targets, signaling pathways and cellular responses. Molecules 2015:185−205.

[84] Kunnumakkara AB, Bordoloi D, Padmavathi G, Monisha J, Roy NK, Prasad S, et al. Curcumin, the golden nutraceutical: multitargeting for multiple chronic diseases. Br J Pharmacol 2017:1325−48.

[85] Kocaadam B, Şanlier N. Curcumin, an active component of turmeric (*Curcuma longa*), and its effects on health. Crit Rev Food Sci Nutr 2017;57(13):2889−95. Available from: http://www.tandfonline.com/doi/full/10.1080/10408398.2015.1077195.

[86] Anand P, Kunnumakkara AB, Newman RA, Aggarwal BB. Bioavailability of curcumin: problems and promises. Mol Pharm 2007;4(6):807−18.

[87] Zou L, Liu W, Liu C, Xiao H, McClements DJ. Utilizing food matrix effects to enhance nutraceutical bioavailability: increase of curcumin bioaccessibility using excipient emulsions. J Agric Food Chem 2015;63(7):2052−62.

[88] Shoba G, Joy D, Joseph T, Majeed M, Rajendran R, Srinivas P. Influence of piperine on the pharmacokinetics of curcumin in animals and human volunteers. Planta Med 1998;64(5):353−6.

[89] Weisberg SP, Leibel R, Tortoriello DV. Dietary curcumin significantly improves obesity-associated inflammation and diabetes in mouse models of diabesity. Endocrinology 2008;149(7):3549−58.

[90] Bradford PG. Curcumin and obesity. BioFactors 2013:78−87.

[91] Aggarwal BB. Targeting inflammation-induced obesity and metabolic diseases by curcumin and other nutraceuticals. Annu Rev Nutr 2010;30:173−99. Available from: http://www.ncbi.nlm.nih.gov/pubmed/20420526%5Cnhttp://www.pubmedcentral.nih.gov/articlerender.fcgi?artid=PMC3144156.

[92] Septembre-Malaterre A, Le Sage F, Hatia S, Catan A, Janci L, Gonthier MP. *Curcuma longa* polyphenols improve insulin-mediated lipid accumulation and attenuate proinflammatory response of 3T3-L1 adipose cells during oxidative stress through regulation of key adipokines and antioxidant enzymes. BioFactors 2016;42(4):418−30.

[93] Shehzad A, Ha T, Subhan F, Lee YS. New mechanisms and the anti-inflammatory role of curcumin in obesity and obesity-related metabolic diseases. Eur J Nutr 2011:151−61.

[94] Priyanka A, Shyni GL, Anupama N, Raj PS, Anusree SS, Raghu KG. Development of insulin resistance through sprouting of inflammatory markers during hypoxia in 3T3-L1 adipocytes and amelioration with curcumin. Eur J Pharmacol 2017;(March):1−9. Elsevier B.V. Available from: https://doi.org/10.1016/j.ejphar.2017.07.005.

[95] Na LX, Yan BL, Jiang S, Cui HL, Li Y, Sun CH. Curcuminoids target decreasing serum adipocyte-fatty acid binding protein levels in their glucose-lowering effect in patients with type 2 diabetes. Biomed Environ Sci 2014;27(11):902−6.

[96] He H-J, Wang G-Y, Gao Y, Ling W-H, Yu Z-W, Jin T-R. Curcumin attenuates Nrf2 signaling defect, oxidative stress in muscle and glucose intolerance in high fat diet-fed mice. World J Diabetes 2012;3(5):94.

[97] Mohammadi A, Sahebkar A, Iranshahi M, Amini M, Khojasteh R, Ghayour-Mobarhan M, et al. Effects of supplementation with curcuminoids on dyslipidemia in obese patients: a randomized crossover trial. Phytother Res 2013;27(3):374−9.

[98] Chuengsamarn S, Rattanamongkolgul S, Phonrat B, Tungtrongchitr R, Jirawatnotai S. Reduction of atherogenic risk in patients with type 2 diabetes by curcuminoid extract: a randomized controlled trial. J Nutr Biochem 2014;25(2):144−50. Elsevier Inc. Available from: http://www.ncbi.nlm.nih.gov/pubmed/24445038.

[99] Ramírez-Boscá A, Soler A, Carrión MA, Díaz-Alperi J, Bernd A, Quintanilla C, et al. An hydroalcoholic extract of *Curcuma longa* lowers the apo B/apo A ratio. Implications for atherogenesis prevention. Mech Ageing Dev 2000;119(1−2):41−7.

[100] Jazayeri-tehrani SA, Rezayat SM, Mansouri S, Qorbani M, Alavian SM, Daneshi-maskooni M. Efficacy of nanocurcumin supplementation on insulin resistance, lipids, inflammatory factors and nesfatin among obese patients with non-alcoholic fatty liver disease (NAFLD): a trial protocol. BMJ Open 2017;7(7):e0169141−8.

[101] Tsao R. Chemistry and biochemistry of dietary polyphenols. Nutrients 2010;2(12):1231−46.

[102] Kumar S, Pandey AK. Chemistry and biological activities of flavonoids: an overview. Sci World J December 2013;2013:162750. Hindawi.

[103] Kim S, Kim CE, Kim MH, Eun C, Hyun M. Flavonoids inhibit high glucose-induced up-regulation of ICAM-1 via the p38 MAPK pathway in human vein endothelial cells. Biochem Biophys Res Commun December 2011;415(4):602−7. Elsevier Inc.

[104] Brusselmans K, Vrolix R, Verhoeven G, Swinnen JV. Induction of cancer cell apoptosis by flavonoids is associated with their ability to inhibit fatty acid synthase activity. J Biol Chem February 2005;280(7):5636−45.

[105] Wedick NM, Pan A, Cassidy A, Rimm EB, Sampson L, Rosner B, et al. Dietary flavonoid intakes and risk of type 2 diabetes in US men and women. Am J Clin Nutr 2012;95(4):925–33.

[106] Schwartz MW, Woods SC, Porte D, Seeley RJ, Baskin DG. Central nervous system control of food intake. Nature April 2000;404(6778):661–71.

[107] Fernandes I, Pérez-Gregorio R, Soares S, Mateus N, de Freitas V. Wine flavonoids in health and disease prevention. Molecules February 2017;22(4):292. Multidisciplinary Digital Publishing Institute.

[108] Tan Y, Chang SKC, Zhang Y. Comparison of α-amylase, α-glucosidase and lipase inhibitory activity of the phenolic substances in two black legumes of different genera. Food Chem January 2017;214:259–68.

[109] Rupasinghe HPV, Sekhon-Loodu S, Mantso T, Panayiotidis MI. Phytochemicals in regulating fatty acid β-oxidation: potential underlying mechanisms and their involvement in obesity and weight loss. Pharmacol Ther September 2016;165:153–63.

[110] Ali F, Ismail A, Kersten S. Molecular mechanisms underlying the potential antiobesity-related diseases effect of cocoa polyphenols. Mol Nutr Food Res January 2014;58(1):33–48.

[111] de la Iglesia R, Loria-Kohen V, Zulet MA, Martinez JA, Reglero G, Ramirez de Molina A. Dietary strategies implicated in the prevention and treatment of metabolic syndrome. Int J Mol Sci November 2016;17(11). Multidisciplinary Digital Publishing Institute (MDPI).

[111a] Larson A, Witman MA, Guo Y, Ives S, Richardson RS, Bruno RS, Jalili T, Symons JD. Acute, quercetin-induced reductions in blood pressure in hypertensive individuals are not secondary to lower plasma angiotensin-converting enzyme activity or endothelin-1: Nitric oxide. Nutr. Res. 2012;32:557–64.

[112] Overman A, Chuang C-C, McIntosh M. Quercetin attenuates inflammation in human macrophages and adipocytes exposed to macrophage-conditioned media. Int J Obes (Lond) 2011;35(9):1165–72.

[113] Chuang C-C, Martinez K, Xie G, Kennedy A, Bumrungpert A, Overman A, et al. Quercetin is equally or more effective than resveratrol in attenuating tumor necrosis factor-{alpha}-mediated inflammation and insulin resistance in primary human adipocytes. Am J Clin Nutr 2010;92:1511–21.

[114] Loke WM, Proudfoot JM, Hodgson JM, McKinley AJ, Hime N, Magat M, et al. Specific dietary polyphenols attenuate atherosclerosis in apolipoprotein e-knockout mice by alleviating inflammation and endothelial dysfunction. Arterioscler Thromb Vasc Biol 2010;30(4):749–57.

[115] Rivera L, Morón R, Sánchez M, Zarzuelo A, Galisteo M. Quercetin ameliorates metabolic syndrome and improves the inflammatory status in obese Zucker rats. Obesity 2008;16(9):2081–7.

[116] Egert S, Bosy-Westphal A, Seiberl J. Quercetin reduces systolic blood pressure and plasma oxidised low-density lipoprotein concentrations in overweight subjects with a high-cardiovascular disease risk phenotype: a double-blinded, placebo-controlled cross-over study. Br J Nutr 2009;102.

[117] Panchal SK, Poudyal H, Brown L. Quercetin ameliorates cardiovascular, hepatic, and metabolic changes in diet-induced metabolic syndrome in rats. J Nutr 2012;142:1026–32.

[118] Arias N, Macarulla MT, Aguirre L, Martínez-Castaño MG, Portillo MP. Quercetin can reduce insulin resistance without decreasing adipose tissue and skeletal muscle fat accumulation. Genes Nutr January 2014;9(1):361. BioMed Central.

[119] Leeya Y, Mulvany MJ, Queiroz EF, Marston A, Hostettmann K, Jansakul C. Hypotensive activity of an n-butanol extract and their purified compounds from leaves of *Phyllanthus acidus* (L.) Skeels in rats. Eur J Pharmacol 2010;649(1–3):301–13.

[120] Knekt P, Kumpulainen J, Järvinen R, Rissanen H, Heliövaara M, Reunanen A, et al. Flavonoid intake and risk of chronic diseases. Am J Clin Nutr September 2002;76(3):560–8.

[121] Clark JL, Zahradka P, Taylor CG. Efficacy of flavonoids in the management of high blood pressure. Nutr Rev 2015:799–822.

[122] Lin X, Zhang I, Li A, Manson JE, Sesso HD, Wang L, et al. Cocoa flavanol intake and biomarkers for cardiometabolic health: a systematic review and meta-analysis of randomized controlled trials. J Nutr November 2016;146(11):2325–33.

[123] Osakabe N, Hoshi J, Kudo N, Shibata M. The flavan-3-ol fraction of cocoa powder suppressed changes associated with early-stage metabolic syndrome in high-fat diet-fed rats. Life Sci September 2014;114(1):51–6.

[124] Davison K, Howe PRC. Potential implications of dose and diet for the effects of cocoa flavanols on cardiometabolic function. J Agric Food Chem November 2015;63(45):9942–7.

[125] Hostetler GL, Ralston RA, Schwartz SJ. Flavones: food sources, bioavailability, metabolism, and bioactivity. Adv Nutr 2017;8(3):423–35.

[126] Singh M, Kaur M, Silakari O. Flavones: an important scaffold for medicinal chemistry. Eur J Med Chem 2014;84:206–39.

[127] Cardenas H, Arango D, Nicholas C, Duarte S, Nuovo G, He W, et al. Dietary apigenin exerts immune-regulatory activity in vivo by reducing NF-κB activity, halting leukocyte infiltration and restoring normal metabolic function. Int J Mol Sci March 2016;17(3):323.

[128] Nicholas C, Batra S, Vargo MA, Voss OH, Gavrilin MA, Wewers MD, et al. Apigenin blocks lipopolysaccharide-induced lethality in vivo and proinflammatory cytokines expression by inactivating NF-κB through the suppression of p65 phosphorylation. J Immunol November 2007;179(10):7121–7.

[129] Hendriks JJA, Alblas J, van der Pol SMA, van Tol EAF, Dijkstra CD, de Vries HE. Flavonoids influence monocytic GTPase activity and are protective in experimental allergic encephalitis. J Exp Med December 2004;200(12):1667–72.

[130] Henkels KM, Frondorf K, Gonzalez-Mejia ME, Doseff AL, Gomez-Cambronero J. IL-8-induced neutrophil chemotaxis is mediated by Janus kinase 3 (JAK3). FEBS Lett January 2011;585(1):159–66.

[131] Arango D, Diosa-Toro M, Rojas-Hernandez LS, Cooperstone JL, Schwartz SJ, Mo X, et al. Dietary apigenin reduces LPS-induced expression of miR-155 restoring immune balance during inflammation. Mol Nutr Food Res April 2015;59(4):763–72.

[132] Nielsen SE, Young JF, Daneshvar B, Lauridsen ST, Knuthsen P, Sandstro B, et al. Effect of parsley (*Petroselinum crispum*) intake on urinary apigenin excretion, blood antioxidant enzymes and biomarkers for oxidative stress in human subjects. Br J Nutr 1999;81(6):447–55.

[133] Janssen PLTMK, Mensink RP, Cox FJJ, Harryvan JL, Hovenier R, Hollman PCH, et al. Effects of the flavonoids quercetin and apigenin on hemostasis in healthy volunteers: results from an in vitro and a dietary supplement study. Am J Clin Nutr 1998;67(2):255–62.

[134] Bundy R, Walker AF, Middleton RW, Wallis C, Simpson HCR. Artichoke leaf extract (*Cynara scolymus*) reduces plasma cholesterol in otherwise healthy hypercholesterolemic adults: a randomized, double blind placebo controlled trial. Phytomedicine 2008;15(9):668–75.

[135] Dalli E, Colomer E, Tormos MC, Cosín-Sales J, Milara J, Esteban E, et al. Crataegus laevigata decreases neutrophil elastase and has hypolipidemic effect: a randomized, double-blind, placebo-controlled trial. Phytomedicine 2011;18(8–9):769–75.

[136] Jiang N, Doseff AI, Grotewold E. Flavones: from biosynthesis to health benefits. Plants June 2016;5(2). Multidisciplinary Digital Publishing Institute (MDPI).

[137] Kim J-A, Kim D-K, Kang O-H, Choi Y-A, Park H-J, Choi S-C, et al. Inhibitory effect of luteolin on TNF-alpha-induced IL-8 production in human colon epithelial cells. Int Immunopharmacol 2005;5(1):209–17.

[138] Ruiz PA, Haller D. Functional diversity of flavonoids in the inhibition of the proinflammatory NF-kappaB, IRF, and Akt signaling pathways in murine intestinal epithelial cells. J Nutr 2006;136(3):664–71.

[139] Khan MK, Dangles O, Zill-E-Huma DO. A comprehensive review on flavanones, the major citrus polyphenols. J Food Compos Anal February 2014;33(1):85–104. Elsevier Inc.

[140] Matsumoto H, Ikoma Y, Sugiura M, Yano M, Hasegawa Y. Identification and quantification of the conjugated metabolites derived from orally administered hesperidin in rat plasma. J Agric Food Chem October 2004;52(21):6653–9. American Chemical Society.

[141] Lee CH, Jeong TS, Choi YK, Hyun BH, Oh GT, Kim EH, et al. Anti-atherogenic effect of citrus flavonoids, naringin and naringenin, associated with hepatic ACAT and aortic VCAM-1 and MCP-1 in high cholesterol-fed rabbits. Biochem Biophys Res Commun June 2001;284(3):681–8.

[142] Choe SC, Kim HS, Jeong TS, Bok SH, Park YB. Naringin has an antiatherogenic effect with the inhibition of intercellular adhesion molecule-1 in hypercholesterolemic rabbits. J Cardiovasc Pharmacol December 2001;38(6):947–55.

[143] Chanet A, Milenkovic D, Claude S, Maier JAM, Khan MK, Rakotomanomana N, et al. Flavanone metabolites decrease monocyte adhesion to TNF-α-activated endothelial cells by modulating expression of atherosclerosis-related genes. Br J Nutr January 2013;110(6):1–12.

[144] Pérez-Jiménez J, Hubert J, Hooper L, Cassidy A, Manach C, Williamson G, et al. Urinary metabolites as biomarkers of polyphenol intake in humans: a systematic review. Am J Clin Nutr October 2010;92(4):801–9.

[145] Dalgård C, Nielsen F, Morrow JD, Enghusen-Poulsen H, Jonung T, Hørder M, et al. Supplementation with orange and blackcurrant juice, but not vitamin E, improves inflammatory markers in patients with peripheral arterial disease. Br J Nutr January 2009;101(2):263–9.

[146] Rangel-Huerta OD, Aguilera CM, Martin MV, Soto MJ, Rico MC, Vallejo F, et al. Normal or high polyphenol concentration in orange juice affects antioxidant activity, blood pressure, and body weight in obese or overweight adults. J Nutr August 2015;145(8):1808–16.

[147] Kurowska EM, Spence JD, Jordan J, Wetmore S, Freeman DJ, Piché LA, et al. HDL-cholesterol-raising effect of orange juice in subjects with hypercholesterolemia. Am J Clin Nutr November 2000;72(5):1095–100.

[148] Miwa Y, Yamada M, Sunayama T, Mitsuzumi H, Tsuzaki Y, Chaen H, et al. Effects of glucosyl hesperidin on serum lipids in hyperlipidemic subjects: preferential reduction in elevated serum triglyceride level. J Nutr Sci Vitaminol (Tokyo) June 2004;50(3):211–8.

[149] Miwa Y, Mitsuzumi H, Sunayama T, Yamada M, Okada K, Kubota M, et al. Glucosyl hesperidin lowers serum triglyceride level in hypertriglyceridemic subjects through the improvement of very low-density lipoprotein metabolic abnormality. J Nutr Sci Vitaminol (Tokyo) December 2005;51(6):460–70.

[150] Buscemi S, Rosafio G, Arcoleo G, Mattina A, Canino B, Montana M, et al. Effects of red orange juice intake on endothelial function and inflammatory markers in adult subjects with increased cardiovascular risk. Am J Clin Nutr May 2012;95(5):1089–95.

[151] Rizza S, Muniyappa R, Iantorno M, Kim J, Chen H, Pullikotil P, et al. Citrus polyphenol hesperidin stimulates production of nitric oxide in endothelial cells while improving endothelial function and reducing inflammatory markers in patients with metabolic syndrome. J Clin Endocrinol Metab May 2011;96(5):E782–92.

[152] Habauzit V, Morand C. Evidence for a protective effect of polyphenols-containing foods on cardiovascular health: an update for clinicians. Ther Adv Chronic Dis 2011;3(2):87–106.

[153] Sharma AK, Bharti S, Ojha S, Bhatia J, Kumar N, Ray R, et al. Up-regulation of PPARγ, heat shock protein-27 and -72 by naringin attenuates insulin resistance, β-cell dysfunction, hepatic steatosis and kidney damage in a rat model of type 2 diabetes. Br J Nutr December 2011;106(11):1713–23.

[154] Mulvihill EE, Allister EM, Sutherland BG, Telford DE, Sawyez CG, Edwards JY, et al. Naringenin prevents dyslipidemia, apolipoprotein B overproduction, and hyperinsulinemia in LDL receptor-null mice with diet-induced insulin resistance. Diabetes October 2009;58(10):2198–210.

[155] Gardana C, Guarnieri S, Riso P, Simonetti P, Porrini M. Flavanone plasma pharmacokinetics from blood orange juice in human subjects. Br J Nutr July 2007;98(1):165–72.

[156] Rangel-Huerta OD, Aguilera CM, Perez-de-la-Cruz A, Vallejo F, Tomas-Barberan F, Gil A, et al. A serum metabolomics-driven approach predicts orange juice consumption and its impact on oxidative stress and inflammation in subjects from the BIONAOS study. Mol Nutr Food Res 2017;61(2):1600120.

[157] Dimmock JR, Elias DW, Beazely MA, Kandepu NM. Bioactivities of chalcones. Curr Med Chem 1999;6(12):1125–49.

[158] Muir SR, Collins GJ, Robinson S, Hughes S, Bovy A, Ric De Vos CH, et al. Overexpression of petunia chalcone isomerase in tomato results in fruit containing increased levels of flavonols. Nat Biotechnol 2001;19(5):470–4. Nature Publishing Group.

[159] Nagarajan GR, Parmar VS. Flavonoids of prunus cerasus. Planta Med. 1977;32(1):50–3.

[160] Liu M, Yin H, Liu G, Dong J, Qian Z, Miao J. Xanthohumol, a prenylated chalcone from beer hops, acts as an α-glucosidase inhibitor in vitro. J Agric Food Chem June 2014;62(24):5548–54. American Chemical Society.

[161] Zhao L-M, Jin H-S, Sun L-P, Piao H-R, Quan Z-S. Synthesis and evaluation of antiplatelet activity of trihydroxychalcone derivatives. Bioorg Med Chem Lett November 2005;15(22):5027–9.

[162] Mahapatra DK, Asati V, Bharti SK. Chalcones and their therapeutic targets for the management of diabetes: structural and pharmacological perspectives. Eur J Med Chem 2015;92:839–65.

[163] Israf DA, Khaizurin TA, Syahida A, Lajis NH, Khozirah S. Cardamonin inhibits COX and iNOS expression via inhibition of p65NF-kappaB nuclear translocation and Ikappa-B phosphorylation in RAW 264.7 macrophage cells. Mol Immunol February 2007;44(5):673–9.

[164] Aoki N, Muko M, Ohta E, Ohta S. C-Geranylated chalcones from the stems of *Angelica keiskei* with superoxide-scavenging activity. J Nat Prod July 2008;71(7):1308–10. American Chemical Society and American Society of Pharmacognosy.

[165] Birari RB, Gupta S, Mohan CG, Bhutani KK. Antiobesity and lipid lowering effects of *Glycyrrhiza* chalcones: experimental and computational studies. Eur J Integr Med 2011;18:795–801.

[166] Sashidhara KV, Palnati GR, Sonkar R, Avula SR, Awasthi C, Bhatia G. Coumarin chalcone fibrates: a new structural class of lipid lowering agents. Eur J Med Chem 2013;64.

[167] Enoki T, Ohnogi H, Nagamine K, Kudo Y, Sugiyama K, Tanabe M, et al. Antidiabetic activities of chalcones isolated from a Japanese herb, *Angelica keiskei*. J Agric Food Chem 2007;55(15):6013–7.

[168] Kuhrts EH. Methods and compositions for treating dyslipidaemia. 20070218155 A1. 2007. p. 1–6.

[169] Mahapatra DK, Bharti SK. Therapeutic potential of chalcones as cardiovascular agents. Life Sci March 2016;148:154–72.

[170] Casaschi A, Maiyoh GK, Rubio BK, Li RW, Adeli K, Theriault AG. The chalcone xanthohumol inhibits triglyceride and apolipoprotein B secretion in HepG2 cells. J Nutr 2004;134(6):1340–6.

[171] Zang BX, Jin M, Si N, Zhang Y, Wu W, Piao YZ. Antagonistic effect of hydroxysafflor yellow A on the platelet activating factor receptor. Acta Pharmacol Sin 2002;37(1):696–9.

[172] Zanotti I, Dall'Asta M, Mena P, Mele L, Bruni R, Ray S, et al. Atheroprotective effects of (poly)phenols: a focus on cell cholesterol metabolism. Food Funct 2015;6(1):13–31. Royal Society of Chemistry.

[173] Vendrame S, Del Bo' C, Ciappellano S, Riso P, Klimis-Zacas D. Berry fruit consumption and metabolic syndrome. Antioxidants September 2016;5(4):34.

[174] Qin Y, Xia M, Ma J, Hao Y, Liu J, Mou H, et al. Anthocyanin supplementation improves serum LDL- and HDL-cholesterol concentrations associated with the inhibition of cholesteryl ester transfer protein in dyslipidemic subjects. Am J Clin Nutr September 2009;90(3):485–92.

[175] Zhu Y, Xia M, Yang Y, Liu F, Li Z, Hao Y, et al. Purified anthocyanin supplementation improves endothelial function via NO-cGMP activation in hypercholesterolemic individuals. Clin Chem November 2011;57(11):1524–33.

[176] Stull A, Cash K, Champagne C, Gupta A, Boston R, Beyl R, et al. Blueberries improve endothelial function, but not blood pressure, in adults with metabolic syndrome: a randomized, double-blind, placebo-controlled clinical trial. Nutrients 2015;7(6):4107–23.

[177] Bertoia ML, Rimm EB, Mukamal KJ, Hu FB, Willett WC, Cassidy A. Dietary flavonoid intake and weight maintenance: three prospective cohorts of 124 086 US men and women followed for up to 24 years. BMJ 2016;352.

[178] Tsuda T. Recent progress in anti-obesity and anti-diabetes effect of berries. Antioxidants April 2016;5(2):13.

[179] Basu A, Du M, Leyva MJ, Sanchez K, Betts NM, Wu M, et al. Blueberries decrease cardiovascular risk factors in obese men and women with metabolic syndrome. J Nutr September 2010;140(9):1582–7.

[180] Zhu Y, Huang X, Zhang Y, Wang Y, Liu Y, Sun R, et al. Anthocyanin supplementation improves HDL-associated paraoxonase 1 activity and enhances cholesterol efflux capacity in subjects with hypercholesterolemia. J Clin Endocrinol Metab February 2014;99(2):561–9.

[181] Boto-Ordóñez M, Urpi-Sarda M, Queipo-Ortuño MI, Tulipani S, Tinahones FJ, Andres-Lacueva C, et al. High levels of bifidobacteria are associated with increased levels of anthocyanin microbial metabolites: a randomized clinical trial. Food Funct July 2014;5(8):1932–8. The Royal Society of Chemistry.

[182] Cardona F, Andrés-Lacueva C, Tulipani S, Tinahones FJ, Queipo-Ortuño MI. Benefits of polyphenols on gut microbiota and implications in human health. J Nutr Biochem August 2013;24(8):1415–22.

[183] Hursel R, Viechtbauer W, Westerterp-Plantenga MS. The effects of green tea on weight loss and weight maintenance: a meta-analysis. Int J Obes 2009;33(9):956–61.

[184] Ortsäter H, Grankvist N, Wolfram S, Kuehn N, Sjöholm A. Diet supplementation with green tea extract epigallocatechin gallate prevents progression to glucose intolerance in db/db mice. Nutr Metab (Lond) February 2012;9:11.

[185] Byun J-K, Yoon B-Y, Jhun J-Y, Oh H-J, Kim E, Min J-K, et al. Epigallocatechin-3-gallate ameliorates both obesity and autoinflammatory arthritis aggravated by obesity by altering the balance among CD4+ T-cell subsets. Immunol Lett 2014;157(1–2):51–9.

[186] Okuda MH, Zemdegs JCS, de Santana AA, Santamarina AB, Moreno MF, Hachul ACL, et al. Green tea extract improves high fat diet-induced hypothalamic inflammation, without affecting the serotoninergic system. J Nutr Biochem 2014;25(10):1084–9.

[187] Wang S, Moustaid-Moussa N, Chen L, Mo H, Shastri A, Su R, et al. Novel insights of dietary polyphenols and obesity. J Nutr Biochem January 2014;25(1):1–18. Elsevier.

[188] Ihm S-H, Jang S-W, Kim O-R, Chang K, Oak M-H, Lee J-O, et al. Decaffeinated green tea extract improves hypertension and insulin resistance in a rat model of metabolic syndrome. Atherosclerosis October 2012;224(2):377–83.

[189] Onakpoya I, Spencer E, Heneghan C, Thompson M. The effect of green tea on blood pressure and lipid profile: a systematic review and meta-analysis of randomized clinical trials. Nutr Metab Cardiovasc Dis August 2014;24(8):823–36.

[190] Yang CS, Zhang J, Zhang L, Huang J, Wang Y. Mechanisms of body weight reduction and metabolic syndrome alleviation by tea. Mol Nutr Food Res January 2016;60(1):160–74. NIH Public Access.

[191] Wang Y, Chung S, Song WO, Chun OK. Estimation of daily proanthocyanidin intake and major food sources in the U. S. diet. J Nutr 2011;141:447–52.

[192] Neilson AP, O'Keefe SF, Bolling BW. High-molecular-weight proanthocyanidins in foods: overcoming analytical challenges in pursuit of novel dietary bioactive components. Annu Rev Food Sci Technol Annu Rev February 2016;7(1):43–64.

[193] Ou K, Gu L. Absorption and metabolism of proanthocyanidins. J Funct Foods March 2014;7:43–53.

[194] Škerget M, Kotnik P, Hadolin M, Hraš AR, Simonič M, Knez Ž. Phenols, proanthocyanidins, flavones and flavonols in some plant materials and their antioxidant activities. Food Chem February 2005;89(2):191–8.

[195] Bladé C, Aragonès G, Arola-Arnal A, Muguerza B, Bravo FI, Salvadó MJ, et al. Proanthocyanidins in health and disease. BioFactors 2016;42(1):5–12.

[196] Lambert JD, Yennawar N, Gu Y, Elias RJ. Inhibition of secreted phospholipase a $_2$ by proanthocyanidins: a comparative enzymological and in silico modeling study. J Agric Food Chem August 2012;60(30):7417–20.

[197] Kutil Z, Temml V, Maghradze D, Pribylova M, Dvorakova M, Schuster D, et al. Impact of wines and wine constituents on cyclooxygenase-1, cyclooxygenase-2, and 5-lipoxygenase catalytic activity. Mediators Inflamm May 2014;2014:178931. Hindawi.

[198] Gil-Cardoso K, Ginés I, Pinent M, Ardévol A, Arola L, Blay M, et al. Chronic supplementation with dietary proanthocyanidins protects from diet-induced intestinal alterations in obese rats. Mol Nutr Food Res March 2017:1601039.

[199] Martinez-Micaelo N, González-Abuín N, Ardèvol A, Pinent M, Blay MT. Procyanidins and inflammation: molecular targets and health implications. BioFactors July 2012;38(4):257–65. Wiley Subscription Services, Inc., A Wiley Company.

[200] Salvadó MJ, Casanova E, Fernández-Iglesias A, Arola L, Bladé C, Pallarès V, et al. Roles of proanthocyanidin rich extracts in obesity. Food Funct 2015;6(4):1053–71. The Royal Society of Chemistry.

[201] Vogels N, Nijs IMT, Westerterp-Plantenga MS. The effect of grape-seed extract on 24 h energy intake in humans. Eur J Clin Nutr April 2004;58(4):667–73. Nature Publishing Group.

[202] Flechtner-Mors M, Biesalski HK, Jenkinson CP, Adler G, Ditschuneit HH. Effects of moderate consumption of white wine on weight loss in overweight and obese subjects. Int J Obes November 2004;28(11):1420–6.

[203] Massolt ET, van Haard PM, Rehfeld JF, Posthuma EF, van der Veer E, Schweitzer DH. Appetite suppression through smelling of dark chocolate correlates with changes in ghrelin in young women. Regul Pept April 2010;161(1–3):81–6.

[204] Tschöp M, Smiley DL, Heiman ML. Ghrelin induces adiposity in rodents. Nature October 2000;407(6806):908–13. Nature Publishing Group.

[205] Pinent M, Cedó L, Montagut G, Blay M, Ardévol A. Procyanidins improve some sisrupted glucose homoeostatic situations: an analysis of doses and treatments according to different animal models. Crit Rev Food Sci Nutr July 2012;52(7):569–84. Taylor & Francis Group.

[206] Jacques PF, Cassidy A, Rogers G, Peterson JJ, Meigs JB, Dwyer JT. Higher dietary flavonol intake is associated with lower incidence of type 2 diabetes. J Nutr September 2013;143(9):1474–80. American Society for Nutrition.

[207] Liu X, Zhou H-J, Rohdewald P. French maritime pine bark extract pycnogenol dose-dependently lowers glucose in type 2 diabetic patients. Diabetes Care 2004;27(3).

[208] Curtis PJ, Sampson M, Potter J, Dhatariya K, Kroon PA, Cassidy A. Chronic ingestion of flavan-3-ols and isoflavones improves insulin sensitivity and lipoprotein status and attenuates estimated 10-year CVD risk in medicated postmenopausal women with type 2 diabetes: a 1-year, double-blind, randomized, controlled trial. Diabetes Care February 2012;35(2):226–32. American Diabetes Association.

[209] Hsu C-H, Liao Y-L, Lin S-C, Tsai T-H, Huang C-J, Chou P. Does supplementation with green tea extract improve insulin resistance in obese type 2 diabetics? A randomized, double-blind, and placebo-controlled clinical trial. Altern Med Rev June 2011;16(2):157–63.

[210] Balzer J, Rassaf T, Heiss C, Kleinbongard P, Lauer T, Merx M, et al. Sustained benefits in vascular function through flavanol-containing cocoa in medicated diabetic patients. A double-masked, randomized, controlled trial. J Am Coll Cardiol 2008;51(22):2141–9.

[211] Mellor DD, Sathyapalan T, Kilpatrick ES, Beckett S, Atkin SL. High-cocoa polyphenol-rich chocolate improves HDL cholesterol in type 2 diabetes patients. Diabet Med November 2010;27(11):1318–21.

[212] Marzocchella L, Fantini M, Benvenuto M, Masuelli L, Tresoldi I, Modesti A, et al. Dietary flavonoids: molecular mechanisms of action as anti-inflammatory agents. Recent Pat Inflamm Allergy Drug Discov September 2011;5(3):200–20.

[213] Sakai T, Kogiso M. Soy isoflavones and immunity. J Med Investig 2008;55(3,4):167–73. The University of Tokushima Faculty of Medicine.

[214] Nielsen ILF, Williamson G. Review of the factors affecting bioavailability of soy isoflavones in humans. Nutr Cancer May 2007;57(1):1–10.

[215] Setchell KD, Brown NM, Desai P, Zimmer-Nechemias L, Wolfe BE, Brashear WT, et al. Bioavailability of pure isoflavones in healthy humans and analysis of commercial soy isoflavone supplements. J Nutr April 2001;131(4 Suppl.):1362S–75S. American Society for Nutrition.

[216] Barnes S. The biochemistry, chemistry and physiology of the isoflavones in soybeans and their food products. Lymphat Res Biol March 2010;8(1):89–98. Mary Ann Liebert, Inc. 140 Huguenot Street, 3rd Floor New Rochelle, NY 10801 USA.

[217] Manach C, Williamson G, Morand C, Scalbert A, Rémésy C. Bioavailability and bioefficacy of polyphenols in humans. I. Review of 97 bioavailability studies. Am J Clin Nutr January 2005;81(1 Suppl.):230S–42S. American Society for Nutrition.

[218] Barros RPA, Gustafsson J-Å, Kearbey JD, Barrett CM, Raghow S, Veverka KA, et al. Estrogen receptors and the metabolic network. Cell Metab September 2011;14(3):289–99. Elsevier.

[219] Vitale DC, Piazza C, Melilli B, Drago F, Salomone S. Isoflavones: estrogenic activity, biological effect and bioavailability. Eur J Drug Metab Pharmacokinet March 2013;38(1):15–25. Springer-Verlag.

[220] Yu J, Bi X, Yu B, Chen D. Isoflavones: anti-inflammatory benefit and possible caveats. Nutrients June 2016;8(6):361. Multidisciplinary Digital Publishing Institute.

[221] Wu SH, Shu XO, Chow W-H, Xiang Y-B, Zhang X, Li H-L, et al. Soy food intake and circulating levels of inflammatory markers in Chinese women. J Acad Nutr Diet July 2012;112(7). 996−1004, 1004−4. Sage Publications, Newbury Park, CA.

[222] Azadbakht L, Kimiagar M, Mehrabi Y, Esmaillzadeh A, Hu FB, Willett WC. Soy consumption, markers of inflammation, and endothelial function. Diabetes Care 2007;30(4).

[223] Nasca MM, Zhou J-R, Welty FK, Bugel S, Koebnick C, Reimann M, et al. Effect of soy nuts on adhesion molecules and markers of inflammation in hypertensive and normotensive postmenopausal women. Am J Cardiol July 2008;102(1):84−6. Elsevier.

[224] Mangano KM, Hutchins-Wiese HL, Kenny AM, Walsh SJ, Abourizk RH, Bruno RS, et al. Soy proteins and isoflavones reduce interleukin-6 but not serum lipids in older women: a randomized controlled trial. Nutr Res 2013;33(12):1026−33.

[225] Acharjee S, Zhou J-R, Elajami TK, Welty FK. Effect of soy nuts and equol status on blood pressure, lipids and inflammation in postmenopausal women stratified by metabolic syndrome status. Metabolism February 2015;64(2):236−43.

[226] Allison DB, Gadbury G, Schwartz LG, Murugesan R, Kraker JL, Heshka S, et al. A novel soy-based meal replacement formula for weight loss among obese individuals: a randomized controlled clinical trial. Eur J Clin Nutr April 2003;57(4):514−22. Nature Publishing Group.

[227] Cederroth CR, Vinciguerra M, Gjinovci A, Kühne F, Klein M, Cederroth M, et al. Dietary phytoestrogens activate AMP-activated protein kinase with improvement in lipid and glucose metabolism. Diabetes 2008;57(5).

[228] Anna RD, Santamaria A, Cannata ML, Interdonato ML, Giorgianni GM, Granese R, et al. Effects of a new flavonoid and Myo-inositol supplement on some biomarkers of cardiovascular risk in postmenopausal women: a randomized trial. Int J Endocrinol January 2014;2014:653561.

[229] Ae Park S, Choi M-S, Cho S-Y, Seo J-S, Jung UJ, Kim M-J, et al. Genistein and daidzein modulate hepatic glucose and lipid regulating enzyme activities in C57BL/KsJ-db/db mice. Life Sci August 2006;79(12):1207−13.

[230] Choi MS, Jung UJ, Yeo J, Kim MJ, Lee MK. Genistein and daidzein prevent diabetes onset by elevating insulin level and altering hepatic gluconeogenic and lipogenic enzyme activities in non-obese diabetic (NOD) mice. Diabetes Metab Res Rev January 2008;24(1):74−81. John Wiley & Sons, Ltd.

Chapter 12

Aging, Telomere Integrity, and Antioxidant Food

Ana Ojeda-Rodriguez[1,2], Lydia Morell-Azanza[1,2], Lucia Alonso-Pedrero[1,2] and Amelia Marti del Moral[1,2,3]

[1]University of Navarra, Pamplona, Spain; [2]IdiSNA (Instituto de Investigación Sanitaria de Navarra), Pamplona, Spain; [3]CIBERobn (Centro de Investigación Biomédica en Red, Fisiopatología de la obesidad y nutrición), Carlos III Health Institute, Madrid, Spain

1. AGING AND CELLULAR SENESCENCE

A major public health aim is the prevention of age-related pathologies, since the proportion of elder population is increasing in almost all countries [1]. Aging is a multifactorial, time-dependent decline in physiological functions of multiple organs and tissues that occurs in biological systems [2]. It is the result of molecular interactions, cellular responses, and protein actions in different tissues and multicellular organisms, associated with mechanisms such as deregulated autophagy, mitochondrial dysfunction, telomere shortening, oxidative stress, systemic inflammation, metabolic dysfunction [3], and senescence (Fig. 12.1). These hallmarks of aging are divided into three categories: the causes of age-associated damage; the responses to the damage; and the consequences of the responses and culprits of the aging phenotype [4]. In the last 2 decades there has been intensively studied the telomere shortening, which is influenced by genetic and lifestyle factors [5]. Aging occurs at all levels (molecular, cellular, and organ levels) and involves a large number of genes [6]. The effects of aging are reflected as deoxyribonucleic acid (DNA) damage in human cells [5].

Cellular senescence is the main aging-related event [4] and can be defined as the irreversible cell cycle arrest (usually in G_0 state), which may contribute to phenotypic changes [3]. Senescence arrest is irreversible because there is no stimulus able to rejoin the cell cycle [6]. Cell cycle arrest requires the overexpression of p53, pRB, p21, or p16[INK4a] [6]. Throughout life humans produce these senescent cells, which are accumulated in mitotic tissues, causing tissue degradation and leading to the aging process [6]. It has been known since 1970 that every time a cell divides, one cell enters randomly into a senescent state and this chance is increased with each division [7].

Hayflick et al. [7a] found 5 decades ago that cells have a limited proliferation in human fibroblasts [6]. Now it is known that the senescence observed by Hayflick and colleagues was due to telomere shortening [8]. Moreover, senescence involves changes in chromatin organization and gene expression, resulting in cells that overproduce a large variety of proinflammatory cytokines, interleukins, chemokines, proteases, and growth factors [7]. This process, called the senescence-associated secretory phenotype (SASP), has potent autocrine and paracrine activity [9], tissue remodeling, and immune cell recruitment [4].

Moreover, many pathologies have been associated with senescence. Some studies have shown that senescent cells could lead to pathological states [3,7], including sarcopenia, atherosclerosis, heart failure, osteoporosis, macular degeneration, pulmonary insufficiency, renal failure, diabetes, neurodegeneration, cancer, and cardiovascular disease, among others [6].

There are two recognized types of cellular senescence: replicative senescence and stress-induced premature senescence (SIPS) [10]. The first refers to telomere attrition, capping the end of chromosomes; and the second is triggered by external factors, mitogenic oncogenes, and irradiation, leading to SIPS [9] which is not related to telomere shortening [10].

Senescence plays its main role in preventing tissue damage and potential oncogenic cells, thus it has a beneficial compensatory response to damage. However, this process should work efficiently as a replacement mechanism for cell clearance and killing [8], and is carried out by the immune system and stimulated by SASP [6]. The immune system

Obesity. https://doi.org/10.1016/B978-0-12-812504-5.00012-X

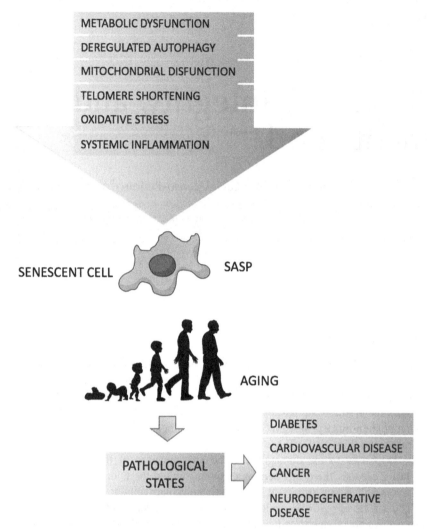

FIGURE 12.1 Senescence and aging-related diseases. The accumulation of senescent cells produced by some mechanisms may lead to SASP (senescence-associated secretory phenotype) and aging-related diseases (cardiovascular disease, cancer, and neurodegenerative disease, among others).

removes these senescent cells by the secretion of proinflammatory agents able to attract defense cells, that are able to phagocyted senescent cells. However, because of immunosenescence these capabilities are reduced in elder subjects and these cells accumulate with age [3]. SASP also causes an immune reaction to stimulate oncogene-expressing cells [6].

To senescent cells can be recognized by certain characteristics: their lack of proliferation cell markers (cell cycle arrest), their increased length, and their flattened morphology [6]. Senescence-associated β-galactosidase was the first marker used to assess senescent cells because it is overexpressed at a near-neutral pH [6]. Nowadays the marker used is p16^{INK4a}, which is a tumor suppressor protein expressed in senescent cells and almost absent in normal cells [6].

Due to the great complexity of the changes produced by the aging process, it is not surprising that there are multiple theories proposed to explain where, how, and why these changes happened. There is no consolidated theory about why aging occurs, but many scientists suggest that it might be caused by cellular damage [10]. Thus it can be assumed that senescence contributes to aging, since the number of senescent cells increases with age [8].

2. OXIDATIVE STRESS AND AGING

Oxidative stress is explained in the free radicals theory, which postulates that free radicals damage the macromolecular components of the cell [11]. Reactive oxygen species (ROS) comprise diverse chemical species containing free radicals: superoxide anion (O_2^-), hydroxyl radical (OH^-), and hydrogen peroxide (H_2O_2) [2]. These ROS activate the homeostatic compensatory response and aggravate the damage associated with aging. In mammals there are many ROS sources, such as mitochondrial respiration, cyclooxygenase and lypoxigenase, cytochrome p450s, xanthine oxidase, nicotinamide adenine dinucleotide phosphate (NADPH) oxidase, nitric oxide (NO) synthase, peroxidase, and endoplasmic reticulum, among other hemoproteins [3].

An important source of ROS is NADPH oxidase, known as the Nox complex. The regulation of the Nox complex is carried out by TNF-α (tumor necrosis factor alpha) and angiotensin receptor 1. activated by angiotensin 2. An increase of ROS generates the inhibition of nuclear factor (erythroid-derived 2)-like 2 by the cross-talk with nuclear factor kappa light-chain enhancer of activated B cells factor, which increases TNF-α; hence TNF-α decreases, aggravating oxidative stress and producing a vicious cycle. This process occurs gradually with aging, and is proportional to cellular dysfunction [3]. However, the main ROS source in human is mitochondria, strongly related to telomere shortening and dysfunctional mitochondria.

The balance in ROS levels (redox balance) is created by antioxidants, which are a set of enzymatic and nonenzymatic complexes with a cellular detoxification function [3]. This redox balance requires an equilibrium between the production of ROS and the production of antioxidant defenses [12]. An imbalance of these complexes produce an oxidative damage status called oxidative stress, which is linked to declined physiological functions [3]. The endogenous antioxidant system has low efficiency in old people, thus this section of the population is more likely to suffer oxidative stress.

Interestingly, the aging process could be accelerated by oxidative stress (Fig. 12.2), ROS, and inflammation caused by both genetic and nongenetic factors (smoking, sedentary lifestyle, alcohol, stress, etc.). These lifestyle factors may affect telomere length (TL) and telomerase [9]. In addition, a diet rich in antioxidants is associated with longer telomeres [13]. Nowadays it is accepted that aging is linked to oxidative stress caused by free radicals and other ROS, which could affect telomere maintenance [10].

Even though ROS have harmful effects, they also have beneficial effects at low concentrations since they regulate responses to anoxia (lack of oxygen), defenses against infectious agents, and induction of a mitogenic response [5].

3. TELOMERES AS MARKERS OF BIOLOGICAL AGE

Telomeres (from the Greek *telos*, end, and *meros*, part) [11] are the noncoding sections located at the end of linear eukaryotes chromosomes, and were discovered by Muller and McClintock in the 1930s. The relationship between telomere shortening and aging was first suggested by Allsopp et al. [11a,14], and they are considered to be good biomarkers of biological age. They are made up of thousands of tandem TTAGGG repeats, with a length from 4 to 15 kb (depending on the tissue type and the age of the individual), and associated with specialized proteins [15]. When telomeres shorten to a critical length, they enter into cellular senescence and finally into apoptosis or oncogenic transformation of somatic cells [11].

A cell divides during mitosis, replicating its full genomic information coded in the DNA, hence with each cell division every daughter cell takes an identical copy of all chromosomes. The leading strand is replicated by the DNA polymerase,

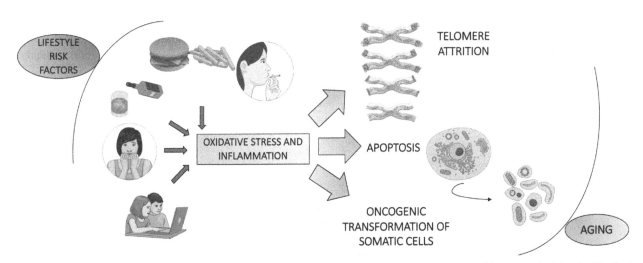

FIGURE 12.2 Oxidative stress and inflammation. Oxidative stress, produced by several risk factors such as smoking, stress, alcohol, unhealthy food, or sedentariness, could trigger DNA damage and repair response, inflammation, and mutagenic signals, producing apoptosis, oncogenic transformation of somatic cells, and telomere attrition [9].

but the lagging strand cannot be entirely replicated by this polymerase, therefore with every cell division telomeres lose hundreds of bases (30–200 nucleotides) due to the limited amount of DNA polymerase, producing damaged checkpoints and cell senescence. This is called the "end-replication problem" [16], and it can be restored by a ribonucleoprotein called telomerase which adds TTAGGG to the end of chromosomes. Harley et al., 20 years ago, discovered the evidence that telomeres get shorter with each cell division [17].

Telomerase is formed by a telomere RNA component (TERC), which is used as a template for telomere replication; and a reverse telomere transcriptase (TERT), used as a catalytic component for elongation [14]. The amount of telomerase depends on the cell type, for instance germ cells, stem cells, and cancer immortal cells have a high level of telomerase activity for lower telomere shortening; but somatic cells have a low amount of telomerase activity, limiting cell division [9]. Thus telomerase acts as a mitotic clock indicating the number of cell divisions [10]. A TERT deficiency accelerates the aging process [2].

Telomeres are involved in the protection of genomic DNA through different mechanisms, preserving chromosome stability and integrity [18]. Another function of telomeres is their role in meiosis, where they cluster on the nuclear envelope during the specialized prophase of meiosis I, meiotic prophase (which starts late in the leptotene stage), and move the diploid genetic material around the nucleus, aligning the chromosomes two by two and efficiently recombining them with precision. The bouquet stage of the meiosis is defined by this clustering, which is universal among life cycles with sexual reproduction. This is an important function resulting in chromosome recombination and segregation defects (including the production of aneuploidy daughter cells or sterility) generated by genetic disruption in meiotic telomere clustering, since it involves motility forces that act across the nuclear envelope via microtubules, actin, or other filamentous systems [16]. The telomere structure includes a telomere (T) loop at the end, and a displacement (D) loop [14]. The guanine (G) bases may combine with one another, forming an unusual structure known as G-quadruplex DNA. The G-rich tail can form "quartets" of G residues, which form a planar structure with four Gs that hydrogen bonds with one another [16]. Telomeres are formed by a complex of six proteins (TRF1, TRF2, RAP1, TIN2, TPP1, and POT1) called shelterin, packed into the T-loop structure (Fig. 12.3). Shelterin inhibits the activation of a DNA repair mechanism at the end of chromosomes and regulates the telomerase activity [15]. Telomere repeat-binding factor 2 (TRF2) acts as a stabilizer of the G repetitive sequences, prevents telomere fusions and cellular senescence, and isolates repressor-activated protein 1 (RAP1), which avoids telomere fusions, causing telomere elongation while it is overexpressed [15,19]. RAP1 also operates out of telomeres as a transcription factor and silences subtelomeric DNA [19]. Both TRF1 and TRF2 interact with the double-strand telomeric DNA [11] and act as a negative regulator of TL. They also inhibit telomerase activity and are involved in two routes, ataxia telangiectasia mutated and Ataxia-telangiectasia-mutated and Rad3-related (ATR), which decrease DNA damage [15]. TIN2 (TRF1-interacting nuclear factor 2) plays an important role in stabilizing TRF2 to telomeres. It connects TRF1 and TRF2 and binds TPP1 (TINF1-interacting protein 2) to TRF1 and TRF2. POT1 (protection of telomeres 1) operates as a protector of telomeres from DNA damage response pathways [11,19].

4. TELOMERE INTEGRITY IN HUMAN STUDIES

The most frequent parameter used to assess biological age is the TL of circulating leukocytes in somatic cells [9]. Leukocyte telomere length (LTL) declines with age, although LTL might not exactly reflect TL in poorly proliferating tissues such as brain, fat, or liver [9]. Unhealthy lifestyle, demographic, and genetic factors could influence this biomarker.

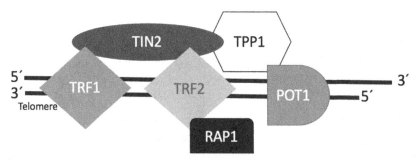

FIGURE 12.3 Shelterin complex. Telomere shortening is led by the 3′ end of the telomere, since it is incompletely reproduced at cell division. The complex includes TRF1 (telomere repeat-binding factor 1), TRF2 (telomere repeat-binding factor 2), RAP1 (repressor-activated protein 1), TIN2 (TRF1-interacting nuclear factor 2), TPP1 (TINF1-interacting protein 2), and POT1 (protection of telomeres 1), associated with TERT, which protects and regulates telomeres.

Hereditary factors affect telomere dynamics [9]. TL is a heritable factor in the range from 30% to 80% [18]. It should be mentioned that heritability could be influenced by a shared environment [20]. Several studies are trying to identify specific genomic regions related with TL, such as GWAS (Genome Wide Association Study), which has demonstrated the association between TL and single-nucleotide polymorphisms (SNPs), including OBFC1 (involved in the replication and capping of telomeres), CTC1 (involved in telomere maintenance), and ZNF66 (whose function is unknown). The biggest GWAS to date evaluated TERC and OBFC1, and showed a novel association between TL and SNPs at 19p12 and 2p16.2 loci [20]. However, only about 1.6% of the intraindividual variation in TL has been explained. Mutations in some telomere components such as TERC or TERT are associated with short telomeres and premature aging, and it has a connection with dyskeratosis congenita (also known as Zinsser–Cole–Engman syndrome), which is a rare congenital disorder. Nevertheless, there are mutations such as that produced in the WRN gene (producing Werner syndrome), which cause premature aging, cardiovascular disease (myocardial infarction), and cancer at a young age. sirtuin (SIRT1), which is a protein of the Nicotinamide adenine dinucleotide (NAD)-dependent protein deacetylase sirtuin family (SIRT1–7), was found to be associated with both TL and longevity in individuals in Louisiana Healthy Aging. Decreased expression of SIRT1 is associated with endothelial dysfunction in arteries from aged mice and humans. An association was also found between the D allele of the angiotensin-converting enzyme insertion/deletion (I/D) polymorphism and short telomeres [9].

There is interindividual and intraindividual TL variation. The strongest predictor so far is age, with 17.5% of the interindividual variation in TL [20]. Other predictors, such as sex or ethnicity, are also linked to TL variation but to a lesser extent [20]. It is known that woman have longer telomeres than men, and that their telomeres decrease slower with age [9]. A study revealed that African Americans have longer telomeres than Caucasians [21]. In an intraindividual way, TL and rate of attrition are strongly associated with different cell types within the same individual [9].

Likewise, sedentariness, especially physical inactivity, is associated with telomere attrition and thus with a vascular function deterioration [21]. Low-density lipoprotein cholesterol may be an important contributing factor to vascular senescence [9], causing latent general inflammatory activity and heightened oxidative stress [22]. In addition, the effects of alcohol consumption on telomere shortening are currently unknown, but might induce oxidative stress and inflammation [9]. With regard to smoking, a study revealed that cellular senescence was clearly related to oxidative damage and markers of inflammation, thus senescence in smokers might be stress induced [9]. Other environmental factors accelerating telomere shortening might be physiological stress, anxiety, physical abuse during childhood, and socioeconomic status, since they are linked to increased oxidative stress [9]. Interestingly, an antioxidant diet could decrease telomere attrition since the content of G is highly sensitive to oxidative stress [23].

5. PRECISION NUTRITION FOR TELOMERE INTEGRITY

The role of nutrients in the prevention of the aging process is crucial. In addition, in an elderly population an inadequate intake of nutrients, mainly vitamins and minerals, is common. Besides age and genetic factors, poor diet could increase the risk of neurodegenerative and cardiovascular diseases associated with aging. Although aging is inevitable, antioxidants may play an important role in slowing down the process and preventing common diseases driven by oxidative stress [24,25].

A bibliographic search was conducted in Pubmed for the last 10 years to gather information on the effect of dietary factors on telomere integrity. The keywords used were: nutrients OR foods OR beverages OR dietary patterns AND telomere length (Tables 12.1–12.4).

5.1 Nutrients

Significant associations between nutrients and telomere length were found in a number of studies (Table 12.1). It has been shown that a deficiency in several antioxidants (vitamins and minerals) can accelerate telomere shortening through their potential role in pathways linked to oxidative stress and inflammation (Table 12.1). Furthermore, the effect of several nutrients on TL may depend on sex and age [59,60]. Several B-group vitamins, including vitamin B9 or folate, vitamin B12 or cobalamin, vitamin B7 or choline, vitamin B2 or riboflavin, and vitamin B6 or pyridoxine, are involved in one-carbon metabolism. The one-carbon metabolism pathway is essential for DNA integrity, and the dietary factors involved in this metabolic pathway could affect telomere length through DNA methylation and synthesis (Fig. 12.4). Folate is a methyl group donor that allows the synthesis of methionine from homocysteine, a process that demand the vitamin B12 cofactor. Methionine is converted to S-adenosyl methionine, the methyl donor for methylation of histones and cytosine in mammalian DNA. Folate is also needed in nucleotide synthesis for the conversion of deoxyuridine monophosphate (dUMP) to deoxythymidine monophosphate. Others B-group vitamins influence this pathway, including

TABLE 12.1 Effect of Nutrient Intake on Leukocyte Telomere Length

References	Study Design	Sample Characteristics	Type of Nutrient	Study Aim	Associations with LTL
Cassidy et al. [26]	Cross-sectional	NHS, USA: 2284 women; 58.9 years (mean)	Energy intake, total protein, carbohydrate, fiber, cereal fiber, whole grains, fatty acids, SFAs, MUFAs, TFAs, PUFAs, linolenic and linoleic acid, vitamin E, vitamin D, fruits, and vegetables	Examine the association between diet, body composition, and lifestyle factors, and the effect on women's LTL	Direct associations: total fiber and cereal fiber; Inverse associations: PUFAs and linoleic acid
Farzaneh-Far et al. [27]	Prospective cohort (5 years)	Heart and Soul Study, California: 608 outpatients with coronary artery disease; 79% males; 66 years (mean)	Omega-3	Investigate the association between blood omega-3 levels and temporal changes in LTL	Direct association: lower blood levels of long-chain n-3 PUFAs and fasted rate of telomere shortening
Marcon et al. [28]	Cross-sectional	Italy: 56 healthy subjects; 55% females; 56 years (mean)	Antioxidant micronutrients: vitamin B1, riboflavin, niacin, vitamin B6, folic acid, retinol, vitamin C, tocopherol, and beta-carotene	Investigate the influence of dietary habits on LTL and the functional consequences of diet-related shortening of telomeres on chromosome stability	Direct associations: retinol, folic acid, vitamin C, tocopherol and beta-carotene
Tiainen et al. [29]	Cross-sectional	HBCS, Finland: 1492 elderly subjects; 54% females; 61.5 years (mean)	Fat and fatty acids: total fat, total SFAs, cis-MUFAs, PUFAs, linoleic acid, alpha-linolenic acid, marine-3 fatty acids	Study the association between fats, fruits, vegetables, and LTL	Inverse associations: total fat and SFAs (men)
Liu et al. [30]	Cross-sectional	NHS, USA: 1715 women; 59.8 years (mean)	Folate, choline, methionine, riboflavin, vitamin B6, vitamin B12	Examine associations between dietary and genetic factors in the one-carbon metabolism pathway and relative peripheral blood LTL	No associations
Song et al. [31]	Cross-sectional	WHI—OS, USA: 4029 postmenopausal women; 62.5 years (mean)	Total fat; fatty acids were categorized into SFAs, MUFAs, and PUFAs. SFAs were further categorized into SMSFAs and LSFAs	Examine the direct relations of total fat and different types of dietary fats and fat-rich foods with peripheral LTL	Inverse associations: total SFAs, SMSFAs (butyric acid, hexanoic acid, octanoic acid, decanoic acid), myristic acid, and palmitic acid
Sen et al. [32]	Cross-sectional	Austrian Stroke Prevention Study, Austria: 786 adults; 58% females; 66 years (mean)	Antioxidant micronutrients: vitamin C, lutein, zeaxanthin, beta-cryptoxanthin, canthaxanthin, lycopene, alpha-tocopherol and gamma-tocopherol, alpha-carotene and beta-carotene, and retinol	Analyze the association between plasma concentrations of antioxidant micronutrients and LTL in older adults	Direct associations: lutein, zeaxanthin, vitamin C

García-Calzón et al. [23]	Cross-sectional	GENOI, Spain: 287 children and teenagers; 55% males; 11.5 years (mean)	Total fat (MUFAs, PUFAs, and SFAs), protein, and carbohydrate	Evaluate the relationship between diet and LTL in a cross-sectional study of children and adolescents	Direct associations: PUFAs
Milne et al. [33]	Cross-sectional	Western Australia: 437 healthy children aged 3, 6, and 9 years; 54% males	Zinc, calcium, magnesium, vitamin B12, folate, vitamin D, selenium, niacin, lutein, retinol, alpha-tocopherol, lycopene, alpha-carotene, and beta-carotene	Determine whether nutritional factors are associated with LTL in children	Inverse association: zinc
Zhu et al. [34]	Cross-sectional	Georgia: 766 healthy teenagers (49% African American); 50% females; 16.1 years (mean)	Sodium intake	Observe the relationship between high sodium intake and LTL, particularly in the context of obesity	Inverse association: sodium intake
Williams et al. [35]	Cross-sectional	NFBC 1966, Finland: 5096 participants; 51.8% females; 31.1 years (mean)	Vitamin D (circulating 25(OH)D)	Investigate the association between 25(OH)D and body mass index with LTL	No association:
Liu et al. [36]	Cross-sectional	NHS, USA: 4780 women; 59.2 years (mean)	Caffeine and TFAs consumption	Examine the association between coffee consumption and LTL	Direct association: caffeine consumption Inverse association: TFAs consumption
Bok et al. [37]	Cross-sectional	NHANES population 1999–2002, USA: 3660 adults; 51.3% females; ≥20 years	Carotenoid levels: provitamin A carotenoids (alpha-carotene, beta-carotene trans + cis, and beta-cryptoxanthin) and nonvitamin A carotenoids (combined lutein/zeaxanthin and translycopene)	Investigate the association between blood carotenoid levels and LTL	Direct association: provitamin A carotenoids
Tucker et al. [38]	Cross-sectional	NHANES population 1999–2002, USA: 5768 adults; 52.8% females; ≥20 years	Vitamin E: alpha-tocopherol and gamma-tocopherol	Determine the association between alpha-tocopherol and gamma-tocopherol and LTL	Inverse association: gamma-tocopherol
Lee et al. [39]	Prospective cohort (10 years)	Korean Genome Epidemiology Study, Republic of Korea: 1958 adults; 52.3% males; 48.2 years (mean)	Vitamins A, B1, B2, B3, B6, B9 (folate), C, and E; calcium, phosphorus, potassium, iron, and zinc	Evaluate the consumption of micronutrients, including antioxidant nutrients and B vitamins, and LTL	Direct associations: vitamin C, folate, and potassium in all subjects; only in middle age (<50 years) was this association significant

25(OH)D, 25-hydroxyvitaminD or 25-hydroxycholecalciferol; GENOI, Navarro Study Group on Childhood Obesity; HBCS, Helsinki Birth Cohort Study; LSFAs, long-chain saturated fatty acids; LTL, leukocyte telomere length; MUFAs, monounsaturated fatty acids; NFBC, Northern Finland Birth Cohort; NHANES, US National Health and Nutrition Examination Survey; NHS, Nurses' Health Study; PUFAs, polyunsaturated fatty acids; SFAs, saturated fatty acids; SMSFAs, short- to medium-chain saturated fatty acids; TFAs, transfatty acids; WHI—OS, Women's Health Initiative—Observational Study.

TABLE 12.2 Effect of Food Consumption on Leukocyte Telomere Length

References	Study Design	Sample Characteristics	Type of Food	Study Aim	Associations with LTL
Bekaert et al. [40]	Cross-sectional	Asklepios study population, Belgium: 2509 volunteers without cardiovascular disease; 51.4% females; 46 years (mean)	Fruits, vegetables and alcohol	Study the association between LTL and cardiovascular risk factors	No associations
Nettleton et al. [41]	Cross-sectional	MESA, USA: 840 white, black, and Hispanic adults; 51.7% males; 61.5 years (mean)	Whole and refined grains, fruit, vegetables, nonfried fish, nuts or seeds, dairy products, red meat, processed meat, fried food, non-diet soft drinks and coffee, dietary patterns for fats and processed meat, and dietary patterns for whole grains and fruit	Study the association between LTL and dietary patterns and foods and beverages associated with markers of inflammation	Inverse association: processed meat
Hou et al. [42]	Case-control	Warsaw, Poland: 300 cases (66.3% males) of gastric cancer and 416 controls; 64.7% males; 21–79 years (range)	Intake of fruits and vegetables	Study the association between LTL and risk of gastric cancer	Direct association: fruit intake
Mirabello et al. [43]	Case-control	CGEMS study, USA: 612 cases of prostate cancer and 1049 controls; 64 years (mean)	Fruits, vegetables, and alcohol	Study the relationship between LTL and smoking, diet, and other variables with the risk of prostate cancer	No associations
Chan et al. [44]	Cross-sectional	China: 2006 subjects; 51.3% females; 72.4 years (mean)	Cereals, meats, poultry, eggs and egg products, fish, milk and milk products, fruits and dried fruits, vegetables, legumes/nuts/seeds, pickled vegetables, dim sum, fast food, and fats and oils for cooking	Examine the association between some food groups and LTL	Inverse associations: fats and oil for cooking (women)
Shiels et al. [45]	Cross-sectional	pSoBid study, Scotland: 382 participants with samples for LTL analysis, stratified with similar distribution across males and females and age groups (35–44, 45–54, 55–64)	Diet score for consumption of fruit and vegetables	Investigate the association between socioeconomic factors, lifestyle, and traditional and novel risk factors with LTL	Inverse association: diet score among the lower 50% of scores

Study	Study design	Population	Dietary factors	Objective	Associations
Marcon et al. [28]	Cross-sectional	Italy: 56 healthy subjects; 55% females; 56 years (mean)	Cereals, vegetables (leafy vegetables, fruiting vegetables, root vegetables, peppers, tomatoes, cabbages, carrots, and spinach) fruits, eggs, milk, yogurt, cheeses, olive oil, seed oil, butter, meat, fish, and alcohol	Investigate the influence of dietary habits on LTL and the functional consequences of diet-related shortening of telomeres for chromosome stability	Direct associations: vegetables, fruiting vegetables, root vegetables, peppers, carrots, and spinach
Tainen et al. [29]	Cross-sectional	HBCS, Finland: 1492 elderly subjects; 54% females; 61.5 years (mean)	Total fats (butter, margarine, oil), vegetables (roots and legumes), and fruits (including berries and juice)	Study the association between fats, fruits, and vegetables and LTL	Direct association: vegetables (women) and fruit (men) Inverse association: butter intake (men)
Song et al. [31]	Cross-sectional	WHI—OS, USA: 4029 postmenopausal women; 62.5 years (mean)	Main foods abundant in SMSFAs	Examine the direct relations of total and types of dietary fats and fat-rich foods to LTL	Inverse associations: milk, non-skim milk, butter, fat added to bread and cheese
García-Calzón et al. [23]	Cross-sectional	GENOI, Spain: 287 children and teenagers; 55% males; 11.5 years (mean)	Dietary total antioxidant capacity, glycemic load, legumes, vegetables, fruits, fish, meat, dairy products, sweetened beverages, cereals, and white bread	Evaluate the relationship between diet and LTL in a cross-sectional study of children and adolescents	Direct associations: dietary total antioxidant capacity and legumes Inverse associations: glycemic load, total cereal consumption, and white bread
Gu et al. [46]	Cross-sectional	WHICAP study, USA: 1743 multiethnic community residents of New York (506 whites, 536 African Americans, 679 Hispanics); 68.3% females; 78.1 years (mean)	Mediterranean diet and its different components	Investigate the association between LTL and Mediterranean diet pattern in a multiethnic study	Direct associations: vegetable consumption in whole population, and dairy and meat consumption among nonHispanic whites Inverse association: cereal intake in whole population
Lee et al. [47]	Prospective cohort (10 years)	Korean Genome Epidemiology Study, Republic of Korea: 1958 adults; 52.3% males; 48.2 years (mean)	Nuts, legumes, seaweed, fruits, dairy, red or processed meat, coffee, and sweetened carbonated beverages	Investigate the association between dietary patterns or consumption of specific foods and LTL	Direct associations: nuts, legumes, seaweed, fruits, and dairy products Inverse associations: red meat and processed meat
García-Calzón et al. [48]	Prospective cohort (5 years)	PREDIMED, Spain: 520 participants with high risk of cardiovascular disease; 55% females; 67 years (mean)	Dietary inflammatory index	Determine the association of the dietary inflammatory index with LTL and examine whether diet-associated inflammation could modify telomere attrition	Inverse association: proinflammatory index
Lian et al. [49]	Case-control	China: 271 hypertensive patients (51% females) and 455 normotensive controls (50.8% males); 60 years (mean)	Vegetables, fruit, eggs, meat, poultry, fish/seafood, milk, soy milk, fried foods, desserts, and salt	Examine the relationship of the 11 items with LTL and the risk of hypertension	Direct association: vegetable intake

Continued

TABLE 12.2 Effect of Food Consumption on Leukocyte Telomere Length—cont'd

References	Study Design	Sample Characteristics	Type of Food	Study Aim	Associations with LTL
Zhou et al. [50]	Cross-sectional	Type 2 diabetes project, Bejing, China: 556 Chinese subjects without diabetes history (156 newly diagnosed diabetes, 197 prediabetes, and 200 normal glucose tolerance); 61.7% females; 53.2 years (mean)	Diet carbohydrates/fat proportion and diet ingredients (daily energy, protein, fat, carbohydrates, cereals and cereal products, tuber crops, legumes, meat, dairy products, seeds and nuts, vegetables, fruits, fish and other seafood, seaweed, and sweetened carbonated beverages)	Explore influence of carbohydrate/fat proportions and dietary ingredients on TL shortening, oxidative stress, and inflammation in adults subjects with different glucose-tolerance status	Direct associations: legumes, nuts, fish, and seaweed consumption
Shivappa et al. [51]	Cross-sectional	NHANES population 1999–2002, USA: 7215 adults; 52.5% females; 49.2 years (mean)	Dietary inflammatory index	Examine the association between the dietary inflammatory index and LTL	Inverse association: proinflammatory index

CGEMS, Cancer Genetic Markers of Susceptibility; *GENOI*, Navarro Study Group on Childhood Obesity; *HBCS*, Helsinki Birth Cohort Study; *LTL*, leukocyte telomere length; *MESA*, Multi-Ethnic Study of Atherosclerosis; *MUFAs*, monounsaturated fatty acids; *NHANES*, National Health and Nutrition Examination Survey; *PREDIMED*, Prevención con Dieta Mediterránea; *pSoBid*, psychological, social, and biological determinants of ill health; *PUFAs*, polyunsaturated fatty acids; *SFAs*, saturated fatty acids; *SMSFAs*, short- to medium-chain saturated fatty acids; *TFAs*, transfatty acids; *WHICAP*, Washington Heights Inwood Community Aging Project; *WHI—OS*, Women's Health Initiative—Observational Study.

TABLE 12.3 Effect of Beverages on Leukocyte Telomere Length

References	Study Design	Sample Characteristics	Type of Beverages	Study Aim	Associations with LTL
Chan et al. [44]	Cross-sectional	China: 2006 subjects; 51.3% females; 72.4 years (mean)	Chinese tea	Examine the association between some food groups and LTL	Direct association: Chinese tea consumption (men)
Pavanello et al. [52]	Case-control	Italy: 457 males, 200 drunk-driving traffic offenders diagnosed as alcohol abusers 257 social drinkers (controls); 38 versus 44 years (mean), respectively	Alcohol	Investigate the effect of alcohol abuse on LTL, and elucidate whether such effect is modified by genetic variants in alcohol metabolic genes	Inverse associations: the condition of being an alcohol abuser, rather than the amount of drinking, is associated with shorter LTL
Strandberg et al. [53]	Prospective cohort (28 years)	Helsinki Businessmen Study, Finland: 499 healthy Caucasian men from the highest social class; 75.7 years (mean)	Alcohol	Investigate the association between alcohol consumption in healthy middle-aged adults and LTL	Inverse association: alcohol consumption in the elderly
Weischer et al. [54]	Prospective cohort (10 years)	Heart Study, Denmark: 4576 healthy adults; 58% females; 54.5 years (mean)	Alcohol	Study the association between shortening of telomeres and alcohol intake as well as other variables	No association: alcohol consumption at enrolment unrelated to TL at baseline or change after follow-up
Leung et al. [55]	Cross-sectional	NHANES, USA: 5309 adults; 51,8% women; 39.7 years (mean)	Sugar-sweetened soda, diet soda, noncarbonated sugar-sweetened soda, 100% fruit juice	Investigate whether LTL maintenance, which underlies healthy cellular aging, provides a link between sugar-sweetened beverage consumption and the risk of cardiometabolic disease	Direct association: 100% fruit juice Inverse association: sugar-sweetened soda
Lee et al. [47]	Prospective cohort (10 years)	Korean Genome Epidemiology Study, Republic of Korea: 1958 adults; 52.3% males; 48.2 years (mean)	Coffee and sweetened carbonated beverages	Investigate the association between dietary patterns or consumption of specific foods and LTL	Direct association: coffee consumption Inverse association: sweetened carbonated beverages
Zhou et al. [50]	Cross-sectional	Type 2 diabetes project, China: 556 Chinese subjects without diabetes history (156 newly diagnosed diabetes, 197 prediabetes, and 200 normal glucose tolerance); 61.7% females; 53.2 years (mean)	Sweetened carbonated beverages	Explore influence of carbohydrate/fat proportions and dietary ingredients on LTL shortening, oxidative stress, and inflammation in adult subjects with different glucose-tolerance status	Inverse association: sweetened carbonated beverages
Liu et al. [36]	Cross-sectional	NHS, USA: 4780 women; 59.2 years (mean)	Coffee	Examine the association between coffee consumption and LTL	Direct association: coffee consumption

LTL, leukocyte telomere length; NHANES, National Health and Nutrition Examination Survey; NHS, Nurses' Health Study.

TABLE 12.4 Effect of Dietary Patterns on Leukocyte Telomere Length

References	Study Design	Sample Characteristics	Type of Dietary Pattern	Study Aim	Associations with LTL
Pellat et al. [56]	Case-control	DALS, USA: two samples, 249 colon cancer cases and 371 controls, and 276 rectal cancer cases and 372 controls; 30–79 years (range)	Prudent Western	Investigate the association between genetics, diet, and lifestyle factors and LTL, and the association between LTL and colorectal cancer	No associations: dietary pattern and some food item such as alcohol, tea, dietary fiber, fruit, red meat and vegetables
Marin et al. [12]	Interventional	Spain: 20 free-living elderly subjects; 50% males; 67.1 years (mean)	Three diets each for a period of 4 weeks; 14 menus made with regular solid food: 1. Mediterranean diet rich in MUFAs 2. SFA-rich diet 3. Low-fat, high-carbohydrate diet rich in n-3 PUFAs	Investigate intracellular reactive oxidative species; cellular apoptosis, and LTL generated by three different diets	Cellular senescence was lower following the Mediterranean diet as compared to the SFA and low-fat, high-carbohydrate diets, as demonstrated by a lower percentage of cells with short telomeres in vitro Mediterranean diet protects against endothelial cell senescence, as shown by lower intracellular oxidative stress, lower shortening of telomeres, and lower apoptosis
Boccardi et al. [57]	Cross-sectional	Italy: 217 elderly subjects; 53% males; 77.9 years (mean)	Mediterranean diet	To investigate the relationship between LTL, telomerase activity and adherence to Mediterranean diet among elderly people	Direct association: adherence to Mediterranean diet DP
Crous-Bou et al. [58]	Cross-sectional	NHS, USA: 4676 women without disease; 59 years (mean)	Mediterranean diet Western prudent healthy	Examine whether adherence to the Mediterranean diet was associated with longer LTL	Direct associations: Mediterranean diet and healthy dietary pattern
Gu et al. [46]	Cross-sectional	WHICAP study, USA: 1743 multiethnic community residents of New York (506 nonHispanic whites, 536 African Americans, 679 Hispanics); 68.3% females; 78.1 years (mean)	Mediterranean diet	Investigate the association between LTL and Mediterranean diet in a multiethnic study	Direct association: Mediterranean diet in white nonHispanics
Lee et al. [47]	Prospective cohort (10 years)	Korean Genome Epidemiology Study, Republic of Korea: 1958 adults; 52.3% males; 48.2 years (mean)	Prudent Western	Investigate the association between dietary pattern or consumption of specific foods and LTL	Direct association: prudent dietary pattern
Liu et al. [36]	Cross-sectional	NHS, USA: 4780 women; 59.2 years (mean)	Mediterranean diet	Examine the association between coffee consumption and LTL	Direct association: alternative Mediterranean diet score

DALS, Diet, Activity, and Lifestyle Study; LTL, leukocyte telomere length; MUFAs, monounsaturated fatty acids; NHS, Nurses' Health Study; PUFAs, polyunsaturated fatty acids; SFAs, saturated fatty acids; WHICAP, Washington Heights Inwood Community Aging Project.

Nucleotide biosynthesis   **Methylation**

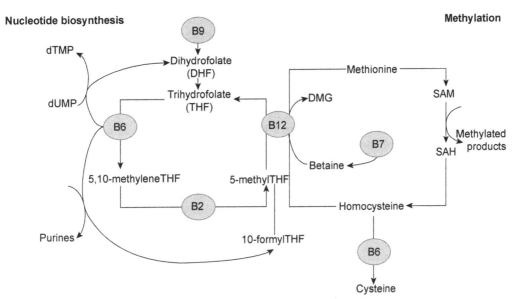

FIGURE 12.4 Role of B-group vitamins in nucleotide synthesis and DNA methylation through the one-carbon metabolism pathway. Vitamin B9 or folate; Vitamin B6 or pyridoxine; Vitamin B2 or riboflavin; Vitamin B12 or cobalamin; Vitamin B7 or choline; Vitamin B6 or pyridoxine. *DHF*, dihydrofolate; *DMG*, dimethyl-glycine; *dTMP*, deoxythymidine monophosphate; *dUMP*, deoxyuridine monophosphate; *SAM*, S-adenosyl methionine; *SAH*, S-adenosylhomocysteine; *THF*, trihydrofolate.

choline, a methyl group donor, and other cofactors such as vitamin B6, involved in metabolism of homocysteine to cysteine, and vitamin B2, which is the cofactor for reduction of 5,10-methylTHF to the predominant form of folate in the circulation (10-formylTHF). DNA methylation is important for the regulation of gene expression and the maintenance of genomic stability and TL. A deficiency of these vitamins, specifically of folate and vitamin B12, can lead to inadequate DNA methylation and may have an important effect on TL attrition in humans [61,62]. In folate deficiency, the accumulation of dUMP and uracil incorporations into DNA in place of thymine lead to DNA mutation associated with telomere dysfunction and attrition [61,63]. The homocysteine accumulation due to vitamin B12, vitamin B6, and folate deficiency shows an inverse association with TL [63−66]. Current evidence suggests that folate and vitamin B12 play an important role in DNA damage and oxidative stress as potential antioxidants [61].

However, inconsistent results have been found about these one-carbon metabolism biomarkers and TL [64,65,67,68]. Liu et al. [67] evaluated this association in 1715 women with an average age of 59.8 years, and found no relation between plasmatic and Food Frequency Questionnaire (FFQ) measurements of folate, choline, riboflavin, vitamins B6 and B12, and TL [30]. Likewise, in children aged 3, 6 and 9 years old, nutrients involved in one-carbon metabolism, including vitamin B12 and folate, were not associated with TL [33]. In contrast, the potential protective effects of B vitamins were evaluated in 1958 middle-aged and older Korean men, and an association of folate and vitamin B2 with TL was found [39].

Vitamin A is known for its antioxidant properties and its roles in the immune system, regulation of gene expression, cell differentiation, and maintaining of normal vision [24]. Vitamin A could influence TL by different mechanisms [28]. It has been postulated that its antioxidant capacity could reduce oxidative stress and, as a consequence, reduce telomere attrition [69,70]. Another hypothesis is that retinol acid, a bioactive metabolite of vitamin A, may contribute to epigenetic modifications binding and activating the cognate nuclear receptors for regulating target genes [69,71]. Some carotenoid precursors of vitamin A, known as provitamin A carotenoids, have been positively associated with longer telomeres [37]. However, it has been suggested that carotenoids which are not provitamin A have greater protective effects on DNA maintenance [72] and have been linked to a significantly greater effect on TL [32].

Vitamin C, also known as ascorbic acid, is one of the most important vitamins because of its multiple actions, including antiinflammatory, immune modulation, antioxidative, lymphocyte proliferation, and apoptosis modulation properties. It has been postulated that the antioxidative properties of vitamin C could improve intracellular redox status and, as a consequence, protect TL [32]. Some studies performed on cell cultures have demonstrated the antioxidative action of vitamin C diminishing telomere attrition [32,73]. In humans a significant relationship between TL and vitamin C has been observed [28,39], and it has been found that the activity of telomerase may be enhanced by vitamin C [74].

Vitamin D and its biologically active form, 1,25-dihydroxyvitamin D (25(OH)D), have been directly associated with TL [67,75−77] and telomerase activity [78]. The mechanism that could explain this relationship is that vitamin D decreases C-reactive protein (CRP), interleukin-6, and other mediators of systemic inflammation, reducing the turnover rate of leukocytes and so attenuating the rate of TL attrition [79]. In human studies, vitamin D serum levels have presented a significant association with TL in premenopausal and postmenopausal women [67,75], and even maternal vitamin D levels during pregnancy have been significantly linked to the TL of offspring [80]. However, the findings in a large population sample of young women and men do not support the hypothesis that 25(OH)D levels and TL are associated [35]. Recent studies have been controversial in evaluating associations between people of different race, age range, and sex. In 373 white females, 278 white males, 338 black females, and 165 black males in the range of 48–93 years old, a deficiency of vitamin D was only associated with longer TL in white subjects [81]. In contrast, Beilfuss et al. [82] suggested that lower vitamin D concentrations were associated with genomic instability, independently of age, sex, and race/ethnicity.

Vitamin E is considered the most effective fat-soluble antioxidant: it protects cell membranes and prevents dissemination of free-radical damage and lipid peroxidation. In aging, vitamin E supplementation could have an important role in enhancing microglial activation [83]. This process may preserve telomeres and reduce cell aging. Indeed, intake [28] and multivitamin use [84] of alpha-tocopherol, the main biologically active form of vitamin E, have been linked to longer telomeres in humans. Unexpectedly, an inverse association between TL and gamma-tocopherol was found in the US National Health and Nutrition Examination Survey population [85].

Selenium is an essential micronutrient for humans: it is a cofactor for the reduction of antioxidant enzymes, and a component of the amino acids selenocysteine and selenomethionine. Selenoproteins, characterized by their antioxidant and antiinflammatory properties, cannot be synthesized in a dietary deficiency of selenium [86,87]. Animal models showed that the efficacy curve of selenium intake was U-shaped, and the optimum selenium level can depend upon different forms of selenium and the genotype [86]. In addition, the beneficial effects of selenium on senescence and aging could be mediated by the increase of telomerase activity [85]. However, in a study performed in children no association between selenium intake and TL was found, suggesting that the shape of dose response has yet to be determined in humans [33,86].

Zinc is a relevant antiinflammatory agent and a regulator of gene expression. This mineral acts as a cofactor for enzymes involved in antioxidant defense systems [88]. A dietary deficiency of zinc is associated with inflammation and oxidative damage [89,90]. There is evidence that zinc supplementation has reduced proinflammatory cytokines [91] and incidence of infections [92]. In addition, it possible that zinc affects TL through its influence on telomerase activity and DNA integrity, and its protective role against oxidative stress [59]. In humans it has been demonstrated that changes in dietary zinc intake affects DNA integrity maintenance [89]. In an elderly population, the number of cells with short telomeres and telomere shortening may impair zinc homeostasis, and therefore the synthesis and zinc metalloprotein activity that protect from ROS and reactive nitrogen species [93]. Controversially, a study in children showed that higher zinc levels are associated with shorter telomeres [33].

Magnesium is an essential cofactor for enzymes involved in DNA processing, and is needed to maintain genomic stability [94]. Magnesium deficiency debilitates membrane integrity and membrane function, increases susceptibility to oxidative stress, and accelerates the aging process [95]. It has been found that a low magnesium level is associated with the CRP inflammatory marker [96] and influences TL by affecting DNA integrity and repair [59]. In older women a direct association between plasma magnesium and TL has been demonstrated [97].

Iron is positively linked to oxidative damage and physiological changes that appear with aging. Iron is a potent prooxidant, and its accumulation increases the risk of RNA and DNA damage [98–100], so high levels of iron in the body could affect telomere integrity and accelerate telomere shortening [100,101]. Interestingly, several studies have shown inverse associations between iron overload (reflected as high transferrin saturation) and shorter telomeres in middle-aged and older participants [102] and in adults over 25 years old [103]. Xu et al. demonstrated in 527 participants (35–74 age range) that subjects with iron supplementation had shorter TL than subjects without iron supplementation [84]. However, a recent study evaluated dietary intake of different micronutrients and TL, and observed no association between iron intake and TL [39].

5.2 Fat Intake

Several studies have evaluated the relation between total fat and individual fatty acids with TL (Table 12.1). This association is very important due to the crucial role of fatty acids in biological processes such as aging. Also, fat consumption has been associated with cardiovascular diseases, which are the most prevalent age-related diseases [104,105].

Saturated fatty acid and transfatty acid intakes are associated with inflammation and oxidative damage, which may lead to telomere shortening. The underlying effects of fat consumption were the influence on lipid profile and the fact that fats are markers of inflammation [106–108]. In elderly men, shorter telomeres were associated with total fat and saturated fatty acid intake, but in women this association was not found [29]. In postmenopausal women it is reported that total saturated fatty acids and small- to medium-chain saturated fatty acid intake was inversely linked to TL. But there was no association between the long-chain saturated fatty acids and TL [31], which could be explained by the effect of specific saturated fatty acids on plasma lipids and lipoproteins levels, possibly linked to telomere shorting [109]. Despite existing scientific evidence about the association between saturated fatty acids and TL, transfat consumption and its possible effect on TL have been poorly investigated. In 4780 females with an average age of 59.2 years, it was observed that those with shorter telomeres had significantly higher transfat consumption [36].

On the other hand, polyunsaturated fatty acids (PUFAs) modulate the production of lipid mediators that regulate inflammation in different ways [110,111], and for this reason they may have different effects on TL. In Spanish children and adolescents, total PUFA intake was positively associated with TL [48]. In contrast, Cassidy et al. [26] observed that total PUFA and linoleic acid intake was inversely associated with TL. This could be explained because different omega-6 fatty acids, such as linoleic acid and arachidonic acid, are an inflammatory component and a substrate for proinflammatory molecules respectively [111], promoting telomere shortening. Nevertheless, omega-3 fatty acids, particularly docohexaenoic and eicosapentaenoic acids, are known for their antioxidant and antiinflammatory properties that could decrease oxidative DNA damage [112]. A set of studies suggests that their intake protects against telomere attrition. In outpatients with coronary artery disease, a direct association between lower blood levels of marine omega-3 fatty acids and the rate of telomere shortening was observed [27]. Additionally, in elderly individuals with mild cognitive impairment, omega-3 fatty acid supplementation attenuated telomere attrition during a 6-month intervention [113].

5.3 Foods and Beverages

Total antioxidant capacity of food describes the ability of the antioxidants in food to remove preformed free radicals. It has been found that antioxidant-rich food has protective effects against inflammation, modulating the synthesis of inflammatory markers such as CRP [114,115] and reducing the rate of telomere shortening and aging [23,48,51].

Several epidemiological studies have supported the hypothesis that antioxidant-rich food consumption is positively associated with TL (Table 12.2). All the nutrients described previously have a positive or negative effect on oxidative stress and inflammation; consequently, they could exert their actions on TL and aging. There are some studies on the association between high consumption of vegetables [29,46,49], mainly fruiting vegetables, roots vegetables, peppers, carrots, spinach [28], and seaweed [47,50], and higher TL, probably for their main antioxidant components (β-carotene, vitamin C, and folic acid). Regarding fruit, another important natural antioxidant source, there is evidence of the positive effect of fruit consumption on TL [42,47]. In a case-controlled study it was demonstrated that in subjects with a low fruit intake, shorter telomeres were associated with gastric cancer risk factors [42]. In contrast, no significant associations were found for fruit and vegetable intake in middle-aged populations in studies to evaluate the association between cardiovascular risk factors [40] or prostate cancer risk factor [43] and TL.

Interestingly, there are other nutrient-rich plant foods that may reduce the risk of oxidative stress and modulate gene expression, and could thus have an important role in telomere integrity [116]. Consumption of legumes and nuts has been related to longer telomeres in several studies [23,47,50]. Antioxidant components found in the outer layer of seeds, and these properties have been associated with reduced oxidative damage and DNA repair [116]. Thus although there is a direct association between fiber cereal intake and TL [26], findings show that shorter telomeres are related to white bread and total cereals intake [23,46]; this may be caused by the refinement process, in which the outer seed layer is eliminated.

Inversely, several studies have extensively indicated a consistent link between consumption of processed meat and red meat and risk of total and cause-specific mortality [117,118]. The nutritional composition of these foods is characterized by high amounts of saturated fat, sodium, cholesterol, and iron, and in the case of processed meat added nitrous preservatives may accelerate the aging process [118,119]. Regarding TL, several studies performed in adults have shown an inverse association with processed meat [41,47,120]. However, evidence is less clear for red meat consumption; indeed a direct association with TL has been found [47], and unexpected positive correlation with TL [121].

The relation between dairy products and TL is also controversial, probably due to the wide range of dairy products with different fatty acids composition, mainly saturated fats. A direct association has been observed between dairy products and TL in adults [46,47], which could be due to some components of these products, such as bioactive peptides, calcium, and vitamin B12, that have beneficial effects on oxidative stress during aging [122].

In relation to beverages, the impact of alcohol consumption on health status is extensively studied (Table 12.3). Excess alcohol consumption leads to increased mortality and morbidity risk factors. However, light to moderate consumption of alcohol has been shown to have protective effects in cardiovascular diseases [123,124]. These health benefits are mainly attributed to polyphenol-rich alcoholic beverages, such as wine and beer. Polyphenols exhibit antioxidant and antiinflammatory properties [125,126]. The ambiguous effects of alcohol on human health are also apparent in TL. Pavanello et al. [52] compared social drinkers and alcohol abusers, and observed that alcohol abusers were associated with shorter telomeres, suggesting premature aging. Also, in healthy middle-aged adults alcohol consumption was inversely associated with TL. In contrast, no association was found between alcohol consumption and TL at baseline or change after 10 years in healthy adults [54].

Other polyphenol-rich beverages, such as tea and coffee, have been evaluated for their antioxidant and antiin-flammatories properties (Table 12.3). Both are potential sources of antioxidant compounds due to their content of poly-phenols and caffeine. For this reason, although few studies have evaluated the effect of consumption of these beverages on TL, they have shown a positive effect on TL [36,44,47]. In contrast, sweetened-beverage intake has been widely linked to high prevalence of obesity, insulin resistance, type 2 diabetes, and increased oxidative stress, inflammation, and vascular dysfunction [127]. Excessive intake of sweetened beverages could accelerate TL shortening, and regular consumption of such beverages might intervene in metabolic disease development through cell aging [47,50,55].

5.4 Dietary Patterns

Increasing evidence suggests that examining the role of dietary patterns, rather than food or nutrient intake in isolation, would facilitate acquiring knowledge about the influence of diet on health, due to the interactions of nutrients and bioactive compounds [128] (Table 12.4).

A Mediterranean diet has been considered as one of the healthiest global patterns, due to its association with a reduction of overall mortality and incidence of chronic disease and, consequently, with greater longevity [129,130]. The main features are the use of olive oil as a main source of fat, a high consumption of fruits, vegetables, whole grains, legumes, nuts, and seeds, a low consumption of saturated fatty acids, red and processed meat, and dairy products, and mild to moderate intake of alcohol [131]. As a result, a Mediterranean diet is considered a great source of antioxidants and therefore an effective dietary approach to reduce oxidative stress and inflammation markers [132]. It is noteworthy that it has a positive effect on telomere integrity [12,36,46,57] and telomerase activity [58]. In elderly subjects who received a Mediterranean diet enriched with monounsaturated fatty acid for 4 weeks, lower intracellular oxidative stress, lower shortening of telomeres, and lower apoptosis in umbilical endothelial cells were found compared to a baseline, a saturated fatty acid diet, and a low-fat, high-carbohydrate diet [12]. However, in a multiethnic study higher adherence to a Mediterranean diet was associated with longer TL in nonHispanic white subjects, but this effect was not found among African Americans and Hispanic subjects [46].

The effects of other dietary patterns on human health have been studied. A prudent dietary pattern based on high intake of fruits, vegetables, legumes, fish and other seafood, poultry, and whole grains is associated with lower inflammation and oxidative stress markers. On the other hand, a Western dietary pattern characterized by higher intake of red and processed meats, sweets, desserts, refined grains, and sweetened beverages is positively linked to circulating markers of inflammation [133—135]. Few studies have examined the effects of these dietary patterns on TL, so the evidence is less robust (Table 12.4). In middle-aged and older adults it was observed that a prudent diet in the past (10 years ago) was associated with TL, but a Western dietary pattern showed a nonsignificant inverse trend [47]. Similarly, other research has evaluated the possible interaction of prudent and Western dietary patterns on TL and no significant results have been observed, supporting the health benefits of a Mediterranean diet [56,58].

6. CONCLUSIONS

The aging process could be affected by oxidative stress, ROS, and inflammation. For this reason, lifestyle factors as smoking, sedentariness, alcohol abuse, poor-quality diet, and stress may affect telomere length and telomerase. In addition, an antioxidant-rich diet has been associated with longer telomeres.

Antioxidants play an important role in precision nutrition since they are able to slow down the aging process and prevent diseases driven by oxidative stress. Different nutrients such as vitamins B12, A, C, and E, selenium, zinc, magnesium, and PUFAs have been associated with DNA protection (telomere integrity). Subjects following dietary patterns characterized by higher intakes of fruits, vegetables, legumes, fish, poultry, and whole grains were reported to have lower inflammation and oxidative stress markers, and longer telomeres.

In conclusion, dietary factors can be an essential tool in precision nutrition for reducing cell damage and oxidative stress, thus ameliorating telomere attrition.

LIST OF ABBREVIATIONS

25(OH)D 1,25-dihydroxy vitamin D
CRP C-reactive protein
DNA Deoxyribonucleic acid
dUMP Deoxyuridine monophosphate
GWAS Genome Wide Association Study
LTL Leucocyte telomere length
POT1 Protection of telomeres 1
PUFA Polyunsaturated fatty acid
RAP1 Repressor-activated protein 1
RNA Ribonucleic acid
ROS Reactive oxygen species
SASP Senescence-associated secretory phenotype
SIPS Stress-induced premature senescence
SNPs Single-nucleotide polymorphisms
TERC Telomere RNA component
TERT Telomerase reverse transcriptase
TIN2 TRF1-interacting nuclear factor 2
TL Telomere length
TNF-α Tumor necrosis factor alpha
TPP1 TINF1-interacting protein 2
TRF1 Telomere repeat-binding factor 1
TRF2 Telomere repeat-binding factor 2

ACKNOWLEDGMENTS

Funding was provided by the Navarra Government (PI 54/209), PIUNA, CIBERobn (project CIBER, CB06/03/1017). AOR, LMA and LAP are fully acknowledged for the fellowship to Asociación de Amigos de la Universidad de Navarra (ADA).

REFERENCES

[1] World Health Organization (WHO). Acción multisectorial para un envejecimiento saludable basado en el ciclo de vida. http://apps.who.int/iris/bitstream/10665/251185/1/B138_16-sp.pdf.

[2] Cui H, Kong Y, Zhang H. Oxidative stress, mitochondrial dysfunction, and aging. J Signal Transduct 2011;2012:1−13.

[3] Almeida AJPO, Ribeiro TP, De Medeiros IA. Aging: molecular pathways and implications on the cardiovascular system. Oxid Med Cell Longev 2017;2017:1−19.

[4] Mchugh D, Gil J. Senescence and aging: causes, consequences, and therapeutic avenues. J Cell Biol 2018:1−13.

[5] Vidaček NŠ, Nanić L, Ravlić S, Sopta M, Gerić M, Gajski G, et al. Telomeres, nutrition, and longevity: can we really navigate our aging? Gerontol Soc Am 2017;0:1−9.

[6] Campisi J. Aging, cellular senescence, and cancer. Annu Rev Physiol 2014:685−705.

[7] Faragher RG, McArdle A, Willows A, Ostler EL. Senescence in the aging process. F1000Research 2017;6:1219.

[7a] Hayflick L. The limited in vitro lifetime of human diploid cell strains. Exp Cell Res. 1965;37:614−36.

[8] López-Otín C, Blasco MA, Partridge L, Serrano M, Kroemer G. The hallmarks of aging. Cell 2013;153:1194−217.

[9] Fyhrquist F, Saijonmaa O, Strandberg T. The roles of senescence and telomere shortening in cardiovascular disease. Reviews 2013;10:274−83.

[10] Yeh J-K, Wang C-Y. Telomeres and telomerase in cardiovascular diseases. Genes (Basel) 2016;7:58.

[11] Marti del Moral A, Zalba Goñi G. Telomeres, diet and human disease. Advances and therapeutic opportunities. CRC Press Taylor & Francis Group; 2017. 178 pp.

[11a] Allsopp RC, Vaziri H, Patterson C, Goldstein S, Younglai EV, Futcher AB, Greider CW, et al. Telomere lenght predicts replicative capacity of human fibroblast. Proc Natl Acad Sci USA 1992;89:10114−8.

[12] Marin C, Delgado-Lista J, Ramirez R, Carracedo J, Caballero J, Perez-Martinez P, et al. Mediterranean diet reduces senescence-associated stress in endothelial cells. Age (Omaha) 2012;34:1309−16.

[13] Freitas-Simoes TM, Ros E, Sala-Vila A. Nutrients, foods, dietary patterns and telomere length: update of epidemiological studies and randomized trials. Metabolism 2016;65:406−15.

[14] Xi H, Li C, Ren F, Zhang H, Zhang L. Telomere, aging and age-related diseases. Aging Clin Exp Res 2013;25:139−46.

[15] Gómez DLM, Armando RG, Farina HG, Gómez DE. Telomerasa y telómero: su estructura y dinámica en salud y enfermedad: Arquitectura funcional de los telómeros. Medicina (Buenos Aires) 2014:69−76.

[16] Krebs JE, Lewin B, Kilpatrick ST, Goldstein ES. Lewin's genes XI. Burlington (MA): Jones & Bartlett Learning; 2014.

[17] Bendix L, Horn PB, Jensen UB, Rubelj I, Kolvraa S. The load of short telomeres, estimated by a new method, universal STELA, correlates with number of senescent cells. Aging Cell 2010;9:383–97.

[18] Blackburn EH, Epel ES, Lin J. Human telomere biology: a contributory and interactive factor in aging, disease risks, and protection. Sci Spec Sect Aging 2015:1193–8.

[19] Denham J, O'Brien BJ, Charchar FJ. Telomere length maintenance and cardio-metabolic disease prevention through exercise training. Sports Med 2016:1–25.

[20] Barrett JH, Iles MM, Dunning AM, Pooley KA. Telomere length and common disease: study design and analytical challenges. Hum Genet 2015;134:679–89.

[21] Zietzer A, Hillmeister P. Leucocyte telomere length as marker for cardiovascular ageing. Acta Physiol 2014;211:251–6.

[22] García-Calzón S, Moleres A, Marcos A, Campoy C, Moreno LA, Azcona-Sanjulián MC, et al. Telomere length as a biomarker for adiposity changes after a multidisciplinary intervention in overweight/obese adolescents: the EVASYON study. PLoS One 2014;9:1–8.

[23] García-Calzón S, Moleres A, Martínez-González MA, Martínez JA, Zalba G, Marti A, et al. Dietary total antioxidant capacity is associated with leukocyte telomere length in a children and adolescent population. Clin Nutr 2015;34:694–9.

[24] Dabhade P, Kotwal S. Tackling the aging process with bio-molecules: a possible role for caloric restriction, food-derived nutrients, vitamins, amino acids, peptides, and minerals. J Nutr Gerontol Geriatr 2013;32:24–40.

[25] Skully R, Saleh AS. Aging and the effects of vitamins and supplements. Clin Geriatr Med 2011;27:591–607.

[26] Cassidy A, De Vivo I, Liu Y, Han J, Prescott J, Hunter DJ, et al. Associations between diet, lifestyle factors, and telomere length in. Am J Clin Nutr 2010;91:1273–80.

[27] Farzaneh-Far R, Lin J, Epel ES, Harris WS, Blackburn EH, Whooley MA. Association of marine omega-3 fatty acid levels with telomeric aging in patients with coronary heart disease. JAMA 2010;303:250–7.

[28] Marcon F, Siniscalchi E, Crebelli R, Saieva C, Sera F, Fortini P, et al. Diet-related telomere shortening and chromosome stability. Mutagenesis 2012;27:49–57.

[29] Tiainen A-M, Männistö S, Blomstedt PA, Moltchanova E, Perälä M-M, Kaartinen NE, et al. Leukocyte telomere length and its relation to food and nutrient intake in an elderly population. Eur J Clin Nutr 2012;66:1290–4.

[30] Liu JJ, Prescott J, Giovannucci E, Hankinson SE, Rosner B, De Vivo I. One-carbon metabolism factors and leukocyte telomere length. Am J Clin Nutr 2013;97:794–9.

[31] Song Y, You N-CY, Song Y, Kang MK, Hou L, Wallace R, et al. Intake of small-to-medium-chain saturated fatty acids is associated with peripheral leukocyte telomere length in postmenopausal women. J Nutr 2013;143:907–14.

[32] Sen A, Marsche G, Freudenberger P, Schallert M, Toeglhofer AM, Nagl C, et al. Association between higher plasma lutein, zeaxanthin, and vitamin C concentrations and longer telomere length: results of the Austrian Stroke Prevention Study. J Am Geriatr Soc 2014;62:222–9.

[33] Milne E, O'Callahan N, Ramankutty P, De Klerl NH, Greenop KR, Armstrong BK, et al. Plasma micronutrient levels and telomere length in children. Nutrition 2015;31:331–6.

[34] Zhu H, Bhagatwala J, Pollock NK, Parikh S, Gutin B, Stallmann-Jorgensen I, et al. High sodium intake is associated with short leukocyte telomere length in overweight and obese adolescents. Int J Obes 2015;39:1249–53.

[35] Williams DM, Palaniswamy S, Sebert S, Buxton JL, Blakemore AIF, Hyppönen E, et al. 25-Hydroxyvitamin D concentration and leukocyte telomere length in young adults: findings from the Northern Finland birth cohort 1966. Am J Epidemiol 2016;183:191–8.

[36] Liu JJ, Crous-Bou M, Giovannucci EL, De Vivo I. Coffee consumption is positively associated with longer leukocyte telomere length in the Nurses' Health Study. J Nutr 2016:1373–8.

[37] Bok K, Jin M, Min Y. Association between leukocyte telomere length and serum carotenoid in US adults. Eur J Nutr 2017;56:1045–52.

[38] Tucker LA. Alpha- and gamma-tocopherol and telomere length in 5768 US men and women: a NHANES study. Nutrients 2017;9:7–10.

[39] Lee JY, Shin C, Baik I. Longitudinal associations between micronutrient consumption and leukocyte telomere length. J Hum Nutr Diet 2017;30:236–43.

[40] Bekaert S, De Meyer T, Rietzschel ER, De Buyzere ML, De Bacquer D, Langlois M, et al. Telomere length and cardiovascular risk factors in a middle-aged population free of overt cardiovascular disease. Aging Cell 2007;6:639–47.

[41] Nettleton JA, Diez-Roux A, Jenny NS, Fitzpatrick AL, Jacobs DR. Dietary patterns, food groups, and telomere length in the Multi-Ethnic Study of Atherosclerosis (MESA). Am J Clin Nutr 2008;88:1405–12.

[42] Hou L, Savage SA, Blaser MJ, Perez-perez G, Dioni L, Pegoraro V, et al. NIH public access. Biomarkers 2010;18:3103–9.

[43] Mirabello L, Huang W, Wong JYY, Chatterjee N, Crawford ED, De Vivo I, et al. The association between leukocyte telomere length and cigarette smoking, dietary and physical variables, and risk of prostate cancer. Aging (Albany NY) 2009;8:405–13.

[44] Chan R, Woo J, Suen E, Leung J, Tang N. Chinese tea consumption is associated with longer telomere length in elderly Chinese men. Br J Nutr 2010;103:107.

[45] Shiels PG, McGlynn LM, MacIntyre A, Johnson PCD, da Batty GD, Burns H, et al. Accelerated telomere attrition is associated with relative household income, diet and inflammation in the pSoBid cohort. PLoS One 2011;6:1–7.

[46] Gu Y, Honig LS, Schupf N, Lee JH, Luchsinger JA, Stern Y, et al. Mediterranean diet and leukocyte telomere length in a multi-ethnic elderly population. Age (Omaha) 2015;37:1–13.

[47] Lee J-Y, Jun N-R, Yoon D, Shin C, Baik I. Association between dietary patterns in the remote past and telomere length. Eur J Clin Nutr 2015;69:1048–52.

[48] García-Calzón S, Zalba G, Ruiz-Canela M, Shivappa N, Hébert JR, Martínez JA, et al. Dietary inflammatory index and telomere length in subjects with a high cardiovascular disease risk from the PREDIMED-NAVARRA study: cross-sectional and longitudinal analyses over 5 y. Am J Clin Nutr 2015;102:897−904.

[49] Lian F, Wang J, Huang X, Wu Y, Cao Y, Tan X, et al. Effect of vegetable consumption on the association between peripheral leucocyte telomere length and hypertension: a case-control study. BMJ Open 2015;5:1−7.

[50] Zhou M, Zhu L, Cui X, Feng L, Zhao X, He S, et al. Influence of diet on leukocyte telomere length, markers of inflammation and oxidative stress in individuals with varied glucose tolerance: a Chinese population study. Nutr J 2015;15:39.

[51] Shivappa N, Wirth MD, Hurley TG, Hébert JR. Association between the dietary inflammatory index (DII) and telomere length and C-reactive protein from the National Health and Nutrition Examination Survey-1999−2002. Mol Nutr Food Res 2017;61:1−7.

[52] Pavanello S, Hoxha M, Dioni L, Bertazzi PA, Snenghi R, Nalesso A, et al. Shortened telomeres in individuals with abuse in alcohol consumption. Natl Inst Health 2012;129:983−92.

[53] Strandberg TE, Strandberg A, Saijonmaa O, Tilvis RS, Pitkälä KH, Fyhrquist F. Association between alcohol consumption in healthy midlife and telomere length in older men. The Helsinki Businessmen Study. Eur J Epidemiol 2012;27:815−22.

[54] Weischer M, Bojesen SE, Nordestgaard BG. Telomere shortening unrelated to smoking, body weight, physical activity, and alcohol intake: 4,576 general population individuals with repeat measurements 10 years apart. PLoS Genet 2014;10:1−11.

[55] Leung CW, Laraia BA, Needham BL, Rehkopf DH, Adler NE, Lin J, et al. Soda and cell aging: associations between sugar-sweetened beverage consumption and leukocyte telomere length in healthy adults from the national health and nutrition examination surveys. Am J Public Health 2014;104:2425−31.

[56] Pellatt AJ, et al. Genetic and lifestyle influence on telomere length and subsequent risk of colon cancer in a case control study. Int J Mol Epidemiol Genet 2012;3:184−94.

[57] Boccardi V, Esposito A, Rizzo MR, Marfella R, Barbieri M, Paolisso G. Mediterranean diet, telomere maintenance and health status among elderly. PLoS One 2013;8(4):4−9.

[58] Crous-Bou M, Fung TT, Prescott J, Julin B, Du M, Sun Q, et al. Mediterranean diet and telomere length in Nurses' Health Study: population based cohort study. BMJ 2014;349:1−11.

[59] Paul L. Diet, nutrition and telomere length. J Nutr Biochem 2011;22:895−901.

[60] Marti A, Echeverría R, Morell-azanza L, Ojeda-Rodríguez A. Telómeros y calidad de la dieta. Nutr Hosp 2017;34:1226−45.

[61] Fenech M. Folate (vitamin B9) and vitamin B12 and their function in the maintenance of nuclear and mitochondrial genome integrity. Mutat Res − Fundam Mol Mech Mutagen 2012;733:21−33.

[62] Hughes CF, Ward M, Hoey L, McNulty H. Vitamin B12 and ageing: current issues and interaction with folate. Ann Clin Biochem 2013;50:315−29.

[63] Bull CF, O'Callaghan NJ, Mayrhofer G, Fenech MF. Telomere length in lymphocytes of older South Australian men may be inversely associated with plasma homocysteine. Rejuvenation Res 2009;12:341−9.

[64] Shin C, Baik I. Leukocyte telomere length is associated with serum vitamin B12 and homocysteine levels in older adults with the presence of systemic inflammation. Clin Nutr Res 2016;5:7−14.

[65] Pusceddu I, Herrmann M, Kirsch SH, Werner C, Hübner U, Bodis M, et al. Prospective study of telomere length and LINE-1 methylation in peripheral blood cells: the role of B vitamins supplementation. Eur J Nutr 2016;55:1863−73.

[66] Richards JB, Valdes AM, Gardner JP, Kato BS, Siva A, Kimura M, et al. Homocysteine levels and leukocyte telomere length. Atherosclerosis 2008;200:271−7.

[67] Liu JJ, Prescott J, Giovannucci E, Hankinson SE, Rosner B, Han J, et al. Plasma vitamin D biomarkers and leukocyte telomere length. Am J Epidemiol 2013;177:1411−7.

[68] Moores CJ, Fenech M, O'Callaghan NJ. Telomere dynamics: the influence of folate and DNA methylation. Ann NY Acad Sci 2011;1229:76−88.

[69] Nomura SJO, Robien K, Zota AR. Serum folate, vitamin B-12, vitamin a, g -tocopherol, a -tocopherol, and carotenoids do not modify associations between cadmium exposure and leukocyte telomere length in the general US adult population 1 − 3. J Nutr 2017:1−11.

[70] Honarbakhsh S, Schachter M. Vitamins and cardiovascular disease. Br J Nutr 2009;101:1113.

[71] McGrane MM. Vitamin A regulation of gene expression: molecular mechanism of a prototype gene. J Nutr Biochem 2007;18:497−508.

[72] Azqueta A, Collins AR. Mutation research/fundamental and molecular mechanisms of mutagenesis carotenoids and DNA damage. Mutat Res − Fundam Mol Mech Mutagen 2012;733:4−13.

[73] Furumoto K, Inoue E, Nagao N, Hiyama E, Miwa N. Age-dependent telomere shortening is slowed down by enrichment of intracellular vitamin C via suppression of oxidative stress. Life Sci 1998;63:935−48.

[74] Wei F, Qu C, Song T, Ding G, Fan Z, Liu D, et al. Vitamin C treatment promotes mesenchymal stem cell sheet formation and tissue regeneration by elevating telomerase activity. J Cell Physiol 2012;227:3216−24.

[75] Richards JB, Valdes AM, Gardner JP, Paximadas D, Kimura M, Nessa A, et al. Higher serum vitamin D concentrations are associated with longer leukocyte telomere length in women. Am J Clin Nutr 2007:1420−5.

[76] Borras M, Panizo S, Sarró F, Valdivielso JM, Fernandez E. Assessment of the potential role of active vitamin D treatment in telomere length: a case-control study in hemodialysis patients. Clin Ther 2012;34:849−56.

[77] Julin B, Shui IM, Prescott J, Giovannucci EL, De Vivo I. Plasma vitamin D biomarkers and leukocyte telomere length in men. Eur J Nutr 2017;56:501−8.

[78] Zhu H, Guo D, Li K, Pedersen-White J, Stallmann-Jorgensen IS, Huang Y, et al. Increased telomerase activity and vitamin D supplementation in overweight African Americans. Int J Obes 2012;36:805−9.

[79] Mazidi M, Kengne AP, Banach M. Mineral and vitamin consumption and telomere length among adults in the United States. Pol Arch Intern Med 2017;127:87−90.

[80] Kim JH, Kim GJ, Lee D, Ko JH, Lim I, Bang H, et al. Higher maternal vitamin D concentrations are associated with longer leukocyte telomeres in newborns. Matern Child Nutr 2018;14:E12475.

[81] Liu JJ, Cahoon EK, Linet MS, Little MP, Dagnall CL, Higson H, et al. Relationship between plasma 25-hydroxymitamin D and leucocyte telomere length by sex and race in a US study. Br J Nutr 2016;116:953−60.

[82] Beilfuss J, Camargo CA, Kamycheva E. Serum 25-hydroxyvitamin D has a modest positive association with leukocyte telomere length in middle-aged US adults 1,2. J Nutr Genom Proteom Metab 2017;25:1−7.

[83] McElroy PD, Beier JC, Oster CN, Beadle C, Sherwood JA, Oloo AJ, et al. Alpha-tocopherol (vitamin E) induces rapid, nonsustained proliferation in cultured rat microglia. Am J Trop Med Hyg 2006;53:669−74.

[84] Xu Q, Parks CG, DeRoo LA, Cawthon RM, Sandler DP, Chen H. Multivitamin use and telomere length in women. Am J Clin Nutr 2009;89:1857−63.

[85] Yu R-A, Chen H-J, He L-F, Chen B, Chen X-M. Telomerase activity and telomerase reverse transcriptase expression induced by selenium in rat hepatocytes. Biomed Environ Sci 2009;22:311−7.

[86] Ferguson LR, Karunasinghe N, Zhu S, Wang AH. Selenium and its' role in the maintenance of genomic stability. Mutat Res − Fundam Mol Mech Mutagen 2012;733:100−10.

[87] Berry MJ, Martin GW, Tujebajeva R, Grundner-Culemann E, Mansell JB, Morozova N, et al. Selenocysteine insertion sequence element characterization and selenoprotein expression. Methods Enzymol 2002;347:17−24.

[88] Marreiro D, Cruz K, Morais J, Beserra J, Severo J, de Oliveira A. Zinc and oxidative stress: current mechanisms. Antioxidants 2017;6:24.

[89] Song Y, Chung CS, Bruno RS, Traber MG, Brown KH, King JC, et al. Dietary zinc restriction and repletion affects DNA integrity in healthy men. Am J Clin Nutr 2009;90:321−8.

[90] Olechnowicz J, Tinkov A, Skalny A, Suliburska J. Zinc status is associated with inflammation, oxidative stress, lipid, and glucose metabolism. J Physiol Sci 2017;68:19−31.

[91] Bao B, Prasad A, Beck F, Fitzgerald J. Zinc decreases C-reactive protein, lipid peroxidation, and implication of zinc as an atheroprotective agent. Am J Clin Nutr 2010;91:1634−41.

[92] Meydani SN, Barnett JB, Dallal GE, Fine BC, Jacques PF, Leka LS, et al. Serum zinc and pneumonia in nursing home elderly.pdf. Am J Clin Nutr 2007;86:1167−73.

[93] Cipriano C, Tesei S, Malavolta M, Giacconi R, Muti E, Costarelli L, et al. Accumulation of cells with short telomeres is associated with impaired zinc homeostasis and inflammation in old hypertensive participants. J Gerontol − Ser A Biol Sci Med Sci 2009;64:745−51.

[94] Hartwig A. Role of magnesium in genomic stability. Micronutr Genom Stab 2001;475:113−21.

[95] Anastassopoulou J, Theophanides T. Magnesium-DNA interactions and the possible relation of magnesium to carcinogenesis. Irradiation and free radicals. Crit Rev Oncol Hematol 2002;42:79−91.

[96] Guerrero-Romero F, Rodríguez-Morán M. Relationship between serum magnesium levels and C-reactive protein concentration, in non-diabetic, non-hypertensive obese subjects. Int J Obes Relat Metab Disord 2002;26:469−74.

[97] O'Callaghan NJ, Bull C, Lenech M. Elevated plasma magnesium and calcium may be associated with shorter telomeres in older South Australian women. J Nutr Health Aging 2014;18:131−6.

[98] Dunaief JL. Iron induced oxidative damage as a potential factor in age-related macular degeneration: the Cogan lecture. Investig Ophthalmol Vis Sci 2006;47:4660−4.

[99] Xu J, Knutson MD, Carter CS, Leeuwenburgh C. Iron accumulation with age, oxidative stress and functional decline. PLoS One 2008;3(8).

[100] Prá D, Franke SIR, Henriques JAP, Fenech M. Iron and genome stability: an update. Mutat Res − Fundam Mol Mech Mutagen 2012;733:92−9.

[101] Kepinska M, Szyller J, Milnerowicz H. The influence of oxidative stress induced by iron on telomere length. Environ Toxicol Pharmacol 2015;40:931−5.

[102] Shin C, Baik I. Transferrin saturation concentrations associated with telomeric ageing: a population-based study. Br J Nutr 2017;117:1693−701.

[103] Mainous AG, Wright RU, Hulihan MM, Twal WO, McLaren CE, Diaz VA, et al. Elevated transferrin saturation, health-related quality of life and telomere length. BioMetals 2014;27:135−41.

[104] Zock PL, Blom WAM, Nettleton JA, Hornstra G. Progressing insights into the role of dietary fats in the prevention of cardiovascular disease. Curr Cardiol Rep 2016;18:111.

[105] Sacks FM, Lichtenstein AH, Wu JHY, Appel LJ, Creager MA, Kris-Etherton PM, et al. Dietary fats and cardiovascular disease: a presidential advisory from the American Heart Association. Circulation 2017;136:e1−23.

[106] Stachowska E, Jamiol D, Chlubek D. Trans fatty acids and their role in inflammation and cardiovascular disease Kwasy tłuszczowe trans i ich rola w zapaleniu i chorobach układu krążenia Streszczenie Absorption of trans fatty acids. Ann Acad Med Stetin 2010;56:30−8.

[107] Smit LA, Katan MB, Wanders AJ, Basu S, Brouwer IA. A high intake of trans fatty acids has little effect on markers of inflammation and oxidative stress in humans. J Nutr 2011;141:1673−8.

[108] Anderson C, Milne GL, Sandler DP, Nichols HB. Oxidative stress in relation to diet and physical activity among premenopausal women. Br J Nutr 2016;116:1416−24.

[109] Hu FB, Stampfer MJ, Manson JE, Ascherio A, Colditz GA, Speizer FE, et al. Dietary saturated fats and their food sources in relation to the risk of coronary heart disease in women. Am J Clin Nutr 1999;70:1001—8.

[110] Kris-etherton PM, Harris WS, Appel LJ, Committee N. AHA scientific statement. 2003. p. 2747—57.

[111] Harris WS, Mozaffarian D, Rimm E, Kris-etherton P, Rudel LL, Appel LJ, et al. Omega-6 fatty acids and risk for cardiovascular disease a science advisory from the American Heart Association Nutrition Subcommittee of the Council on Nutrition, Physical Activity, and Metabolism; Council on Cardiovascular Nursing; and Council on Epidemiology and Prevention. Circulation 2009:902—7.

[112] Martínez-Fernández L, Laiglesia LM, Huerta AE, Martínez JA, Moreno-Aliaga MJ. Omega-3 fatty acids and adipose tissue function in obesity and metabolic syndrome. Prostaglandins Other Lipid Mediat 2015;121:24—41.

[113] O'Callaghan N, Parletta N, Milte CM, Benassi-Evans B, Fenech M, Howe PRC. Telomere shortening in elderly individuals with mild cognitive impairment may be attenuated with ω-3 fatty acid supplementation: a randomized controlled pilot study. Nutrition 2014;30:489—91.

[114] Valtueña S, Pellegrini N, Franzini L, Bianchi MA, Ardigo D, Del Rio D, et al. Food selection based on total antioxidant capacity can modify antioxidant intake, systemic inflammation, and liver function without altering markers of oxidative stress. Am J Clin Nutr 2008;87:1290—7.

[115] Brighenti F, Valtueña S, Pellegrini N, Ardigò D, Del Rio D, Salvatore S, et al. Total antioxidant capacity of the diet is inversely and independently related to plasma concentration of high-sensitivity C-reactive protein in adult Italian subjects. Br J Nutr 2005;93:619.

[116] Bohn SK, Myhrstad MC, Thoresen M, Holden M, Karlsen A, Tunheim SH, et al. Blood cell gene expression associated with cellular stress defense is modulated by antioxidant-rich food in a randomised controlled clinical trial of male smokers. BMC Med 2010;8:54.

[117] Wang X, Lin X, Ouyang YY, Liu J, Zhao G, Pan A, et al. Red and processed meat consumption and mortality: dose—response meta-analysis of prospective cohort studies. Public Health Nutr 2016;19:893—905.

[118] Kouvari M, Tyrovolas S, Panagiotakos DB. Red meat consumption and healthy ageing: a review. Maturitas 2016;84:17—24.

[119] Linseisen J, Rohrmann S, Norat T, Gonzalez CA, Iraeta MD, Gómez PM, et al. Dietary intake of different types and characteristics of processed meat which might be associated with cancer risk — results from the 24-hour diet recalls in the European Prospective Investigation into Cancer and Nutrition (EPIC). Public Health Nutr 2006;9:449—64.

[120] Fretts AM, Howard BV, Siscovick DS, Best LG, Beresford SA, Mete M, et al. Processed meat, but not unprocessed red meat, is inversely associated with leukocyte telomere length in the Strong Heart Family Study. J Nutr 2016;146:2013—8.

[121] Kasielski M, Eusebio M-O, Pietruczuk M, Nowak D. The relationship between peripheral blood mononuclear cells telomere length and diet — unexpected effect of red meat. Nutr J 2016;15:1—7.

[122] Camfield DA, Owen L, Scholey AB, Pipingas A, Stough C. Review article dairy constituents and neurocognitive health in ageing. Br J Nutr 2017;106:159—74.

[123] Fernández-Solà J. Cardiovascular risks and benefits of moderate and heavy alcohol consumption. J Nat Rev Cardiol 2015;12:576—87.

[124] Ronksley PE, Brien SE, Turner BJ, Mukamal KJ, Ghali WA. Association of alcohol consumption with selected cardiovascular disease outcomes: a systematic review and meta-analysis. BMJ 2011;342:1—13.

[125] Arranz S, Chiva-Blanch G, Valderas-Martínez P, Medina-Remón A, Lamuela-Raventós RM, Estruch R. Wine, beer, alcohol and polyphenols on cardiovascular disease and cancer. Nutrients 2012;4:759—81.

[126] Ramos S. Cancer chemoprevention and chemotherapy: dietary polyphenols and signalling pathways. Mol Nutr Food Res 2008;52:507—26.

[127] Malik VS, Hu FB. Fructose and cardiometabolic health what the evidence from sugar-sweetened beverages tells us. J Am Coll Cardiol 2015;66:1615—24.

[128] Jacobs DR, Gross MD, Tapsell LC. Food synergy: an operational concept for understanding nutrition. Am J Clin Nutr 2009;89:1543—8.

[129] Trichopoulou A. Traditional Mediterranean diet and longevity in the elderly: a review. Public Health Nutr 2004;7:943—7.

[130] Roman B, Carta L, Martínez-González MA, Serra-Majem L. Effectiveness of the Mediterranean diet in the elderly. Clin Interv Aging 2008;3:97—109.

[131] Willett WC, Sacks F, Trichopoulou A, Drescher G, Ferro-Luzzi A, Helsing E, et al. Mediterranean diet pyramid: a cultural model for healthy eating. Am J Clin Nutr 1995;61:1402e6.

[132] Bonaccio M, Di Castelnuovo A, Bonanni A, Costanzo S, De Lucia F, Pounis G, et al. Adherence to a Mediterranean diet is associated with a better health-related quality of life: a possible role of high dietary antioxidant content. BMJ Open 2013;3:1—16.

[133] Lopez-Garcia E, Schulze MB, Fung TT, Meigs JB, Rifai N, Manson JE, et al. Major dietary patterns are related to plasma concentrations of markers of inflammation and endothelial dysfunction. Am J Clin Nutr 2004;80:1029—35.

[134] Giugliano D, Ceriello A, Esposito K. The effects of diet on inflammation. Emphasis on the metabolic syndrome. J Am Coll Cardiol 2006;48:677—85.

[135] Wood AD, Strachan AA, Thies F, Aucott LS, Reid DM, Hardcastle AC, et al. Patterns of dietary intake and serum carotenoid and tocopherol status are associated with biomarkers of chronic low-grade systemic inflammation and cardiovascular risk. Br J Nutr 2014;112:1341—52.

Chapter 13

Antioxidant Supplements in Obesity and Metabolic Syndrome: Angels or Demons

Rafael A. Casuso and Jesús R. Huertas
University of Granada, Granada, Spain

1. INTRODUCTION

The causes of oxidative stress are increased production of reactive oxygen species (ROS), a default of antioxidant defense mechanisms, or both. In any case, damage to deoxyribonucleic acid (DNA), lipids, and proteins of cell structures takes place; depending on the severity of the damage, it can be irreversible and play a key role in the genesis of several diseases of inflammatory origin, such as cancer, cardiovascular diseases, hypertension, diabetes mellitus, and obesity.

It is difficult to clarify the role oxidative stress in obesity because, among other issues, it is not clear if oxidative stress is a cause or a consequence of obesity. Some researchers attribute oxidative stress to a higher cell consumption of oxygen with a subsequent increase in mitochondrial production of ROS, a decrease of antioxidant capacity, and finally an increase in fat deposits. Other researchers justify this association by considering obesity and metabolic diseases in general as a state of chronic inflammation. In this case, inflammatory cytokines (interleukin-6, tumor necrosis factor alpha) and the C-reactive protein predominate over antiinflammatory factors, contributing together to a prooxidant obesogenic environment. Both models can be more pronounced in situations of physical-exercise-induced oxidative stress. In such situations, ROS production exceeds antioxidant mechanisms when the intensity exceeds the anerobic threshold.

Regardless of whether oxidative stress is a cause or a consequence of noncommunicable chronic inflammatory diseases, including obesity, a series of strategies to block ROS production using very different antioxidant therapies have been developed. These strategies include an increased intake of antioxidants by adjusting the diet or through supplements, caloric restriction, and sports training to strengthen the body's natural defense mechanisms.

These antioxidant strategies are under continuous evaluation, with conflicting results depending on type of antioxidant, amount, target population, age, physical activity, etc. Understanding of ROS function as cell signals has increased in recent years [1]. Actually, ROS are required in very small amounts (Fig. 13.1) as mediators of expression of critical genes for establishing an active and healthy phenotype (e.g., in athletes) (Fig. 13.2). Moreover, many subjects with overweight/obesity or diabetes undertaking physical activity to lose weight or increase insulin sensitivity could not obtain the expected results if they take antioxidant supplements, as these supplements might inhibit the expression of key proteins such as the glucose transporter type 4 (GLUT-4).

In this chapter we review the dark face of ROS, and their role as mediators of the expression of key genes for the remission of inflammatory diseases where oxidative stress is a key factor and where antioxidant supplements could prevent this function.

2. OXYGEN, REACTIVE OXYGEN SPECIES, AND OXIDATIVE STRESS

Oxygen is critical for life in an atmosphere rich in this molecule. The ability to metabolize oxygen allowed evolution from unicellular to multicellular organisms. However, during oxygen metabolism the superoxide anion ($O_2^{\cdot-}$) is produced by the reduction of one of the unpaired electrons of molecular oxygen. A series of ROS and nitric oxide synthase (NOS) are produced from the superoxide anion. These species are highly reactive, and for their stabilization they require the donation

Obesity. https://doi.org/10.1016/B978-0-12-812504-5.00013-1

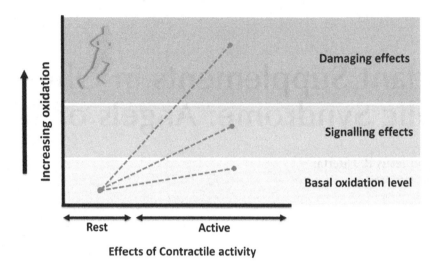

FIGURE 13.1 Hypothetical model depicting muscle responses to increasing oxidation of redox-sensitive components due to increased ROS exposure. Low levels of ROS change the cellular redox state to increase the redox-sensitive signaling pathways. *ROS*, reactive oxygen species. *Adapted from Powers SK, Jackson MJ. Exercise-induced oxidative stress: cellular mechanisms and impact on muscle force production. Physiol Rev 2008;88(4):1243−76.*

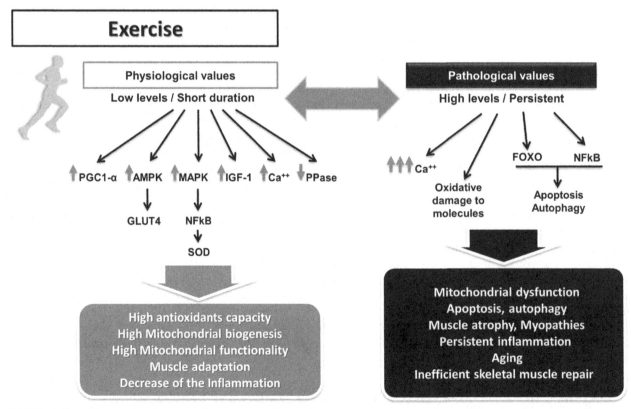

FIGURE 13.2 ROS are required in very small amounts as mediators of expression of critical genes for establishing an active and healthy phenotype. *AMPK*, adenosine monophosphate-activated protein kinase; *FoxO*, forkhead box O; *GLUT4*, glucose transporter type 4; *IGF-1*, insulin-like growth factor 1; *MAPK*, mitogen-activated protein kinase; *NF-κB*, nuclear factor kappa B; *PGC-1α*, peroxisome proliferator-activated receptor gamma coactivator 1 alpha; *PPases*, phosphatases; *ROS*, reactive oxygen species; *SOD*, superoxide dismutase. *Adapted from Barbieri E, Sestili P. Reactive oxygen species in skeletal muscle signaling. J Signal Transduct 2011;2012:1−17.*

of electrons from other molecules; this process is known as oxidative damage. In normal physiological conditions the body has many antioxidant mechanisms maintaining balanced oxidation-reduction (redox) processes, and thus preventing oxidative damage [2].

Movement is an inherent ability in humans that has allowed us to survive over thousands of years in a hostile environment. For this reason, skeletal muscle is one of the main sites of ROS and NOS production as a result of a large use of oxygen as substrate. Trained skeletal muscle has the acquired ability to react quickly to high levels of ROS derived from its activity and prevent oxidative damage using enzymatic and nonenzymatic antioxidants [3,4]. Moreover, a skeletal muscle adapted to training maintains basal ROS production at levels that are physiologically beneficial. Among the many functions of ROS, they are in charge of mitochondrial adaptations, control of muscle mass, and glucose uptake. The beginning of metabolic disease is characterized by an increase of ROS that cannot be counteracted by the endogenous antioxidant systems. In addition, this increase of ROS affects structures such as the mitochondria, causing irreversible damage to them and leading to higher production of mitochondrial ROS [5]. Thus ROS play a key role in the development of metabolic disease that could lead to alterations in glucose uptake, type 2 diabetes, dyslipidemia, cardiovascular disease, or cancer (Fig. 13.3). In this chapter we address the role of ROS in metabolic disease and how supplementation with antioxidants can alter these processes.

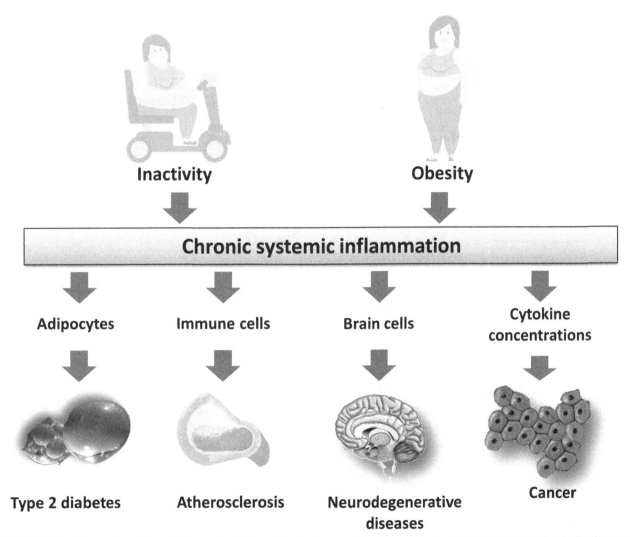

FIGURE 13.3 Inflammation and chronic diseases. Inactivity and obesity trigger persistent, low-grade systemic inflammation linked to the development of many chronic diseases such as insulin resistance, type 2 diabetes, atherosclerosis, neurodegenerative diseases (Alzheimer's, Huntington's, Parkinson's), cancer, etc. *Adapted from Handschin C, Spiegelman BM. The role of exercise and PGC1alpha in inflammation and chronic disease. Nature 2008;454(7203):463–9.*

3. OBESITY AND DIABETES "PANDEMIC"

We live in a very busy society in which we have almost no time for activities other than everyday work. This fast-paced lifestyle, mainly seen in occidental societies, implies neglect of nutrition and an increasingly sedentary lifestyle. The lack of time has led to overeating of fast food that, in general, has a high content of fat, salt, and sugar. This increased intake of hypercaloric diets in conjunction with the increased sedentary lifestyle has led to unprecedented levels of obesity in occidental society (Fig. 13.4). For example, the journal *The Lancet* published a study that compared obesity levels in the United Kingdom for the period between 1980 and 2013. Results showed that 67% of men and 55% of women aged

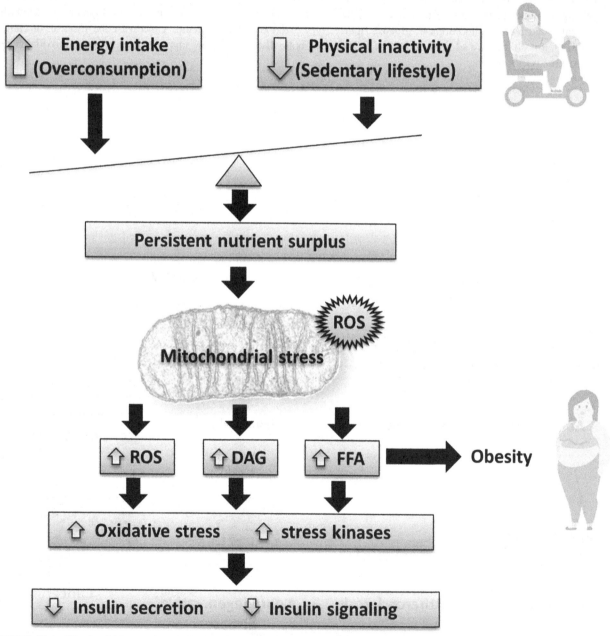

FIGURE 13.4 Mitochondrial stress in type 2 diabetes and obesity. Persistent nutrient surplus as a consequence of overconsumption and physical inactivity determines mitochondrial stress that can trigger oxidative stress and activation of stress-sensitive kinases. Impaired insulin secretion and sensitivity occur as a result of stress-induced β-cell dysfunction and insulin resistance. *DAG*, diacylglycerol; *FFA*, free fatty acid; *ROS*, reactive oxygen species. *Adapted from Cheng Z, Almeida FA. Mitochondrial alteration in type 2 diabetes and obesity: an epigenetic link. Cell Cycle 2014;13(6):890—7.*

between 40 and 60 years presented as overweight in 2013. Notably, the study found 26% of boys and 29% of girls were overweight or obese, compared to 17.5% and 21% in 1980 [6].

In addition, this increase of obesity triggers a maintained chronic inflammation state. This inflammatory state in some tissues leads to a series of metabolic diseases: for example, the inflammatory response of immune system cells can trigger atherosclerosis; in the brain it has been associated with Alzheimer's; and the systemic increase of proinflammatory cytokines has been linked with the development of certain cancers (Fig. 13.3) [7]. However, due to its incidence and relevance, it should be highlighted that inflammatory cytokines released by the adipose tissue are related to insulin resistance, which can lead to type 2 diabetes. Thus uncontrolled fat storage is directly linked to metabolic syndrome and type 2 diabetes.

Insulin resistance and type 2 diabetes are a public health problem in developed countries. The magnitude of this problem was characterized in a study published in 2001 in the prestigious journal *Diabetes Care*: the researchers predicted that 29 million Americans would present with type 2 diabetes by 2050. However, this number was reached in 2012, and more recent data suggests that 9% Americans suffer from type 2 diabetes [8]. Updated calculations suggest that one out of three Americans will have type 2 diabetes by 2050. The International Diabetes Federation also predicts that 642 million people worldwide will suffer type 2 diabetes by 2040. Thus type 2 diabetes is currently an uncontrolled pandemic, and unfortunately it seems that public health systems are taking no action against it.

To date, some epidemiological studies conducted in subjects with metabolic syndrome (prediabetic) have investigated the changes in lifestyle during the disease development [9–11]. In general, these studies have changed the diet and/or physical activity of the subjects over periods of 3–6 years. The results show that the physical exercise is able to decrease the incidence of type 2 diabetes in 45% of cases and dietary changes can improve the incidence in 30% of cases. Moreover, the combination of diet and exercise can decrease the incidence of disease up to 60%. Notably, administration of the drug metformin reduces the incidence of the disease by 30%. Dietary changes in conjunction with a more active lifestyle seem to be the more sensible interventions to decrease the incidence of the disease.

4. REACTIVE OXYGEN SPECIES PRODUCTION, MITOCHONDRIA, AND ADAPTATION

We are therefore facing the paradox that an adaptation which has helped us to survive for millennia, the ability to store fat, is nowadays killing us. It is noteworthy that studies conducted in humans and rodents suggest that subcutaneous adipose tissue can also have an endocrine effect. Indeed, it has been demonstrated in rodents that adipose tissue transplanted from active mice to sedentary mice improves not only the lipid profile but also the glucose uptake [12]. A significant adaptation produced by exercise is the phenotypic change of subcutaneous fat. In this process, adipokines secreted by fat modulate more beneficially the inflammation, glucose metabolism, blood pressure, and atherosclerosis. It has been shown, for example, that regular exercise is able to transform white fat into brown fat by specific molecular mechanisms. One of the main features of brown fat is that adipocytes are much smaller than those found in white fat. In addition, brown fat shows a high content of mitochondria; thus it is a tissue with a high metabolism. This property helped researchers to discover the main regulator of mitochondrial biogenesis, the peroxisome proliferator-activated receptor gamma coactivator 1-alpha (PGC-1α) [13].

PGC-1α seems to be critical not only for the phenotypic change of subcutaneous fats but also for correct functioning of the metabolism. Pioneering studies by Mootha et al. in 2003 [14] showed that subjects with metabolic syndrome presented problems expressing PGC-1α in skeletal muscle. Moreover, these subjects showed a reduced ability to express key genes of oxidative metabolism; and this was directly related to lower aerobic performance. A few years later it was found that PGC-1α responds to physiological stimuli to control biogenesis and the mitochondrial function when acting as transcriptional coactivator of genes directly related to these processes.

In response to an increase in nutrient supply, mitochondrial biogenesis is activated to increase the number of mitochondria. If this supply is maintained at high levels for long periods of time, biogenesis and the functional capacity of mitochondria decrease. Thus nutrients are necessary to trigger beneficial mitochondrial adaptations, but hypercaloric diets reverse this effect. Indeed, mitochondrial biogenesis is regulated by energy sensors such as cAMP-response-element binding (CREB), adenosine monophosphate-dependent kinase (AMPK), and sirtuin 1 (SIRT1), which are cell sensors at the levels of cAMP, adenosine monophosphate (AMP)/adenosine triphosphate (ATP) ratio, and NAD/NADH ratio, respectively. All these signaling pathways converge in the expression of PGC-1α, which can also be expressed by epigenetic mechanisms since hypomethylation of the DNA seems to regulate its expression. Subjects with metabolic syndrome, obesity, or type 2 diabetes show levels of DNA methylation much higher than that in healthy subjects. This effect has been associated with decreased expression of PGC-1α and a loss of mitochondrial function [15]. This relation of DNA methylation—mitochondrial dysfunction has also been found in subjects presenting cardiovascular risk. Importantly, subjects with metabolic syndrome showed high levels of mitochondrial fission. In this process, where mitochondria are fragmented until degradation, an overproduction of ROS has also been found [16]. However, it is not fully understood if the high levels of ROS found in patients showing high levels of mitochondrial fission are a cause or a consequence of this dysfunction. This makes it difficult to know whether supplementation with antioxidants could improve this mitochondrial pathology.

Within the mitochondria itself there are many different sites for ROS production, although the best characterized are complex I and complex III of the mitochondrial electron transport chain. However, it is worth noting that other mitochondrial ROS are produced, such as those produced by the NADPH oxidase system and found in the sarcoplasmic reticulum, transverse tubules, and sarcolemma [17]. During transitory periods of cell stress, such as that resulting from exercise, all these sites of ROS production are very active in the exercised skeletal muscle, producing ROS at levels above the basal. In addition, large amounts of ROS are produced by the xanthine oxidase system at very high exercise intensities or exercise involving repeated phases of ischemia reperfusion. To balance the production of ROS, the muscle contains copper and zinc superoxide dismutase (CuZnSOD), catalase, and glutation peroxidase (GPx) in the sarcoplasma and manganese SOD (MnSOD) and GPx in the mitochondrial matrix, in addition to other enzymatic systems such as thioredoxin, thioredoxin reductase, and peroxiredoxins. Nonenzymatic antioxidants include vitamins E and C, ubiquinone (coenzyme Q10), lipoic acid, and glutation.

All these enzymatic and nonenzymatic antioxidants help prevent ROS produced during high metabolism from triggering irreversible oxidative damage. It is unclear which signals are transduced by the cell to allow the tissues to identify whether a specific ROS emission is beneficial or harming. However, certain proteins act as transducers of this signal and trigger a beneficial molecular signaling cascade. In response to exercise, PGC-1α should be highlighted again, since in response to muscle contraction it can trigger the expression of antioxidant enzymes such as MnSOD by a molecular pathway mediated by sirtuin 3 [18]. It is not clear how the oxidative stress produced during the muscle contraction activates PGC-1α, but it is likely that p38 mitogen-activated protein kinase is in charge of controlling this antioxidant pathway in response to exercise.

Taking into account all this data, it is necessary to maintain the correct amount of ROS for biologic function (Figs. 13.1 and 13.2): it is harmful to have high levels of ROS, like those produced in metabolic disease, but equally unhealthy to have ROS levels below the physiological minimum [19]. This hormetic response has been tested under different circumstances, including the study of supplementation with antioxidants during exercise. As described above, a large amount of ROS is produced during exercise through several independent pathways; thus tests have been conducted for some years to see if the intake of antioxidants could prevent certain processes related to oxidative damage, such as inflammation and the associated sarcomere damage. It was found that the intake of antioxidants before strenuous exercise can prevent muscle damage associated with ROS production. These findings led to supplementation with antioxidants being extended to athletes. However, the chronic effect of the combination of exercise and supplementation with antioxidants was not considered. It was not until well into the 2000s that a series of studies used animal and human models to test how the intake of antioxidant supplements interferes in chronic adaptation to training. Among the observed effects there was a performance decrease, which was associated with a decrease in mitochondrial function and biogenesis by preventing the expression of PGC-1α [20]. The concept of mitohormesis was thus extended: a minimum of mitochondrial oxidative stress is key for adaptation, but the total suppression of ROS as well as a sustained increase of ROS is harmful (Fig. 13.5) [21]. There is still much to elucidate and research in this regard; for example, the discovery of antioxidants blocking particular pathways of ROS production could help to individualize pharmacological treatments for particular diseases. Diseases such as type 2 diabetes, cardiovascular diseases, cancer, and Alzheimer's have been associated with an overproduction of ROS. In almost all these diseases exercise seems to produce a beneficial effect, among other mechanisms by controlling the production of ROS. Nevertheless, the intake of antioxidants seems to prevent these improvements; this is very evident in subjects with a risk of developing type 2 diabetes. In these subjects, supplementation with antioxidants prevented the beneficial effects of exercise on insulin signaling [22].

5. INSULIN RESISTANCE, DIABETES, AND REACTIVE OXYGEN SPECIES

During conditions of a large availability of substrates, such as after food intake, the pancreas acts as a sensor of glucose levels, triggering insulin secretion by β cells. Insulin, through self-regulatory mechanisms, produces the activation of protein kinase B (AKT) kinase. This acts as a central nucleus in regulation of glucose homeostasis by promoting the release of glucose transporter 1 (GLUT-4) from intracellular vesicles to the plasma membrane. At the same time, AKT inhibits the synthesis of glycogen, enabling the availability of a glucose reservoir through glycogenolytic mechanisms (Fig. 13.6).

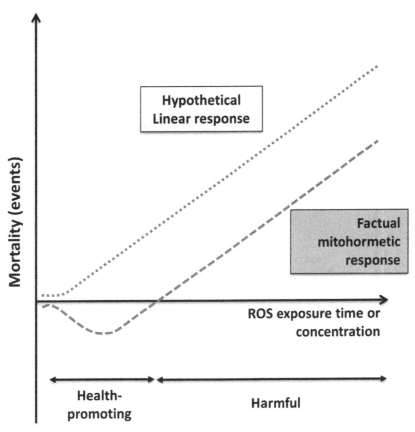

FIGURE 13.5   The mitohormetic response (*dashed line*) is in conflict with the free-radical theory of aging, which hypothesizes a linear response to ROS (*dotted line*) and suggests that any exposure to ROS (even at low doses) may be harmful. Nevertheless, in the mitohormetic response, low levels of ROS promote healthy effects. *ROS*, reactive oxygen species. *Adapted from Ristow M. Unraveling the truth about antioxidants: mitohormesis explains ROS-induced health benefits. Nat Med 2014;20(7):709−11.*

GLUT-4 is one of the 13 glucose transporters encoded by the genome, and is most abundant in adipose tissue, cardiac tissue, and skeletal muscle. During exercise the increase in the transport of glucose is mainly mediated by the translocation of GLUT-4 from intracellular sites to sarcolemma and T tubules [23]. Actually, glucose metabolism is improved both during and after exercise. However, adaptations produced by exercise are not easy to interpret. For example, some studies have shown that when analyzing the capacity of glucose uptake before and after moderate-intensity training, at the same relative intensity, the trained muscle absorbs less glucose. Moreover, during very intense exercises the training increases glucose flow to exercised muscles. Thus GLUT-4 may facilitate glucose metabolism in response to intense exercises which would not only improve the performance of the muscles involved but also increase the capacity of postexercise glycogen storage.

GLUT-4 helps to introduce a glucose molecule through the sarcolemma. This glucose molecule is phosphorylated to glucose-6-phosphate (G-6-P) in a reaction catalyzed by the hexokinase II enzyme (HKII). This step is also critical for glucose metabolism during exercise: G-6-P acts as an inhibitor of HKII, so during exercise with a sudden entry of glucose to the muscle cell there is a consequent inhibition of the HKII−G-6-P pathway. However, as the exercise continues the concentration of G-6-P decreases and glucose can metabolize again to G-6-P through HKII. Thus HKII and GLUT-4 are the main regulators of glucose metabolism during exercise: GLUT-4 controls the entry of glucose through the sarcoplasmic membrane, while HKII regulates glucose phosphorylation based on energy needs [23].

The metabolic signals regulating the glucose uptake by the muscle have been widely studied. The first in vitro studies showed that caffeine triggered an increase in glucose uptake [23]. This fact led researchers to suggest that calcium (caffeine is a potent releaser of calcium) could be related to glucose uptake. However, subsequent studies showed that the regulation through calcium was not due to direct mechanisms but was caused by other proteins. It was concluded that AMPK is the main regulatory protein of muscle glucose uptake in a mechanism that is initially triggered by calcium release from the sarcoplasmic reticulum [24].

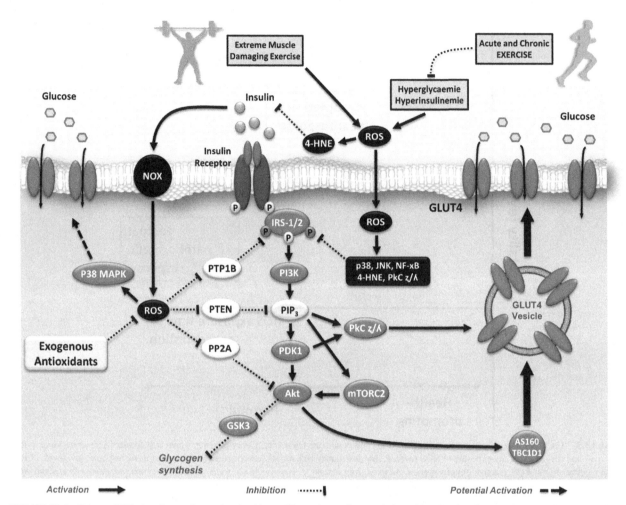

FIGURE 13.6 Primary ROS signaling pathways involved in positive and negative regulation of insulin signaling. *4-HNE*, 4-hydroxynonenal; *AKT*, protein kinase B; *AS160*, AKT substrate of 160 kDa; *GLUT4*, glucose transporter type 4; *GSK3*, glycogen synthase kinase 3; *IRS-1/2*, insulin receptor substrates 1 and 2; *JNK*, c-Jun N-terminal kinases; *mTORC2*, mechanistic target of rapamycin complex 2; *NF-κB*, nuclear factor kappa B; *NOX*, nicotinamide adenine dinucleotide phosphate oxidase; *p38MAPK*, p38 mitogen-activated protein kinase; *PDK1*, phosphoinositide-dependent kinase-1; *PI3K*, phosphatidylinositol-3 kinase; *PIP3*, phosphatidylinositol (3,4,5)-trisphosphate; *PKC*, protein kinase C; *PP2A*, protein phosphatase 2; *PTEN*, phosphatase and tensin homolog; *PTP1B*, protein tyrosine phosphatase 1B; *ROS*, reactive oxygen species. *Adapted from Parker L, Shaw CS, Stepto NK, Levinger I. Exercise and glycemic control: focus on redox homeostasis and redox-sensitive protein signaling. Front Endocrinol 2017;8:87.*

It should be highlighted that the activation of AMPK depends on the cell redox state due to the regulation of sirtuin 1, a protein dependent on the NADP/NADPH gradient. However, the regulation of insulin signaling and glucose uptake through redox mechanisms is a complex process because ROS can have a stimulator or inhibitor effect on glucose uptake. Sustained activation of stress-activated protein kinase in the overproduction of ROS implies a sustained phosphorylation of insulin-receptor substrates (IRSs)-1/2, which prevents the activity of phosphatidylinositol-3 kinase (PI3Kl) and results in an inhibition of insulin metabolism (Fig. 13.6). Importantly, preventing the degradation of IRS by the administration of antioxidants can restore glucose uptake by insulin-dependent mechanisms [25]. However, this process is not fully defined, since other studies have shown that phosphorylation of IRS can be necessary for normal glucose uptake. This data suggests that both excessive oxidative stress (such as that produced in chronic sedentary states) and the total blocking of ROS production can prevent the correct performance of insulin by altering IRS function.

In addition, there are certain proteins that require the action of oxidative mechanisms. The protein tyrosine phosphatase (PTP) has a residue which is susceptible to reversible oxidation by ROS. The oxidation of PTPs keeps IRS in a dephosphorylated state, maintaining activated PIK3 and AKT and unaltered insulin-dependent glucose uptake processes [25]. A correct functioning of antioxidant enzymes maintains ROS at physiological levels that prioritize their activities on PTPs. Insulin can stimulate ROS production by NADP oxidase.

Another important molecule produced in the skeletal muscle is nitric oxide (NO), which is produced by NOS. During exercise NOS increases its activity, producing an increase in NO (Fig. 13.6). Among the effects attributed to NO is an increase in glucose uptake in fast muscle fibers [26]. In addition, NO is one of the main angiogenic factors, and can help directly to improve vascularization in diabetic patients by improving blood flow and decreasing the associated cardiovascular risk.

The regulation of glucose uptake thus uses mechanisms depending on the cell redox state and the ROS. In addition, the NADP/NADH ratio regulates a SIRT1—AMPK—GLUT-4 axis that seems to be key in glucose uptake during exercise [24]. It has been suggested that AMPK can present three states based on the redox state: oxidized (inactive), reduced (activatable), and reduced and phosphorylated (active) [27]. Recently it has been suggested that the intake of antioxidants during very intense exercises phosphorylates serine 485 and 491 residues of AMPK, and this prevents the activation of AMPK (phosphorylation of threonine 172 residue) [27]. In humans it has been suggested that the administration of antioxidants during exercise prevents some adaptations regulated by the SIRT1—AMPK axis. However, there is no direct evidence that supplementation with antioxidants can prevent the increase of GLUT-4 occurring during exercise. It is reasonable to suggest that in response to AMPK inhibition by supplementation with antioxidants, the skeletal muscles use alternative pathways to ensure the cell glucose supply. However, it is clear that supplementation with high amounts of antioxidants during exercise does not produce additional beneficial effects on GLUT-4.

It should be noted that recent data suggests a new regulation pathway for glucose uptake by mechanisms related to insulin. Several studies have shown a relationship between hypoxia-inducible factor 1 (HIF1) activation and GLUT-4 expression [28]. This metabolic pathway relates directly the cell levels of oxygen and the expression of GLUT-4. When the oxygen available for the cell decreases, the mitochondria increases its production of ROS, and these mitochondrial ROS seem to be responsible for HIF1 activation. It has been claimed that supplementation with vitamin C blocks mitochondrial ROS produced during exercise. Thus the metabolic pathway HIF1—GLUT-4 can help to elucidate if antioxidants can alter exercise-induced GLUT-4 expression.

Several studies conducted in humans suggest that the intake of 1000 mg vitamin C daily can alter the cell redox state reached in a regular training. In addition, the intake of a daily cocktail of 1000 mg vitamin C and 400 IU vitamin E during training alters the beneficial effects that exercise has on insulin metabolism. This data collectively suggests that the intake of antioxidants prevents the induction of molecular regulators of insulin sensitivity, likely by preventing ROS production (Fig. 13.7). However, as previously described, it is still unclear whether the intake of antioxidants can directly prevent the expression of GLUT-4.

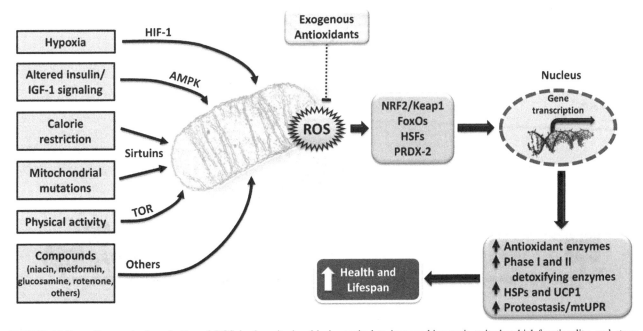

FIGURE 13.7 mall amount of production of ROS in the mitochondria is required to increase biogenesis, mitochondrial functionality, and stress resistance, as well as cellular responses that can extend health and lifespan. *AMPK*, AMP-activated protein kinase; *FoxOs*, forkhead box O proteins; *HIF-1*, hypoxia-inducible factor-1; *HSFs*, heat shock factors; *HSPs*, heat shock proteins; *IGF-1*, insulin-like growth factor-1; *Keap1*, Kelch-like ECH-associated protein 1; *mtUPR*, mitochondrial unfolded protein response; *NRF2*, nuclear factor-like 2; *PRDX-2*, peroxiredoxin-2; *ROS*, reactive oxygen species; *UCP1*, uncoupling protein 1. *Adapted from Ristow M. Unraveling the truth about antioxidants: mitohormesis explains ROS-induced health benefits. Nat Med 2014;20(7):709—11.*

6. CANCER AND ANTIOXIDANTS

Large increases in ROS production have been found at both cellular and systemic levels during the development of cancer. At first it was believed that these ROS were a consequence of the disease itself. However, current data seems inconsistent with that hypothesis. It should be noted that during the first phase of development and growth of cancer cells there is a huge increase of ROS. Few studies have investigated the intake of antioxidants during this phase of the disease because of the implicit methodological complexity, so data is not conclusive regarding the use of antioxidants during the first phase of cancer development.

Most studies have focused on the investigation of supplementation with antioxidants during tumor progression. Results suggest that supplementation with antioxidants reduces the ROS production and DNA damage. These effects are added to a decrease in the expression of genes involved in endogenous antioxidant defense. However, the intake of antioxidants was directly associated with a faster proliferation of tumor cells. Some studies have shown that tumor cells promote the encoding of oncogenes, and one of the functions of these genes is to decrease the level of ROS to promote tumor proliferation [29]. This data suggests that ROS produced during tumor proliferation can have a key signaling effect to try to prevent the progression of the disease.

In the key metabolic pathways that activate ROS is found p53 (Fig. 13.8). The protein p53 is considered a tumor suppressor and is activated by high levels of ROS. When there is a high intake of antioxidants there is an inhibition of the expression of p53 in tumor cells. It is of particular relevance that when tumor cells treated with antioxidants show a

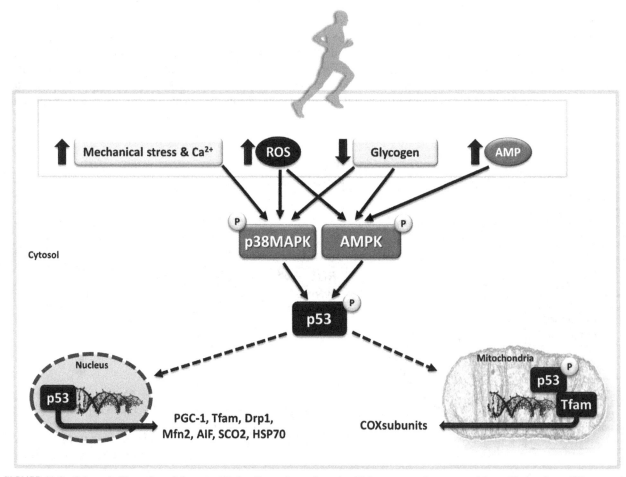

FIGURE 13.8 Schematic illustration of the potential signaling pathway through which acute exercise may modulate p53 signaling. *AIF*, apoptosis-inducing factor; *AMP*, adenosine monophosphate; *AMPK*, 50AMP-activated protein kinase; *ATP*, adenosine triphosphate; *COX*, cytochrome c oxidase; *Drp1*, dynamin-related protein 1; *HSP70*, heat shock protein 70; *Mfn2*, mitofusion 2; *P*, phosphorylation; *p38MAPK*, p38 mitogen-activated protein kinase; *PGC-1a*, peroxisome proliferator-activated receptor gamma coactivator 1a; *ROS*, reactive oxygen species; *SCO2*, synthesis of cytochrome c oxidase 2; *Tfam*, mitochondrial transcription factor A; *solid lines* represent activation and *dashed lines* represent translocation. *Adapted from Bartlett JD, Close GL, Drust B, Morton JP. The emerging role of p53 in exercise metabolism. Sports Med. 2014; 44(3):303–309.*

previous inhibition of p53, proliferation of tumors induced by antioxidants stops. Thus the increase in tumor proliferation found when supplementing with antioxidants seems be caused by the inability of ROS to activate p53. This data is consistent with the data discussed above suggesting that supplementation with antioxidants prevents the activation of PGC-1α by preventing ROS signaling (Fig. 13.8). Indeed, recently it has been found that p53 seems to be a regulator of mitochondrial biogenesis by controlling, among others, PGC-1α signaling [30].

7. MEDITERRANEAN DIET AND OBESITY

A balanced diet rich in fruit, vegetables, extravirgin olive oil, pasta, legumes, and fish seems to have a beneficial effect on overall health. The Mediterranean diet follows these recommendations and has been related to the improvement of a large number of metabolic diseases. Indeed, some experts have linked a lower incidence of cardiovascular events in Mediterranean countries to dietary habits. Recent studies have demonstrated that following a Mediterranean diet with supplements of extravirgin olive oil improves the lipid profile and decreases blood pressure, insulin resistance, and inflammatory levels [31]. Another study assessed more than 7000 subjects who followed a Mediterranean diet for 6 years. The findings showed that the Mediterranean diet can decrease the incidence of breast cancer [32]. The researchers highlighted that a high consumption of extravirgin olive oil is key for this prevention.

Extravirgin olive oil when consumed in high amounts in the context of a Mediterranean diet modulates the activity of some antioxidant enzymes in subjects with metabolic syndrome. This effect has been associated with improvements in high-density lipoprotein function in individuals with a high risk of coronary disease [33]. Among its effects, it is worth noting better metabolism of cholesterol, systemic inflammatory state, and vasodilator capacity. This data suggests that improvement of the antioxidant state through general dietary changes such as intake of extravirgin olive oil can improve the metabolism of patients at risk of suffering cardiovascular events, type 2 diabetes, and cancer. The mechanisms by which the intake of particular foods rich in antioxidants may produce a healthy effect are unknown. Further studies should focus on the analysis of key nutrients present in healthy food and then on the interaction of these nutrients and their isolated effects in populations with metabolic disease. This may help to elucidate why supplementation with isolated antioxidants seems not to have beneficial effects whereas antioxidant food such as olive oil seem produce beneficial effects.

8. CONCLUSIONS

In conclusion, maintaining ROS at physiological levels is a key aspect for a normal function of the metabolism and for maintaining the control of systemic inflammation. ROS production follows a hormetic pattern: high levels can induce oxidative damage in proteins and DNA, while suppression of ROS production prevents basic molecular signaling. Supplementation with isolated antioxidants seems to prevent this molecular signaling at both mitochondrial and sarcomeric levels.

Regular moderate physical exercise has very beneficial effects on the systemic inflammatory state, which impact directly on improvement in insulin resistance and glucose uptake, cardiovascular function, lipid profile, and cancer incidence. This overall health improvement mediated by exercise is achieved through very specific molecular mechanisms in which mitochondria and nucleus are in continues interaction. This interaction depends on ROS emitted at both mitochondrial and sarcolemmal levels, with PGC-1 as a key coactivator. Chronic supplementation with isolated antioxidants can maintain ROS production at too low levels to execute the necessary signaling of PGC-1. This prevents some key adaptations that are achieved with exercise through this protein. In addition, basal levels of ROS are required for glucose uptake by mechanisms related to insulin through redox-sensitive processes involving reversible oxidation of PTPs. Thus in subjects without particular clinical needs the intake of antioxidants is not recommended, since the beneficial effects produced by exercise require ROS formation.

It is advisable that, in conjunction with moderate physical activity, subjects follow a balanced diet rich in fruit, vegetables, extravirgin olive oil, pasta, legumes, and fish, which can provide the necessary antioxidants to meet requirements. The authors of the present chapter would like to highlight that the Mediterranean diet meets these requirements. A Mediterranean diet adjusted to individual energy requirements can provide the necessary antioxidants to prevent excessive production of ROS but allow the ROS-dependent beneficial effects. The particular mechanisms by which supplementation with antioxidants alone cannot result in overall health benefits are unknown, but following a diet rich in antioxidants such as extravirgin olive oil seems to improve cholesterol metabolism, cardiovascular disease, insulin resistance, and cancer. Possibly these antioxidants found in original food sources can interact with other nutrients to give a synergic healthy effect, but basic nutrition studies generating data applicable to studies in the population at clinical risk are required to test this hypothesis.

LIST OF ACRONYMS AND ABBREVIATIONS

4-HNE 4-hydroxynonenal
AIF Apoptosis inducing factor
AKT Protein kinase B
AMP Adenosine monophosphate
AMPK Adenosine monophosphate-activated protein kinase
AS160 AKT substrate of 160 kDa
ATP Adenosine triphosphate
COX Cytochrome c oxidase
DAG Diacylglycerol
Drp1 Dynamin-related protein 1
FoxOs Forkhead box O proteins
GLUT4 Glucose transporter type 4
GSK3 Glycogen synthase kinase 3
HIF-1 Hypoxia-inducible factor-1
HSFs Heat shock factors
HSP Heat shock proteins
HSP70 Heat shock protein 70
IGF-1 Insulin-like growth factor-1
IRS-1/2 Insulin receptor substrates 1 and 2
JNK c-Jun N-terminal kinases
Keap1 Kelch-like ECH-associated protein 1
MAPK Mitogen-activated protein kinase
Mfn2 Mitofusion 2
mTORC2 Mechanistic target of rapamycin complex 2
mtUPR Mitochondrial unfolded protein response
NF-κB Nuclear factor kappa B
NOS Nitric oxide synthase
NOX Nicotinamide adenine dinucleotide phosphate oxidase
NRF2 Nuclear factor-like 2
$O_2^{\cdot-}$ Superoxide anion
p38MAPK p38 mitogen-activated protein kinase
PDK1 Phosphoinositide-dependent kinase-1
PGC-1α Peroxisome proliferator-activated receptor gamma coactivator 1 alpha
PI3K Phosphatidylinositol-3 kinase
PIP3 Phosphatidylinositol (3,4,5)-trisphosphate
PKC Protein kinase C
PP2A Protein phosphatase 2
PPases Phosphatases
PRDX-2 Peroxiredoxin-2
PTEN Phosphatase and tensin homolog
PTP1B Protein tyrosine phosphatase 1B
ROS Reactive oxygen species
SCO2 Synthesis of cytochrome c oxidase 2
SOD Superoxide dismutase
Tfam Mitochondrial transcription factor A
UCP1 Uncoupling protein 1

REFERENCES

[1] Sies H. Hydrogen peroxide as a central redox signaling molecule in physiological oxidative stress: oxidative eustress. Redox Biol 2017;11:613–9.

[2] Sies H, Berndt C, Jones DP. Oxidative stress. Annu Rev Biochem 2017;86:715–48.

[3] Casuso RA, Aragón-Vela J, López-Contreras G, Gomes SN, Casals C, Barranco-Ruiz Y. Does swimming at a moderate altitude favor a lower oxidative stress in an intensity-dependent manner? Role of nonenzymatic antioxidants. High Alt Med Biol 2017;18(1):46–55.

[4] Huertas JR, Al Fazazi S, Hidalgo-Gutierrez A, López LC, Casuso RA. Antioxidant effect of exercise: exploring the role of the mitochondrial complex I superassembly. Redox Biol 2017;13:477–81.

[5] Acin-Perez R, Enriquez JA. The function of the respiratory supercomplexes: the plasticity model. Biochim Biophys Acta April 2014;1837(4):444–50.

[6] Ng M, Fleming T, Robinson M, Thomson B, Graetz N, Margono C, et al. Global, regional and national prevalence of overweight and obesity in children and adults 1980—2013: a systematic analysis. Lancet 2014;384(9945):766—81.

[7] Handschin C, Spiegelman BM. The role of exercise and PGC1alpha in inflammation and chronic disease. Nature 2008;454(7203):463—9.

[8] Boyle JP, Honeycutt AA, Narayan KM, Hoerger TJ, Geiss LS, Chen H, et al. Projection of diabetes burden through 2050: impact of changing demography and disease prevalence in the U.S. Diabetes Care 2001;24(11):1936—40.

[9] Pan XR, Li GW, Hu YH, Wang JX, Yang WY, An ZX, et al. Effects of diet and exercise in preventing NIDDM in people with impaired glucose tolerance. The Da Qing IGT and Diabetes Study. Diabetes Care 1997;20(4):537—44.

[10] Tuomilehto J, Lindström J, Eriksson JG, Valle TT, Hämäläinen H, Ilanne-Parikka P, et al. Prevention of type 2 diabetes mellitus by changes in lifestyle among subjects with impaired glucose tolerance. N Engl J Med 2001;344(18):1343—50.

[11] Knowler WC, Barrett-Connor E, Fowler SE, Hamman RF, Lachin JM, Walker EA, et al. Reduction in the incidence of type 2 diabetes with lifestyle intervention or metformin. N Engl J Med 2002;346(6):393—403.

[12] Stanford KI, Goodyear LJ. Muscle-adipose tissue cross talk. Cold Spring Harb Prespect Med 2017, May 15. https://doi.org/10.1101/cshperspect.a029801 [Epub ahead of print].

[13] Scarpulla RC, Vega RB, Kelly DP. Transcriptional integration of mitochondrial biogenesis. Trends Endocrinol Metabol 2012;23(9):459—66.

[14] Mootha VK, Lindgren CM, Eriksson KF, Subramanian A, Sihag S, Lehar J, et al. PGC-1alpha-responsive genes involved in oxidative phosphorylation are coordinately downregulated in human diabetes. Nat Genet 2003;34(3):267—73.

[15] Cheng Z, Almeida FA. Mitochondrial alteration in type 2 diabetes and obesity: an epigenetic link. Cell Cycle 2014;13(6):890—7.

[16] Yu T, Robotham JL, Yoon Y. Increased production of reactive oxygen species in hyperglycemic conditions requires dynamic change of mitochondrial morphology. Proc Natl Acad Sci USA 2006;103:2653—8.

[17] Jackson MJ. Redox regulation of muscle adaptations to contractile activity and aging. J Appl Physiol 2015;119(3):163—71.

[18] Kong X, Wang R, Xue Y, Liu X, Zhang H, Chen Y, et al. Sirtuin 3, a new target of PGC-1α, plays an important role in the suppression of ROS and mitochondrial biogenesis. PLoS One 2010;5:e11707.

[19] Ristow M. Unraveling the truth about antioxidants: mitohormesis explains ROS-induced health benefits. Nat Med 2014;20(7):709—11.

[20] Gomez-Cabrera MC, Domenech E, Romagnoli M, Arduini A, Borras C, Pallardo FV, et al. Oral administration of vitamin C decreases muscle mitochondrial biogenesis and hampers training-induced adaptations in endurance performance. Am J Clin Nutr 2008;87:142—9.

[21] Merry TL, Ristow M. Mitohormesis in exercise training. Free Radic Biol Med 2016;98:123—30.

[22] Ristow M, Zarse K, Oberbach A, Klöting N, Birringer M, Kiehntopf M, et al. Antioxidants prevent health-promoting effects of physical exercise in humans. Proc Natl Acad Sci USA 2009;106(21):8665—70.

[23] Richter EA, Hargreaves M. Exercise, GLUT4, and skeletal muscle glucose uptake. Physiol Rev 2013;93(3):993—1017.

[24] Lira VA, Soltow QA, Long JH, Betters JL, Sellman JE, Criswell DS. Nitric oxide increases GLUT4 expression and regulates AMPK signalling in skeletal muscle. Am J Physiol Endocrinol Metab 2007;293(4):E1062—8.

[25] Parker L, Shaw CS, Stepto NK, Levinger I. Exercise and glycemic control: focus on redox homeostasis and redox-sensitive protein signaling. Front Endocrinol 2017;8:87.

[26] Hong YH, Betik AC, McConell GK. Role of nitric oxide in skeletal muscle glucose uptake during exercise. Exp Physiol 2014;99(12):1569—73.

[27] Morales-Alamo D, Calbet JAL. AMPK signalling in skeletal muscle during exercise: role of reactive oxygen and nitrogen species. Free Radic Biol Med 2016;98:68—77.

[28] Sakagami H, Makino Y, Mizumoto K, Isoe T, Takeda Y, Watanabe J, et al. Loss of HIF-1α impairs GLUT4 translocation and glucose uptake by the skeletal muscle cells. Am J Physiol Endocrinol Metab 2014;306(9):E1065—76.

[29] Sayin VI, Ibrahim MX, Larsson E, Nilsson JA, Lindahl P, Bergo MO. Antioxidants accelerate lung cancer progression in mice. Sci Transl Med 2014;6(221):221ra15.

[30] Bartlett JD, Close GL, Drust B, Morton JP. The emerging role of p53 in exercise metabolism. Sports Med 2014;44(3):303—9.

[31] Estruch R, Martínez-González MA, Corella D, Salas-Salvadó J, Ruiz-Gutiérrez V, Covas MI, et al. Effects of a Mediterranean-style diet on cardiovascular risk factors: a randomized trial. Ann Intern Med 2006;145(1):1—11.

[32] Toledo E, Salas-Salvadó J, Donat-Vargas C, Buil-Cosiales P, Estruch R, Ros E, et al. Mediterranean diet and invasive breast cancer risk among women at high cardiovascular risk in the PREDIMED trial: a randomized clinical trial. JAMA Intern Med 2015;175(11):1752—60.

[33] Hernáez Á, Castañer O, Elosua R, Pintó X, Estruch R, Salas-Salvadó J, et al. Mediterranean diet improves high-density lipoprotein function in high cardiovascular-risk individuals: a randomized controlled trial. Circulation 2017;135(7):633—43.

[34] Powers SK, Jackson MJ. Exercise-induced oxidative stress: cellular mechanisms and impact on muscle force production. Physiol Rev 2008;88(4):1243—76.

[35] Barbieri E, Sestili P. Reactive oxygen species in skeletal muscle signaling. J Signal Transduct 2011;2012:1—17.

Index

'*Note:* Page numbers followed by "f" indicate figures, "t" indicate tables.'

Printed in the United States
By Bookmasters